The Biomechanics of Back Pain

Commissioning Editor: *Alison Taylor*
Development Editor: *Veronika Watkins/Clive Hewat*
Project Manager: *Sruthi Viswam*
Designer/Design Direction: *Miles Hitchen*
Illustration Manager: *Jennifer Rose*

The Biomechanics of Back Pain

Third Edition

Michael A. Adams BSc PhD

Professor of Biomechanics, Centre for Comparative and Clinical Anatomy, University of Bristol, Bristol, UK

Nikolai Bogduk BSc(Med) MB BS MD PhD DSc DipAnat DipPainMed FAFRM FAFMM FFPM(ANZCA)

Professor of Pain Medicine, University of Newcastle and Head, Department of Clinical Research, Royal Newcastle Hospital, Newcastle, New South Wales, Australia

Kim Burton OBE DO PhD Hon FFOM

Director, Spinal Research Unit, Centre for Health and Social Care Research, University of Huddersfield, Huddersfield, UK

Patricia Dolan BSc PhD

Reader in Spine Biomechanics, Centre for Comparative and Clinical Anatomy, University of Bristol, Bristol, UK

Brian J C Freeman MB BCh BAO DM(Nottm) FRCS(Tr & Orth) FRACS
Professor of Spinal Surgery, University of Adelaide and Head of Spinal Services, Royal Adelaide Hospital, Adelaide, South Australia, Australia

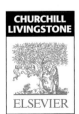

CHURCHILL LIVINGSTONE

ELSEVIER

Edinburgh   London   New York   Oxford   Philadelphia   St Louis   Sydney   Toronto   2013

ELSEVIER
CHURCHILL
LIVINGSTONE

First edition 2002
Second edition 2006

ISBN 9780702043130

British Library Cataloguing in Publication Data
A catalogue record for this book is available from the British Library

Library of Congress Cataloging in Publication Data
A catalog record for this book is available from the Library of Congress

Notices
Knowledge and best practice in this field are constantly changing. As new research and experience broaden our understanding, changes in research methods, professional practices, or medical treatment may become necessary.

Practitioners and researchers must always rely on their own experience and knowledge in evaluating and using any information, methods, compounds, or experiments described herein. In using such information or methods they should be mindful of their own safety and the safety of others, including parties for whom they have a professional responsibility.

With respect to any drug or pharmaceutical products identified, readers are advised to check the most current information provided (i) on procedures featured or (ii) by the manufacturer of each product to be administered, to verify the recommended dose or formula, the method and duration of administration, and contraindications. It is the responsibility of practitioners, relying on their own experience and knowledge of their patients, to make diagnoses, to determine dosages and the best treatment for each individual patient, and to take all appropriate safety precautions.

To the fullest extent of the law, neither the Publisher nor the authors, contributors, or editors, assume any liability for any injury and/or damage to persons or property as a matter of products liability, negligence or otherwise, or from any use or operation of any methods, products, instructions, or ideas contained in the material herein.

ELSEVIER your source for books, journals and multimedia in the health sciences
www.elsevierhealth.com

Working together to grow
libraries in developing countries

www.elsevier.com | www.bookaid.org | www.sabre.org

ELSEVIER   BOOK AID International   Sabre Foundation

The publisher's policy is to use **paper manufactured from sustainable forests**

Printed in China

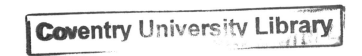

Contents

Preface
to the 3rd Edition

As the *Biomechanics of Back Pain* moves into its third edition, a prospective reader may wonder at the authors' motivation for carrying on. Do we have anything new to say? Are we creatures of habit? In fact we were uncertain of the value of a third edition until recent events helped us to make up our minds.

At long last, research into back pain seems to be paying off, with important clinically-relevant advances being reported in the last three years. For example, large population-based imaging studies now confirm beyond doubt that intervertebral disc degeneration has a strong association with severe and chronic back pain. The latest 'twins' studies show that genetic inheritance and environmental influences are equally important determinants of spinal pathology and pain, with some fascinating interactions. Other interesting and potentially useful therapeutic advances include an injection-based treatment for discogenic back pain with a 92% 'satisfaction' rating after two years, and a new generation of prosthetic intervertebral discs with highly encouraging short-term results. It remains to be seen if these apparent breakthroughs will stand the test of time, but certainly this is an invigorating period for back pain research.

These recent advances suggest a shift in perspective, from trying to understand and reverse age-related spinal degeneration, to tackling directly the tissue causes of pain. Securing perpetual youth for our backs may not be achievable, but we are learning how to identify and deal with the sensitised neurons which ultimately cause most back pain. This is the main reason for this new edition: to emphasise the new perspective, and to show how research is finally leading to clinical advances. This has required a complete re-writing of the final Summary chapter.

There are other reasons for carrying on. The book remains popular, and has been translated into several foreign languages, including Chinese. Although conceived as an undergraduate text, it has become accepted as an authoritative reference for teachers, researchers, clinicians, and those working in the medico-legal arena. With that comes a responsibility: it must be updated or replaced at regular intervals. Accordingly, every chapter and most paragraphs have been revised, and more than 350 new references incorporated. It was our intention to remove as much as we added, to keep the text concise, but we were equally concerned to preserve the best research from before the digital era, because access to this literature is often denied to young researchers. As a result, the book has grown slightly, but we suggest that the extra weight is 'meat' rather than 'fat'.

Other improvements include an all-colour format with many additional diagrams and photographs. Additional chapters are devoted to 'Sensorimotor Control' and 'Cervical Spine Biomechanics'. Not all of the material in these two chapters is new, but it should now be easier to find. The online content now allows the reader to download Figures, and to access PowerPoint slide shows summarising much of the core material. We hope that this new content will assist those who, like us, teach as well as learn.

Additional On-line Information

Besides the plethora of information found in the latest edition of *The Biomechanics of Back Pain*, this book comes with a bank of material which is available at www.biomechanicsofbackpain.com.

We have used this website for posting additional material which includes two extensive Power-Point presentations which are suitable for senior undergraduate/post graduate teaching purposes – *Forces on the Spine* and *Back Pain*.

The site also includes instructive material about the *Psychosocial Flags Framework* and a short promotional video entitled *Get Back Active* [The Stationery Office, UK, 2009]. This DVD, which is based on *The Back Book*, was the winner of the 'Creative Excellence' award at the US International Film and Video Festival, and delivers evidence-based advice on overcoming back pain through a mixture of activities and positive thinking.

Finally, the now full-colour artwork program found within the book is available to download from the site and can be used for teaching purposes free of charge.

For full access to these additional resources on this website please register at www. biomechanicsofbackpain.com.

Chapter | 1 |

Introduction

MECHANICAL LOADING AND BACK PAIN

Mechanical loading is good for your back. The bones, muscles, ligaments and discs of the spine are all capable of adapting to physical exercise by becoming stronger and this makes them less vulnerable to injury. Old notions concerning the harmful effects of physical exercise are gradually being discredited, as is the use of bed rest as a treatment for back pain. Instead, current research emphasises the importance of exercise in maintaining the health of the musculoskeletal system. The new threats to spinal health are considered to be genetic inheritance, which exerts a strong influence on the risk of intervertebral disc degeneration, and the human personality, which influences all aspects of back pain behaviour, including recovering from it. The 'back pain revolution' is how one leading expert has summarised these changes in attitudes.[1507]

However, it would be wrong to assume that genetic influences on spinal pathology somehow reduce the importance of mechanical or biochemical factors: on the contrary, genes exert their influence by affecting the mechanical, biochemical and metabolic properties of spinal tissues. Likewise it is a mistake to assume that psychosocial factors such as depressive tendencies and work dissatisfaction are important causes of back pain; infact they explain people's responses to pain rather than the pain itself. Recent pain provocation studies have not only located the anatomical origins of severe back pain, they have also confirmed that patients' characteristic back pain is often reproduced when the affected tissue is mechanically stimulated. These considerations have also been acknowledged[1507]: 'The balance of back pain research has perhaps swung too far towards these psychosocial issues, to the neglect of the physical. . . . Hopefully, the pendulum will swing back'.

PURPOSE OF THIS BOOK

The purpose of this book is not just to push the pendulum back again, but to help bring it to rest in a balanced position where all of the factors which influence back pain are given due attention. The title *The Biomechanics of Back Pain* does not imply a bias towards mechanical explanations of back pain; it merely reflects the fact that mechanical factors are the most obvious and preventable influences in a complex natural history which involves biological and psychological processes as well as mechanical ones (hence 'biomechanics'). The title is also intended to imply a mechanistic approach to back pain, in which our knowledge of the biological and physical sciences is applied to explaining the various chains of events which lead to back pain. Back pain is certainly a difficult and multifaceted problem, but it is not so difficult that we must abandon the normal scientific method in favour of some vague holistic approach. Back pain should be explained, not explained away. The varied background of the authors of this book reflects a desire by them, and by the publishers, to produce a balanced and integrated text which incorporates all of the recent scientific advances in our understanding of back pain.

THE AUTHORS

Mike Adams graduated in natural philosophy (physics) before studying for a PhD in spinal mechanics. Much of his research has involved mechanical testing of cadaveric spines and articular cartilage, but this strong biomechanics influence has been moderated by 20 years of teaching musculoskeletal biology to science students. His primary interest in back pain is to explain the interactions between mechanical and biological (cell-mediated) events which lead to degenerative changes within spinal tissues.

Nik Bogduk began studies into back pain while still an undergraduate medical student. He investigated the nerve supply of the lumbar spine with the view to establishing the possible sources of back pain. After graduating .in medicine, he pursued a PhD in neurology in which he developed diagnostic procedures for back pain and for neck pain, based on his anatomical studies. His work subsequently progressed to apply those diagnostic procedures and others to determine the relative prevalence of different sources of back pain and neck pain, and to evaluate neuroablative surgical procedures for the treatment of pain. In the course of these clinical studies he continued to contribute to basic sciences on the anatomy of spinal muscles and the kinematics of spinal movement.

Kim Burton graduated as an osteopath before moving into research and undertaking a PhD in the biomechanics and epidemiology of back pain. Subsequent research involved epidemiological studies of different occupational groups, with a focus on the relative influence of psychosocial and ergonomic factors on disability due to back pain. More recently his research has been in the clinical environment, developing and testing interventions addressing psychosocial factors as obstacles to recovery. He has been involved in the development of the UK primary care and occupational health guidelines for the management of low-back pain, as well as the European guidelines on prevention in low-back pain. He is an Honorary Fellow of the Faculty of Occupational Medicine, and is the Editor-in-Chief of *Clinical Biomechanics*.

Trish Dolan graduated in biological sciences before concentrating on exercise and muscle physiology for her PhD. This was followed by postdoctoral experience in a biomechanics tissue-testing laboratory, and her subsequent research has continued to straddle the boundaries of physiology and biomechanics. Her primary research interests include the assessment of spinal loading in vivo, quantification and analysis of muscle function, sensorimotor control mechanisms and vertebral augmentation.

WHO SHOULD READ THIS BOOK?

The book has evolved from seminars in musculoskeletal tissues given by two of the authors (MA and TD) to final-year undergraduate students in anatomical science, and to postgraduate students of physiotherapy, orthopaedic surgery and ergonomics. This knowledge base has been augmented by the anatomical, epidemiological and clinical expertise of the other authors. The book is intended primarily for those who treat back pain, including physiotherapists, osteopaths, chiropractors, general practitioners, spine surgeons, occupational health professionals and nurses. It may also interest advanced undergraduate science students, ergonomists and those involved in personal injury litigation.

Very little previous knowledge of musculoskeletal tissue biology or biomechanics is required, because introductory chapters are included to explain the concepts and terminology used later in the book. However, in order to do justice to the many controversies regarding back pain, certain areas of the research literature have been analysed in more detail, and with more rigour, than is customary in undergraduate texts.

INTRODUCTION TO INDIVIDUAL CHAPTERS

Later sections of Chapter 1 define all biomechanical terminology used later in the book. Chapters 2–4 then describe the functional anatomy of the spine, including the overlying muscles and fascia. Structure and function are conveniently described together, but where a particular function is considered to be controversial or difficult to understand, reference is made to the relevant sections later in the book.

The provocative question 'where does back pain come from?' is tackled in Chapter 5. A satisfactory answer could be offered on the basis of pain provocation and pain-blocking studies alone, but additional sections in this and the previous chapter attempt to link back pain to the underlying neuroanatomy, and to common diagnostic syndromes. The evidence from this chapter justifies the emphasis placed on intervertebral discs in subsequent sections of the book.

Chapter 6 reviews the epidemiological evidence concerning the causes of spinal pathology, pain and disability. This information is essential to understand the relative importance of mechanical and other influences in the aetiology of back pain. It is a key chapter, which justifies the title and scope of the entire book.

The biology of spinal tissues is considered in Chapter 7. Some knowledge of the interactions between cell metabolism and mechanical loading is required to appreciate why loading is sometimes beneficial to the spine, and sometimes harmful. This chapter also introduces concepts and terminology which are used in later sections on spinal growth, ageing and degeneration.

Chapter 8 describes how the spine develops before birth, grows to maturity and then declines into old age. Care is taken to discuss only those changes which are inevitable (and therefore 'constitutional') so that they might later be distinguished from spinal 'degeneration' (Ch. 15) which afflicts some people much more than others, usually in middle age.

Before considering how the spine responds to mechanical loading, it is necessary to consider the origins and magnitude of the forces applied to it during the activities of daily living. Spinal loading is analysed in Chapter 9.

The normal response of the thoracolumbar spine to non-damaging forces is described in Chapter 10. This indicates how each spinal structure has a specific job to do, and is a prerequisite to understanding mechanical dysfunction and failure. Wherever possible, qualitative descriptions are supported by experimental measurements, because it is generally true that you do not really understand a mechanism until you have measured it. To give an example, the observation that intervertebral discs bulge radially outwards when compressed may seem to be of some clinical interest – until, that is, you learn that the bulge is generally a small fraction of 1 mm, even when the compressive force is several times body weight!

Chapter 11 describes mechanisms of injury and fatigue failure in each spinal structure. It is the largest chapter, and primary focus of the book. Intervertebral disc failure is treated in particular detail, and numerous illustrations are included to give the reader a feel for normal and dysfunctional discs.

Cervical spine anatomy and biomechanics are considered briefly in Chapter 12. Much less is known about the cervical spine compared to the lumbar spine, so this chapter necessarily lacks detail. However, it is instructive to compare the two regions in order to give insight into cervical pathology and pain.

Many clinicians will require little convincing that back pain can arise in the apparent absence of injury or degenerative changes. Chapter 13 suggests that 'functional pathology' arises from high localised stresses within innervated tissues, and it shows how stress concentrations can be generated by small changes in posture, and intensified by time-dependent 'creep' loading.

The important and growing topic of sensorimotor control is introduced in Chapter 14. Muscles are required to move, stabilise and protect the underlying spine, but their function can be compromised by factors such as soft-tissue creep, muscle fatigue and pain.

Chapter 15 describes the various manifestations of spinal degeneration, including intervertebral disc degeneration, apophyseal joint osteoarthritis and osteoporosis.

Attempts are made to explain the relative contributions of genetic inheritance, cell metabolism and mechanical loading to the key process of intervertebral disc degeneration, and how disc failure can lead on to a 'degenerative cascade' involving other spinal tissues.

This leads directly to possibilities for preventing back pain (Ch. 16) and for treating it conservatively (Ch. 17). The evidence from recent clinical and epidemiological research is shown to be consistent with the basic science presented in previous chapters. The old view that mechanical loading is always bad for the back is exposed as a fallacy, and the potential benefits of various physical, biological and psychosocial interventions are described, with detailed reference to the latest published international guidelines. As an antidote to the nihilism of the guidelines, Chapter 17 ends with some practical advice from the authors for preventing (and coping with) back pain.

The conceptual benefits and drawbacks of spinal surgery are outlined in Chapter 18, and a detailed review of current procedures is given in Chapter 19. This latter chapter has been contributed by a leading spine surgeon who is renowned for his willingness to submit surgical practice to scientific scrutiny.

Financial compensation and personal injury litigation are considered by some experts to be a natural consequence of chronic back pain coupled with ineffective treatment. Others view them as an important cause of back pain reporting, and subsequent disability. Chapter 20 shows that there is some truth in both points of view, but concludes nevertheless that certain spinal disorders, including disc prolapse, can often be attributed to mechanical loading of vulnerable tissues. The nature of tissue 'vulnerability', and its medicolegal implications, is a key issue in this chapter.

The concluding Chapter 21 summarises and emphasises the main themes of the book. It suggests that cell-mediated degenerative changes are often a consequence rather than a cause of tissue failure, and it attempts to explain why the links between spinal pathology and pain are so complex.

BIOMECHANICAL TERMS AND CONCEPTS

Certain words and concepts used later in the book are explained here for ease of reference. These notes are intended to provide helpful explanations for typical readers of the book, rather than rigorous definitions for the specialist.

Force

Force is an action exerted on a body which causes it to deform or to move. It is a **vector** quantity which has a magnitude (the size of the force) and a direction. The unit

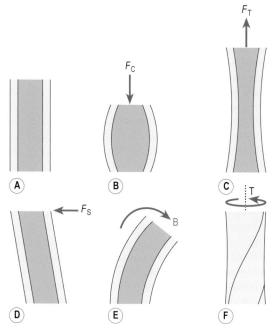

Figure 1.1 The effects of different types of forces acting on a solid object. (A) No forces acting; (B) compressive force, F_C; (C) tensile force, F_T, (D) shear force, F_S, (E) bending moment, B; (F) torsional moment, or torque, T.

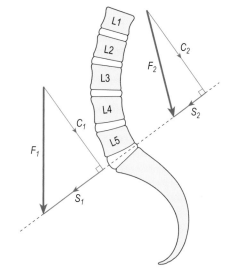

Figure 1.2 F_1 and F_2 represent the abdominal and back muscle forces acting on the lumbar spine. Because F_1 and F_2 act in slightly different directions, they cannot simply be added together to give the overall resultant force on the spine. To calculate the resultant, it is necessary to represent each force by two components, C and S, which act in two directions at 90° to each other. The components are added up to give the total force acting in these two directions (i.e. $C_1 + C_2$, and $S_1 + S_2$). Then the overall resultant force, R (not shown), acting on the L5–S1 disc, is given by: $R^2 = (C_1 + C_2)^2 + (S_1 + S_2)^2$. When adding forces in this manner, it is useful to calculate components in two meaningful directions, in this case, perpendicular to and parallel to the L5–S1 intervertebral disc.

of force is the newton (N). Approximately, 9.81 N = 1 kg = 2.2 lb.

A force is **compressive** if it compacts an object, **tensile** if it pulls it apart, and **shear** if it acts to deform the object without compacting or stretching it (Fig. 1.1).

A force can be represented (in two dimensions) by two **components** which act in convenient directions, usually at right angles to each other, as shown in Figure 1.2. 'Resolving' forces into components is a useful means of adding together two (or more) forces which act in different directions: the component forces can easily be summed, and then used to reconstruct the 'resultant' of the two original forces.

Mass

The mass of an object is the quantity of matter it contains, and represents the resistance of that body to being moved quickly (i.e. being accelerated). Mass simply has a magnitude, and so is a **scalar** quantity. The unit of mass is the kilogram (kg).

Weight

The weight of an object is the force exerted on it by the gravitational pull of the Earth. According to Newton's second law of motion:

$$\text{Force} = \text{mass} \times \text{acceleration} \qquad \boxed{1}$$

so the weight of an object is given by $(m \times g)$, where m is its mass, and g the acceleration due to gravity. g depends on the height above sea level, falling to zero in outer space. Therefore, the weight of an object also diminishes with height above sea level. For this reason, weight should not be confused with mass. Equation [1] enables the unit of force (N) to be expressed in terms of the more familiar unit of mass (kg): 9.81 N = 1kg. This is approximate only, because the acceleration due to gravity is not exactly 9.81 m/s².

Stress

This is the intensity of loading, equal to the force exerted divided by the area over which it is applied. The unit of stress is the mega-pascal (MPa): 1 MPa = 1 N/mm². 1 MPa is equivalent to a 10-kg weight being applied to an area the size of a fingernail. A **shear stress** is equal to the shear force divided by the area over which it is applied.

Fluid

A fluid is a substance with such little rigidity that it deforms to take the shape of its container. In a fluid, shear stresses are very small, so there is little resistance to the substance spreading out to equalise the pressure within it. In a static fluid, pressure does not vary with direction (e.g. vertically or horizontally) or with location.

Pressure (or hydrostatic pressure)

This is the intensity of loading within a fluid. It has the same units (MPa) as stress and so the two are often confused, but they should not be, because stress refers to solids and pressure to fluids. In a healthy intervertebral disc, the nucleus behaves like a fluid whereas most of the annulus behaves like a fibrous solid. Therefore the intensity of loading throughout the nucleus can be given by a single scalar quantity, the intradiscal pressure, whereas the intensity of loading within the annulus must be described by stresses which vary with location and direction.

Displacement

Displacement defines the location of one point relative to another. It is a vector quantity which has a magnitude (the **distance** between the two points) and a direction. Units are metres (m), millimetres (mm), micrometres (µm) or nanometres (nm). 1000 nm = 1 µm; 1000 µm = 1 mm; 1000 mm = 1 m. Approximately, 25.4 mm = 1 inch.

Velocity

This is the rate of change of displacement with time. Again, it is a vector quantity with a magnitude (the **speed**) and a direction. Units are metres/second (m/s).

Acceleration

This is the rate of change of velocity with time. It is another vector quantity with magnitude (acceleration) and a direction. Units are metres/second/second (m/s^2).

Strain

This is the amount an object deforms when a force is applied to it.

$$\text{Strain} = \text{change in length/original length} \qquad \boxed{2}$$

Strain can be expressed as a fraction or as a percentage, so if the length of an object was increased by half, the strain would be 0.5 or 50%. Small deformations of stiff materials such as bone can be expressed in microstrains, where 10000 microstrains is equivalent to a strain of 1%.

Energy

Energy and **work** are essentially the same thing. If a force f is applied to an object in order to move it a distance d, then the work done is equal to $f \times d$. If the object is raised vertically against gravity, then it gains energy (in this case, potential energy) equal to the work done in moving it. If the object is allowed to fall, its potential energy is converted to energy of movement, or kinetic energy. (In fact, the kinetic energy of an object of mass m moving at a velocity v is equal to $\frac{1}{2}mv^2$.) Energy can transform itself into many other forms, including heat, and the unit of energy (the joule) is defined in terms of heat rather than forces and distances.

Momentum

Momentum is the mass of an object multiplied by its velocity. Bodies with a lot of momentum require a lot of stopping!

Bending moment

This is a measure of the turning or bending effect of a force which is applied to an object. It is equal to the size of the force (in newtons) multiplied by the lever arm (in metres) between the force and the chosen centre of rotation, so its units are newton metres (Nm). Note that any location can be chosen as the centre of rotation, and that the bending moment of a given force about each centre of rotation will be different (Fig. 1.3). For example, when a person bends forwards, the weight of the person's upper body (a force!) exerts a different bending moment about the centre of each of the intervertebral discs. A bending moment can be specified relative to the centre of rotation of the disc, or relative to its geometric centre, or indeed relative to any other point.

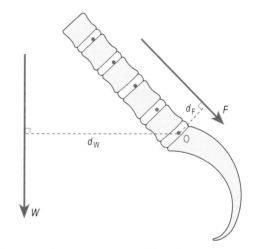

Figure 1.3 The moment generated by a force is equal to the magnitude of that force multiplied by the length of its lever arm. In this example, body weight W exerts a flexor moment of $W \times d_W$ about the centre of rotation O. No movement occurs if this is balanced by the extensor moment $F \times d_F$, generated by the back muscle force F. Moments can be calculated relative to any point whatsoever, but it is usual to select a point which coincides with a physical pivot, such as the centre of rotation within each intervertebral disc.

Torque

This is the equivalent to a bending moment except that the applied force acts to twist a body (Fig. 1.1) rather than to bend it. Its units are also newton metres (Nm).

Stiffness and strength

Stiffness is a measure of how strongly an object resists being deformed. It is normally measured as the deforming force (in newtons) divided by the deformation it causes (in millimetres) so a convenient unit of stiffness is the newton/millimetre (N/mm). If a biological tissue is referred to as being 'non-linear' it means that its stiffness increases as the applied load increases, so that a graph of deformation against applied force is curved, as shown in Figure 1.4. Stiffness is then measured as the gradient of the graph at any specified level of force (or deformation). Strength is the force (or stress) at which an object is damaged. Because the stiffness of most biological tissues depends on the force applied (Fig. 1.4), it cannot be used to predict strength, and stiffness and strength should not be confused.

Damage

Damage can be defined as a permanently impaired resistance to deformation, and is indicated on a force deformation graph by the first fall in stiffness (reduction in gradient). The point on the graph at which this occurs is the 'elastic limit' (Fig. 1.4). Any deformation occurring beyond the elastic limit is 'plastic' (non-recoverable) deformation which remains as a 'permanent set' when the object is unloaded. Sometimes, an 'ultimate strength' is defined as the force (or stress) at which the stiffness (gradient) not only reduces, but falls to zero. Warning! These concepts were developed to explain engineering materials, and 'permanent' changes can sometimes be reversed in living tissues.

Modulus

Young's modulus is a measure of how stiff a material is, and is equal to applied stress divided by strain. Unlike stiffness, which describes an object, modulus is independent of specimen size.

Strain energy, hysteresis and toughness

The work done in deforming an object is indicated by the area under a force deformation graph (Fig. 1.5). This work

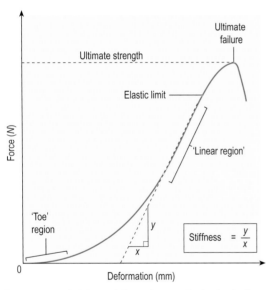

Figure 1.4 Typical force deformation graph obtained when stretching or compressing a biological tissue. In the toe region, deformation increases rapidly with increasing force, indicating that the stiffness of the specimen is low. (In some tissues, this region of low stiffness is attributable to straightening out the crimp structure of collagen fibres.) At higher loads, there is often a linear region in which the stiffness is approximately constant. The elastic limit marks the point where stiffness begins to fall, and this usually indicates that the specimen is starting to be damaged. Ultimate failure occurs when the stiffness falls to zero, and the force at this point is the (ultimate) strength of the specimen.

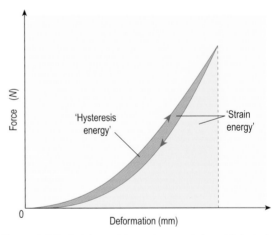

Figure 1.5 Typical force deformation graph for a biological tissue which is subjected to a non-damaging loading cycle. The unloading part of the curve (indicated by the downwards-pointing arrow) is below the loading curve, indicating that specimen deformation is greater for the same applied load. The area under the loading curve has units of energy (force × distance moved) and in fact this area represents the work done in deforming the specimen, or strain energy. Most of the strain energy is returned when the specimen is unloaded, but a small proportion is lost as heat. This small fraction is the hysteresis energy and is indicated by the hatched area between the loading and unloading curves.

is stored by the object as 'strain energy', and any body which can absorb a lot of strain energy before it is damaged is called 'tough'. A tin can is tough because it is strong and deformable, whereas a wine glass is the opposite ('brittle') because it cannot deform sufficiently to absorb much strain energy. When the deforming force is released, the object returns towards its original shape, and the strain energy is released. If the object is perfectly 'elastic', then the original shape is exactly regained, and all of the strain energy is recovered. However, many biological tissues exhibit a certain amount of inelastic deformation, in which some of the stored strain energy is lost as heat, and the original shape is not regained immediately. The non-recovered strain energy is referred to as 'hysteresis energy', and can be measured as the area between the loading and unloading curves (Fig. 1.5). Hysteresis energy is responsible for warming up any object that is repeatedly deformed and released: think of a squash ball after a hard game, or a small packet of butter after being squeezed repeatedly.

Creep

'Creep' is time-dependent deformation (or strain) under constant load (Fig. 1.6). In most soft biological materials, creep occurs because water is slowly expelled from the loaded tissue. However, other mechanisms of creep exist, and the lead on a church roof creeps over many years

because of gradual relative slipping of adjacent atoms within the rigid material. Creep arising from fluid flow can usually be reversed: when the loading is reduced, the expelled fluid is sucked back in again, rapidly at first, but then slowing down later.

Tissues such as annulus fibrosus and articular cartilage are termed **poroelastic** because they can behave rather like an elastic body if they are loaded quickly (i.e. they spring back to shape as soon as the load is removed) but when loaded slowly, they creep, as fluid is expelled through tiny pores in the tissue. The term **biphasic** is also used to describe these tissues, because their fluid phase (water) is capable of moving relative to its solid phase (collagen and proteoglycans). Note, however, that articular cartilage and annulus fibrosus do not contain any macroscopic pores filled with fluid: the solid and liquid phases are mixed at the molecular level to form a fibrous solid, and the intensity of loading within these tissues must be characterised by stresses, not a pressure. Importantly, cells within these tissues do not simply experience a fluid pressure. On the contrary, they are deformed by unequal stresses acting in different directions.

Fatigue failure

A structure can be damaged by applying a high force to it once, or a smaller force to it many times. Small forces can create microscopic damage, perhaps in the form of tiny cracks, or a small plastic deformation, which would pass unnoticed if the force was applied and removed only once. However, after a large number of loading cycles, the microscopic damage can accumulate until the entire weakened structure fails, even though the applied loading remains relatively low. This is 'fatigue failure', and the process is often referred to as 'fatigue'. Fatigue failure can occur after only a few loading cycles if the applied load is greater than 60% of the strength of the structure, or it may require millions of loading cycles if the load is below 30% (Fig. 1.7). Sometimes a structure or material has a 'fatigue limit': a force below which fatigue failure never occurs, no matter how many loading cycles are applied. Fatigue explains how engine vibrations can eventually cause aeroplane wings to fall off, and why athletes can suffer so-called 'stress fractures' of bones during intense training or competition.

Cube-square law

If a solid object is scaled up in size, its volume (and therefore its weight) will increase approximately in proportion to its length cubed. However, its area or 'footprint' will increase in proportion to its length squared, so the compressive stress (weight per unit area) acting on the base of the object will steadily increase. If the scaling-up continues, the object will eventually crush itself. This general principle of scaling-up explains why polystyrene can be used to make a model bridge, but not a real bridge, and

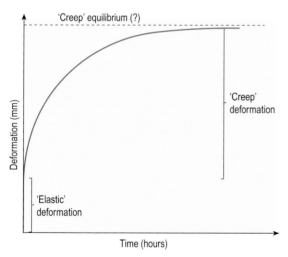

Figure 1.6 Creep curve for a typical biological specimen. When a constant force is initially applied, there is an immediate elastic deformation. If the force is not removed, then further creep deformation occurs as water is expelled from the specimen. Creep is rapid at first, but usually approaches an equilibrium as the water expulsion slows down. The word 'creep' can be used to denote the time-dependent deformation itself, or the process which causes it.

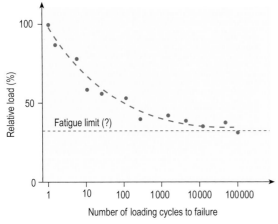

Figure 1.7 Typical fatigue curve showing how the strength of biological specimens decreases markedly with the number of loading cycles applied. The relative load (or stress) is the percentage of the load required to cause failure in a single loading cycle. In some (but not all) specimens there is a fatigue limit, which defines a threshold load below which fatigue failure never occurs, no matter how many loading cycles are applied.

why an elephant cannot fall as far as a mouse without hurting itself. The cube-square law is far from accurate, but it is often useful when attempting to interpret the significance of animal experiments to human beings. In general, large structures must be made from stronger materials than small structures.

Biomechanics and aesthetics

Biomechanical principles determine that the main bulk of each limb muscle should lie near the top of the limb or limb segment, so that the proximal tendon is much shorter than the distal (Fig. 1.8). The weight of the distal limb is therefore minimised, and so can be moved more quickly. This is why ballet shoes must be extremely light. A curious consequence of this principle is the widespread aesthetic judgement that slim ankles and wrists are desirable, whereas thighs and calves should have good shape. A well-tapered leg is best suited to rapid movements, to survival, and hence to attractiveness in a mate!

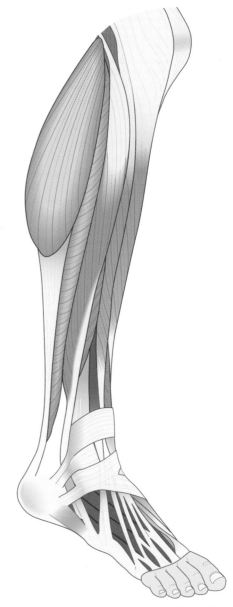

Figure 1.8 The calf muscle (gastrocnemius) has a long distal tendon (the Achilles tendon) but only a short proximal tendon, so most of the mucle bulk lies high up the leg, near the knee. Other limb muscles are similarly asymmetrical, ensuring that distal limb mass is minimised, so feet and hands can be moved more quickly. In this way, biomechanical benefits may provide a darwinian explanation for the widespread aesthetic appreciation of 'a shapely leg'!

Chapter | 2 |

The vertebral column and adjacent structures

When endowed with muscles and other surrounding tissues, the vertebral column is converted into a structure known as the spine. The vertebral column, therefore, constitutes the skeleton of the spine. The following account is based primarily on the thoracolumbar spine, but is mostly applicable to the cervical spine also. Some anatomical differences in the cervical spine are described in Chapter 12.

DESIGN FEATURES

In mechanical terms, the vertebral column is a device that:
- provides axial rigidity to the trunk
- enables certain movements between the skull and pelvis.

Secondarily, the vertebral column:
- affords an origin for muscles of the trunk and limbs.

The individual components of the vertebral column, in one way or another, are designed to contribute to one or other of these functions. Conversely, disorders of the spine may present with impairment of one or other of these functions. It is, therefore, pertinent to appreciate how the elements of the spine are designed to subserve their functions, not only to understand normal anatomy but also to understand the effects of pathology.

Rigidity

Axial rigidity is the cardinal feature that distinguishes vertebrates from soft-bodied molluscs. In biomechanical terms, rigidity means stiffness, or resistance to bending or collapse. This property is essential for the ability of humans to walk upright in the Earth's gravitational field.

In order to provide rigidity, the vertebral column consists largely of bone, in the form of vertebrae, named by number, from above downwards. If rigidity was its sole function, a single bone would suffice, acting as a strut between the skull and pelvis. A single bone, however, would not allow mobility. For that reason multiple bones form the skeleton of the spine.

The notion of a single bone is, however, not totally absurd, because for a variety of reasons some individuals undergo surgical fusion of their spine, usually at one or two lumbar levels, but in some instances at up to five levels. Such patients effectively have their lumbar vertebral column converted to a single bone. Rigidity is maintained and, indeed, increased, but the cost is loss of mobility.

Separation

The essential component of each vertebra is its vertebral body. This is a block of bone, rectangular in profile in a side view, with flat superior and inferior surfaces (Fig. 2.1A), and semicolumnar in top view, with curved anterior and lateral surfaces but a flat posterior surface (Fig. 2.1B). Because of the height of each vertebral body, the vertebral column is endowed with length, and thereby achieves separation of the skull from the pelvis. Separation is essential in order to provide space through which the skull can move relative to the pelvis. Without separation, the thoracic cage, for example, would clash against the pelvic brim and movement would be obstructed. The taller the vertebral bodies the greater the length of the spine, and the greater the possible range of movement.

Although the cervical, thoracic and lumbar regions of the vertebral column most commonly comprise seven, twelve and five vertebrae, respectively, variations do occur. For example, some individuals have four lumbar vertebrae; others have six. Changing the number of vertebrae changes the length of the lumbar spine and the potential mobility of the thorax. The clinical relevance of vertebral number lies in the naming of the last lumbar vertebra. Normally this is L5, but in a shorter lumbar spine it will be L4; in a longer lumbar spine it will be L6. In individuals with an abnormal number of lumbar vertebrae, disorders that normally befall L5 will affect L4 or L6 accordingly.

Compression

In fish, which live in a buoyant environment and are oblivious to the Earth's gravitational field, rigidity, separation and mobility are the only mechanical design requirements of the spine. However, any animal that ventures to be upright in the Earth's gravitational field inherits a liability resulting from the separation of the skull from the pelvis. Under the influence of gravity, the weight of the thorax, and of any load carried in the upper limbs, will exert a compression load on the vertebral column. Moreover, these loads are amplified by the contraction of the back muscles that control the position of the upright spine (Chs 3 and 9). Consequently, the vertebrae are designed to sustain axial compression loads.

Each vertebral body consists of an outer shell of cortical bone, much like a box (Fig. 2.2). Although strong, this shell is not strong enough to sustain the axial loads that are habitually exerted on the spine. Therefore, the vertebral bodies are reinforced internally by narrow struts of bone called trabeculae (Fig. 2.2). Basically, these are arranged in vertical and horizontal arrays (Fig. 2.3). The vertical trabeculae act like columns that transmit compression loads from the upper surface of the vertebral body to its

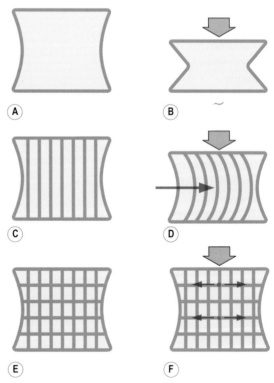

Figure 2.2 Reconstruction of the internal architecture of the vertebral body. (A) With just a shell of cortical bone, a vertebral body is like a box, and collapses (B) when a load is applied. (C, D) Internal vertical struts brace the box. (E) Transverse connections prevent the vertical struts from bowing, and increase the load-bearing capacity of the box. (F) Loads are resisted by tension in the transverse connections. *(From Bogduk (1997), with permission.)*

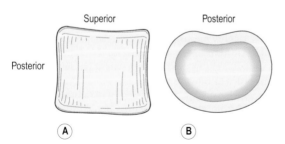

Figure 2.1 Side view (A) and top view (B) of a lumbar vertebral body.

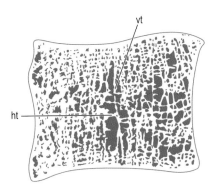

Figure 2.3 A sketch of a sagittal section through a lumbar vertebral body showing the appearance of its vertical (vt) and horizontal (ht) trabeculae.

lower surface. The horizontal trabeculae serve to reinforce the vertical trabeculae by preventing them from buckling sideways under large compression loads.

Absence of horizontal trabeculae weakens the vertebral body. Under load, the vertical trabeculae buckle and can fracture. Lacking the support of the vertical trabeculae, the cortical shell and, therefore, the entire vertebral body can subsequently be easily crushed. This phenomenon is of particular relevance to the condition of spinal osteoporosis (Fig. 8.7).

Mobility

In order to be mobile, the spine requires joints. The principal joints occur between the vertebral bodies. These joints have no formal name (other than 'the intervertebral amphiarthroses', which few people use), but they can be conveniently referred to as the interbody joints. They occur between the inferior surface of one vertebral body and the superior surface of the next. Each is a secondary cartilaginous joint, in which the vertebral bodies are separated by an intervertebral disc. The structure of these joints is such that they allow bending, twisting and sliding movements between vertebral bodies, and the total mobility of the spine is the sum of the mobilities of its joints.

INTERVERTEBRAL DISCS

The intervertebral discs are designed to separate consecutive vertebrae, thereby producing a potential space between them into which the vertebral bodies can dip and execute bending movements. In order to separate the vertebral bodies, each intervertebral disc must have height, but in order to allow movement, the tissue of the disc must be pliable. Meanwhile, the tissue must also be stiff and strong in order to sustain the compression loads between the vertebral bodies.

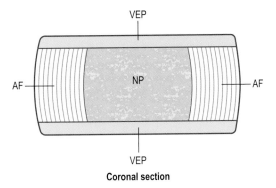

Coronal section

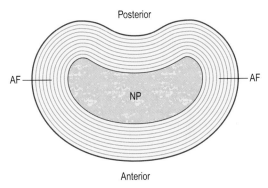

Transverse section

Figure 2.4 The basic structure of a lumbar intervertebral disc. The disc consists of a nucleus pulposus (NP) surrounded by an annulus fibrosus (AF), both sandwiched between two cartilaginous vertebral endplates (VEP). *(From Bogduk (1997), with permission.)*

The essential component of the intervertebral disc is the annulus fibrosus. This consists of some 10–20 sheets of collagen, called lamellae, tightly packed together in a circumferential fashion around the periphery of the disc (Fig. 2.4). While packed tightly together, these lamellae are stiff, and can sustain considerable compression loads. A suitable analogy is the stiffness of a telephone directory that is wrapped into a cylindrical shape and stood end-on. Nevertheless, being collagenous, the annulus fibrosus is sufficiently pliable that it can deform and thereby enable bending movements between vertebral bodies. However, herein lies the liability of the annulus fibrosus. If it buckles it loses its stiffness, and is less able to sustain compression loads. To prevent this, the annulus fibrosus requires the second component of the intervertebral disc – the nucleus pulposus.

The nucleus pulposus is a hydrated gel located in the centre of each disc (Fig. 2.4). When compressed, this semifluid mass expands in a radial fashion. On the one hand this radial expansion is resisted by the surrounding annulus fibrosus, but on the other hand, the expansion braces the annulus fibrosus from the inside, thereby preventing it from buckling inwards and losing its stiffness. Cooperatively, the nucleus pulposus and annulus fibrosus maintain the stiffness of the disc against compression loading, but both tissues are sufficiently compliant that they allow some degree of movement between vertebral bodies.

The third components of the intervertebral disc are the superior and inferior vertebral endplates. These are plates of hyaline cartilage that cover the superior and inferior aspects of the disc, and bind the disc to their respective vertebral bodies (Fig. 2.4). Each endplate covers almost the entire surface of the adjacent vertebral body; only a narrow rim of bone, called the ring apophysis, around the perimeter of the vertebral body is left uncovered by cartilage.

That portion of the vertebral body to which the cartilaginous vertebral endplate is applied lacks a formal name, but can be referred to as the subchondral bone (of the vertebral body) or the bony vertebral endplate. It is, however, a component of the vertebral body and not a component of the disc, as is the cartilaginous vertebral endplate. Notwithstanding this distinction in nomenclature, mechanical disorders that affect the region of the endplate typically involve both the osseous and cartilaginous endplates simultaneously.

In addition to enabling bending movements between vertebral bodies, the intervertebral disc allows for twisting and sliding movements of small amplitude. These are resisted by tension developed in the collagen fibres of the annulus fibrosus, and their amplitude is a function of the elasticity and tensile stiffness of the annulus.

Microstructure

The annulus fibrosus consists mostly of type I and type II collagen. The concentration of type I collagen is greater towards the periphery of the annulus, while that of type II collagen is reciprocally greater towards the centre of the disc. This distribution of type I collagen matches the greater tensile role of the outer annulus fibrosus.

Within each lamella of the annulus fibrosus, the collagen fibres are arranged in parallel. They pass obliquely from one vertebral body to the next, at an angle of about 65° to the sagittal plane. However, as a rule, the fibres in each successive lamella are oriented in an opposite sense, with one layer inclined to the left, the next layer inclined to the right, and so on (Fig. 2.5). This alternating arrangement precludes any cleavage plane developing through the annulus, through which nuclear material might seep or burst, and is critical to the integrity of the disc. Moreover, the alternating orientation allows the annulus to resist tension in a variety of directions.

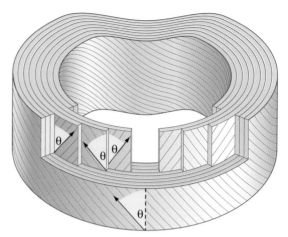

Figure 2.5 The architecture of the annulus fibrosus. Collagen fibres are arranged in 10–20 concentric, circumferential lamellae. The orientation of fibres alternates in successive lamellae, but their orientation with respect to the vertical (θ) is approximately the same, and measures about 65°. *(From Bogduk (1997), with permission.)*

Sliding movements between the vertebral bodies will be resisted by all those collagen fibres that are inclined in the direction of movement (Fig. 2.6A). Similarly, twisting movements will be resisted by those fibres inclined in the direction of movement (Fig. 2.6B). All fibres will contribute to resisting separation of the vertebral bodies (Fig. 2.6C).

In this regard, it is the outermost fibres of the annulus fibrosus that contribute most to resisting these movements. To that end, they are attached directly to bone, around the ring apophysis, and for that reason they are referred to as the ligamentous portion of the annulus fibrosus (Fig. 2.7). The inner fibres of the annulus do not attach to bone but insert into the vertebral endplate. Within the endplate they can be traced forming a continuous envelope around the nucleus pulposus. For this reason they are, at times, referred to as the capsular portion of the annulus fibrosus.

The nucleus pulposus consists largely of proteoglycans, which are large molecules consisting of complex sugars and protein (Fig. 7.13). They have the valuable property of being able to imbibe and retain large amounts of water. It is this property that endows the nucleus pulposus with its hydrodynamic properties. If the nucleus loses its proteoglycans, it can no longer hold its water, and the nucleus can no longer properly brace the annulus fibrosus. If that function is lost, the disc can no longer resist compression loads, and will be progressively compressed and narrowed under the loads of daily living.

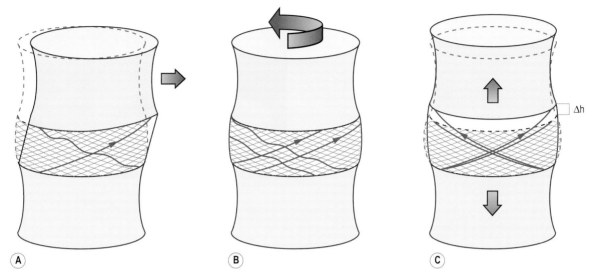

(A) (B) (C)

Figure 2.6 Mechanics of the annulus fibrosus. (A) Sliding movements between vertebral bodies are resisted by tension developing in those fibres of the annulus that are inclined in the direction of movement. Other fibres are relaxed by the displacement. (B) Twisting movements are resisted by those fibres lengthened by the movement. Other fibres are relaxed. (C) Separation of the vertebral bodies (Δh) is resisted by all fibres, regardless of their orientation. *(From Bogduk (1997), with permission.)*

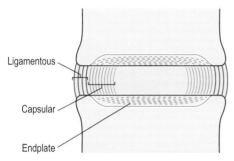

Figure 2.7 Detailed structure of the annulus fibrosus. The peripheral fibres attach to the ring apophysis and constitute the tensile, ligamentous portion of the annulus. The inner fibres surround the nucleus pulposus and constitute the capsular portion. They can be traced into the cartilage of the vertebral endplate, thereby forming a complete envelope around the nucleus. Because of these fibres the superficial parts of the endplate are fibrocartilage. The deeper parts are hyaline cartilage.

Disc height

Each lumbar intervertebral disc is 5–10 mm in height. Thoracic discs are somewhat narrower. Collectively, the intervertebral discs contribute approximately 25% to the length of the spine. During activities of daily living, when an individual is upright, water is squeezed out of the discs, and they each lose height. After rest in a recumbent position this height is restored, as water is re-imbibed. Disc height is fully restored at night, during sleep.

Disc height is preserved with age. Discs do not narrow because of age. Discs of the elderly have even been reported to be slightly higher than average,[1445] although this refers to the nucleus pulposus, which can sink into adjacent vertebrae if they are osteoporotic. However, disc narrowing can occur in certain disorders of the disc. Any disorder that disrupts or degrades the proteoglycans of the nucleus pulposus will impair their water-binding capacity, and compromise the ability of the disc to restore and maintain its height.

THE ESSENTIAL LUMBAR VERTEBRAL COLUMN

Five vertebral bodies and their respective discs constitute the essential components of the lumbar vertebral column (Fig. 2.8). From above downwards, the five vertebral bodies are named numerically as lumbar one to five, i.e. L1, L2, L3, L4 and L5. The intervertebral discs are numbered according to the vertebral bodies that each separates, i.e. L1–2, L2–3, L3–4, L4–5, and the last disc is known as the lumbosacral disc, or L5–S1.

Collectively the vertebral bodies and discs form a column that provides rigidity and length, and permits movements. The vertebral bodies and intervertebral discs strongly resist compression, and easily bear the loads of the thorax and upper limbs. Forward bending is achieved by each intervertebral disc being compressed slightly,

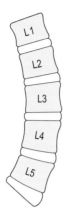

Figure 2.8 The essential lumbar vertebral column consists of the five lumbar vertebral bodies and their intervertebral discs.

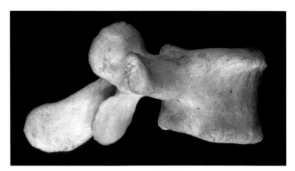

Figure 2.10 A typical lumbar vertebra, comprising the vertebral body (VB) and the neural arch (NA).

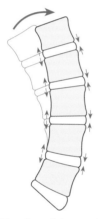

Figure 2.9 Forward bending of the vertebral column is achieved by compression of the anterior ends of the intervertebral discs, and resisted by tension in the posterior annulus fibrosus.

anteriorly, and is resisted by tension developed in the posterior annulus fibrosus (Fig. 2.9). Extension and lateral flexion are achieved by corresponding events in the opposite direction and in the coronal plane, respectively. Rotation of the lumbar spine is achieved by each disc allowing a small degree of twist, and is resisted by tension developed in the annulus fibrosus.

However, the vertebral bodies and discs are not the complete structure of the lumbar vertebral column. Alone these structures are relatively unstable and susceptible to injury. The annulus fibrosus is not strong enough, on its own, to resist excessive torsion of the lumbar spine without being damaged. Nor can the vertebral bodies and discs alone maintain a straight, or upright, posture; the discs are sufficiently compliant that the slightest axial load will tend to bend the column. In order to maintain stability, and to

afford control of movements, the essential lumbar vertebral column requires additional elements. These are the posterior elements of the lumbar vertebrae.

POSTERIOR ELEMENTS

The posterior elements of the lumbar vertebrae (Fig. 2.10) are designed to control the position of the vertebral bodies. Forces may be exerted directly by muscles acting on the posterior elements, or indirectly by loads on the thorax trying to bend or twist the lumbar spine.

Towards the upper end of its posterior surface, each lumbar vertebral body is endowed with a pair of stout pillars of bone called the pedicles (Fig. 2.11B). These support the posterior elements, and transmit forces from them to the vertebral body, and vice versa.

From each pedicle, a plate of bone, called the lamina, projects towards the midline, in the manner of a sloping roof (Fig. 2.11D). At the midline, the two laminae fuse seamlessly. In a top view, the pedicles and laminae can be perceived as forming an arch, known as the neural arch, which together with the posterior surface of the vertebral body encloses a space and channel, behind the vertebral body, known as the vertebral foramen (Fig. 2.11E). By convention, the laminae are perceived to form the roof of the foramen, and the vertebral body to form the floor.

At the junction of its two laminae in the midline, each lumbar vertebra bears a spinous process which projects dorsally in the shape of the blade of an axe (Fig. 2.11A). Projecting laterally from the junction of the pedicle with its lamina on each side is a long, rectangular, flattened bar of bone called the transverse process (Fig. 2.11C). On its posterior surface, near its root, each transverse process bears a thick but narrow spike of bone called the accessory process (Fig. 2.11D). These several processes serve as sites of attachment for muscles that control the lumbar vertebral column, and endow these muscles with lever arms.

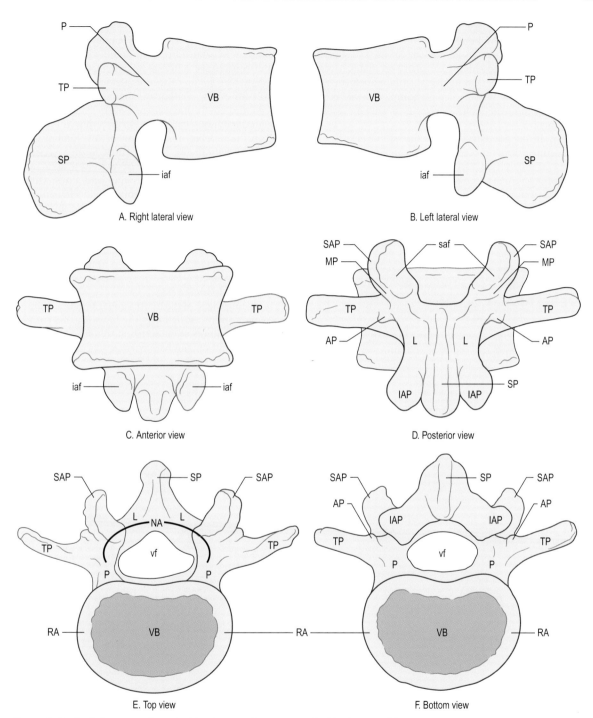

Figure 2.11 (A–F) The parts of a typical lumbar vertebra. VB, vertebral body; P, pedicle; TP, transverse process; SP, spinous process; L, lamina; SAP, superior articular process; IAP, inferior articular process; saf, superior articular facet; iaf, inferior articular facet; MP, mamillary process; AP, accessory process; vf, vertebral foramen; RA, ring apophysis; NA, neural arch. *(From Bogduk (1997), with permission.)*

From its superior, lateral corner, the lamina gives rise to an extension of bone called the superior articular process (Fig. 2.11E). On its medial surface, the superior articular process presents an articular facet that is covered by articular cartilage. On its dorsal surface, each superior articular process bears a small bump, known as the mamillary process, which serves as a site for muscle attachments.

From its inferior, lateral corner, the lamina gives rise to an inferior articular process that bears an articular facet on its lateral surface (Fig. 2.11B). The superior articular processes of one vertebra receive the inferior articular processes of the vertebra above to form synovial joints known as the zygapophyseal joints. These joints serve to enable certain movements of the lumbar vertebral column but to limit or prevent others.

THE COMPLETE LUMBAR VERTEBRAL COLUMN

When the posterior elements of the lumbar vertebrae are added to the essential vertebral column, they provide a series of interlocking bony elements behind the vertebral bodies and discs (Fig. 2.12). The laminae of consecutive vertebrae are separated from one another by a short interval, but consecutive vertebrae are articulated through the zygapophyseal joints. The complete lumbar vertebral column sits on the sacrum, articulating with it anteriorly through the L5–S1 intervertebral discs, and posteriorly through the lumbosacral (L5–S1) zygapophyseal joints.

When the vertebral foramina of the five lumbar vertebrae are longitudinally aligned, they form a series of arcades surrounding what can be perceived as a canal running behind the vertebral bodies and discs. This is known as the vertebral canal. Amongst other elements, the vertebral canal transmits the lower end of the spinal cord and the roots of the lumbar, sacral and coccygeal nerves (see Ch. 4). Routes of access to the vertebral canal occur in the form of passages between consecutive pedicles, behind each intervertebral disc and in front of the zygapophyseal joints at each level. These passages are called the intervertebral foramina (Fig. 2.12).

The resting shape of the intact lumbar vertebral column is a curve concave posteriorly. The basis for this curve is tension in the joints of the vertebral column and the ligaments that bind the lumbar vertebrae together.

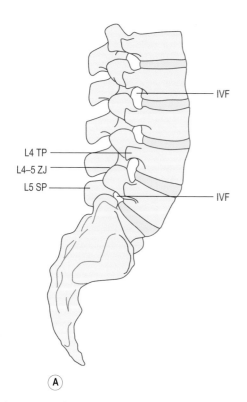

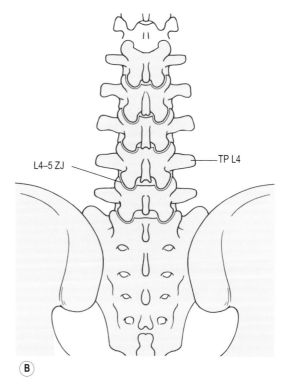

Figure 2.12 The complete lumbar vertebral column. (A) Side view; (B) rear view. TP, transverse process; SP, spinous process; ZJ, zygapophyseal joint; IVF, intervertebral foramen.

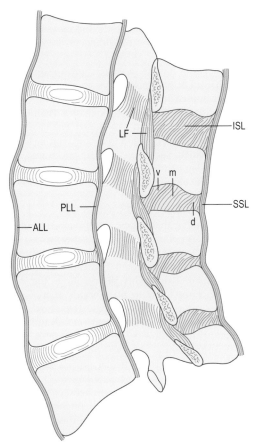

Figure 2.13 A median sagittal section of the lumbar spine to show its various ligaments. ALL, anterior longitudinal ligament; PLL, posterior longitudinal ligament; SSL, supraspinous ligament; ISL, interspinous ligament; v, ventral part; m, middle part; d, dorsal part; LF, ligamentum flavum, viewed from within the vertebral canal, and in sagittal section at the midline. *(From Bogduk (1997), with permission.)*

LIGAMENTS

Many of the structures called ligaments in the lumbar spine are not truly ligaments. Either they do not connect two bones, or they are too feeble to serve as ligaments.

The most definitive ligament is the ligamentum flavum (Fig. 2.13). It consists of fibres of elastin that connect the lower end of the internal surface of one lamina to the upper end of the external surface of the lamina below, and closes the gap between consecutive laminae. This is a very extensible ligament that stretches when the lumbar vertebral column bends forwards. It consists of elastin in order that, upon resumption of the neutral posture of the lumbar spine after flexion, the fibres of the ligamentum

flavum can recoil and shorten without buckling. A ligament made of collagen could just as well resist flexion as does the ligamentum flavum, but it could not shorten. As a result it would buckle inwards towards the neural elements within the vertebral canal, with the risk of compressing them. The virtue of an elastic ligamentum flavum is that it ensures that the neural elements are always presented with a smooth flat surface.

The transverse processes are connected by thin sheets of collagen fibres. Although called the intertransverse ligaments, these structures are too insubstantive to function as ligaments. Rather, they constitute membranes that separate the ventral muscle compartment of the lumbar spine from its dorsal muscle compartment (Ch. 3).

The opposing edges of spinous processes are connected by collagen fibres referred to as the interspinous ligaments (Fig. 2.13). Although the ventral portions of these ligaments are distinctly ligamentous, their dorsal portions actually constitute tendinous fibres of the erector spinae muscle (Ch. 3).

A supraspinous ligament has traditionally been recognised, but this structure is not a ligament. It consists of tendinous fibres of various muscles (Ch. 3), and is lacking below L3.

In addition to the ligaments of the posterior elements, the lumbar vertebral column is reinforced by ligaments that connect the vertebral bodies. The posterior longitudinal ligament covers the floor of the vertebral canal (Fig. 2.13). Its fibres are attached to the posterior aspects of the lumbar vertebral bodies and to the intervertebral discs. It has short fibres that span consecutive vertebra, and longer fibres that span several vertebrae. The anterior longitudinal ligament covers the anterior aspects of the vertebral bodies and discs (Fig. 2.13). Its fibres are attached to the edges of the vertebral bodies. Many of its fibres, however, are not truly ligamentous, but constitute the prolonged tendons of the crura of the diaphragm.

The strongest ligament attached to the lumbar vertebral column is the iliolumbar ligament. Its fibres arise from the tip and borders of the transverse process of the fifth lumbar vertebra, and pass backwards and laterally to the ilium. They serve to anchor the L5 vertebra on the pelvic girdle, to prevent it from sliding forwards and from rotating.

ZYGAPOPHYSEAL JOINTS

The zygapophyseal joints provide an important locking mechanism between consecutive lumbar vertebrae. They are designed to block axial rotation and forward sliding of the lumbar vertebrae. By blocking axial rotation the joints protect the intervertebral discs from excessive torsion. By blocking forward slide they prevent the vertebral bodies from dislocating under the weight of the trunk when the spine is flexed forwards.

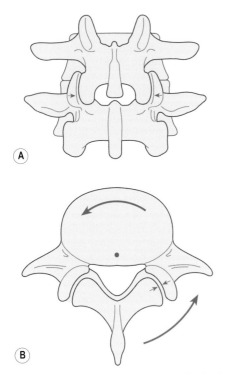

Figure 2.14 (A) A sketch of a posterior view of a lumbar zygapophyseal joint showing how the superior articular processes clasp the inferior articular processes laterally. (B) A top view showing how the superior articular processes block rotation of the inferior articular processes.

Axial rotation of the lumbar vertebrae occurs around a longitudinal axis that passes through the posterior third or so of the vertebral bodies and intervertebral discs. When rotation occurs about this axis, the posterior elements of the moving vertebra swing laterally, in a direction opposite to that of the rotation. To block this rotation, the zygapophyseal joints are arranged in such a way as to block the lateral displacement of the posterior elements.

Each pair of superior articular processes clasps the inferior articular processes of the vertebra above (Fig. 2.14A). The flat, medially facing facet of each superior articular process apposes the laterally facing facet of the inferior articular process. If the upper vertebra attempts to rotate to the left, its right inferior articular process will ram into the apposing superior articular process (Fig. 2.14B). This locking mechanism limits axial rotation at each intervertebral joint, and protects the intervertebral disc from torsion (Fig. 11.10).

In order to prevent forward slide, the inferior articular processes act as hooks. Projecting downwards from the pedicles, the inferior articular processes extend below the bottom of the vertebral body and engage the superior articular processes of the vertebra below, from behind (Fig. 2.15A). Consequently, if the upper vertebra attempts to

slide forwards, its inferior articular processes hook on to the superior articular processes which oppose the motion and thereby prevent forward sliding. In order to exert resistance to the inferior articular processes, the superior articular processes have to face backwards to some extent. This is achieved in one of several ways.

When examined in a top view, the superior articular processes exhibit one of three basic shapes. Their articular facets may be flat, C-shaped or J-shaped. Flat facets afford resistance to axial rotation and to forward sliding by being obliquely oriented, such that they face backwards as well as medially (Fig. 2.15B). C-shaped and J-shaped facets offer a posterior end that faces medially and opposes axial rotation, and an anterior end that faces posteriorly and opposes forward slide (Fig. 2.15C and D).

Notwithstanding their shape in top view, the superior articular facets are flat in a longitudinal sense, as are the apposing inferior articular facets. This shape allows for unrestricted gliding movement between the facets in a superoinferior direction. This gliding allows the inferior articular processes freely to lift upwards as its vertebral body flexes on the one below (Fig. 2.16). Thus, whereas the zygapophyseal joints restrict axial rotation and forward slide, they permit flexion between their vertebrae. Extension is permitted in the same way but is limited in range as the tips of the inferior articular processes impact the lamina of the vertebra below (Fig. 2.16).

To facilitate the gliding movement between the articular processes, the facets of the zygapophyseal joints are covered by articular cartilage, which in turn is lubricated by a film of synovial fluid. The fluid is retained by a synovial membrane that attaches to the edges of the articular cartilage, and the membrane is supported by a joint capsule (Fig. 2.17). Posteriorly the joint capsule is fibrous, with short, tight fibres running transversely between the articular processes. Superiorly and inferiorly the fibrous capsule is lax in order to accommodate the displacement of the articular processes during flexion and extension movements. Anteriorly the fibrous capsule is replaced by the most lateral fibres of the ligamentum flavum.

As the inferior articular process in a zygapophyseal joint slides across the apposing superior articular facet during flexion, it subluxates, i.e. while the lower half of its articular facet remains in contact with the facet of the superior articular process, its upper half loses contact, and is effectively exposed. Similarly, the lower half of the superior articular facet is exposed. In order to protect these exposed surfaces, and to maintain a film of synovial fluid over their articular cartilages, the zygapophyseal joints are endowed with intra-articular meniscoids. These fibroadipose structures are crescentic wedges, located at the superior and inferior poles of the joint, with a base attached to the joint capsule, and a tapering apex that projects into the joint cavity (Fig. 2.17). In the neutral position of the joint, the meniscoids project between the articular cartilages. As the inferior articular process slides upwards across the

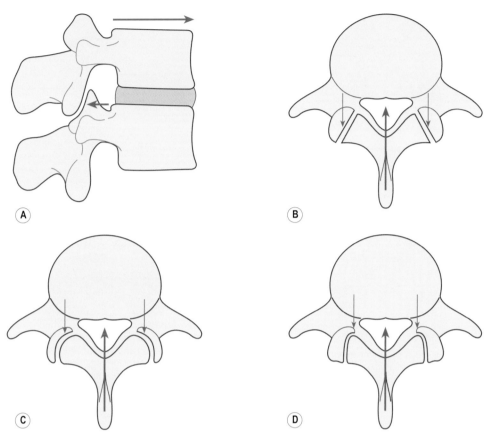

Figure 2.15 (A) A sketch of a lateral view of a lumbar zygapophyseal joint showing how the inferior articular processes hook behind the superior articular processes. The external surface of the superior articular process has been cut away in order to reveal the internal features of the joint. (B) A top view of a flat zygapophyseal joint showing how it resists forward sliding of the inferior articular processes. (C) A top view of a C-shaped zygapophyseal joint showing how its anterior end resists forward sliding of the inferior articular processes. (D) A top view of a J-shaped zygapophyseal joint showing how its narrow anterior end resists forward sliding of the inferior articular processes.

superior articular process, it leaves the inferior meniscoid applied to the exposed surface of the superior articular facet, and takes the superior meniscoid with it to protect its own exposed surface.

THE SACRUM

The sacrum is a block of bone that supports the lumbar vertebral column. However, it is also an integral component of the pelvic girdle, and thereby serves to transmit forces between the vertebral column and the lower limbs.

In front and rear views the sacrum is triangular in shape, with a broad upper end tapering to a blunt point inferiorly (Figs 2.18 and 2.19). In profile the sacrum is curved, with a smooth, concave anterior surface and a rough, convex posterior surface (Fig. 2.20). Superiorly it presents features

designed to receive the lumbar vertebral column. Laterally, it is designed to articulate with the ilium on each side.

Intrinsically the sacrum consists of five segments that are fused together, each representing a rudimentary vertebra. On the anterior surface of the sacrum the superior and inferior edges of the vertebral bodies are represented as transverse ridges (Fig. 2.18). Between these ridges a narrow block of bone replaces what might have been an intervertebral disc. In longitudinal sections of the sacrum (Fig. 2.20), rudimentary discs may be found deep within the substance of the bone, particularly between the first and second sacral segments.

Projecting laterally from the vertebral bodies are the lateral masses of the sacral segments (Fig. 2.18). These represent the transverse processes, but instead of remaining separate, the tips of these transverse processes are fused together laterally to form a single mass of bone. However, fusion does not occur more medially where between

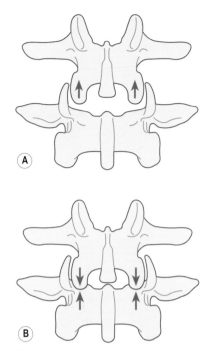

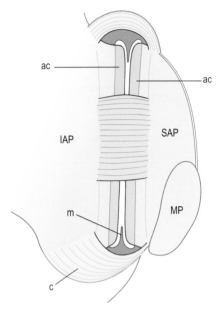

Figure 2.16 Posterior views of a lumbar zygapophyseal joint. (A) During flexion the inferior articular processes are free to glide upwards across the superior articular processes. (B) During extension the inferior articular processes glide downwards across the superior articular processes but are arrested by impaction against the lamina below.

Figure 2.17 A posterior view of the components of a right, lumbar zygapophyseal joint. The facets of the superior articular process (SAP) and inferior articular process (IAP) are covered by articular cartilage (ac). The capsule (c) is loose and abundant at the superior and inferior poles of the joint. Dorsally it consists of transverse fibres. These have been resected superiorly and inferiorly to reveal the fibroadipose meniscoids (m) that lie between the articular cartilages at the superior and inferior poles.

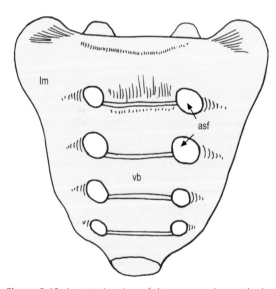

Figure 2.18 An anterior view of the sacrum. vb, vertebral body; lm, lateral mass; asf, anterior sacral foramina. *(From Bogduk (1997), with permission.)*

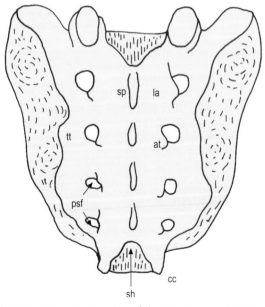

Figure 2.19 A posterior view of the sacrum. sp, spinous process; la, lamina; tt, transverse tubercle; psf, posterior sacral foramen; at, articular tubercle; sh, sacral hiatus; c, cornu. *(From Bogduk (1997), with permission.)*

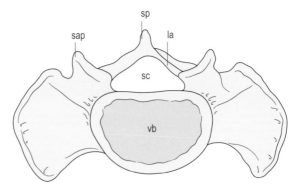

Figure 2.21 A superior view of the sacrum. vb, vertebral body; sap, superior articular process; sp, spinous process; la, lamina; sc, sacral canal. *(From Bogduk (1997), with permission.)*

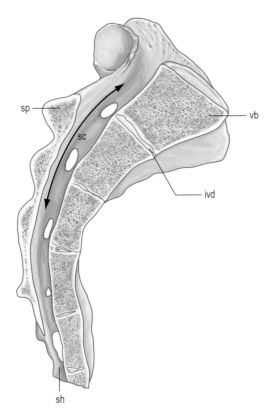

Figure 2.20 A longitudinal section through the sacrum. sc, sacral canal; sh, sacral hiatus; sp, spinous process; vb, vertebral bodies; ivd, remnant of an intervertebral disc. *(From Bogduk (1997), with permission.)*

consecutive transverse processes foramina are formed. The foramina seen on the anterior surface of the sacrum transmit the anterior rami of the sacral spinal nerves, and are known as the anterior sacral foramina.

Posteriorly, each of the sacral segments exhibits components homologous to the posterior elements of the lumbar vertebrae. Prominent in the midline are the spinous processes (Fig. 2.19). Beside these are the laminae, which are fused between consecutive segments. A lamina and spinous process are lacking from the fifth sacral segment, leaving a hole, known as the sacral hiatus. This hiatus constitutes the inferior opening of the sacral canal, which passes longitudinally through the sacrum, and represents the continuation of the lumbar vertebral canal. Laterally, the transverse processes of the sacral segments are fused and surround the posterior sacral foramina, which transmit the posterior rami of the sacral spinal nerves. The tip of each transverse process is marked by a small prominence, each known as a transverse tubercle. Medial to each posterior sacral foramen is a small bump that represents

what might have been a zygapophyseal joint, for which reason the bump is known as the articular tubercle. The fifth sacral segment presents a pair of definitive articular processes which articulate with the coccyx. They flank the sacral hiatus like horns, for which reason they are known as the sacral cornua.

The superior end of the sacrum presents a central surface that resembles the superior surface of a lumbar vertebral body (Fig. 2.21). It receives the L5–S1 intervertebral disc. Laterally, the transverse process is long and thick, and is known as the ala (wing) of the sacrum. From its posterior surface on each side projects a superior articular process which receives the inferior articular process of the L5 vertebra.

In the upright position, the sacrum is inclined forwards, such that its upper surface slopes below horizontal at an angle of about 50° (Fig. 2.22). This orientation compromises the base for the lumbar vertebral column, for it invites the lumbar vertebral column to slip forwards and downwards across the sloping superior surface of the sacrum. Three design features militate against this tendency. First, the L5–S1 intervertebral disc is wedge-shaped, by about 16°, so as to lessen the angle between the top of the sacrum and the bottom of the L5 vertebral body. Secondly, the superior articular processes of the sacrum face backwards, at between 45° and 90° to the sagittal plane. As a result, the inferior articular processes of L5 hook securely on to the sacrum, and prevent the lumbar vertebral column from sliding forwards. Finally, the L5 transverse processes are strongly secured to the ilium on each side by the iliolumbar ligaments. These large ligaments prevent forward displacement of the L5 vertebra in relation to the sacrum and pelvis.

The lateral surface of the sacrum presents a large ear-shaped articular surface, known either as the articular surface or the auricular surface, and a roughened

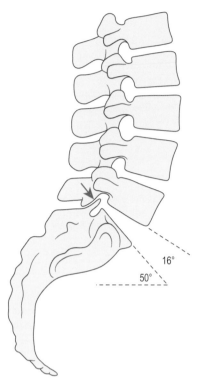

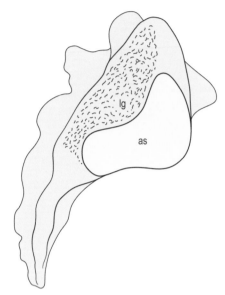

Figure 2.23 A lateral view of the sacrum. as, auricular surface; lg, ligamentous surface. *(From Bogduk (1997), with permission.)*

Figure 2.22 A side view of the lumbosacral junction in the upright standing position. The superior surface of the sacrum slopes downwards at about 50° below horizontal. The L5–S1 intervertebral disc is wedge-shaped. The inferior articular processes of L5 hook behind the superior articular processes of the sacrum, so as to prevent slipping of the L5 vertebra on the sloping surface of the sacrum.

ligamentous area behind it (Fig. 2.23). These are designed to lock the sacrum into the pelvic ring through the sacro-iliac joint.

SACROILIAC JOINT

Unlike the typical joints of the limbs, or even those of the lumbar vertebral column, the sacroiliac joint is not designed to accommodate substantial ranges of movement. Indeed, its mobility is limited to about 2°. Moreover, there are no muscles that act to produce active physiological movements of this joint. Rather, the sacroiliac joint is designed to act as a stress-relieving joint in the pelvic girdle.

During gait, the pelvic girdle is subjected to complex twisting forces, the nature of which can be likened to the effect of taking a ring and twisting it towards the shape of a figure of eight. The stresses applied to the pelvic girdle are such that if it were a solid ring of bone, it would crack.

Intriguingly, this phenomenon occurs in elderly individuals in whom the sacroiliac joints are fused as a result of age changes or disease. If they remain mobile, their pelvic girdle fails by fractures that develop parallel to the line of the sacroiliac joints. By having sacroiliac joints, the pelvic girdle avoids cracking. For this purpose the sacroiliac joint is endowed with strong ligaments that absorb the stresses applied to the pelvic girdle during gait.

The sacroiliac joint is a synovial joint between the auricular surface of the sacrum and the articular surface of the ilium. The auricular surface of the sacrum is not flat, but presents a depression opposite the second sacral segment, and prominences opposite the first and third segments. These undulations articulate with reciprocal surfaces on the ilium, such that the sacrum is locked between the two ilia of the pelvic girdle (Fig. 2.24). Provided the ilia are kept pressed against the sacrum, the sacrum is prevented by the locking mechanism from being driven downwards by the weight of the trunk, or from rotating forwards. The ilia are attached to the sacrum by the interosseous sacroiliac ligament.

This ligament is short but thick. It arises from the ligamentous area of the sacrum and inserts into an opposing area of the ilium (Fig. 2.25). Tension within the ligaments on both sides keeps the ilia pressed against the sacrum. Injuries that tear this ligament, or conditions that slacken it, such as pregnancy, can compromise the integrity of the sacroiliac joint by relaxing the pressure of the ilium against the sacrum.

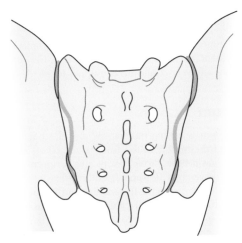

Figure 2.24 A posterior view of the sacroiliac joints, showing the sinuous shape of the joint space, and how the undulating surface of the sacrum locks into reciprocal surfaces of the ilium. *(From Bogduk (1997), with permission.)*

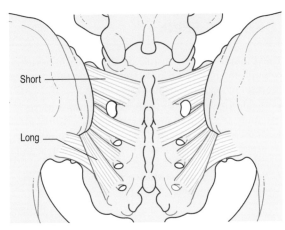

Figure 2.26 The posterior sacroiliac ligaments. *(From Bogduk (1997), with permission.)*

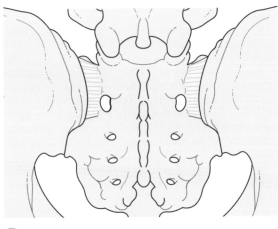

(A)

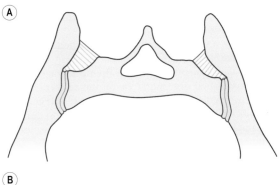

(B)

Figure 2.25 The interosseous sacroiliac ligament. (A) Posterior view. (B) Axial view. *(From Bogduk (1997), with permission.)*

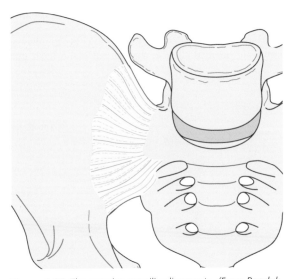

Figure 2.27 The anterior sacroiliac ligaments. *(From Bogduk (1997), with permission.)*

Additional ligaments reinforce the sacroiliac joint. Posteriorly, the long and short posterior sacroiliac ligaments connect the ilium to the posterior surface of the sacrum (Fig. 2.26). Anteriorly, the capsule of the joint is thickened to form the anterior sacroiliac ligament (Fig. 2.27). It serves to prevent the anterior edges of the sacrum and ilium from separating. Remote from the sacroiliac joint, the sacrospinous and sacrotuberous ligaments anchor the sacrum to the spine of the ischium and the tuberosity of the ischium, respectively. They serve to prevent forward rotation of the sacrum.

THORACIC SPINE

The thoracic spine consists of the thoracic vertebral column, the ribs and the sternum. It is pertinent to the function of the lumbar spine in so far as:

- loads from the upper trunk are transmitted to the lumbar spine from the thoracic spine
- muscles that act on the lumbar spine reach into the thoracic region and attach to thoracic vertebrae and ribs
- abdominal muscles, which act on the lumbar spine, arise from the ribs.

Thoracic vertebral column

In general terms, the thoracic vertebrae resemble lumbar vertebrae (Fig. 2.28). When stacked, the thoracic vertebrae form a curve that is concave forwards, and this is known as thoracic kyphosis. A concave curve increases the antero-posterior diameter and, therefore, the volume of the thoracic cavity.

At most thoracic levels, the thoracic zygapophyseal joints are oriented close to the coronal plane, such that

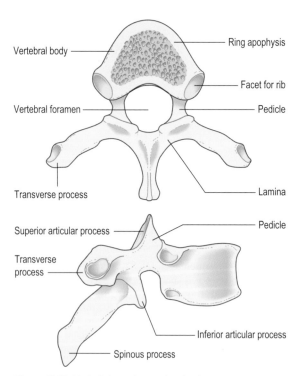

Figure 2.28 Typical thoracic vertebra in the transverse (upper) and sagittal planes. *(Adapted from Bogduk N In: Rheumatology, 4th edn. Hochberg et al. (eds) Elsevier.)*

Labels for upper figure: Vertebral body, Ring apophysis, Facet for rib, Vertebral foramen, Pedicle, Transverse process, Lamina

Labels for lower figure: Superior articular process, Pedicle, Transverse process, Inferior articular process, Spinous process

their superior articular processes face backwards; but at lower levels the joints exhibit a gradual transition towards a more lumbar orientation, towards the sagittal plane. This arrangement prevents axial rotation at lower thoracic levels but allows it at middle and upper levels.

Sternum

The sternum is a long but narrow and flat bar of bone located in the middle of the front of the chest. Along its lateral edges it bears facets that receive connections form the upper seven ribs. Its upper lateral corners are expanded and thickened to receive the medial end of the clavicle. Through the sternoclavicular joint, certain loads are transmitted from the upper limb to the thorax and then through the ribs to the vertebral column.

Ribs

The ribs form the skeleton of the thoracic cage. They are narrow curved bones of different lengths. They are short at upper levels; become progressively longer to middle levels; and then progressively shorter at lower levels of the thorax.

At its medial end each rib is expanded to form a head. A short distance laterally along its shaft each typical rib bears a bump known as the tubercle. That portion of the rib between its head and its tubercle is known as the neck of the rib. A short distance laterally beyond the tubercle the rib changes its curvature. This point is known as the angle. In effect, that region medial to the angle belongs to the back, and is involved in spinal functions, whereas the remainder of the rib, laterally, pertains to respiratory functions.

At its anterior end each rib is prolonged by a shaft of cartilage known as the costal cartilage. The costal cartilages of the upper seven ribs reach the sternum, with which they form sternocostal joints. The costal cartilages of the eighth, ninth and 10th ribs join the costal cartilages above. The tips of the 11th and 12th ribs float freely, without forming any articulations.

Medially, a typical rib articulates with the thoracic vertebral column through two joints. The head of the rib forms a costovertebral joint with the posterior corner of the intervertebral disc and facets on the adjacent corners of the two vertebral bodies joined by the disc (Fig. 2.28). The tubercle of the rib articulates with a facet on the anterior surface of the tip of the transverse process, to form a costotransverse joint. Various ligaments bind the head, neck and costal tubercles of the rib to the vertebral bodies and transverse process.

The first rib differs in that its head articulates exclusively with the first thoracic vertebra. The 11th and 12th ribs differ in that their tubercles form rudimentary or no joints with their transverse processes.

Muscle surface

When fully articulated, the thoracic vertebral column and ribs present a posterior surface on to which various muscles attach. Intrinsic muscles of the thoracic spine attach between the spinous processes in the roots of the transverse processes. Certain respiratory muscles suspend each rib to the transverse process above. Certain muscles of the neck take root on upper thoracic transverse processes.

Otherwise, various muscles descend from thoracic levels to act on the lumbar spine. These arise from:

• the posterior surface of the lateral end of each transverse process

• the adjacent surface of each lateral to the tubercle
• the posterior surface of the angle of each rib.

Additionally, various abdominal muscles arise from the external and internal surfaces of the lower six ribs or their costal cartilages.

FURTHER READING

Bogduk N. Clinical anatomy of the lumbar spine and sacrum. 3rd ed. Edinburgh: Churchill Livingstone; 1997.

Chapter | 3 |

Muscles and fascia of the lumbar spine

Whereas the joints and ligaments of the vertebral column endow it with a certain amount of intrinsic stability, they protect it only passively from excessive movement. For the control of movement, the column is endowed with muscles. Muscles are the principal tissues that surround the lumbar vertebral column.

Topographically, the muscles of the lumbar spine are located in three distinct groups: (1) the tiny, intersegmental muscles that connect consecutive spinous processes or transverse processes; (2) the anterolateral muscles; and (3) the posterior muscles. Within and between groups, individual muscles differ with respect to their functions in relation to the lumbar vertebral column.

INTERSEGMENTAL MUSCLES

The interspinales are thin, rectangular sheets of fibres that connect the edges of apposing spinous processes (Fig. 3.1). The intertransversarii are small muscles that are attached to the transverse processes of the lumbar vertebrae (Fig. 3.1). The intertransversarii mediales are tiny slips that pass essentially from an accessory process to the mamillary process below. The intertransversarii laterales dorsales are similar slips that pass from an accessory process to the transverse process below. The intertransversarii lateral ventrales are fibres that pass from the lower edge of one transverse process to the superior edge of the transverse process below.

These muscles are too small to be responsible for the execution of movements of the lumbar vertebrae. However, they are densely endowed with muscle spindles. For this reason they are believed to play an important role in proprioception from the lumbar spine.

ANTEROLATERAL MUSCLES

Two muscles cover the lumbar vertebral column anterior to the transverse processes and lateral to the vertebral bodies. The first is a muscle that takes an adventitious origin from the lumbar vertebral column in order to act on the hip. It has no primary action on the lumbar spine. The second is a respiratory muscle that sends some fibres to the lumbar vertebral column, but whose action on the lumbar spine is minor.

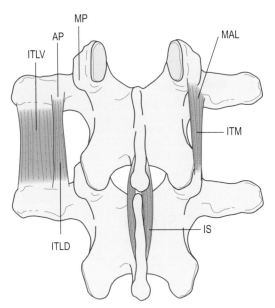

Figure 3.1 The short, intersegmental muscles. ITLV, intertransversarii laterales ventrales; ITLD, intertransversarii laterales dorsales; ITM, intertransversarii mediales; IS, interspinales; AP, accessory process; MP, mamillary process; MAL, mamillo-accessory ligament. *(From Bogduk (1997), with permission.)*

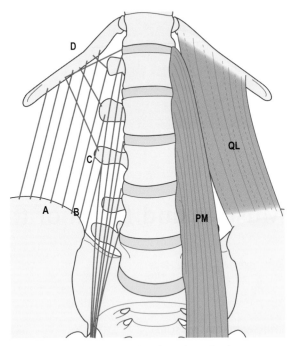

Figure 3.2 Psoas major (PM) and quadratus lumborum (QL). At each segmental level psoas major attaches to the transverse process, the intervertebral disc and adjacent vertebral margins. The attachments of quadratus lumborum are to the iliac crest (A), the iliolumbar ligament (B), the transverse processes (C) and the 12th rib (D). *(From Bogduk (1997), with permission.)*

Psoas major

Psoas major covers the lateral aspects of the lumbar vertebral bodies and the proximal quarter of the anterior aspects of the transverse processes (Fig. 3.2). Its fibres arise from the transverse processes and from the intervertebral discs and the superior and inferior margins of the vertebrae adjacent to each disc. From these sites, the fibres stream inferiorly and slightly laterally to join a tendon that passes over the brim of the pelvis to reach the lesser trochanter of the femur. The essential action of the psoas is to flex the hip, for which purpose the lumbar vertebral column constitutes a solid base. However, the psoas has no intrinsic action on the lumbar spine. Its fibres run too close to the axes of movement of the lumbar vertebrae to be able to exert any substantial moment that might bend the lumbar spine forwards, backwards or sideways.[166] However, although not able to execute movements of the lumbar spine, the psoas can exert very large compressive forces on the lumbar discs, when it flexes the hip, or when it is used in the action of sit-ups.[166]

Quadratus lumborum

The quadratus lumborum covers the anterior surfaces of the transverse processes and extends laterally beyond the tips of these processes (Fig. 3.2). Most of its fibres pass directly from the ilium and iliolumbar ligament to the 12th rib. They are joined by other fibres that stem from the lumbar transverse process and also pass to the 12th rib. For this reason the principal function of the quadratus lumborum is held to be to brace the 12th rib, in order to provide a steady base from which the lower thoracic fibres of the diaphragm can act.

Additional fibres pass from the ilium to the L1–4 transverse processes. However, these fibres are irregular in number, frequency and development. In some individuals they are large; in others they are quite feeble or absent. The forces that they exert on the lumbar spine are very small.[1131]

POSTERIOR BACK MUSCLES

The posterior muscles of the lumbar spine are massive (Fig. 3.3), and are the principal, if not only, muscles responsible for controlling its movements. They are arranged in three columns and two layers. From medial to

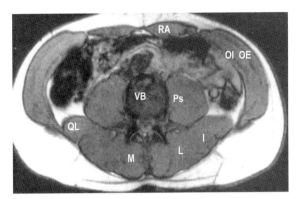

Figure 3.3 Magnetic resonance imaging cross-section (T₁-weighted image) through the trunk at the level of the L4 vertebral body (VB) showing the major back muscles multifidus (M), longissimum lumborum (L) and iliocostalis lumborum (I). Also shown are psoas major (Ps), quadratus lumborum (QL), rectus abdominis (RA), obliquus externus (OE) and obliquus internus (OI). Note how the vertebral body lies equidistant from the surface of the back, and abdomen. *(From Fleckenstein JL, Crues JV, Reimers CD 1996 Muscle imaging in health and disease, with permission of Springer-Verlag, New York, Inc.)*

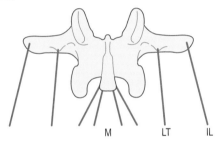

Figure 3.4 A sketch of the systematic attachments of the lumbar back muscles. Each lumbar vertebra is subtended by fibres of the iliocostalis lumborum (IL) stemming from the transverse processes, by fibres of longissimus thoracis (LT) stemming from the accessory processes and by multiple fibres of the multifidus (M) radiating from the spinous process.

lateral, the three columns are formed by multifidus, longissimus thoracis and iliocostalis lumborum, which systematically arise from the lumbar spinous processes, the accessory processes and the transverse processes, respectively (Fig. 3.4). The longissimus thoracis and iliocostalis lumborum, however, are each formed by two parts. The deeper parts of each muscle arise from the lumbar vertebrae, and lie in the same plane as the multifidus. The superficial parts of each arise from thoracic vertebrae and ribs, and cover their respective lumbar parts. Moreover, the tendons of the thoracic parts of these muscles form the erector spinae aponeurosis, which covers the multifidus and thereby completes the superficial layer of the posterior lumbar back muscles.

Multifidus

The fibres of multifidus are centred on each of the lumbar spinous processes. From each spinous process, fibres radiate inferiorly in a systematic order to assume a variety of attachments inferiorly[869] (Fig. 3.5). The arrangement of fibres is such as to pull downwards on each spinous process, thereby either causing the vertebra of origin to extend, or controlling its movement into flexion.[868]

At each level, short fibres arise from the lamina and inferior edge of the spinous process and pass to the mamillary process of the vertebra two levels below. These are flanked by fibres from the inferior corner of the spinous process that pass to mamillary processes three, four and five levels below. Fibres that extend below the L5 vertebra lack mamillary processes into which to insert. Instead, they find anchorage on the ilium and on the posterior surface of the sacrum.

The fibres of multifidus are arranged in laminated bands. The fibres from L1 cover those from L2 laterally and posteriorly. Those from L3 cover those from L4, and so on. This arrangement allows the multifidus to act on each spinous process individually and separately.

By some authorities in the past the multifidus has been regarded as a rotator of the lumbar spine. It has no such action. The obliquity of the fibres provides them with only a minor transverse action; the predominant action of the multifidus is to pull downwards on the spinous processes.

Longissimus thoracis pars lumborum

This is a relatively slender muscle that lies immediately lateral to multifidus.[871] Its fibres arise from the tips of the L1–4 accessory processes and converge to a common tendon, flattened in the sagittal plane, and known as the lumbar intermuscular aponeurosis, that inserts into the ilium just above and medial to the posterior superior iliac spine (Fig. 3.6). These fibres are joined by a bundle of fibres from the posterior surface of the L5 transverse process that insert into the ilium just ventral to the site of insertion of the common tendon.

These fibres pull downwards and slightly backwards on the transverse processes, thereby being able to extend the lumbar vertebrae, or control their flexion. Acting unilaterally, these muscles contribute to controlling lateral bending of the lumbar spine.

Iliocostalis lumborum pars lumborum

The fibres of this muscle arise from the tips of the L1–4 transverse processes.[871] Fibres are lacking from L5, having been incorporated into the posterior division of the iliolumbar ligament. In addition, at each level, fibres arise from the posterior surface of the middle layer of

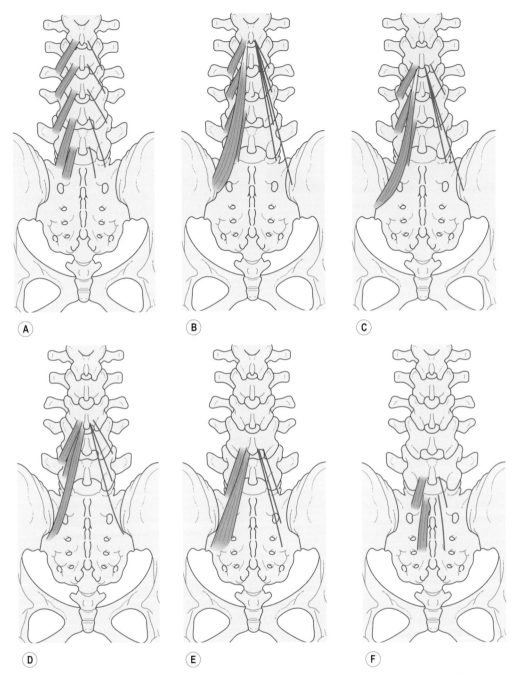

Figure 3.5 The component fascicles of multifidus. (A) The laminar fibres of multifidus. (B–F) The fascicles from the L1 to L5 spinous processes respectively. *(From Bogduk (1997), with permission.)*

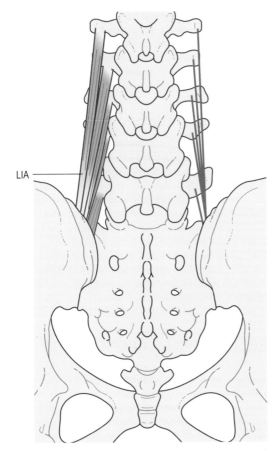

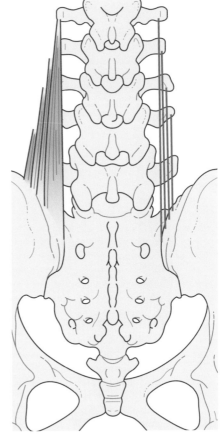

Figure 3.6 The longissimus thoracis pars lumborum. On the left, the five fascicles of the intact muscle are drawn. The formation of the lumbar intermuscular aponeurosis (LIA) by the lumbar fascicles of longissimus is depicted. On the right, the lines indicate the attachments and span of the fascicles. *(From Bogduk (1997), with permission.)*

Figure 3.7 The iliocostalis lumborum pars lumborum. On the left, the four lumbar fascicles of iliocostalis are shown. On the right, their span and attachments are indicated by the lines. *(From Bogduk (1997), with permission.)*

thoracolumbar fascia that attaches to the transverse processes. From these origins the fibres pass inferiorly as flat sheets, in a laminated fashion, those from L1 covering those from L2 and so on, to insert into the crest of the ilium distal to the posterior superior iliac spine (Fig. 3.7). These fibres pull downwards and backwards on the transverse processes, thereby being able to extend the lumbar vertebra, or control their flexion. Acting unilaterally, they contribute to controlling lateral bending of the lumbar spine.

Longissimus thoracis pars thoracis

This muscle consists of a series of aggregated muscle bellies that arise at thoracic levels.[871] Individual bellies

arise from the tip of the transverse processes from T1 or T2 to T12. Additional bellies arise from the posterior surfaces of the ribs adjacent to the transverse processes from T4 to T12. Each belly is some 1–2 cm wide and 9–12 cm long, and ends in a long caudal tendon. These tendons pass into the lumbar region where they are aggregated side to side to form the medial half of what is known as the erector spinae aponeurosis, which covers the multifidus and the longissimus thoracis pars lumborum. The individual tendons are inserted systematically to the lumbar and sacral spinous processes, across the lower end of the sacrum, and on to the posterior segment of the iliac crest (Fig. 3.8). The tendons from muscle bellies arising from the highest thoracic levels insert into the L1 spinous process. Tendons from lower muscle bellies insert at progressively lower levels. The tendons from T12 reach the posterior superior iliac spine.

31

The fibres of this muscle are arranged to extend the thorax in relation to the pelvis, or to control flexion of the trunk. They do not act directly on the lumbar vertebra but those that span the entire lumbar spine can exert an extension moment on it, acting like the string of a bow to bend it.

Iliocostalis lumborum pars thoracis

This muscle consists of a series of small, overlapping muscle bellies located in the thoracic region.[871] The bellies arise from the angles of the lower eight ribs. From each belly a long caudal tendon extends into the lumbar region. These tendons are aggregated side to side to form the lateral part of the erector spinae aponeurosis, which covers the iliocostalis lumborum pars lumborum, and inserts into the iliac crest (Fig. 3.9).

These muscles are arranged to extend the thorax on the pelvis, or control forward or lateral flexion of the trunk. They do not act directly on the lumbar vertebrae but exert a bowstring effect on them.

ERECTOR SPINAE APONEUROSIS

Traditional anatomical textbooks describe the erector spinae aponeurosis as a large flat tendon arising from the lumbar and sacral spinous processes, the sacrum and the ilium, that gives rise to the erector spinae muscle that assumes a variety of insertions into the lumbar and thoracic vertebrae. This description disguises the true anatomy of this region.

The erector spinae aponeurosis is, indeed, a broad, flat tendon that covers the lumbar region posteriorly (Fig. 3.10). However, its fibres consist exclusively of the caudal tendons of the muscle bellies of longissimus thoracis pars thoracis and iliocostalis lumborum pars thoracis, that lie in the thoracic region.[871] The tendons simply cover underlying muscles, and offer no attachment to them.

In sequence, from medial to lateral, lying deep to the erector spinae aponeurosis are the multifidus, longissimus thoracis pars lumborum and iliocostalis lumborum pars lumborum. These muscles arise from various elements of the lumbar vertebrae and anchor them to the sacrum and ilium.

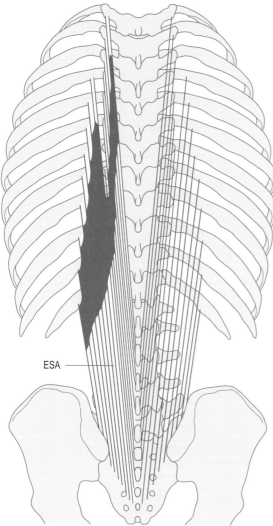

ESA

Figure 3.8 The longissimus thoracis pars thoracis. The intact fascicles are shown on the left. The darkened areas represent the short muscle bellies of each fascicle. Note the short rostral tendons of each fascicle, and the long caudal tendons, which collectively constitute most of the erector spinae aponeurosis (ESA). The span of the individual fascicles is indicated on the right. *(From Bogduk (1997), with permission.)*

As the tendons reach the lumbar spinous processes they form a longitudinal bundle of fibres running dorsal to the tips of the spinous processes. This bundle constitutes the deep part of what is known as the supraspinous ligament. However, this structure lacks the features of a ligament. Its component fibres are clearly tendons. The deepest tendinous fibres curve into the interspinous space to find insertion on to the superior border of a spinous process. These fibres form the dorsal parts of the interspinous ligament.

FORCES AND LINE OF ACTION

No single force or line of action can be ascribed to any one of the lumbar back muscles. These muscles act on or across each of the five lumbar vertebrae, and each muscle consists of several individual fascicles. In this regard, a fascicle is defined as a bundle of muscle fibres that share

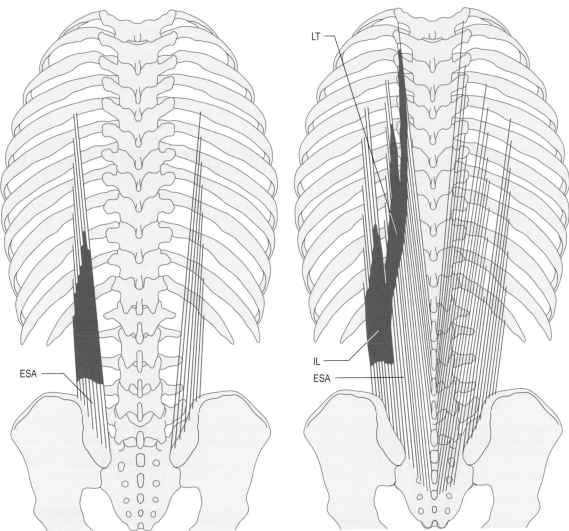

Figure 3.9 The iliocostalis lumborum pars thoracis. The intact fascicles are shown on the left, and their span is shown on the right. The caudal tendons of the fascicles collectively form the lateral parts of the erector spinae aponeurosis (ESA). *(From Bogduk (1997), with permission.)*

Figure 3.10 The erector spinae aponeurosis (ESA). This broad sheet is formed by the caudal tendons of the thoracic fibres of longissimus thoracis (LT) and iliocostalis lumborum (IL). *(From Bogduk (1997), with permission.)*

the same origin and insertion, such that they exert forces on the same bones. The forces exerted on a given lumbar vertebra will be those exerted by the fascicles that attach to it and by those fascicles that cross that vertebra but without attaching to it.

The force exerted by a given fascicle is determined by its orientation, its size and its degree of activation. The extent to which a fascicle is activated requires information about its electromyographic activity. To date, it has not been possible to obtain electromyographic data on each and every

fascicle of the back muscles. However, dissection studies have determined the size and orientation of each fascicle. These data can be used to provide estimates of the maximum possible force exerted by any fascicle, using the relationship that maximum force is the product of the physiological cross-sectional area of the fascicle and a force coefficient. The physiological cross-sectional area is the volume of the fascicle divided by its length, and is a better estimate of the force exerted by the fascicle than an anatomical cross-section taken at an arbitrary point along

33

the fascicle. The force coefficient that has been found to apply to the back muscles[164] is about 0.46 N/mm^2. In order to determine the force exerted by a fascicle in any given plane, the maximum force is corrected trigonometrically according to the orientation of that fascicle with respect to that plane.

The orientation of the fascicle is critical with respect to not only the vertebra from which it arises, but also its line of action with respect to any vertebrae that it crosses. This arises because the lumbar vertebral column is not a single bone but a series of five vertebrae, each with a different orientation in the lumbar lordosis. Consequently, the force exerted on a distant vertebra will not necessarily be the same as that exerted by the same fascicle on an intervening vertebra.

The multifidus essentially consists of 11 fascicles on each side. At each segmental level a fascicle (ms) arises from the lateral aspect of the spinous process, and three arise from the tip of the spinous process (mt1–3). Those fascicles from L1 each assume a separate insertion and, therefore, need to be considered separately. The ms fascicle from L1 inserts into the L3 mamillary process, and the mt fascicles insert respectively into the mamillary processes of L4, L5 and S1. From the L2 spinous process, the ms and

mt1 fascicles insert into the L4 and L5 mamillary processes, but the mt2 and mt3 fascicles both insert into the sacrum and can be treated together for biomechanical purposes (Fig. 3.11). The ms fascicle from L3 reaches the L5 mamillary process, but all three mt fascicles insert into the sacrum and can be treated collectively. From L4 all fascicles insert into the sacrum and can be treated collectively, as can the fascicles from L5.

There are five fascicles of the longissimus thoracis pars lumborum, each arising from a separate accessory process, and named by number according to the segment of origin. All reach the ilium. There are four fascicles of iliocostalis lumborum pars lumborum, which arise from the first four lumbar transverse processes and insert into the ilium. A fascicle from L5 is lacking.

Twelve fascicles of longissimus thoracis pars thoracis arise from thoracic levels and insert systematically into the lumbar spinous processes, across the base of the sacrum and the posterior segment of the iliac crest. Eight fascicles of iliocostalis lumborum arise from the lower eight ribs and insert into the iliac crest.

In a posterior view, the fascicles of multifidus all exhibit a downward and lateral orientation (Fig. 3.11A). The lateral obliquity is about 15° at L1, increasing to about

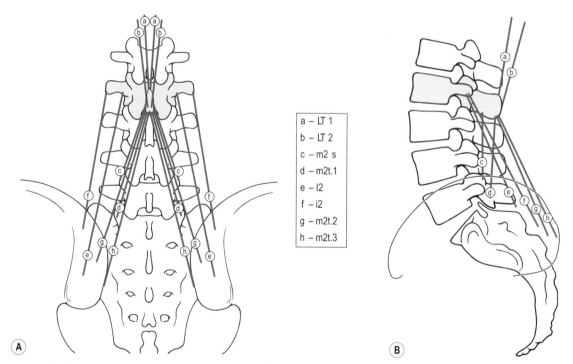

a – LT 1
b – LT 2
c – m2 s
d – m2t.1
e – l2
f – i2
g – m2t.2
h – m2t.3

Figure 3.11 The attachments and lines of action of the individual fascicles of multifidus, iliocostalis lumborum and longissimus thoracis that attach to the L2 vertebra. (A) Posterior view; (B) lateral view. m2s, fascicles of multifidus that arise from the caudal edge of the L2 spinous process; m2t.1–m2t.3, the three fascicles of multifidus that arise from the tip of the L2 spinous process; i, fascicles of iliocostalis lumborum; l, lumbar fascicles of longissimus thoracis; LT, thoracic fascicles of longissimus thoracis.

20° at L2 and L3 as the multifidus widens over the sacrum, but decreasing to 16° at L4 and 6° at L5.[870] This obliquity reduces the force exerted by the fascicle in the sagittal plane in proportion to the cosine of its obliquity, but the angle is so small that virtually all of the force of each fascicle is exerted in the sagittal plane.

In a lateral view, the fascicles of multifidus exhibit a variety of orientations (Fig. 3.11B). Those from upper lumbar segments pass downwards and ventrally to their mamillary processes, whereas those from lower spinous processes pass downwards but dorsally to reach the sacrum. The orientation of fascicles varies from 11° ventral to the long axis of the vertebra of origin to 23° dorsal to this axis.[164] These differences in orientation affect the moment arm of each fascicle on each vertebra. Any accurate determination of the force and moments exerted by multifidus requires precise attention to the orientation of each fascicle.[164]

In a posterior view (Fig. 3.11A), the fascicles of longissimus thoracis pars lumborum assume an increasing obliquity from above downwards, with the fascicles from L1 and L2 being oriented at about 5° to the sagittal plane, and that of L5 at some 27° to the sagittal plane.[872] The fascicles of iliocostalis lumborum pars lumborum are uniformly oriented at only 5° to the sagittal plane,[872] except for the fascicle from L4, which assumes an angle of 15°. However, these inclinations are so small that virtually all of the force of each fascicle is exerted in the sagittal plane.

In a lateral view (Fig. 3.11B), the L2–4 fascicles of longissimus thoracis pars lumborum are oriented at about 30° to the long axis of their vertebra of origin. The fascicle from L1 is inclined some 10° less, and that from L5 some 10° more. The fascicles of iliocostalis lumborum pars lumborum are all oriented at about 20° to the long axis of their vertebra of origin.

The thoracic fascicles of longissimus thoracis and iliocostalis lumborum run essentially along a sagittal plane, deviating not more than about 4–8° from this plane (Fig. 3.12). In lateral projection, these fascicles all run essentially parallel to the lumbar spine. Consequently, essentially all of the force exerted by any of these fascicles is directed parallel to the long axes of the lumbar vertebrae.[164]

Table 3.1 records the physiological cross-sectional areas of the fascicles of the posterior lumbar back muscles, together with the maximum force exerted by each fascicle in the sagittal plane, the moment arms of each fascicle for each segment, as measured to the average location of the instantaneous axis of rotation of each lumbar vertebra, and the maximum moment exerted by each fascicle on each segment.[164] These data, which apply to the upright, standing position, show that half or more of the extension moment exerted on any lumbar segment is provided by the thoracic fibres of longissimus thoracis and iliocostalis lumborum. The remainder is provided by the lumbar fibres of these muscles and the multifidus, in almost equal proportions.

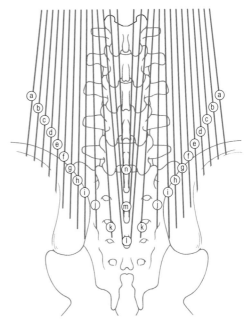

a – IT12	e – IT8	i – LT12	m – LT 8
b – IT11	f – IT7	j – LT11	n – LT 7
c – IT10	g – IT6	k – LT10	
d – IT9	h – IT5	l – LT 9	

Figure 3.12 The lines of action and caudal attachments of the thoracic parts of longissimus thoracis and iliocostalis lumborum.

Upon flexion of the lumbar spine, the orientation of the fascicles of the back muscles changes, but not in a uniform manner. Some decrease their obliquity with respect to the longitudinal axis of the lumbar vertebral column; others increase their obliquity. Some increase their moment arm; others decrease their moment arm. The net effect is that there is only a small reduction in the total moments exerted on each lumbar segment.[874] Nor is there any appreciable change in the compression load exerted by the back muscles on any lumbar segment. However, there are major changes in the posterior shear forces exerted by the multifidus and lumbar parts of longissimus and iliocostalis.

In the upright position, these muscles exert a posterior force on L1–4 but paradoxically an anterior force on L5. This arises because of the shape of the lumbar lordosis and the lumbosacral angle. Essentially, maximum contraction of the back muscles draws the upper lumbar vertebrae backwards but also drives them downwards under compression. As a result of this compression, the L5 vertebra is forced forwards across the sloping upper surface of the sacrum. Upon flexion, the lumbar spine is straightened, and the posterior shear force on the upper lumbar

Table 3.1 The physiological cross-sectional areas (PCSA) of the fascicles of the lumbar back muscles, their maximum force in the sagittal plane (F_{sag}), their moment arms and the maximum moments exerted on individual segments. Maximum forces and moments are expressed in terms of a force coefficient, K, which is the maximum force that can be generated by unit cross-sectional area of muscle. An indicative value of K is 0.46 (N/mm²). Absent values occur where the fascicle does not act on the segment in question. Negative values obtain for those fascicles of longissimus thoracis pars thoracis that insert into lumbar spinous processes and, therefore, pull upwards on those vertebrae

Muscle and fascicle	PCSA (cm²)	F_{sag} (N)	Moment arm (cm) by segment					Maximum moment (Nm) by segment				
			L1–2	L2–3	L3–4	L4–5	L5–S1	L1–2	L2–3	L3–4	L4–5	L5–S1
Multifidus												
L1ms	0.40	39.5K	4.4	4.2	3.5	–	–	1.7K	1.7K	1.4K	–	–
Lmt1L	0.42	41.6K	5.5	5.1	4.2	2.8	–	2.3K	2.1K	1.8K	1.2K	–
L1mt2	0.36	35.7K	5.5	5.6	5.2	4.0	2.5	2.0K	2.0K	1.8K	1.4K	0.9K
L1mt3	0.60	59.4K	5.3	6.4	7.0	6.8	6.0	3.1K	3.8K	4.2K	4.1K	3.6K
L2ms	0.39	38.2K	–	4.6	4.2	3.0	–	–	1.7K	1.6K	1.2K	–
L2mt1	0.39	38.4K	–	5.6	5.2	4.0	2.5	–	2.2K	2.0K	1.5K	0.9K
L2mt2–3	0.99	97.1K	–	5.3	6.3	6.5	6.0	–	5.2K	6.2K	6.4K	5.8K
L3ms	0.54	52.0K	–	–	4.5	3.9	2.8	–	–	2.4K	2.4K	1.4K
L3mt1–3	1.57	151.8K	–	–	5.2	6.0	5.9	–	–	7.9K	9.0K	8.9K
L4 all	1.86	179.2K	–	–	–	4.9	4.7	–	–	–	8.7K	8.5K
L5 all	0.90	88.5K	–	–	–	–	4.2	–	–	–	–	3.7K
Total								9.1K	18.7K	29.3K	35.9K	35.9K
LTpL												
L1	0.79	78.8K	3.3	4.8	5.8	6.1	5.6	2.6K	3.8K	4.6K	4.8K	4.4K
L2	0.91	90.7K	–	3.6	4.9	5.5	5.2	–	3.2K	4.4K	4.9K	4.7K
L3	1.03	102.7K	–	–	3.5	4.6	4.8	–	–	3.6K	4.7K	4.9K
L4	1.10	108.6K	–	–	–	3.3	4.2	–	–	–	3.5K	4.5K
L5	1.16	115.7K	–	–	–	–	2.8	–	–	–	–	3.3K
Total								2.6K	7.0K	12.8K	17.9K	21.8K
ILpL												
L1	1.08	107.4K	3.5	5.0	6.2	5.7	5.7	3.8K	5.6K	6.7K	6.7K	6.1K
L2	1.54	153.8K	–	3.6	4.6	4.8	4.2	–	5.6K	7.1K	7.4K	6.5K

L3	1.82	181.8K	—	—	3.5	4.1	3.8	—	—	6.4K	7.4K	7.0K
L4	1.89	188.6K	—	—	—	3.2	3.5	—	—	—	6.0K	6.6K
Total								3.8K	11.2K	20.3K	27.5K	26.2K
LTpT												
T1	0.29	28.7K	5.3	—	—	—	—	2.0K	22.1K	—	—	—
T2	0.57	56.4K	5.3	—	—	—	—	3.9K	24.1K	—	—	—
T3	0.56	55.4K	5.3	4.7	6.2	—	—	3.8K	4.0K	24.0K	—	—
T4	0.45	44.6K	5.3	5.7	6.2	—	—	3.1K	3.2K	3.2K	23.0K	—
T5	0.44	43.6K	5.3	5.7	6.2	—	—	3.0K	3.1K	3.2K	23.0K	—
T6	0.64	63.4K	5.3	5.7	6.2	5.7	—	4.4K	4.6K	4.6K	4.3K	23.8K
T7	0.78	77.2K	5.3	5.7	6.2	5.7	4.5	5.3K	5.5K	5.6K	5.3K	4.6K
T8	1.25	123.8K	5.3	5.7	6.2	5.7	4.5	8.5K	8.9K	9.0K	8.5K	7.4K
T9	1.46	144.5K	5.3	5.7	6.2	5.7	4.5	9.9K	10.3K	10.4K	9.9K	8.6K
T10	1.60	160.0K	4.6	5.7	6.2	5.7	4.5	10.4K	11.2K	11.8K	11.7K	10.3K
T11	1.67	167.0K	3.8	4.9	6.2	5.7	4.5	10.4K	11.7K	12.5K	12.5K	11.6K
T12	1.38	138.0K	3.1	4.0	5.2	5.7	4.5	8.2K	9.6K	10.5K	10.4K	9.9K
Total								65.9K	72.9K	66.8K	56.6K	48.6K
ILpT												
T5	0.23	22.8K	5.3	5.7	6.2	5.7	6.8	1.5K	1.6K	1.7K	1.6K	1.6K
T6	0.31	30.7K	5.3	5.7	6.2	5.7	5.7	2.1K	2.2K	2.3K	2.2K	2.1K
T7	0.39	38.6K	5.3	5.7	6.2	5.7	4.5	2.5K	2.7K	2.8K	2.8K	2.6K
T8	0.34	33.7K	5.3	5.7	6.2	4.6	3.6	2.2K	2.4K	2.5K	2.4K	2.3K
T9	0.50	49.5K	5.3	5.7	5.2	4.6	2.6	2.9K	3.1K	3.3K	3.2K	2.8K
T10	1.00	99.0K	5.3	4.9	5.2	4.6	2.6	5.8K	6.3K	6.6K	6.4K	5.6K
T11	1.23	121.8K	3.1	4.0	5.2	4.6	2.6	5.7K	6.7K	6.7K	6.4K	5.1K
T12	1.47	147.0K	3.1	3.0	4.3	3.6	2.6	4.7K	5.3K	5.6K	5.3K	3.8K
Total								27.4K	30.3K	31.5K	30.3K	25.9K
Total for all muscles acting on each segment (on each side)								116K	133K	161K	168K	158K

ms, fascicles of multifidus that arise from the caudal edge of the spinous process indicated; mt1–mt3, the first to third fascicles of multifidus that arise from the tip of the spinous process indicated; LTpL, longissimus thoracis pars lumborum; ILpL, iliocostalis lumborum pars lumborum; LTpT, longissimus thoracis pars thoracis; ILpT, iliocostalis lumborum pars thoracis. (After Bogduk N, Macintosh JE, Pearcy MJ. A universal model of the lumbar back muscles in the upright position. Spine 1992;17:897-913.)

vertebrae is reduced; but at L5, the force is reversed to become a posterior shear force.[874]

With respect to axial rotation, the back muscles contribute little action. They are oriented far too longitudinally to produce rotatory moments. At best, they can exert about 2 Nm, which is only 5% of the maximum torque exerted during rotation of the trunk.[875]

THORACOLUMBAR FASCIA

The muscles of the lumbar spine are enveloped by three layers of fascia known as the thoracolumbar fascia (Fig. 3.13). The anterior layer covers the quadratus lumborum and is formed by the deep fascia of that muscle. The other two layers are misnamed because they are not fascial in nature. A fascia consists of collagen fibres oriented in a variety of directions, with no particular orientation predominating. In contrast, an aponeurosis consists of

collagen fibres derived from the tendon of a muscle and that assume a conspicuous predominant orientation.

The middle layer of thoracolumbar fascia intervenes between the quadratus lumborum and the iliocostalis lumborum, and is continuous with the intertransverse membranes. It consists of tendinous fibres of the transversus abdominis. Whereas the upper fibres of transversus abdominis arise from the costal margin, and whereas its lower fibres arise from the ilium and inguinal ligament, its middle fibres spring from the tips of the middle lumbar transverse processes. Between the transverse processes these tendons interlace to form the middle layer of thoracolumbar fascia.

The posterior layer of thoracolumbar fascia is formed by the aponeurosis of latissimus dorsi. The caudal tendons of the latissimus dorsi cover the erector spinae aponeurosis as they descend obliquely towards the lumbar spinous processes. In the midline they interlace with the tendons from the opposite side to form the superficial layer of the so-called supraspinous ligament. From the midline the

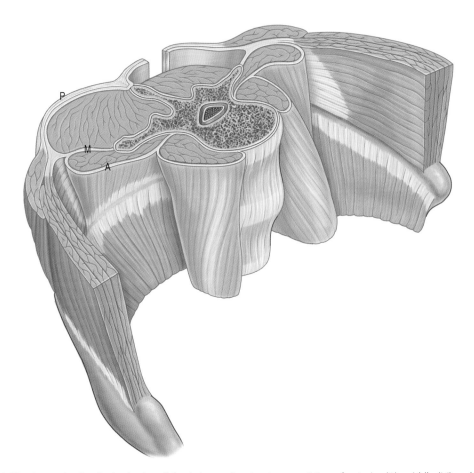

Figure 3.13 The thoracolumbar (or lumbodorsal) fascia is a major structure consisting of anterior (A), middle (M) and posterior (P) layers. *(From Standring S (ed.) 2005 Gray's anatomy 39th edn, with permission of Churchill Livingstone, Edinburgh.)*

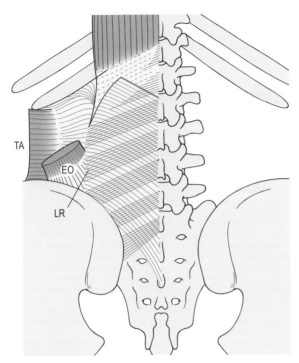

Figure 3.14 The structure of the posterior layer of thoracolumbar fascia. Fibres of the superficial lamina pass downwards and medially to the midline. Fibres of the deep lamina pass downwards and laterally from the spinous processes. Both laminae fuse in the lateral raphe (LR) lateral to the iliocostalis. To the lateral raphe are attached the middle fibres of transversus abdominis (TA) and the most posterior fibres of external oblique (EO).

tendons can be traced into the opposite side. As a result of this arrangement the posterior layer of thoracolumbar fascia obtains a bilaminar structure (Fig. 3.14). The superficial layer is formed by the tendons of the ipsilateral latissimus dorsi, passing caudally and medially. The deep layer is formed by the tendons of the contralateral latissimus dorsi, passing downwards and laterally. Lateral to the iliocostalis lumborum, the two laminae are fused with the middle layer of thoracolumbar fascia along a seam known as the lateral raphe. From the lower end of this raphe, some of the most posterior fibres of external oblique take origin, in some individuals.

The latissimus dorsi exerts no direct action on the lumbar vertebral column. Rather, it uses the lumbar spine and pelvis as a wide base from which to exert its actions on the upper limb. When the upper limb is braced, however, as in climbing, the latissimus dorsi uses its attachments to the lumbar spine and ilium to lift the trunk as a whole. But it does not bend or move the lumbar spine.

Nevertheless, the posterior layer of thoracolumbar fascia acts as a retinaculum around the posterior back muscles, ostensibly helping to keep them applied to the lumbar

vertebral column. The criss-cross arrangement of fibres in the posterior layer allows them to exert an extension moment on the lumbar spine, if the lateral raphe is tensed laterally by the transversus abdominis. However, this effect is trivial, amounting to no more than about 3–6 Nm,[873] compared to the 200 Nm required to sustain a moderately heavy lift.[363]

ABDOMINAL MUSCLES

Although primarily designed to contain the viscera of the abdomen, the muscles of the abdominal wall exert certain actions on the lumbar spine. They do so by acting between the pelvis and the ribs. By pulling on the ribs, the muscles can move the thorax in relation to the pelvis and, thereby, indirectly move the lumbar spine. The ribs endow the muscles with long lever arms so that the moments exerted by the abdominal muscles can be large.

The rectus abdominis (Fig. 3.3) forms a broad strap either side of the midline of the abdomen. Its fibres arise from the anterior surfaces of the medial ends of the fifth to seventh costal cartilages, and insert into the top of the pubic bone and public symphysis. The longitudinal orientation of the muscle and its anterior location allow it to be a powerful flexor of the thorax and, therefore, of the lumbar spine.

The obliquus externus (Fig. 3.3) arises from the lateral surface of the thorax: from the external surfaces of the lower eight ribs. Its fibres pass medially and inferiorly across the abdomen. The upper and middle fibres form an aponeurosis that covers the front of the rectus abdominis, and interlaces with the aponeurosis from the opposite side, forming the linea alba. Lower fibres assume a variety of insertions. The most posterior fibres insert into the iliac crest. Slightly higher fibres form the inguinal ligament and insert into the pubic tubercle. The remaining lower fibres insert into the pubic bone. The attachments and orientation of the obliquus externus allow it to flex the thorax or to rotate it.

The obliquus internus (Fig. 3.3) arises from the iliac crest and inguinal ligament. Its fibres pass medially and superiorly, deep to obliquus externus. The more posterior fibres insert into the inferior borders of the lower three ribs. Middle fibres pass across the abdomen and form an aponeurosis that splits into layers that pass anterior and posterior to the rectus abdominis and insert into the linea alba. The lowest fibres arch inferiorly to insert into the pubic bone. Acting on the thorax, the posterior fibres of obliquus internus can flex or rotate the thorax and, therefore, the lumbar spine. Its middle fibres can act in concert with the opposite obliquus externus to flex or rotate the thorax, but its lower fibres have no action on the spine because they arise from and insert into the pelvis on the same side.

The transversus abdominis has a variety of origins. Its upper fibres arise from the inner surfaces of the lower six ribs. Its lower fibres arise from the iliac crest and inguinal ligament. Its middle fibres arise from the lateral raphe of the thoracolumbar fascia. Most of its fibres pass transversely to form an aponeurosis behind rectus abdominis. The lowest fibres arch from the inguinal ligament into the pubic bone. None of these attachments endows transversus abdominis with an action on the lumbar spine. Only the very middle fibres, which arise from the thoracolumbar fascia, might have an indirect action on the lumbar spine, by tensing the fascia, but this action is very weak.

LATISSIMUS DORSI

The latissimus dorsi is sometimes included amongst the muscles that can exert forces on the lumbar spine. This is a misconception. Very few of the fibres of latissimus dorsi cross the lumbar spine, and the forces and moments that they exert, on the pelvis or through the thoracolumbar fascia, are virtually trivial.[161]

FURTHER READING

Bogduk N. Clinical anatomy of the lumbar spine and sacrum. 3rd ed. Edinburgh: Churchill Livingstone; 1997.

Chapter 4

Nerves and blood supply to the lumbar spine

VERTEBRAL CANAL

The vertebral canal is a well-protected channel used by the nervous system to transmit nerves to and from the lower limb and pelvis. Its floor is formed by the posterior surfaces of the lumbar vertebral bodies and the intervertebral discs. Along the floor, like a carpet, lies the posterior longitudinal ligament. The roof is formed by the laminae of the lumbar vertebrae, and the ligamenta flava. The lateral walls are formed by the pedicles of the lumbar vertebrae. Between the pedicles, the intervertebral foramina constitute windows through which nerves may enter or leave the vertebral canal.

The spinal cord reaches into the lumbar vertebral canal, terminating opposite the L1–2 intervertebral disc. Anchored to the spinal cord are the ventral and dorsal roots of the lumbar, sacral and coccygeal spinal nerves. Systematically, these descend from the spinal cord to their respective intervertebral foramina (Fig. 4.1A). Nerve roots of a given segmental number are directed to the intervertebral foramen below the vertebra of the same segmental number. Because the several nerve roots resemble the fibres of a horse's tail, they are known collectively as the cauda equina.

The spinal cord and cauda equina are enclosed in a sac of meningeal tissue – the dural sac, which contains cerebrospinal fluid that bathes and nourishes the nerve roots (Fig. 4.1B). By this sac and fluid, the delicate nerves are protected from the hazards of movements of the lumbar vertebrae. Where pairs of nerve roots leave the dural sac to enter their intervertebral foramen they take a sleeve of dura mater with them that constitutes the dural sleeve of the nerve roots. Typically, the nerve roots and their dural sleeve curve around the medial aspect of the pedicle above the intervertebral foramen to which they are destined (Fig. 4.2).

As long as the vertebrae, their joints and their ligaments remain normal in shape, the nerve roots in the vertebral canal remain immune to injury. However, alterations in the smooth internal surface of the vertebral canal threaten the nerves. Common alterations in this regard include osteophytes from the edges of the vertebral bodies or zygapophyseal joints, herniations of disc material, bulges of the ligamentum flavum and cysts of the zygapophyseal joints.

SPINAL NERVES

The lumbar spinal nerves are short nerves lying in the intervertebral foramina. They are slightly longer than the intervertebral foramen is wide (Fig. 4.2). Each is a mixed nerve, containing sensory and motor fibres. Those at L1 and L2 also contain preganglionic sympathetic axons. Each spinal nerve is connected to the spinal cord by a dorsal root and a ventral root. Each is enclosed by the tapering apex of the dural sleeve of the nerve roots.

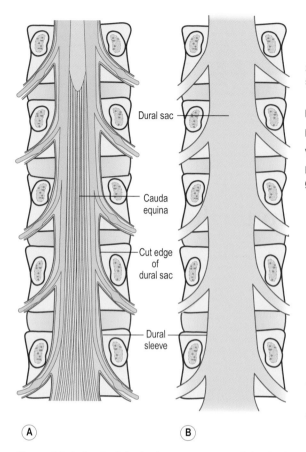

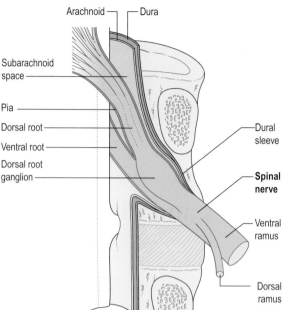

Figure 4.2 A sketch of a lumbar spinal nerve, its roots and meningeal coverings. The nerve roots are invested by pia mater, and covered by arachnoid and dura as far as the spinal nerve. The dura of the dural sac is prolonged around the roots as their dural sleeve, which blends with the epineurium of the spinal nerve. (From Bogduk (1997), with permission.)

Figure 4.1 A sketch of the lumbar nerve roots and the dural sac. **(A)** The posterior half of the dural sac has been removed to reveal the lumbar nerve roots as they lie within the dural sac, forming the cauda equina. **(B)** The intact dural sac is depicted as it lies on the floor of the vertebral canal. (From Bogduk (1997), with permission.)

The spinal nerves lie obliquely in their intervertebral foramina. Each passes downwards and laterally across the back of the lower corner of the vertebral body below the pedicle, skirting across the upper edge of the lateral end of the posterior surface of the intervertebral disc, just as it leaves the intervertebral foramen. At this point the spinal nerve divides into ventral and dorsal rami.

Ventral rami

The ventral rami of the lumbar spinal nerves are destined to supply structures in the ventral compartment of the lumbar region and the lower limb. Upon leaving the intervertebral foramina they enter the substance of the psoas major muscle (Fig. 4.3), in which they communicate with one another, forming the lumbar plexus of nerves.

Deep branches of this plexus innervate the psoas and quadratus lumborum. Peripheral branches emerge from the lateral, ventral and medial surface of the psoas major.

The iliohypogastric and ilioinguinal nerves and the lateral cutaneous nerve of the thigh emerge from the lateral surface of psoas. The former two supply the muscles and skin of the lower abdominal wall and groin. The latter supplies the skin over the lateral thigh.

The genitofemoral nerve emerges from the ventral surface of the psoas, and supplies the cremaster muscle in the groin, and the skin over the femoral triangle of the thigh.

The femoral nerve emerges from the lateral surface of psoas, and the obturator nerve emerges from its medial surface. Also emerging from the medial surface is the lumbosacral trunk, which provides fibres of the L4 and L5 spinal nerves to the sacral plexus, which innervates the lower limb.

The intimate relationship between these nerves and the psoas major means that the nerves can be secondarily involved in pathological processes that affect the psoas, such as infections and spread of spinal tumours. Back pain associated with neurological abnormalities in the lower abdominal wall or proximal thigh strongly implies some such process.

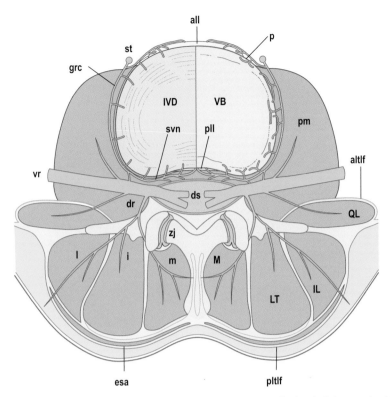

Figure 4.3 Innervation of the lumbar spine. A cross-sectional view incorporating the level of the vertebral body (VB) and its periosteum (p) on the right and the intervertebral disc (IVD) on the left. PM, psoas major; QL, quadratus lumborum; IL, iliocostalis lumborum; LT, longissimus thoracis; M, multifidus; altlf, anterior layer of thoracolumbar fascia; pltlf, posterior layer of thoracolumbar fascia; esa, erector spinae aponeurosis; ds, dural sac; zj, zygapophyseal joint; pll, posterior longitudinal ligament; all, anterior longitudinal ligament; vr, ventral ramus; dr, dorsal ramus; m, medial branch; i, intermediate branch; l, lateral branch; svn, sinuvertebral nerve; grc, grey ramus communicans; st, sympathetic trunk. *(From Bogduk (1997), with permission.)*

Dorsal rami

The dorsal rami of the lumbar spinal nerves are tiny branches that leave the spinal nerves at the intervertebral foramina and pass dorsally over the transverse processes to enter the posterior compartment of the spine, which includes all those structures that lie behind the plane of the transverse processes (Fig. 4.3). Here they divide into lateral, intermediate and medial branches. The lateral branches innervate the iliocostalis lumborum. Those from L1, L2 and L3 also furnish cutaneous branches that emerge from the iliocostalis, penetrate the erector spinae aponeurosis and thoracolumbar fascia and cross the iliac crest to supply the skin over the upper and lateral regions of the buttock. Collectively these nerves are known as the superior clunial nerves. The intermediate branches of the lumbar dorsal rami end in the longissimus lumborum pars lumborum, which they supply.

The medial branches of the lumbar dorsal rami cross the root of the transverse process and hook medially around the base of the superior articular process, at each level. They send articular branches to the zygapophyseal joints above and below their course, and finally ramify in the multifidus and interspinalis muscles. Their distribution is segmental. Each medial branch supplies only those muscle fibres that arise from the spinous process of the vertebra below which emerges the spinal nerve that gives rise to the medial branch. In this way, the nerve of a particular lumbar vertebra innervates only the muscles that act directly on that same vertebra.

INNERVATION OF THE DISC

Each lumbar intervertebral disc receives an innervation from multiple sources (Fig. 4.3). Anteriorly and laterally the annulus fibrosus receives nerves from a plexus of fine nerves that covers the vertebral column, and is derived from branches of the sympathetic trunks and its grey rami

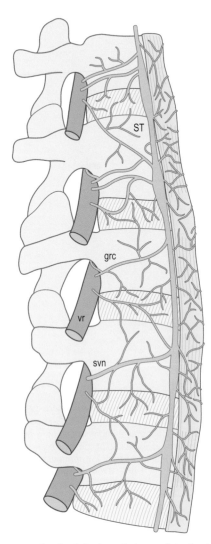

Figure 4.4 A sketch of the lateral plexus of the lumbar spine and its sources. The plexus innervates the lateral aspects of the vertebral bodies and discs. The plexus is formed by branches of the grey rami communicantes (grc) and branches of the ventral rami (vr). Posteriorly the lateral plexus is continued as the sinuvertebral nerves (svn) entering the intervertebral foramina. Anteriorly the plexus blends with the anterior plexus and sympathetic trunks (ST). *(From Bogduk (1997), with permission.)*

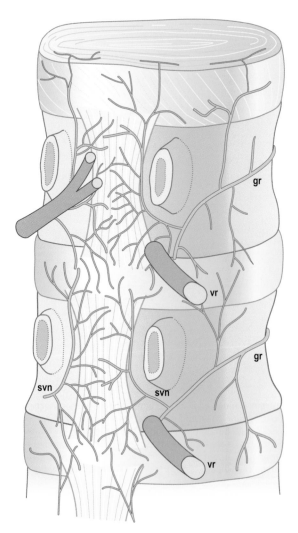

Figure 4.5 The mixed sinuvertebral nerve (svn) arises in the intervertebral foramen from fibres derived from the grey rami communicantes (gr) of the autonomic nervous system, and from the lumbar ventral rami (vr) of the somatic nervous system. The sinuvertebral nerve forms a plexus within the posterior longitudinal ligament. Some fibres penetrate the outer lamellae of the annulus fibrosus. *(Adapted from an original by N Bogduk.)*

communicantes (Fig. 4.4). Posteriorly the annulus receives branches from a plexus that covers the floor of the vertebral canal, and which is derived from the sinuvertebral nerves (Fig. 4.5).

The sinuvertebral nerves are the recurrent meningeal branches of the lumbar ventral rami. Each is formed by a somatic root from the ventral ramus and an autonomic root from the grey ramus communicans. Often the sinuvertebral nerve is represented by a single trunk that enters the intervertebral foramen just below the pedicle. Such a trunk may be accompanied by smaller filaments, or be replaced by multiple small filaments that enter the intervertebral foramen. Upon entering the vertebral canal the nerve divides into branches that ramify over the back of the disc at that level and branches that pass cranially towards the disc above (Fig. 4.5). In addition to innervating the annulus fibrosus, the sinuvertebral nerves innervate the posterior longitudinal ligament, the dural sac and blood vessels in the vertebral canal.

Within the annulus fibrosus, nerve fibres are abundant in the outer third, notably in the ligamentous portion of the annulus (Fig. 4.3).[297,893,1175,1618] They are fewer in the middle third and absent from the inner third and from the nucleus pulposus except in degenerated discs (p. 204). Some of these nerves accompany blood vessels but others end freely amongst the collagen fibres of the annulus. Most of the nerve endings in the annulus fibrosus are free nerve endings, but encapsulated and complex unencapsulated endings occur, particularly in the superficial layers of the lateral annulus. The complex receptors are believed to subserve a proprioceptive function, as do similar endings in other joints of the body. The free nerve endings are believed to subserve a nociceptive function on the grounds that they contain the same neuropeptides as do nociceptive fibres elsewhere in the body. However, the cardinal evidence for a nociceptive function of at least some of the nerves in the annulus fibrosus is that needling the annulus, during the performance of discography, evokes pain (Ch. 5).

Studies have also demonstrated nerve endings in the subchondral bone of the vertebral endplates of lumbar discs.[202] These fibres are probably derived from nerves that accompany blood vessels into the vertebral bodies. Their function is not known, but they could well be nociceptive.

BLOOD VESSELS

Vertebral bodies and muscles of the lumbar spine receive a rich blood supply. Lumbar arteries arise from the back of the aorta and pass dorsally around the waists of the lumbar vertebral bodies towards the intervertebral foramina (Fig. 4.6). En route they furnish penetrating branches that enter the vertebral bodies from their anterior and lateral surfaces. Outside the intervertebral foramina they divide into external and spinal branches. The external branches basically follow the branches of the spinal nerves to supply the muscles of the ventral and dorsal compartments of the lumbar spine. The branches of the ventral compartment also contribute to the supply of the posterior abdominal wall. The spinal branches enter the vertebral canal in company with the sinuvertebral nerves (Fig. 4.5). They supply the nerve roots, and enter the vertebral bodies from behind. Nerves derived from the anterior, lateral and posterior sympathetic plexuses surrounding the lumbar vertebral column accompany penetrating blood vessels deep into the vertebral bodies.

The veins of the lumbar spine emanate from the vertebral bodies and form extensive plexuses around the vertebral bodies. An anterior internal vertebral venous plexus covers the floor of the vertebral canal, and an anterior

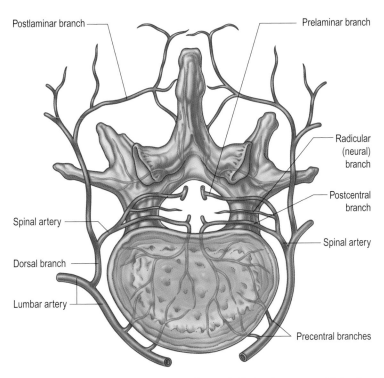

Figure 4.6 The blood supply to the lumbar spine. *(From Standring S (ed.) Gray's anatomy, 39th edn, with permission of Churchill Livingstone, Edinburgh.)*

external vertebral venous plexus covers the anterolateral aspects of the lumbar vertebral column. A similar pair of plexuses covers the internal and external aspects of the roof of the vertebral canal. Ultimately all these plexuses drain to the ascending lumbar veins that pass longitudinally in front of the roots of the transverse processes.

NUTRITION OF THE DISC

The lumbar intervertebral discs receive a relatively poor blood supply. No arteries enter the disc. Their blood supply is limited to tiny vessels that ramify over the external surface of the annulus, derived from the external arteries that supply the adjacent vertebral bodies. Otherwise, the nearest other arteries lie inside the vertebral bodies, separated from the disc by the vertebral endplates and their subchondral bone.

Lacking a direct blood supply, the discs rely mostly on diffusion for their nutrition. Some 50% of this supply stems from the vessels around the periphery of the annulus. The remainder comes through the vertebral endplates from within the vertebral bodies. Nutrients such as glucose and oxygen pass into the disc down concentration gradients, and waste products such as lactic acid and carbon leave the disc in a reciprocal manner, but passage is slow and limited because of the density of proteoglycans in the disc. Nutrition is improved and aided by movement, for movement causes bulk flow of water into and out of the disc, and this bulk flow carries nutrients with it (p. 82).

FURTHER READING

Bogduk N. Clinical anatomy of the lumbar spine and
    sacrum. 3rd ed. Edinburgh: Churchill Livingstone; 1997.

Back pain

In principle, any of the structures of the lumbar spine that receives an innervation could be a source of back pain. Accordingly, back pain could arise from any of the ligaments, muscles, fasciae, joints or discs of the lumbar spine. Moreover, it is quite easy to invent an explanation of how any of these structures could be affected by injury or disease in order to become painful. It is another matter, however, to prove that such explanations are realistic and obtain in a given patient.

EXPERIMENTAL STUDIES

Experimental studies in normal volunteers and patients have shown that noxious stimulation of the back muscles,[729] interspinous ligaments,[420,730] dura mater,[394,1338] zygapophyseal joints[459,937,996] and the sacroiliac joint[434] can produce local and referred pain similar in quality and distribution to that seen in patients. These data corroborate that these structures can indeed be a source of back pain, but alone they do not prove what causes pain in a particular patient. The distribution of pain in a given patient does not imply any particular source.

It has been more difficult to demonstrate in normal volunteers that the discs can be painful. In individuals with intact, normal discs, discography is not painful, as a rule.[1526] The intact laminae of the inner annulus fibrosus prevent the outer, innervated lamina from being distended by increased nuclear pressure. It is only in patients in whom the disc is internally disrupted that provocation discography is painful. However, probing the posterior annulus fibrosus in patients undergoing laminectomy under local anaesthesia evokes back pain.[797,1557] Indeed, the posterior annulus is the most potent source of back pain under these conditions.[797] Thus, the disc can be a source of pain, if it is affected by pathology that involves or compromises the sensitive, outer annulus.

RED-FLAG DISORDERS

Tumours and infections can affect any of the spinal and paraspinal tissues of the back. They are, however, quite uncommon as causes of back pain in primary care. The prevalence of tumours is 0.7%[344] and that of infections less than 0.01%.[345]

Fractures can befall the lumbar vertebral bodies or any of their processes, but are also uncommon causes of back pain in individuals without a reason for a fracture. Such reasons are moderate to severe trauma, or a risk factor for osteoporosis, such as age or use of corticosteroids.

The vast majority of patients with back pain do not have any of these red-flag disorders, so named because they pose a threat to the general health of the patient, and should be recognised as soon as possible. Most patients have some other disorder that is the basis of their pain. However, although many contentions abound, few have been validated.

LIGAMENT SPRAIN

Ligament sprain is an attractive explanation for acute low-back pain following exertion or effort. However, the criteria prescribed for this diagnosis by the International Association for the Study of Pain (IASP)[976] require that the ligament be specified, and that the diagnosis be made by reliable and valid tests specific for that ligament. In contemporary practice these criteria cannot be satisfied. There are no reliable and valid clinical tests. Palpation for tenderness is not specific for sprain of an underlying ligament, and no active or passive motion test has been shown to be specific for ligament sprain in the lumbar spine.

Selective injection of the suspected ligament with local anaesthetic is an attractive, target-specific test for ligament pain, but it has not been rigorously evaluated. Some studies report a 14%[1359] or 10%[1562] prevalence of interspinous ligament pain, diagnosed by local anaesthetic blocks, but no such studies have been controlled for false-positive responses. No other ligaments of the lumbar spine have been so investigated. If ligament sprain is a cause of back pain, it is uncommon.

MUSCLE SPRAIN

Excessive or unusual use of muscles can lead to over-stretching of the tissue, usually near the musculotendinous junction, and give rise to delayed-onset muscle soreness, as described on page 71. It appears likely that the back muscles could be affected in this manner, especially during forward-bending movements when they contract eccentrically to prevent excessive flexion, although there is a lack of reliable evidence for this.

The IASP criteria for muscle sprain require that the muscle be specified and that sprain be diagnosed by reliable and valid tests.[976] Tenderness over muscles is an insufficient sign, for it is neither reliable nor valid. Such tenderness may be quite non-specific. Motion tests are not specific for muscle sprain. Virtually any cause of low-back pain could impair motion in the same way.

MUSCLE SPASM

Muscle spasm is a diagnosis that is both unreliable and invalid. Interobserver agreement on the detection of muscle spasm is extremely poor,[1516] and there is no independent objective correlate of muscle spasm against which the diagnosis might be validated. Studies have failed to demonstrate electromyographic or other features that independently correlate with pain from the allegedly affected muscle.[70]

TRIGGER POINTS

Myofascial pain is an attractive explanation for back pain that is widely entertained. However, it lacks both reliability and validity. Interobserver agreement about the presence of trigger points in the back muscles, quadratus lumborum and gluteus medius is poor,[70,856,1516] and there are no objective correlates for this entity. Its pathophysiology is unknown.

ILIAC CREST SYNDROME

Tenderness over the superomedial aspect of the posterior superior iliac spine is a common feature in patients with back pain.[293] Moreover it is readily recognised. Interobserver agreement is quite good for this sign.[1050] However, there are no objective data as to its significance. It has variously been interpreted by different authors as a sign of muscle sprain, sprain of the iliolumbar ligament or non-specific tenderness.

SEGMENTAL DYSFUNCTION

Although recognised by the IASP,[976] this entity is relatively ambiguous. It amounts to physical examination indicating that something is wrong at a particular spinal segment. However, the nature of the abnormality is entirely speculative or non-specific. It may amount to zygapophyseal joint pain, discogenic pain, muscle tightness, or any combination of these or other conjectures. Objective evidence is lacking. Moreover, no studies have shown that two observers can consistently agree on this diagnosis.

DURAL PAIN

Although it is well established that the dura mater can be a source of back pain and referred pain, there are no data on the pathology that might cause dural pain. Dural tethering has not been validated by any objective investigations, and no clinical test has been shown to be reliable or valid for dural pain. It is conceivable that the dura could be involved in inflammatory reactions to prolapsed disc material in the epidural space, but this model has not been explored.

SPONDYLOLYSIS

Spondylolysis is an acquired defect in the pars interarticularis, usually affecting the L5 or L4 vertebra. It arises most commonly as a result of fatigue failure of the pars following repeated extension or flexion, or in twisting movements of the lumbar spine (p. 162). However, it is present in some 7% of asymptomatic individuals.[1003] Its radiographic presence, therefore, is not diagnostic of the cause of pain. The condition is more common in athletes, in whom the imperative lies in diagnosing the condition before fracture occurs, i.e. while the pars is being stressed and first becoming painful. Bone scan is the singular means of diagnosing this phase of the condition. In patients with frank fracture of the pars, painful fractures can be distinguished from painless, incidental defects by anaesthetising the defect.

SACROILIAC JOINT PAIN

Traditional clinical tests for sacroiliac joint pain have been shown to be very reliable but quite invalid.[373] The only proven means of diagnosing this condition are intra-articular sacroiliac joint blocks. Using such blocks, controlled studies have shown that the prevalence of sacroiliac joint pain is about 20% in patients with chronic low-back pain below L5–S1.[889,1279] Its prevalence amongst patients with acute back pain is unknown.

Data on the pathology of sacroiliac joint pain are meagre. Inflammatory disorders are uncommon. In patients with ostensibly mechanical sacroiliac joint pain, there is a suggestion that sprain or rupture of the anterior sacroiliac ligament is the most likely pathology.[1279]

ZYGAPOPHYSEAL JOINT PAIN

Despite several studies, no clinical test, or combination of tests, has been shown to be diagnostic of pain stemming from the lumbar zygapophyseal joints.[159,1280,1282,1283] However, these are a potent source of low-back pain. Controlled studies using diagnostic blocks of these joints have shown that, in an elderly population, the prevalence of zygapophyseal joint pain is about 40%.[1283] In younger,

injured workers, the prevalence is only about 10–15%.[1280] This figure is nonetheless substantial.

There are no data that directly link zygapophyseal joint pain with any demonstrable pathology. There are no features evident on computed tomography (CT) that correlate with the joint being painful.[1284] However, biomechanics studies and postmortem studies indicate what might be the underlying pathology (Ch. 11).

Forced extension of the lumbar spine causes injuries to the zygapophyseal joints, in which the joint capsule is disrupted by posterior rotation of the inferior articular process.[1605] Torsion injuries to the lumbar spine can cause impaction fractures on the contralateral side, and avulsions of the capsule on the ipsilateral side.[413] In patients with a history of lumbar trauma who undergo postmortem, capsular injuries and small fractures have been demonstrated in the zygapophyseal joints.[1407,1448] Such lesions are absent in subjects with no history of trauma. The challenge remains, however, to demonstrate such lesions in living patients with proven painful zygapophyseal joints.

DISCOGENIC PAIN

Discogenic pain cannot be diagnosed clinically with any degree of certainty. Conventional medical examination offers no signs that are specific for lumbar discogenic pain.[1281] Testing for centralisation and peripheralisation of pain offers positive correlations with proven discogenic pain,[370] but the correlations fall short of being diagnostic.[162] They offer a positive likelihood ratio barely greater than 2, which means that the odds in favour of the diagnosis before the test is performed are increased by only a factor of 2 if and once the test is positive. In this instance, the pretest prevalence of internal disc disruption is 40%,[1281] which amounts to a pretest odds of 40:60. A likelihood ratio of 2 converts the odds to 80:60, which amounts to a diagnostic confidence of only 57%.

The mainstay for diagnosing discogenic pain is disc stimulation and discography. This is achieved by injecting the nucleus pulposus of the target disc with contrast medium (see Fig. 15.5). The critical component of the test is whether or not injection reproduces the patient's accustomed pain. Secondarily, the contrast medium outlines the shape of the nucleus and the interior of the disc. The recommended criterion for discogenic pain is that the patient's pain is reproduced by disc stimulation provided that stimulation of adjacent discs does not reproduce the pain.[976] This form of control is necessary to avoid false-positive interpretations of single-level disc stimulation. Disc stimulation criteria have been used recently to identify patients with discogenic pain in a major clinical trial,[1122] although there is now some concern over the possibly harmful effects of discography on human discs.[254]

Internal disc disruption (IDD) appears to be the cardinal pathological basis for lumbar discogenic pain. This condition is characterised by disruption of the internal architecture of the disc in the form of radial fissures extending from the nucleus to the outer annulus.[155] The further the radial extent, the more likely the disc is to be painful.[1474,1494] The pathology, however, is confined to the interior of the disc. Its outer perimeter remains essentially intact. Population studies, using multivariate analysis, have shown that general age-related disc degeneration does not correlate with discogenic pain, but radial fissures do.[994] This is discussed on page 203.

IDD can be diagnosed on the basis of a positive response to controlled disc stimulation, coupled with the demonstration of radial fissures on CT discography. According to these criteria, the prevalence of IDD is at least 40% in patients with chronic low-back pain.[1281]

Two features evident on magnetic resonance imaging strongly indicate the presence of painful IDD. One is known as a high-intensity zone (HIZ), which appears as a spot of bright signal in the posterior annulus, on T2-weighted magnetic resonance images (Fig. 15.5). The other is known as a Modic lesion (p. 206). Type 1 Modic lesions are areas of oedema in the vertebral body adjacent to the affected disc. These appear as bright signals on T2-weighted images but dark signals on T1-weighted images. Type 2 Modic lesions are areas of fatty infiltration in the vertebral bodies, and appear as bright signals on both T2 and T1 images.

Studies have differed as to the sensitivity of HIZ lesion but are uniform about its specificity (Table 5.1). This means that the sign is not always present, but when present it strongly correlates with the affected disc being painful. Similarly, Modic lesions have low sensitivity but are highly specific for the disc being painful (Table 5.2).

The aetiology of IDD remains in dispute. IDD may arise as a result of degradation of the nuclear matrix following fracture of a vertebral endplate.[155] Perhaps as a result of an inflammatory reaction, or as a result of a disturbance to the pH of the nucleus, the proteoglycans of the nucleus deaggregate, and the water-binding and load-bearing capacity of the nucleus is compromised. More stress is transferred to the annulus (p. 143). Radial fissures develop either as a result of mechanical stress in the disc (p. 154), or as a result of peripheral extension of the degradation of the nuclear matrix. The disc becomes painful as a result of a combination of inflammation about the peripheral end of the radial fissure, and increased strain in the few remaining intact laminae of the outer annulus fibrosus.[155]

Discs painful on discography exhibit abnormal stress profiles.[670,962] Loads applied to the disc are not borne uniformly. Stress concentrations in the nucleus are erratic and low, but are high in the annulus fibrosus, particularly posteriorly.[962] Similar patterns of stress distribution can be produced experimentally by subjecting the disc to compression loading which fractures the vertebral endplate (Fig. 11.8).[22,41] Coincident with this failure is a sudden increase in loading of the posterior annulus fibrosus. These data suggest that IDD is an acquired lesion most likely due to fatigue failure of the vertebral endplate.

Table 5.1 The results of studies on the validity of high-intensity zone lesions as a sign of painful lumbar intervertebral disc

SENSITIVITY	SPECIFICITY	LIKELIHOOD RATIO	SOURCE
0.71	0.89	6.5	Aprill and Bogduk 1992[80]
0.27	0.95	5.4	Saifuddin et al. 1998[1236]
0.52	0.90	5.2	Ito et al. 1998[670]
0.81	0.79	3.9	Lam et al. 2000[801]
0.57	0.84	3.6	Kang et al. 2009[712]
0.31	0.90	3.1	Smith et al. 1998[1334]
0.78	0.74	3.0	Schellhas et al. 1996[1261]
0.45	0.84	2.8	Carragee et al. 2000[256]
0.56	0.70	1.9	Lim et al. 2005[832]
0.27	0.85	1.8	Weishaupt et al. 2001[1549]
0.09	0.93	1.3	Ricketson et al. 1996[1194]

Table 5.2 The results of studies on the validity of Modic lesions as a sign of painful lumbar intervertebral disc

SENSITIVITY	SPECIFICITY	LIKELIHOOD RATIO	SOURCE
0.38	1.00	∞	Modic et al. 1988[988]
0.15	0.98	8.1	Thompson et al. 2009[1417]
0.23	0.97	7.7	Braithwaite et al. 1998[177]
0.22	0.95	4.4	Ito et al. 1998[670]
0.23	0.86	1.6	Sandhu et al. 2000[1243]
0.14	0.87	1.1	Kang et al. 2009[712]
0.09	0.83	0.52	Lim et al. 2005[832]

DISC PROLAPSE

Discogenic pain and IDD need to be distinguished from disc prolapse. Discogenic pain means pain arising as a result of stimulation of nociceptive nerve endings in the intervertebral disc. It requires and implies a pathological process confined to the disc which is capable of stimulating its intrinsic nerve fibres. IDD is one such condition. Another is discitis. In both conditions, the external contour of the disc is essentially normal, for the pathology lies within the substance of the disc. In IDD, although the structure of the annulus fibrosus is disrupted, the outer annulus is intact, at least macroscopically. In particular, the annulus fibrosus does not bulge outwards, and no nuclear material is displaced beyond the normal perimeter of the disc.

Disc prolapse involves relative displacement of nucleus relative to annulus (p. 201). Usually a mixture of nuclear and annular material is displaced beyond the normal perimeter of the disc, typically into the vertebral canal or intervertebral foramen (Fig. 11.19). Nuclear material is displaced through a radial fissure in the annulus fibrosus, where it gathers debris from the annulus. The prolapse may be contained, in that it remains covered by a layer of annulus fibrosus or by the posterior longitudinal ligament; or the prolapsed material may breach this covering layer, in which case it is sometimes described as an extrusion. If the prolapsed material loses continuity with material still within the disc, it is described as a sequestrated fragment.

Disc prolapse may be totally asymptomatic. It has been reported in some 24% of asymptomatic individuals,[151,686] and with increasing frequency with advancing age,[686] although it is not clear if these imaging studies are able to distinguish between a disc that is prolapsed (as defined above) and one that is merely showing increased radial bulging of the annulus with advancing age. If disc prolapse does become symptomatic, it does so by compromising a spinal nerve or its roots. The classical symptom is radicular pain (sciatica). This pain is perceived as a shooting or lancinating pain in the lower limb, and is quite distinct from either back pain or somatic referred pain in the lower limb. Radicular pain is also usually, but not necessarily, associated with objective neurological signs (of weakness or numbness) in the distribution of the nerve roots affected.

Radicular pain is caused by inflammation of the affected nerve roots, by compression of the dorsal root ganglion or its blood supply, or by microscopic damage to the nerve roots. Compression of the roots is not a critical factor for the genesis of pain, for radicular pain can occur in the absence of frank compression, and pain may be relieved despite the persistence of compression.

Patients with radicular pain may complain of back pain. However, their cardinal complaint is of pain in the lower limb. Indeed, a classical feature of disc prolapse is pain in the lower limb worse than in the back. The back pain has traditionally been ascribed to the disc prolapse, but the relationship is both imperfect and specious.

There is a positive correlation between disc prolapse and back pain,[168] but the relationship is weak, for reasons discussed on page 205. Some disc prolapses are associated with back pain but the majority are not. Meanwhile, most patients with back pain do not have disc prolapses.

In patients with a disc prolapse, back pain can arise in a variety of possible ways, none of which involves inflammation or compression of nerve roots. The prolapsed disc material may irritate the dura of the nerve root sleeve, in which case the back pain arises from stimulation of nociceptive nerves in the dura mater. If the prolapsed material is contained, it may cause pain by stretching the overlying annulus fibrosus or posterior longitudinal ligament. Alternatively or additionally, the back pain that the patient suffers may be unrelated to the actual disc prolapse and arises from the IDD that may have preceded the prolapse.[370] The latter is most concordant with clinical experience that records that excision of prolapsed disc material is very effective for the relief of leg pain but offers no guarantee for the relief of back pain.

VERTEBRAL BODY PAIN

Painful vertebral body fractures are common in elderly people with osteoporosis (p. 211). In younger people, there is increasing evidence that relatively minor lesions to a vertebral endplate, with or without inflammatory changes within the vertebral body, are frequent causes of back pain.[57,1118,1639]

SYNOPSIS

Although many lesions have been implicated as the cause of low-back pain, few are supported by objective evidence. Tumours, infections and fractures are rare. Ligament sprains and muscle sprains are attractive explanations for acute low-back pain, but there are no clinical features by which these conditions might be reliably and validly diagnosed. Muscle spasm and trigger points are neither reliable nor valid diagnoses. Spondylolysis is most often asymptomatic, but is perhaps a cause of back pain in athletes. Data are lacking on the diagnosis and prevalence of dural pain.

The best available data implicate the sacroiliac joint, the zygapophyseal joints and the intervertebral discs as the leading sources of chronic low-back pain. Sacroiliac joint pain accounts for some 20% of patients, but its pathology remains unknown. Zygapophyseal joint pain accounts for some 10–15% of patients. Small fractures or tears of the joint capsule are the most likely lesions in injured patients. Discogenic pain caused by IDD accounts for some 40% of patients. This condition can be diagnosed by CT discography. Circumstantial evidence favours fatigue failure of the vertebral endplate or annulus as the cause of this condition.

Chapter | 6 |

Epidemiology of back trouble

INTRODUCTION

The epidemiology of low-back trouble (LBT) is a huge subject which could fill a book on its own. The following selective account aims to summarise the evidence which is most pertinent to the title of this book, and in particular to indicate the relative importance of mechanical, biological and psychological influences to the phenomenon of back pain.

Epidemiology has been defined as 'the study of how diseases occur in different groups of people, and why'.[290] It serves to put a problem into perspective; it provides information on a number of aspects that are necessary to understand the problem and inform possible solutions. That information may include the magnitude and consequences of the problem, its natural history and the identification of its major risk factors.

The value of epidemiology cannot be overstated. The epidemiological patterns can indicate, for instance, the areas in which risk factors may be found or, indeed, where they are unlikely to be found. As well as the fine detail of specific risk factors, epidemiological evidence also helps to build the big picture and enables a condition to be put into perspective, both medically and socially. It is a complex discipline that has developed and enlarged in recent years from descriptive studies, through hypothesis testing to intervention studies and clinical epidemiology. Like all scientific fields, epidemiology is not always perfectly conducted and reported,[1137] so care is needed in interpreting and applying the knowledge it brings – see also the STROBE statement that aims to strengthen the reporting of observational studies in epidemiology (www.strobe-statement.org: accessed January 2011). Nevertheless, there is now a wealth of sound epidemiological data on LBT, which puts things into context and should be used to underpin other fields such as prevention and treatment.

Symptoms, pathology and disability

The title of this chapter, with the word 'trouble' replacing the more usual 'pain', needs some explanation. It reflects some of the difficulties faced when discussing the epidemiology of low-back problems which do not constitute a single identifiable disease. Before the population 'at risk' can be characterised, it is necessary to establish just what is being studied.

The individual experience of low-back pain (LBP) is highly variable, manifesting as discomfort, pain, neurological symptoms and incapacity. The term 'low-back trouble' is a convenient umbrella term covering a range of symptoms and pathology which are not necessarily closely related to each other. Temporally, the experience of LBT ranges from occasional twinges to persistent symptoms with a wide range of consequences, including disability, work absence and litigation. So epidemiology needs to consider not only the reported symptoms, but also their effects on life. The difficulty, in epidemiological terms, is compounded by the fact that LBT usually has no clinical diagnosis (or disease process) that can be identified reliably as the source of symptoms. There are, of course, various pathological states that occur in spinal structures (Ch. 15) but often they do not readily fit a traditional disease model, which further complicates epidemiological study.

The basic epidemiology of LBT will be considered under three main headings: (1) symptoms (pain in the lower back and/or legs); (2) pathology (disc disorders and other degenerative changes); and (3) disability (limitation of daily activities and/or work). Each of these may variously be associated with care-seeking. Four additional sections will then consider the influence of specific risk factors for LBT (other than age and gender), grouped under the following headings: genetic, individual, environmental and psychosocial. Social influences will not be covered in detail, and specific disease processes such as infection, tumours, osteoporosis and spondylolysis lie outside the scope of this chapter.

Epidemiological terminology

Two key concepts in epidemiology are incidence and prevalence. Incidence is the percentage of individuals in a given population who develop a disease during a specified period of time. Prevalence is the percentage of individuals in a given population who have a disease during a specified period of time. Typical period prevalence rates are lifetime, 1-month and 1-year prevalence, with point prevalence being the percentage with the disease at a given moment in time.

Various measures of association are used to summarise comparisons of disease rates between populations; usually the comparison is between 'exposed' and 'unexposed' people, with the variable of interest being some suspected risk factor or protective factor. The most common measures likely to be encountered in epidemiological studies of back pain are relative risk (RR) (ratio of the disease in exposed persons to that in unexposed persons) and odds ratios (OR) (the odds of a disease in exposed persons divided by the odds of a disease in unexposed persons).

The practical meaning of these measures, which are quite similar, should be interpreted related to the overall prevalence rates for the disease in the population. It is also important to consider the methodology of the study in which epidemiological findings are reported: a cross-sectional study may give a high OR but causation cannot be inferred.

In the case of a continuous variable such as body height, it is customary to define the OR in terms of two different values: for example, it could refer to the increased risk associated with having a body height equal to the mean of the population plus one standard deviation, compared to having a height equal to the mean minus one standard deviation. An OR of 4.5 means that risk is increased by a factor of 4.5, which is equivalent to saying that the risk is increased by 350%.

If a risk factor is relatively rare in the population studied, then it is usual to express its influence in terms of an OR or RR, but if the risk factor is common, then its influence is more likely to be expressed in terms of R^2 (this being the proportion of variance in the dataset explained by the multiple linear regression model). An R^2 value of 0.56 means that 56% of variability in the disease prevalence is statistically associated with the risk factor in question. This could mean that the risk factor is entirely responsible for the disease in 56% of people, or that it contributes 56% of the risk in each person, or anything in between. If a risk factor is rare, but decisive whenever it does occur, then it will have a low R^2 but high OR and RR.

Statistical significance is expressed in terms of a probability, P. It is conventional to accept a relationship between two variables as being 'significant' if there is a less than 1-in-20 (5%) chance that it is simply due to chance ($P<0.05$). Note that P does not indicate how important or strong the relationship is: a large epidemiological survey may be able to detect small influences (small R^2) with high probability (small P) simply because data were collected from a large number of subjects. For example, smoking is a highly significant but relatively unimportant risk factor for intervertebral disc degeneration (Ch. 15).

The nature of epidemiological evidence

Rarely can an epidemiological study be designed and conducted to remove all possible confounding factors and sources of bias, certainly for a topic such as back pain. It would be unsafe and probably erroneous to draw firm conclusions or base decision-making on a single study. More specifically, epidemiological studies need to define diseases, predictor variables and outcomes carefully if valid and useful conclusions are to be reached.[1137] It is all too easy to fail to find a statistical relationship between two variables if they are not quantified very well, even though the study itself is well designed. For example, it would be difficult to establish a statistical association between disc degeneration and back pain if the term 'degeneration' was used to include any age-related changes visible on magnetic resonance imaging (MRI), and if 'back pain' was used to include self-reporting of even the mildest symptoms. (Nearly everyone would have both conditions!) So, the results of a number of studies are more likely to provide a balanced view of how the world really is, but there remains the problem of selecting the studies of interest and determining their quality.

The increasing interest in, and reliance on, evidence-based medicine has led to more rigorous assessment of scientific papers with a rapid growth in the publication of systematic reviews. These reviews assemble the evidence in a given subject area from previously published source papers, which are systematically identified and graded for methodological quality according to preset criteria. Systematic reviews are particularly well suited to evaluate the results from clinical trials of treatments where the randomised controlled trial (which is the scientifically preferred methodology) readily permits the assessment of the quality of the original studies against set criteria. However, systematic reviews are less well suited to examining other types of evidence, especially where it is difficult to specify acceptable investigative methodologies and exclusion criteria. Systematic reviews are less likely to introduce bias than narrative reviews, but they can come to inconsistent findings that are not entirely due to the variable quality of the papers reviewed.[461] In the field of back pain, systematic reviews and meta-analyses (which pool and analyse data from multiple studies) must consider studies of varying quality, and have a tendency to come to somewhat nihilistic conclusions. Furthermore, it is possible that interesting, hypothesis-building findings from the occasional innovative source paper will be swamped by findings from more mundane studies, or may be excluded on the grounds of perceived methodological limitations, some of which might have only a slight bearing on the results presented.

The discussion presented in this chapter will be based largely on recent systematic reviews and guidelines because this is the most appropriate way of summarising a large body of evidence in an impartial manner, while at the same time giving due attention to its methodological quality. However, several well-focused and incisive source papers are also discussed, because they can give additional insights, emphasis and direction in certain areas. More recent studies, not included in the reviews, will also be cited where they add to or support ideas and concepts.

SYMPTOMS

Back pain and sciatica in adults

It is important to appreciate that pain is a symptom which may reveal little or nothing about the nature of any underlying disorder or disease. Thus, in large part, epidemiological studies of LBP tell us about the people who experience the symptom, and how they experience it. Of necessity, the data collection method is restricted to questionnaires in which the precise wording of the questions influences the responses, and leads to difficulties when comparing surveys. For example, descriptions of the location of back pain differ between surveys, as does its definition. Some studies take the precaution of specifying the type of pain (e.g. 'low-back pain other than the normal aches and pains after, say, gardening'), but others simply ask about 'pain in the back'. As a result, some studies record what may be considered troublesome symptoms while others will include trivial discomfort. By way of example, some physical risk factors have been found to be significant predictors of 'serious' LBP (which involved medical consultation or time off work) but not of more trivial backache,[36] so the definition of pain is important.

In addition, studies use different target populations, ranging from community surveys to investigation of specialised groups. Not surprisingly, the literature reports differing incidence and prevalence rates for back pain in different populations. However, comprehensive reviews have found some overall consistency in that international studies of adult back pain report a point prevalence of 15–30%, a 1-month prevalence of 19–43% and a lifetime prevalence of 60–70%.[381,1023] Whilst the international evidence does not suggest that back pain (as a symptom) is increasing[1507,645a], there are a couple of intriguing reports from the UK that suggest increases may have occurred at a local level. The first was a comparison of two surveys conducted 10 years apart on samples drawn from general practitioners' lists, which found that the annual prevalence of back pain rose by more than 12% between 1988 and 1998. Interestingly, the disability due to back pain did not increase, and the authors suggested the increase in symptoms was due to cultural changes leading to more awareness of minor back symptoms and willingness to report them.[1093] The more recent report concerns two population surveys 40 years apart, the first of which was in the 1950s. The results showed that in the northwest region of the UK the prevalence of back pain (and shoulder pain and widespread pain) increased quite markedly between the two surveys; the change was unlikely to be entirely due to methodological or environmental differences but, like Palmer et al.,[1093] the authors considered it more likely that the rise resulted from increased reporting or awareness of such symptoms.[570]

Most of the epidemiological studies on LBP have been undertaken in the developed world, leading to the suggestion that it may be related to some aspect(s) of industrialised lifestyle. A study of back pain in an urban population of Turkey found similar rates to those from more developed countries, and noted the prevalence was higher than in other developing countries,[496] which might appear to suggest a prevalence gradient related to level of industrial development. Seemingly, though, LBP is not simply a condition experienced in developed countries. A study from southwest Nigeria found the prevalence rates for LBP to be very similar to those from more industrialised nations, though it was not considered to constitute a major cause of sickness absence.[1078] A large survey of back pain among adult villagers in rural Tibet found point prevalence and 12-month prevalence rates to be at the upper level of the ranges reported from industrialised countries, and some 20% of villagers had substantial functional disability.[635] Similarly, the experience of back pain among Australian Aboriginals is not substantially different in terms of symptom prevalence, but cultural factors mean that it is not readily discussed or reported.[625]

Another example of cultural factors influencing the back pain experience comes from the Turkish study; they found that being religious did not influence the prevalence of back pain but did predict restricted activity related to back pain.[496] Differences can exist between similarly developed countries, and these have been demonstrated in studies using identical designs. One survey found that past and current back pain was more frequent among German participants than British, and that there were differences between East and West Germany; the difference in prevalence rates could not be explained by differing risk profiles.[1186] Another study looking at an identical occupational group found 'reported' back pain to be higher among Belgian nurses than Dutch nurses, which was not explained by a difference in working practices but seemed to be related to psychosocial factors.[222]

The fact that between 40% and 90% of people with back pain also report pain in other (perhaps unrelated) regions suggests that back pain should not necessarily be considered a local pain problem.[1019,1190,1539] The lifetime prevalence of back pain in adults does not seem to increase substantially with age.[1190] So far as the elderly are concerned, a systematic review determined that back pain has not been extensively investigated in this group.[180] More recently, there have been some studies with somewhat inconsistent findings. A study of elderly Danish twins found back pain (and neck pain) to be a common intermittent symptom, the prevalence of which varies little over time or between age groups.[573] Others consider there is some evidence that the prevalence decreases slightly in older people[1019] compared with working-age people. Indeed centenarians, despite general diminished physical functioning, have been found to report less back pain than younger elderly people,[1289] yet the symptom remains highly prevalent in old age.[574a]

The 'true' incidence rate (first ever onset) for back pain is especially difficult to determine, partly because of the high but poorly recalled prevalence in adolescence (see below). One 18-year follow-up study in Canada, concerning 4–16-year-old children, found an incident rate for a first episode of back pain to be 7.5%.[1014] The incidence rate for new *episodes* of back pain is more easily determined, but again estimates vary. Robust evidence in the UK comes from the South Manchester Back Pain Study, which found a 1-year incidence rate of 36%, with 40% of these being reported as the first-ever episode.[309] A somewhat lower

1-year incidence of 24% has been reported for a new episode in Sweden.[1190] In the USA, a study of Veterans Affairs outpatients, who were free of LBP for 4 months and followed for 3 years, found a 3-year incidence rate of 67%, with depression at baseline having the highest OR.[681] Looking specifically at newly employed workers, new-onset LBP was reported by 19% of subjects at both 12 and 24 months.[569] Overall, the available evidence suggests that something of the order of a quarter of the population can expect to experience a new episode of LBP each year.

The symptom of sciatica should be considered separately, but robust epidemiological data are scarce. Whilst leg pain (as a referred symptom associated with back pain) is not uncommon – perhaps occurring in about 35% of cases – the lifetime prevalence of true sciatica as determined by strict diagnostic criteria is far lower, amounting to between 2% and 5%, with a slight preponderance in males.[1023] Sciatica is strongly associated with herniated lumbar discs, peaking between the ages of 40 and 45 years. Obesity is predictive only when patients are considerably overweight.[1019]

Back pain in children

Adolescents seem to have prevalence rates similar to those for adults, although the pain is readily forgotten, and disability is rare.[217,697] The lifetime prevalence in children rises from 12% at age 11 to 50% at age 15, when the point prevalence reaches 13%; the overall experience is episodic yet benign.[217] However, others have suggested that, although acute back pain in children may be common, the presence of recurrence can be related to disabling consequences[700] and clinicians may need to pay special attention to recurrent significant back pain in children. In this age range, genetic influences on back pain are slight.[393] Back pain prevalence rates in developing or undeveloped countries, whilst somewhat lower than industrialised regions, are still substantial at between 14% and 30% by adolescence,[128,1161] and in Tunisia back pain is a common reason for school absence.[128]

Because of the recurrent nature of back pain, it is to be expected that there will be an association between childhood and adult back pain. For example, 20% of a cohort of children/adolescents followed to young adulthood reported back pain at all three follow-up points used during the 13-year follow-up.[179] Nevertheless, it is quite unclear if there is any direct relationship, and the evidence does not support the notion that adult back pain can be attributed to some (physical) event during childhood. Indeed, the reverse may be true: high physical activity in childhood seems to protect against LBP and mid-back pain in early adolescence.[1542] Radiological abnormalities in adolescence were not found to be predictive of adult back pain during a 25-year follow-up.[571] However, early degenerative changes in the lower lumbar discs visualised on MRI scans[1239] does predict the reporting of persistently recurrent symptoms up to age 23 years. A Canadian follow-up of 4–16-year-old children specifically looked at childhood predictors of a first episode of back pain in early adulthood. Following adjustment for age, sex, childhood conditions and health status, and early adult health behaviour, socioeconomic status and work environment, the risk of incident back pain was moderately associated with psychological distress, low childhood socioeconomic status and childhood emotional and behavioural disorders.[1014]

Numerous risk factors for back pain in childhood have been advanced, but there is scant and inconsistent epidemiological evidence for many.[247] There has been widespread interest in the putative risk from carrying school books in backpacks, but a major review found little persuasive scientific support for the concept, from either a biomechanical or epidemiological perspective.[247] Interestingly, a survey of emergency department attendances with backpack-related injuries in school-aged children found that the back ranked sixth (11%) behind head/face (22%), hand, wrist/elbow, shoulder and foot/ankle (~12% each), and the most common mechanisms associated with the injuries were tripping over the backpack (28%), wearing it (13%) and getting hit by the backpack (13%)[1558] – seemingly the dangers of backpacks go well beyond carrying and back pain! The importance of familial factors is somewhat inconsistently reported; some studies find parental experience of back pain associated with childhood reporting of the symptom whilst others suggest educational and social associations.[128,785,815,1019]

The time course of back pain

Back pain is conventionally described as acute, subacute or chronic. Wood and Badley[1589] proposed a simple taxonomy based on their review of the epidemiology in the late 1970s, in which there are three classes: (1) the transient twinges experienced by most people; (2) acute episodes of pain experienced by many; and (3) persistent back pain and disability afflicting a minority. The authors raised the interesting (but unanswered) question: are chronic backs chronic from the beginning, or do they develop from an unfavourable response to acute pain? It is now becoming apparent that the overall picture of the complaint is that of a recurrent, intermittent and episodic phenomenon, leading to a new epidemiological concept of looking at the pattern of pain over long periods of the individual's life.[1023,1507]

This view is well supported by the evidence. In the short term, 24% of patients in primary care were found to have not recovered by 3 months.[534] A longer prospective study suggests that that short-term view may be overly optimistic: 75% of patients presenting to primary care had failed to recover completely in terms of pain and disability after 1 year, leading the authors to suggest that we should

stop characterising LBP as a series of acute problems, and accept it as a chronic problem.[309] Another study, this time in manipulative practice, found that 70% of patients reported multiple episodes during the follow-up period of 4 years.[221] A study in primary care looked at patients who had recovered uneventfully from the presenting spell before 6 weeks, and followed them for 12 months.[1356] Recurrence was found to be dependent on the definition of an episode of recurrence, but the authors suggested that some 75% of primary care patients whose episode of acute pain resolves in a timely fashion will not have a recurrence during the following 12 months.[1356] The length of follow-up, as well as the course of the initial/previous episode, is clearly an important factor in predicting the likelihood of recurrence. A 5-year prospective population study led the authors to conclude that LBP should not be considered transient since the condition seems rarely self-limiting; rather it manifests as periodic attacks and temporary remission.[597]

Longitudinal studies of specific occupational groups with recognised high physical demands, such as nurses[934] and scaffolders,[395] reveal patterns displaying a dynamic process characterised by recurrence rather than displaying a progressive nature. It is difficult to give precise estimates for rates of recurrence since they are highly sensitive to various definitions and data sources (e.g. claims-based, care-based and disability-based rates differ substantially), but a 2-year follow-up may be sufficient to identify more than 85% of recurrences.[1532] An undoubted impediment to quantifying recurrence rates is the difficulty in defining a universally used or accepted definition of an episode.[1356] This has now been addressed by an international multi-disciplinary group who came up with the following arbitrary, yet well-considered, definitions: an episode of LBP was defined as a period of pain lasting for more than 24 hours, preceded and followed by a period of at least 1 month without LBP. An episode of care for LBP was defined as a consultation or series of consultations for LBP, preceded and followed by at least 3 months without consultation for LBP. An episode of work absence due to LBP can be defined as a period of work absence due to LBP, preceded and followed by a period of at least 1 day at work. It is apparent that even persistent (chronic) presentations may be characterised by a fluctuating level of symptoms and disability, rather than constant progression to a dismal state.[934] The course of chronic and recurrent back pain has been studied at the population level, providing information about the stability of the descriptive clusters identified in primary care studies.[1401] The same clusters were identified (severe persistent, moderate persistent, mild persistent and fluctuating): as might be expected, the clusters differed significantly in terms of pain and disability, with a considerable proportion of the 'fluctuating' group changing their classification over time.

This conceptualisation of adult back pain is illustrated diagrammatically in Figure 6.1, which depicts 'typical'

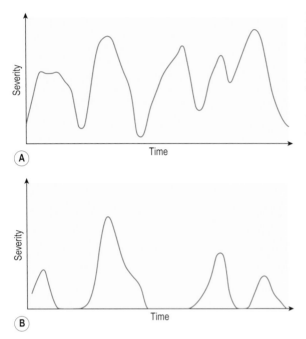

Figure 6.1 Conceptual pattern of low-back pain over a period of years. **(A)** Fluctuating severity of symptoms with no truly painfree periods. **(B)** Fluctuating severity of symptoms with episodic pattern. *(After Croft et al.,*[308] *Deyo,*[343] *Waddell*[1507] *and Weber and Burton*[1541]*.)*

lifetime patterns of fluctuating symptoms of varying severity. The key feature suggested by the epidemiology is one that Croft and colleagues described as 'a chronic problem with an untidy pattern of grumbling symptoms and periods of relative freedom from pain and disability interspersed with acute episodes, exacerbations and recurrences'[309]; this is incompatible with frequently voiced claims that 80–90% of episodes of back pain end in complete recovery. The description by Croft and colleagues neatly accommodates the fact that the best single predictor of future back pain is a previous history of back pain; this has been consistently demonstrated and substantially outweighs any other predictor.[36,903,1104,1019,1190,1355,1510]

LBT, then, can be considered a common health problem affecting most people at some point in their lives, and for the majority will be a recurrent event. This depiction is somewhat generalist (for that is the nature of the evidence) and it is accepted that for some individuals the pattern may be different, as is true for any disease or disorder. The reasons for such differing patterns of back pain are obscure.

CARE-SEEKING

The extent to which the experience of LBT provokes care-seeking helps to put the problem into perspective. A large-scale Swedish study of a working-age population found that approximately 5% of the population sought care for back pain over a 3-year period, and few of the care seekers became symptom-free during the 2-year follow-up period.[1496] A community survey in the UK[1537] found that only about 50% of people with back pain sought treatment for it during a 12-month period. Consultation for episodes lasting less than 2 weeks was associated with greater than median pain; consultation for episodes lasting more than 2 weeks was associated with increased disability; and consultation for episodes lasting more than 3 months was associated with increased depression.[1537] Even for those consulting their general practitioner, only about 10% continue to attend beyond 3 months, despite the fact that they are experiencing symptoms and disability.[309] By contrast, care-seeking can be common for recurrences of back pain: most patients attending an osteopathic clinic generally returned to the same osteopath with recurrences during a 4-year follow-up period.[221] The same has been reported for patients visiting chiropractors.[249] Hadler has suggested that the recurrent/chronic nature of the back pain experience is an indication that what many patients are saying when they consult is not simply 'My back hurts', rather 'My back hurts, but the reason I'm here is that I can't cope on my own any longer'.[549]

PATHOLOGY

Various pathologies affecting the lumbar spine, and potential sources of pain, are considered briefly in Chapter 15. The present section considers the epidemiology of only the most common conditions, including intervertebral disc herniation and degeneration, zygapophyseal joint osteoarthrosis, spinal stenosis, spondylolisthesis and segmental instability. It should be remembered that most patients who present to primary healthcare with simple backache (by far the largest proportion of complaints) have no objectively identified pathology to account for that pain.[157,432] This may, of course, be either a reflection of a failure by current clinical methods to identify a causative pathology, or a true absence of significant pathology.

Intervertebral disc herniation and degeneration

Unlike symptoms, certain types of pathology constitute a 'hard' (objective) outcome measure that may be easier to link to causative risk factors. (Hence the epidemiologists' joke about the hardest of all outcome measures: 'where there's death, there's hope!'). Disc herniation (or extrusion – as opposed to simple protrusion or bulge) is one such hard outcome, because it can be visualised on MRI with a fair degree of reproducibility, and it is not consistently associated with any other age-related findings on MRI scans.[680,1489] Evidently, it is a pathological entity in its own right. Nevertheless, the epidemiology of back pathology remains at the mercy of the variable methodological designs of reported studies[1439] and the problem of interpreting spinal images,[74] which may lead to uncertainties and inconsistencies. Furthermore, a clear distinction between disc herniation and disc degeneration cannot always be made, even though it is of prime clinical and medicolegal importance. Radiologists can find it difficult to distinguish between a bulging disc (which is a normal sign of ageing, but may be exaggerated in degeneration) and a disc herniation (which involves relative displacement of nucleus and annulus, as described in Chapter 15). If herniations are defined as discs bulging more than 5 mm on MRI scans, then they can be identified in 1.6% of lumbar discs from men aged 35–69 years.[1488] If the criterion is a bulge of 0–5 mm, then 5.4% of lumbar discs were herniated. For comparison, 15.1% of lumbar discs were deemed to be 'bulging'.

Disc herniation is the major cause of nerve root pain, most commonly experienced as sciatica. However, disc herniation does not necessarily produce symptoms. MRI scans reveal disc herniations in many asymptomatic volunteers: Boden et al.[151] found at least one herniated disc in 20% of those aged 60 years or less, and in 36% of older subjects, while Boos et al.[168] reported a prevalence of 76% among 46 subjects aged 20–50 years. Nevertheless, the prevalence was increased to 96% in a symptomatic group matched for age, sex and work-related risk factors,[168] emphasising that the MRI finding of a disc prolapse is not clinically irrelevant. A 5-year follow-up of asymptomatic subjects showed that disc herniations and neural compromise did not worsen, whereas disc degeneration progressed in 41.5%,[169] as indicated by small reductions in height (<1%) and increased bulging (<2%).[1490] The prevalence of asymptomatic disc herniation in children is unknown, but symptomatic herniation does occur and may represent between 0.8% and 3.2% of all disc protrusions or herniations.[175] Arguably, the lifetime prevalence of 'true sciatica' (i.e. between 2% and 5%: see above) may be taken to represent the lifetime prevalence of symptomatic disc herniation,[1023] which is similar to the prevalence of 'extrusions' (6%), largely uninfluenced by age, reported by Jarvik and Deyo,[680] and is consistent with the prevalence of discs bulging more than 5 mm (see above).

Intervertebral disc degeneration can be visualised on MRI, and inferred from certain radiographic changes such as height loss. Inconsistencies in the definition of disc degeneration have impeded epidemiological research[117] and, if any age-related changes are included, then 'disc degeneration' is extremely common, of little clinical relevance, and difficult to relate to any risk factor other than age. Generally, disc degeneration is more severe, and starts earlier, at the L5 and L4 levels compared to upper lumbar levels.[74,273] Lumbar disc degeneration has been reported in 31% of 15-year-old schoolchildren,[1238] with prevalence rising to 40% in the age range 18–30 years and to over 90% at 50–55 years.[273] Thoracic discs are rarely degenerated, with only 5–9% being assessed as moderately to severely narrowed in men aged 35–70 years.[1046] Mid-thoracic discs are more likely to be affected than lower thoracic, although posterior bulging is relatively rare at all thoracic levels.[1046] Radiographically defined severe disc degeneration is more common in westernised societies than in certain native populations.[409] This has been attributed to a protective effect from the increased spinal mobility[695] and habitual flexed squatting postures characteristic of native populations,[408] although factors such as genes and diet could also play a role. A prospective MRI study indicated that physical job characteristics and psychological aspects of work are more powerful than MRI-identified disc abnormalities in predicting the need for back pain-related medical consultation and resultant work incapacity.[169] Associations between disc degeneration and back pain are considered in detail in Chapter 15.

Other spinal pathology

Spondylolysis, spondylolisthesis, spina bifida, transitional vertebrae, spondylosis and Scheuermann's disease do not appear to be associated with LBP.[1439] In view of perceived methodological deficiencies in many of the reported studies, it was concluded that there is no firm evidence for the presence or absence of a causal relationship between radiographic findings and LBP.[1439] The term 'lumbar spondylosis' should be reserved to refer to vertebral osteophytes secondary to disc degeneration. Thus, the epidemiology of spondylosis follows closely that for disc degeneration: it increases markedly with age, but seems to occur somewhat later, and is uncommon below 45 years of age.[74] The prevalence of zygapophyseal (facet) joint osteoarthrosis also increases with increasing age; it seems to be related to disc degeneration and the indication is that discs degenerate before zygapophyseal joints.[74]

DISABILITY

Disability is restricted functioning – limitation of activities and restriction of participation in life situations.[1556a] Disability often accompanies LBP, varies in extent and may be temporary or essentially permanent. Much of the available information comes from surveys in which disability is self-reported, so there is no objective evidence or pathological basis for the following figures. Approximately 7–14% of adults in the USA experience disabling back pain during the course of a year, and just over 1% will be permanently disabled.[1507] In the UK, 11% of adults experience back pain-related restrictions of their daily activities during a month, and 8% resorted to bed rest during a 12-month period.[1507] The lifetime prevalence of disability tends to rise with age, and the extent of disability may be slightly greater in males: a UK population survey that used clinical measures of disability revealed that the 1-year prevalence of a disability score of 50% or more was 5.4% for men and 4.5% for women, whereas the lifetime prevalence was 16% and 13% respectively.[1525]

Accurate information on work loss is particularly difficult to obtain, being dependent on social policy and local issues such as compensation systems and job availability. Taking the UK as an example, a 1-year prevalence of time off work due to back pain has been reported as 11% for men and 7% for women, with a lifetime prevalence of 34% and 23%.[1525] A Norwegian looking at sick leave among care seekers found, not unexpectedly, that the annual prevalence was somewhat higher (around 15%) than that in the general working population, though that still leaves sickness absence a relatively rare event.[1496] Approximately 85% of those off work with back pain are absent for short periods (a week or so) and they account for only about half the lost work time – the remainder being accounted for by the 15% who are off work for more than 1 month.[1507] It is this small proportion who account for the greatest societal costs and are a major target for interventions since the longer someone is off work with back pain, the less likely he or she is ever to return to work.[1507] A UK study noted that estimates of the economic impact of LBP on work depend on various factors, and it seems to be higher than previously thought when data on reduced duties are combined with work absence, and if the additional impact of unemployment is included.[1593] What is clear is that sickness absence due to LBP is far from the rule, and many people remain at work, or return to work quite rapidly. However, that situation may not be static. If the prevalence of back pain reports is increasing, as suggested by Palmer and colleagues,[1093] that may represent a cultural shift rendering back pain more acceptable as a reason for absence; the corollary being that the solution to the growing economic burden from back pain may lie more in modifying people's attitudes and beliefs rather than interventions aimed at reducing physical exposures.[1093] Also of relevance, certainly in the UK, are attitudes and beliefs of health professionals towards certification of sick leave.[1255] The balance of the epidemiological data suggests that patients could often be issued with a 'fit' note rather than a sick note! Indeed, the statutory Statement of Fitness for Work, also termed the fit note, has been introduced in the UK (www.dwp.gov.uk/fitnote: accessed January 2011), though it is too early at the time of writing to know its effects on sickness absence rates. These issues will be discussed further in Chapters 16 and 17.

Disability related to back pain, as reflected in the prevalence of 'compensated' back pain, increased exponentially in most industrialised countries through the latter part of the 20th century (Fig. 6.2), though there are signs that this curve is levelling off, at least in the UK,[1507] where mild to moderate mental health problems have overtaken musculoskeletal disorders to become the reason for the greatest proportion of incapacity benefits.[1511] The social

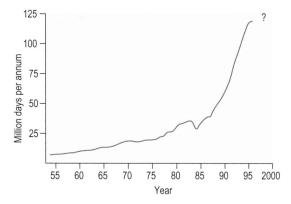

Figure 6.2 The exponential rise in the back pain problem shows recent signs of flattening out. *(From Waddell[1507] with permission.)*

context needs to be considered, and a clear distinction made between the 'epidemiological sea' of low-back symptoms and the small proportion of those who receive long-term sickness benefits.[1507] Predicting who will go on to long-term incapacity is complex, and involves a balance of sociodemographic risk markers acting with clinical and psychosocial factors,[1515] and is beyond the scope of this book.

An overview of the epidemiological evidence on back pain was included in the UK *Occupational Health Guidelines for the Management of Low-back Pain at Work*.[257] These guidelines were based on a comprehensive review,[1509,1510] and presented a synthesis of the evidence reported in a variety of previous reviews, supplemented with individual studies where reviews were unavailable. The guidelines documentation represents the output from the Blue Circle Industries, Faculty of Occupational Medicine and British Occupational Health Research Foundation project on occupational health aspects of LBP. It is convenient to reproduce here some of the relevant evidence statements presented in that review. (Full text for the guidelines and evidence review can be found at www.facoccmed.ac.uk/pubspol/pubs.jsp: accessed January 2011). The star rating against each statement represents the strength of the evidence (*** = strong evidence; ** = moderate evidence; * = limited or contradictory evidence – = no scientific evidence). The following evidence statements relating to disability are taken from that review.

**There is moderate evidence that patients who are older (particularly >50 years), have more prolonged and severe symptoms, have radiating leg pain, whose symptoms impact more on activity and work, and who have responded less well to previous therapy are likely to have slower clinical progress, poorer response to treatment and rehabilitation and more risk of long-term disability.[74,98,266,554,584,664,802,1067]

***There is strong epidemiological evidence that most workers with LBP are able to continue working or to return to work within a few days or weeks, even if they still have some residual or recurrent symptoms, and that they do not need to wait until they are completely painfree.[74,220,354,548,572]

RISK FACTORS

Risk factors for LBT can be grouped in various ways. Figure 6.3 gives a 'taxonomy' in which there are two key domains (genes and environment) with four main drivers of risk (genetic, individual, physical and psychosocial factors) that interact with each other in complex ways. This sort of approach to risk has clear similarities to the biopsychosocial model of disability and incorporates the multifactorial nature of LBT.

Genetic risk factors are risks associated with specific genes inherited from parents. They can be studied by comparing disease prevalence in unrelated people and in identical twins, and the confounding influence of childhood environment can be controlled for if the comparison is between identical and non-identical twins. It is relatively easy to show the overall influence of genetic inheritance on a given disease, but the techniques of molecular biology are required to identify which particular gene or genes are responsible for the increased risk. Individual risk

factors such as body height, weight and spinal mobility are considered separately because they are partly genetic and partly environmental: for example, you might be born with a predisposition to obesity which nevertheless requires access to sufficient food to be fully realised. Individual risk factors are of practical importance because most are easy to quantify, and so could conceivably be employed in the workplace to identify those at risk of LBT. Environmental risk factors for LBT mostly concern the physical environment, such as occupation and sporting activities, but also include nutritional factors, smoking and social policy. Psychosocial risk factors include clinical factors such as depressive mood and somatisation, attitudes and beliefs about the activity/pain/damage relationship and occupational psychosocial interactions.

Biomechanical risk factors need not be environmental. The inheritance of small intervertebral discs, for example, or short spinous processes (Fig. 9.2), could increase the compressive stress acting on the discs. Alternatively, the inheritance of defective collagen or proteoglycans could weaken spinal tissues so that they are more vulnerable to injury.

Genetic risk factors

Identical-twin studies have shown that, after major environmental factors have been controlled for, approximately 50% of intervertebral disc degeneration is associated with genetic factors.[113,117,896] The genetic contribution depends on how degeneration is defined and on the population studied, and it can exceed 75% in women who do not undergo heavy manual work.[1240] Genes explain 'who gets disc degeneration?' rather than 'which discs become degenerated?' and the fact that degeneration mostly affects discs in the lower lumbar spine[273] suggests greater environmental influences, including mechanical. When these factors are taken into account, the heritability of disc degeneration in the lower lumbar spine of men falls to approximately 35%.[116] Disc prolapse in the lower lumbar spine also has a much weaker dependence on genes than other aspects of disc degeneration.[113] In a 5-year follow-up MRI study on twins,[1490] genetic inheritance explained approximately 17% of progressive disc narrowing and 0% of posterior disc bulging, again emphasising that risks for disc herniation differ from risks for disc degeneration.

Genetic inheritance similarly influences spinal pain. In middle-aged women the heritability of back and neck pain is approximately 60% and 45%, respectively, with genetic determinants being associated with structural disc degeneration and an inherited tendency toward psychological distress.[867] For men, the heritability of back pain is somewhat lower (30–46%) but is likewise linked to disc degeneration.[115] A much lower heritability for back pain reported in a Scandinavian twin study[574] may be attributable to their advanced age, which allows more scope for random

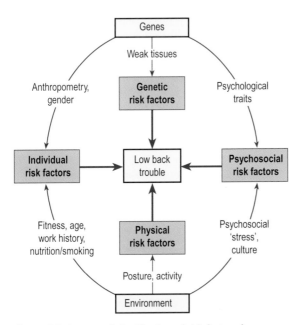

Figure 6.3 Suggested classification of risk factors for low-back trouble, indicating possible relationships to each other.

environmental influences to dominate. Conversely, a Dutch study on twins aged 12–41 years found that early shared environment made a major contribution to back pain in young people.[596] Another twin study looked at whether high physical workload was associated with LBP and/or neck/shoulder pain when taking account of genetic and shared environmental factors.[1054] It transpired that high physical workload was associated with LBP and/or neck/shoulder pain, even after taking account of genetic and shared environmental factors, whilst it was only for concurrent back and neck pain that the genetic and shared environmental factors influenced the association with high physical workload. However, since the data were cross-sectional, there can be no direct implication that the high physical workload was causative: it may simply be that people with high physical demands at work are more aware of backache and that is reflected in the data.

Only a few of the genes responsible for disc degeneration have so far been identified: they include variants in the genes for the vitamin D receptor,[722,1491] for proteoglycans,[723] for collagen type IX[1091] and for other matrix proteins.[1288] The combined action of all identified gene variants explains only a few per cent of the variance in disc degeneration, raising concerns over the ability of twin studies to explain common diseases such as disc degeneration and arthritis.[910] Osteoarthrosis, which affects the zygapophyseal joints in 90% of individuals aged over 45,[824] is influenced by similar genetic risk factors,[1031] suggesting that unfavourable genes may lead to tissues that are mechanically inferior, although this has been confirmed only for collagen type IX.[56]

Individual risk factors

Several large prospective studies have sought to establish links between future LBT and individual factors such as height, weight, flexibility, strength, fatigability and fitness. Generally, the results have been inconsistent, and this may be due, in part, to differing definitions of back trouble. Overall, back muscle strength and general levels of fitness appear to be of little significance[36,111,138,236] and although easily fatigued back muscles were associated with more back pain in men, the same was not found for women.[138] Other studies have found small but variable influences of fatigability on back pain risk.[36,904] There is no persuasive evidence of substantial or meaningful differences in prevalence rates for back pain dependent on gender and leg length discrepancy.[1019] Methodological differences between studies (as well as methodological weaknesses such as poor follow-up rates) will contribute to inconsistent findings, leading to the tendency for summary statements of systematic reviews to indicate weak links between individual characteristics and LBT.

However, a prospective study with 90–99% follow-up rates has shown that certain physical and psychological risk factors are significant predictors of future back pain.[36] Of particular interest is the high risk associated with

having poor lumbar mobility, and a long back, in young healthcare workers who are newly exposed to heavy physical work: these two individual factors explained almost 12% of future back pain in this population.[36] Presumably tall people with long backs tend to lift weights at the end of greater lever arms (Fig. 9.2) and this may explain why tall people have a greater risk of disc prolapse as well.[590]

The UK *Occupational Health Guidelines for the Management of Low-back Pain at Work* review[1510] offered the following evidence statements:

**There is moderate evidence that examination findings, including in particular height, weight, lumbar flexibility and straight-leg raising test, have little predictive value for future LBP or disability.[74,438]

**There is now moderate evidence that the level of general (cardiorespiratory) fitness has no predictive value for future LBP.[74]

*There is limited and contradictory evidence that attempting to match physical capability to job demands may reduce future LBP and work loss.[74,75,474,475]

***There is strong evidence that X-ray and MRI findings have no predictive value for future LBP or disability.[142,169,1195,1252,1393,1439]

Environmental (physical) risk factors

The risks of a physically demanding workplace are best quantified if the risk exposure (the magnitude and intensity of spinal loading) is also quantified,[422] and if the outcome measure is objective (e.g. some pathology or dysfunction[923]) rather than subjective (e.g. pain). Even though they are not fully supported by systematic reviews (see below), there have been numerous individual studies reporting relatively high risks for various outcomes from physical activities at work. These have included activities such as lifting heavy weights from the ground while in a twisted position (for disc prolapse[732,1011]), activities involving a combination of rapid bending and twisting (for back pain[417] and dysfunction[923]) and extreme forward bending (for lumbar disc herniation[1287]). In addition, incidents that require sudden muscular efforts[899] are associated with back pain.[886] If vague job descriptions are used to assess risk exposure, then larger population-based studies are required, and they show significant but modest influences of occupational activity on disc degeneration.[1012]

On the other hand, a prospective study showed little correlation between perceived 'minor trauma', subsequent back pain and changes in spinal pathology, suggesting that psychosocial factors and compensation claims were better predictors of future back pain.[251] Night shift work and perceived lack of support from superiors, in addition to frequent mechanical exposures, are associated with an increased risk of intense low-back symptoms and sick leave in nurses' aides.[399] Similarly, in a cohort of newly employed workers, several non-mechanical aspects of the workplace environment (stressful and monotonous work) were important in predicting new-onset LBP.[569] The influence of some physical exposures may only be realised in the presence of some comorbidity: a relationship between cumulative exposure to weight-lifting or carrying and lumbar disc herniation was found with, but not without, concomitant osteochondrosis or spondylosis.[1287] An intriguing study on nurses suggests that a useful distinction can be made according to the speed of onset of LBP: sudden onset was associated with exposure to specific patient-handling tasks, but LBP of gradual onset showed little relationship with patient-handling.[1330]

Some care is required to reconcile these individual studies with the evidence from a series of systematic reviews which adhere to the Bradford–Hill aspects (sometimes termed criteria) for determining a causal relationship.[605] The aspects were established as a framework for use in epidemiological research to minimize the possibility that important public health decisions are made on the basis of incomplete or flawed evidence. The aspects are: strength of association (OR); consistency; specificity; temporal relationship (temporality); biological gradient (dose–response relationship); plausibility (biological plausibility); coherence; experiment (reversibility); and analogy (consideration of alternate explanations). The authors noted that, whilst some aspects may be fulfilled for a given question, others are not. Their final conclusions were therefore duly cautious and mostly conclude that the physical stressors studied are not independently causative agents. The main findings of the series were:

- Occupational bending or twisting in general is unlikely to be independently causative of LBP.[1520]
- Occupational lifting is unlikely to be independently causative of LBP, but simple association for types of lifting, and lifting 25–35 kg, was apparent.[1522]
- There is strong evidence of no association between awkward occupational postures and LBP: there is no dose–response.[1211]
- There is strong and consistent evidence against both an association and a temporal relationship between occupational carrying and LBP.[1521]
- It appears unlikely that workplace manual handling or assisting patients is independently causative of LBP (assisting ambulation may be an exception).[1215]
- Strong and consistent evidence does not support occupational sitting being independently causative of LBP.[1213]
- It is unlikely that occupational pushing or pulling is independently causative of LBP in the populations of workers studied.[1212]
- It is unlikely that occupational standing or walking is independently causative of LBP.[1214]

This series of systematic reviews generated considerable debate across a number of disciplines. An important and

pertinent point is that the reviews excluded all biomechanical and basic science *experiments* (which investigate *causation*) leaving only selected epidemiological *surveys* (which investigate *association*). Furthermore, they assumed that a simple dose-response relationship suggests causality, even though a consideration of skeletal tissue biology (Ch. 7 and p. 64) suggests that too little physical activity can be as harmful as too much. To make sense of the apparent contradictions it is necessary to recognise that the epidemiological studies had pain and disability as their main outcomes, rather than objectively demonstrable injury or damage (and we know the correlation between symptoms and pathology is inconsistent). So the reviews are really telling us something about the extent to which physical stressors are "independently causative" agents for symptoms and their consequences. There can be little doubt that certain physical exposures can result in some form of tissue insult, possibly leading to pathological changes. This series of reviews does nothing to challenge that. What they do show is that it is difficult to implicate physical occupational exposures as major independent causes of low back *pain*, with the corollary that simply reducing physical exposures is unlikely to have a widespread preventive effect. That, though, is not to say that a proportion of injury and pathology cannot be avoided: it can, and attempts to do so are justified. We just need to be realistic about what we expect to be preventable.

Turning to objective evidence of primary mechanical overload damage, disc height can be severely and significantly decreased in workers exposed to exceedingly heavy manual work (much more arduous than current regulations would permit), but vertebral height decrease seems rare.[187] In the same study, substantial exposure to whole-body vibration on unsprung operators' seats (but not on sprung seats) was associated with a reduction in disc height. Previous injury to a vertebral body has been found to lead to disc degeneration several years later in a high proportion of subjects, although this degeneration was rarely painful.[739] The main value of that small study was that the subjects were aged between 9 and 21 years at follow-up, so there was little disc degeneration in the age-matched control group.

The conclusions put forward in the UK *Occupational Health Guidelines for the Management of Low-back Pain at Work* review[1510] seemingly remain valid: the following evidence statements were offered to reflect what was seen as the balance of the evidence:

***There is strong evidence that physical demands of work (manual materials handling, lifting, bending, twisting and whole-body vibration) are a risk factor for the incidence (onset) of LBP, but overall it appears that the size of the effect is less than that of other individual, non-occupational and unidentified factors.[36,214,354,422,866]

***There is strong epidemiological evidence that physical demands of work (manual materials handling, lifting, bending, twisting and whole-body vibration) can be associated with increased reports of back symptoms, aggravation of symptoms and 'injuries'.[74,174,212,214,354,422,924,1048,1561]

Note: the above two statements are not incompatible. Whilst the epidemiological evidence shows that low-back symptoms are commonly linked to physical demands of work, that does not necessarily mean that LBP is caused by work. Although there is strong scientific evidence that physical demands of work can cause individual attacks of LBP, overall that only accounts for a modest proportion of all LBP occurring in workers.

*There is limited and contradictory evidence that the length of exposure to physical stressors at work (cumulative risk) increases reports of back symptoms or of persistent symptoms.[212,226,866,924,1048,1053]

**There is moderate scientific evidence that physical demands of work play only a minor role in the development of disc degeneration.[113,1487]

***There is strong epidemiological and clinical evidence that care-seeking and disability due to LBP depend more on complex individual and work-related psychosocial factors than on clinical features or physical demands of work.[214,354,1105,1507]

Evidence on the role of sports and leisure activities as risk factors for LBT is somewhat inconsistent, with sports participation variously being reported as having a protective effect, a detrimental effect or no effect on prevalence rates. Vigorous sports such as weight-lifting and gymnastics can carry an increased risk of disc degeneration[1389,1495] and vertebral damage,[1390] some of which is symptomatic.[1389,1390] Running carries no increased risk of back pain or spinal degeneration.[1495] Athletes in general have no more back pain than non-athletes, suggesting that vigorous physical activity can increase resistance to back pain.[1495] There are, of course, substantial physiological benefits from physical fitness, and there is some evidence that physically fit individuals recover more rapidly from episodes of back pain[71] and that exercise programs are an effective prevention intervention.[842] There is limited evidence that sports participation may represent an additional hazard for first-onset back pain when superimposed on another physical hazard,[217] whilst sports participation over and above normal school sport may be a hazard in 15-year-old schoolboys (but not in girls or younger children).[217]

It should not be assumed that the risk of LBT increases uniformly with the spine's exposure to high physical loading. On the contrary, there is evidence that reported LBT is common in sedentary workers,[575,591,876] although this does not imply that the pain is caused by sitting. Whilst accepting the generally high prevalence of back pain in the population, two systematic reviews have failed to find support for the popular notion that sitting while

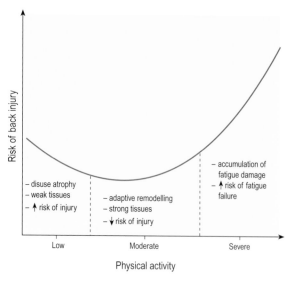

Figure 6.4 Proposed U-shaped relationship between mechanical loading and low-back trouble.

working is a risk factor for LBP.[270,575] Whilst it is accepted that whole-body vibration is a risk factor for back pain (see evidence statements above), there is only limited evidence from prospective studies favouring a dose–response (duration of driving) relationship.[792] Car driving may nevertheless carry an increased risk of disc prolapse,[733] which could be related to vibration, to reduced muscle protection of the spine following prolonged flexion[1344] (Fig. 14.4) or to fatigued muscles having a reduced ability to protect the spine.[359] It may be that there is a U-shaped relationship between spinal loading and risk of back injury, with too little exposure being almost as detrimental as too much[593] (Fig. 6.4). This can be explained in terms of the ability of spinal tissues to adapt to increased or decreased mechanical demands (see Ch. 7). Those who avoid vigorous activity run the risk of developing a weak back which is then vulnerable to injury during slips and falls.

The different rates at which spinal tissues are able to adapt to increased mechanical demands could lead to an increased risk of injury to poorly vascularised tissues (such as intervertebral discs and ligaments) when levels of physical activity are suddenly increased, perhaps as a result of a new job or sporting activity (p. 85). In cross-sectional epidemiological studies, people who have survived in a heavy job without developing back pain will often, but not necessarily, be overrepresented compared to those who have had to give up their job because of back pain. The true impact of mechanical loading on LBP can, therefore, be higher than cross-sectional studies suggest, and will only be quantified accurately when controlled prospective studies are carried out. Already, the physical dangers of a new job are suggested by several longitudinal studies,[36,756] and the effects can occur with only short-term exposure.[1026] Another prospective study of nurses found that time spent in nursing without suffering an attack of LBP was negatively correlated with future episodes of LBP,[903] suggesting some protective adaptation over time to the increased spinal loading.

Other environmental risk factors include cigarette smoking, which accounts for approximately 2% of disc degeneration,[113,114] slightly increases the risk of disc prolapse[731] and predicts hospitalisation for intervertebral disc disorders.[705] Presumably, smoking interferes with the precarious supply of metabolites to the centre of the disc (Fig. 7.21), yet a systematic review concluded that smoking should be considered a weak risk indicator and not a cause of back pain.[812]

Psychosocial influences

The relationship between back pain and psychological and psychosocial factors has received much attention in recent years. The tendency for the terms 'psychological' and 'psychosocial' to be used interchangeably can lead to confusion. There is an argument that the term 'psychological' should be reserved for those factors that embody a clear-cut psychological construct, and the term 'psychosocial' should be used to describe factors having a social element (e.g. work stress), but it is generally convenient to use the term 'psychosocial' to embody both concepts.

Psychosocial influences are related more to what people do about their back trouble than what caused it. Nevertheless, there is some evidence that psychosocial factors can predict up to 3% of reports of new onsets of LBP.[903,1105] It seems that psychosocial influences can have a profound effect at the population level. It has been noted from a number of German health surveys before and after reunification of the country that the wide gap in the prevalence of back pain (in which the prevalence rates were higher in West Germany) consistently decreased until it reached nearly zero.[1185] This led the authors to suggest that back pain may be a communicable symptom if 'communicable' is used to refer to something being transmitted by sharing or exchanging information – they concluded that this hypothesis was supported by experimental research showing that back beliefs, attitudes and subsequent behaviour (reporting patterns) can be influenced by media campaigns and the like.[1185]

It is difficult to draw strong causal inferences, yet employees' reactions to psychosocial work characteristics such as job satisfaction and job stress are more consistently related to LBP reporting than the psychosocial work characteristics themselves (e.g. job demands and social support).[324] In addition, it seems that there is an interaction between physical and psychosocial risk factors to increase the risk of low-back disorders.[340] Psychosocial stress can increase spinal loading due to muscle tension,

suggesting a mechanical explanation for some of the related back pain.[920] However, the psychosocial influences on LBP are usually considered in relation to outcomes: that is, they may predict reporting patterns, attribution of cause, care-seeking, response to treatment and the development of chronicity. Recently, psychosocial factors have been viewed in terms of them acting as 'obstacles to recovery'[216,219,735,914,1511] both in occupational settings as well as clinical environments. Financial compensation for back injury also can act as an obstacle to recovery, but settlement of the claim seemingly does not reduce long-term morbidity.[530] The associations between psychosocial issues and outcomes, especially work-related psychosocial factors and sickness absence, suggest they should be useful screening tools. Seemingly, they are and they aren't: a prospective study of over 4500 workers found that a battery of carefully chosen measures of work-related psychosocial factors predicted the occurrence of absence during 15-month follow-up but did not predict the duration of absence.[105] The duration of sickness absence (or return-to-work time) is clearly subject to other influences (possibly biological) as well as psychosocial factors, with implications for absence management and rehabilitation.[1434,1511]

A systematic review of the role of specific psychological factors as predictors of unfavourable outcome in back pain concluded that there was good evidence to implicate distress/depressive mood and somatisation in the development of chronicity (persisting symptoms and/or disability). Acceptable evidence generally was not found to link other psychological factors to back pain chronicity, although weak links emerged for catastrophising as a coping strategy. There was a basic lack of information on the potentially important role played by fear avoidance beliefs.[1132] The influence of these variables was found to be generally consistent across environments (primary care, clinics and workplace) and have been reported by other reviewers.[840,1434] Considering specifically non-return to work due to LBP, additional predictive factors have been found to include subjective negative appraisal of one's ability to work, and job satisfaction[1434] and the importance of confounders (e.g. age and education) have been stressed.[212,1515] Certainly, attribution of back pain to work is common. In a UK survey, nearly 80% of those with musculoskeletal symptoms identified a work task (or tasks) as leading to their complaint.[699] For LBP, the most commonly perceived causes were manual handling (66%) and posture (33%), along with workload/pace, and lack of social support.[699] Perhaps surprisingly, attribution to work remained high even for symptoms that started after ceasing work.[699]

The UK *Occupational Health Guidelines* review[1510] considered the evidence on psychosocial influences and offered the following evidence statements:

***For symptom-free people, there is strong evidence that individual psychosocial findings are a risk factor for the incidence (onset) of LBP, but overall the size of the effect is small.[36,310,1507]

***There is strong evidence that low job satisfaction and unsatisfactory psychosocial aspects of work are risk factors for reported LBP, healthcare use and work loss, but the size of that association is modest.[167,324,1048]

***There is strong evidence that individual and work-related psychosocial factors play an important role in persisting symptoms and disability, and influence response to treatment and rehabilitation. Screening for 'yellow flags' can help to identify those workers with LBP who are at risk of developing chronic pain and disability. Workers' own beliefs that their LBP was caused by their work and their own expectations about inability to return to work are particularly important.[250,422,429,474,802,1051,1244,1507]

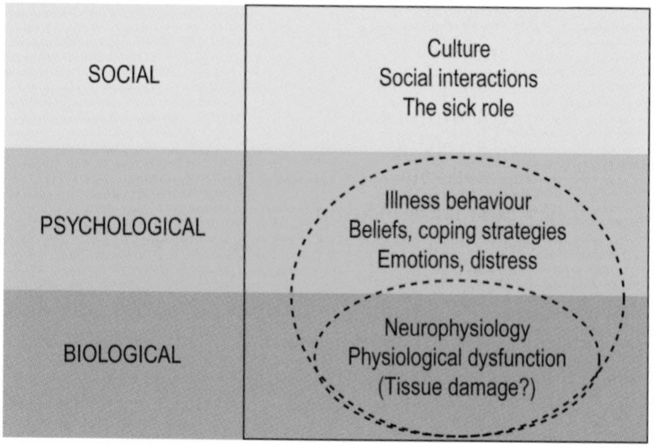

Figure 6.5 The biopsychosocial model of back pain disability. *(Adapted from Waddell and Burton[1511] with permission.)*

CONCLUDING REMARKS

LBT involves tissue changes, symptoms and social consequences. The epidemiology encourages its description as a common health problem[1511] (sometimes termed subjective health complaints,[1460] or regional (pain) disorders). Common health problems are characterised by: high prevalence rates; symptoms but no permanent impairment; episodic, with most episodes settling uneventfully; no work interference for most people; long-term incapacity is not inevitable. People with common health problems, including LBT, are essentially 'whole people' with a manageable health problem.[1511] Within that general description there is, of course, scope for individuals to have much more severe problems, possibly arising from specific pathology, but epidemiology is about populations, not individuals. LBT has a variety of consequences that are of importance variously to the individual and society:

- presence of symptoms
- reporting of symptoms
- seeking healthcare
- spinal pathology
- disc herniation
- degeneration
- attribution to work
  - work-caused
  - work-irritated
- sickness absence
- long-term incapacity.

The epidemiological evidence shows that these consequences have differing determinants in different combinations, and the role of physical stress in each of them is complex.

A simple intuitive 'injury/damage' model for the phenomenon of LBT would suggest that high exposure to physical stressors results in some form of damage to spinal tissues, and that further exposure leads to further damage and/or impeded recovery. However, it is apparent from the epidemiological evidence that such a simple model does not adequately explain what is observed. An alternative injury model might be that there is a U-shaped relationship between exposure and injury (Fig. 6.4). Whilst links between injury and pain are undoubtedly complex, and may involve pain sensitisation phenomena (p. 205), it is becoming obvious that many aspects of back pain and its consequences are not adequately accounted for by a purely mechanistic model.

The biopsychosocial model (Fig. 6.5) was proposed in 1987 to fill this gap,[1506] and it remains supported by more recent research.[1434] This model accounts for all of the epidemiological evidence reviewed above, including the enduring course of much LBP (Fig. 6.1). In essence, it accepts that a proportion of back trouble results from (some sort of) physical insult leading to (some sort of) spinal pathology and (some level of) pain. However, that pain should resolve within a relatively short period of time (perhaps following appropriate treatment/management), as is the case with many other musculoskeletal disorders. That the problem does not resolve for many people suggests that alternative explanations are required. To date, the most promising explanation, guided primarily by the epidemiology, appears to involve a substantial influence from psychosocial factors acting as obstacles to recovery.[219,735,1511] This has significant implications when trying to find solutions, some of which will be discussed in Chapters 16 and 17.

The overall view of back pain shared by the authors of this book is entirely compatible with the epidemiological evidence reviewed above, and with the biopsychosocial model. Evidently, certain types of physical stress are linked to spinal pathology and pain, and the experience of pain appears to interact with psychological characteristics, and with social incentives and constraints, to explain the common manifestations of back pain behaviour.

Chapter | 7 |

Biology of spinal tissues

INTRODUCTION

One purpose of this book is to describe the mechanisms by which spinal tissues can be injured by excessive mechanical loading. The concepts used to describe these mechanisms, such as 'fatigue failure' and 'elastic limit', are derived from mechanical studies of engineering materials, and this terminology might lead the unwary into thinking of biological structures as inert and passive. This would be unfortunate, because the same mechanical loading which deforms and damages spinal tissues also stimulates their cells to repair any damage, and to strengthen the extracellular matrix as a precaution against future damage. The outcome of repetitive loading applied to living tissues can therefore vary from fatigue failure, on the one hand, to hypertrophy and strengthening, on the other. Furthermore, the metabolic rate of different spinal tissues varies greatly: at one extreme is muscle, which has a rich blood supply and a remarkable ability to increase or decrease its strength in a matter of weeks; and on the other extreme are the intervertebral discs, the largest avascular structures in the body, which are able to respond only slowly, and perhaps incompletely, to changes in their mechanical environment. Large imbalances in the ability of spinal tissues to respond to applied loading mean that different tissues could be at risk of damage depending on how quickly the applied loading changes.[15] Therefore the risk of fatigue damage to the spine, and the location of that damage, depends on factors such as the number and severity of loading cycles, the time scale over which they are applied, and the age and health of the individual whose tissues are being loaded. Clearly, it is essential to consider the 'mechanobiology' of spinal tissues when attempting to understand mechanical failure of the spine.

The following sections review the biology of spinal tissues. The description of each tissue starts with the composition and structure of the extracellular matrix, then considers cellular metabolism, including adaptive remodelling in response to external loading, and healing in response to injury. Muscle is considered first, because it applies most of the mechanical loading to the other tissues. Bone comes next, because its responses to changes in applied loading have been studied most, and are best understood. Less is known about the mechanobiology of articular cartilage, tendons, ligaments and intervertebral discs, and in these sections it will be necessary to interpret some preliminary data by drawing analogies with bone. From a histological perspective, different regions of the intervertebral disc resemble several of the other tissues, so discs are considered last. The final section compares the biological activity of these spinal tissues, and considers some likely consequences of mismatches between them.

MUSCLE

Skeletal or striated voluntary muscle is a tissue specialised for forceful contraction, which enables it to produce movement and maintain posture. It has a rich blood supply, and contains a variety of nerve endings capable of monitoring tissue stress and strain. Nociceptive nerve endings capable of signalling pain are mostly located in the collagenous sheaths within and surrounding muscle.

Structure and composition

A human skeletal muscle is composed of bundles of contractile muscle fibres, separated by sheaths of collagenous connective tissue which coalesce at each end into tendons or aponeuroses for attachment to bone (Fig. 7.1). Each individual muscle fibre is a multinucleated cell with its own cell membrane, the sarcolemma. Invaginations along the length of the sarcolemma form a transverse series of tubules, the t-tubules, which are continuous with the

exterior of the muscle fibre and are filled with extracellular fluid. Running longitudinally along the muscle fibre is another series of channels, the sarcoplasmic reticulum, which stores calcium ions in high concentrations. A delicate layer of reticular fibres, the basal lamina, lies outside the sarcolemma, and this is surrounded by a thin connective tissue sheath, the endomysium. The endomysial tissue around each cell is continuous with that of adjacent cells, forming an array of endomysial tubes (Fig. 7.2) in which the muscle fibres are housed.[1431] Groups of muscle fibres are bound into bundles or fascicles by the perimysium. This is the most abundant connective tissue within muscle and is composed of a cross-ply arrangement of crimped collagen I fibres which reorient as the muscle lengthens.[1168] Tension in the perimysium contributes to muscle tension during eccentric contractions, and it protects the muscle fibres from overstretching. Surrounding the whole muscle is a third connective tissue sheath, the epimysium, and lying superficial to this is the fascia, which binds and compartmentalises individual muscles into functional groups. Capillaries penetrate the various connective tissue sheaths to provide muscle fibres with oxygen and remove waste products. Small quiescent muscle precursor cells, termed 'satellite' cells, lie just below the basal lamina of the muscle fibre. These cells are a type of stem cell that are capable of proliferation in response to growth stimuli or muscle damage (see below). Healthy muscles contain very little extracellular matrix, apart from the collagenous sheaths.

Each muscle cell or fibre is packed with numerous myofibrils which are composed of a series of repeating sarcomeres. The sarcomere is the functional unit of muscle, and is composed of parallel arrays of fibrous proteins, actin and myosin that are held in position by filamentous protein structures found in the Z-line at the ends of the sarcomere and in the M-line in the centre of the sarcomere (Fig. 7.3). When an action potential travels along the muscle fibre, calcium ions released from the sarcoplasmic reticulum initiate cross-bridge formation between actin and myosin, which are then able to move relative to each other and thus cause the muscle to contract. Individual muscle fibres can be oriented parallel, or at an angle, to the long axis of the muscle, and this architectural arrangement confers different mechanical properties upon the muscle. Parallel-fibred muscles, which tend to be long and thin with fibres extending the full length of the muscle, are able to contract the greatest distance. Greater forces (but smaller contractions) can be generated by pennate muscles which consist of bundles of relatively short muscle fibres oriented at an angle to the line of pull (Fig. 7.4). This arrangement ensures a larger physiological cross-sectional area and hence a greater capacity for force production. Individual muscle fibres are tapered at their ends, where microscopic interdigitations serve to strengthen the interface between each muscle fibre and its tendon.

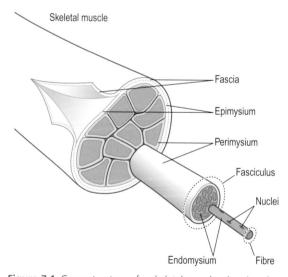

Figure 7.1 Gross structure of a skeletal muscle, showing the collagenous sheaths which surround muscle fibres, fibre bundles (fasciculi) and the whole muscle. Compare with Figure 7.2.

Skeletal muscle

Fascia

Epimysium

Perimysium

Fasciculus

Nuclei

Endomysium   Fibre

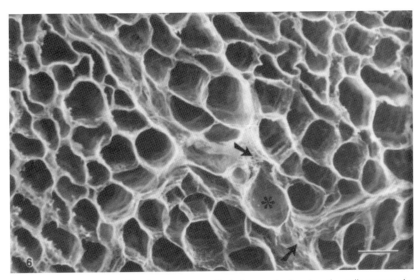

Figure 7.2 Scanning electron micrograph of bovine sternomandibularis muscle showing the collagenous sheaths (endomysium) which surround each individual muscle cell, and the coarser connective tissue (perimysium, indicated by arrows) which surrounds the muscle bundles or fasciculi. Contractile proteins have been enzymatically removed, as described in Trotter and Purslow.[1432] Bar = 50 μm. *(Reproduced from Trotter,[1431] with permission.)*

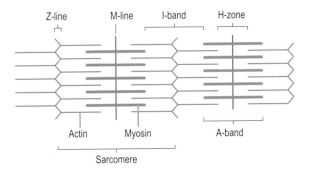

Figure 7.3 Diagram showing the arrangement of actin and myosin within sarcomeres which comprise the contractile machinery within skeletal muscle cells. Contraction is achieved by the myosin molecules moving along the actin molecules by means of cross-bridges which repeatedly form, change orientation and then break. The various lines and bands can be visualised by electron microscopy. Compare with Figure 7.6.

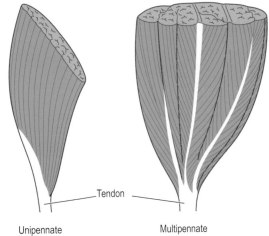

Figure 7.4 Typical arrangement of muscle fibres in unipennate and multipennate muscles.

The mechanism by which muscles generate force has been defined by the 'sliding-filament hypothesis,'[653-654] which is sufficiently well known that it need not be described here. However, several details of muscle mechanics are directly relevant to this book. Firstly, the maximum 'active' tension that a muscle can generate increases with muscle length up to an optimum length (L_o), and then decreases (Fig. 13.13). This can be explained in terms of the optimum interactions between actin and myosin. On the other hand, 'passive' tension in a stretched but relaxed muscle increases greatly with muscle length, because stretching generates tension in the connective tissue sheaths described above, and within the muscle fibres themselves. During eccentric muscle contractions, active and passive processes can combine to generate peak forces considerably larger than the maximum active tension. Forces are particularly high if the muscle is stretched rapidly. This explains why rapid forward-bending movements can generate such high forces within the lumbar erector spinae (p. 108).

Metabolism

Skeletal muscle contains three main types of fibre (Fig. 7.5) which have different mechanical and metabolic properties (Table 7.1). Type I ('slow') muscle fibres rely heavily on oxidative metabolism, have large numbers of mitochondria and high concentrations of enzymes involved in oxidative metabolism, and are supplied by an extensive

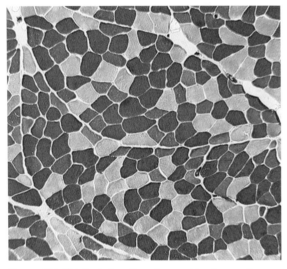

Figure 7.5 Histological section of normal lumbar erector spinae muscle tissue, with staining for muscle enzymes. Collagenous tissue is white, and the three types of muscle fibre are type I (dark), type IIA (light) and type IIB (mid).

capillary network. These fibres contract slowly and are fatigue-resistant. Type IIX ('fast glycolytic') fibres rely mostly on anaerobic metabolism, have lower concentrations of oxidative enzymes, fewer mitochondria and a less dense capillary network than type I fibres, but have higher concentrations of glycolytic enzymes and higher myosin ATPase activity. They produce fast, powerful contractions but fatigue rapidly. Type IIA ('fast oxidative') fibres are intermediate between types I and IIX. A fourth type of fibre, type IIC, is generally found only in neonatal muscle but has been observed, in some animals, in regenerating adult muscle before becoming fully differentiated into one of the main adult phenotypes. It is generally accepted that genetic programming largely determines the relative proportions of type I and II fibres in human muscle at birth. However, changes in gene expression, especially of myosin heavy-chain genes, in response to longitudinal growth (stretch) and mechanical loading will have an effect on the adult phenotypes.[397]

Each muscle cell normally lives for the entire life of the individual, with new cells being produced only following acute traumatic disruption of muscle cell membranes. During growth, muscle cells grow in length when they are stretched such that there is an increase in the functional length of the sarcomeres.[302,594,769] The 'sensing' system that detects this increase in sarcomere length may possibly involve cytoskeletal proteins such as titin which attaches myosin to the Z-line of the sarcomere.[631] Radioactive tracer studies have shown that muscle lengthening occurs primarily by the addition of new sarcomeres to the fibre near the musculotendinous junction, so that each muscle fibre becomes longer.[1574–1576] This longitudinal growth of muscle keeps pace with skeletal growth in order to maintain substantial overlap of the actin and myosin filaments at resting sarcomere lengths. At puberty, muscles also show significant increases in girth which are particularly marked

Table 7.1 Characteristics of the main fibre types found in human skeletal muscle. A fourth type (IIC) can be distinguished in regenerating muscle. Fibre types are defined on the basis of their histochemical staining properties

	Type I	Type IIA	Type IIX
Aerobic capacity	High	Intermediate	Low
Mitochondrial density	High	Intermediate	Low
Capillary density	High	High	Low
Anaerobic capacity	Low	Intermediate	High
Speed of contraction	Slow	Fast	Fast
Force of contraction	Low	Intermediate	High
Fatigue resistance	High	Intermediate	Low
(Based on Lane[803].)			

in boys due to the influence of male sex hormones such as testosterone. This increase in girth is achieved by an increase in the cross-sectional area of individual muscle fibres (hypertrophy) rather than an increase in fibre number (hyperplasia). In young adult muscle tissue, the rate of protein turnover is so rapid that the half-life of contractile proteins is probably between 7 and 15 days.[506] Consequently, muscle can adapt to altered mechanical requirements much more rapidly than other tissues.

How muscle responds to changes in mechanical loading is influenced greatly by the type of exercise performed. Repeated contractions at low force levels (endurance training) produce changes that increase the muscle's capacity for oxidative phosphorylation, enabling the muscle to contract for longer before it becomes fatigued. In response to endurance training, type I fibres show increased vascularisation,[629] increased size and number of mitochondria[1530] and an increased concentration of oxidative enzymes.[508,1530] Depending upon the intensity and duration of endurance training, similar changes may also occur in other fibre types. An experiment on dogs has suggested that vigorous aerobic training can cause transformation of type II to type I fibres.[1172] In human muscle, any transformation resulting from endurance training probably occurs between the type IIX and IIA fibre population,[241,787,1530] although an increased proportion of type I fibres has been reported following long-term endurance training.[1415]

Strength or power training, in which high forces are generated for short periods of time, produces the greatest changes in the fast-twitch (type II) fibres. This type of exercise does not normally create more muscle fibres,[507] but appears to cause some transformation between type IIA and IIX fibres[527] as well as an increase in their diameter.[284,507,527,1410] Such mechanically induced hypertrophy is caused by changes in gene expression that result in increased synthesis of specific proteins, including actin and myosin.[997] Increased activity of myokinase, which helps maintain a high ATP/ADP ratio, has also been reported in response to strength training,[1419] although this finding is not universal.[1410]

Physical inactivity reduces muscle mass (muscle atrophy), with protein synthesis falling within hours. If muscle is immobilised in a shortened position then its length is reduced along with its girth, and the proportion of collagen to contractile protein in the muscle increases.[1577] The muscle becomes stiffer and less extensible.[509] This may explain the reductions in joint mobility which are often reported following injury and/or disuse.

Changes in muscle size and performance have been quantified in many studies. Typically, complete immobilisation of the leg reduces the cross-sectional area of the quadriceps by 15–20% in 6 weeks, with most of this loss being due to type I fibre atrophy resulting from a reduction in protein synthesis rather than an increase in protein catabolism.[492,494] Similarly, the capacity of muscle to respond to increased levels of loading is also marked: it is

a common experience that the maximum weight that can be lifted repeatedly during weight-training exercises can increase by 100% in 12 months. Some of this is attributable to increased endurance, and some to improvements in neuromuscular activation increasing the proportion of muscle fibres that can fire at the same time, but a considerable proportion is attributable to hypertrophy. Animal experiments indicate that muscles overloaded in the stretched position can increase their muscle mass by as much as 30% in just 4 days.[506] This figure will include increases in muscle fibre length as well as girth, but it serves as a useful yardstick by which to judge the adaptive ability of the skeletal tissues which must withstand the increased muscle forces.

The precise mechanical stimulus for muscle hypertrophy is controversial, although high stress, high strain and high strain rate have all been implicated. Excessive or unusual muscle activity, especially when eccentric contractions are involved, is effective in producing exertion-induced damage and subsequent repair and hypertrophy.[829] The damage initiated by this type of activity is characterised by changes in the sarcoplasmic reticulum,[83] disruption of the cell membrane,[963] and a disturbance of normal sarcomere structure,[243,491,696,1041,1042] as shown in Figure 7.6.

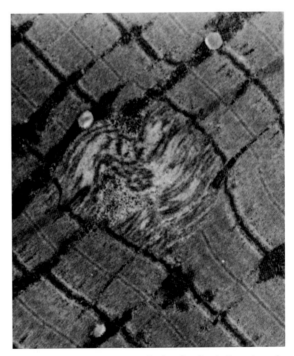

Figure 7.6 Electron micrograph showing focal disruption of sarcomeres in skeletal muscle, resulting from eccentric contractions. The myofilaments are disorganised in this region, and the Z-lines are displaced. Magnification ×19 000. *(From Newham et al.[1042] with permission.)*

Damage to the sarcoplasmic reticulum can affect calcium homeostasis, resulting in decreased excitation of muscle cells and hence a reduction in force-generating capacity that persists for several days.[1040,1245] Disruption of the muscle cell membrane allows proteins such as creatine kinase and histamine to leak out gradually into the extracellular environment, where they can stimulate nociceptors and cause delayed-onset muscle soreness and swelling 24–72 hours after exercise.[696,1245] Muscle damage can be detected in biopsies taken within an hour of completing the exercise, but the damage often worsens over the following few days. Type II fibres are reported to be more susceptible to this type of damage than type I fibres,[449,696,828] although the opposite effect has also been observed.[83]

The damage that occurs during or immediately after exercise has been attributed to protein degradation initiated by non-lysosomal proteases, such as calpain.[131] Together with other proinflammatory mediators, calpain is thought to initiate an inflammatory response that begins 2–6 hours after injury. This results in an infiltration of macrophages and other phagocytic cells into the damaged muscle tissue, where they remove cell debris and release proteases that rapidly break down the damaged myofibrils. These cells also produce cytokines that stimulate cellular repair and initiate the proliferation and migration of satellite cells.[131,242,244] Once at the site of injury, satellite cells differentiate into myoblasts which fuse to form myotubes that repair damaged cells or develop into new multinucleated muscle cells if the original fibres are completely necrosed (Fig. 7.7). Collagenous tissue also regenerates, and if the damage is severe, this can proliferate to such an extent that it interferes with normal muscle function. These repair processes generally take place over a matter of days or weeks[341] and result in muscle hypertrophy. If damage is severe then recovery times are longer, being dependent on the extent of damage to nerves and blood vessels. In a rabbit model involving complete muscle division by laceration, the wound healed by extensive scar formation; after a healing period of 12 weeks, 50% of muscle strength was regained, at which time the muscle's ability to shorten was 80% of normal.[479] Some residual weakness may persist at the musculotendinous junction where overuse injury often involves the rupture of attachments between the perimysium and tendon. In such cases, healing is slow, and resembles that of tendon (p. 80).

Fortunately, most stretch-induced muscle injuries lead not only to effective repair, but also to tissue adaptation so that a similar bout of exercise performed within a few weeks of the first produces much less damage. This rapid adaptation has been attributed to an increased number of sarcomeres (end to end) in the muscle fibre, so that a similar amount of muscle stretch produces less strain in each sarcomere and consequently less risk of injury.[1162] In addition, there is some evidence that in the adapted muscle, sarcomere strength is more homogeneous than in untrained muscle, so that there are fewer weak sarcomeres

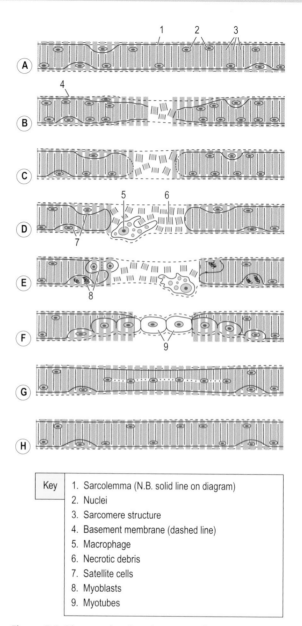

Key	1. Sarcolemma (N.B. solid line on diagram)
	2. Nuclei
	3. Sarcomere structure
	4. Basement membrane (dashed line)
	5. Macrophage
	6. Necrotic debris
	7. Satellite cells
	8. Myoblasts
	9. Myotubes

Figure 7.7 Diagram showing the stages of repair to a damaged skeletal muscle fibre. (A) Healthy intact fibre. (B) Fibre becomes disrupted. (C) Sarcolemmal membrane proliferates to compartmentalise damage. (D) Macrophages phagocytose cell debris. (E) Activated satellite cells migrate to damage and proliferate to form myoblasts. (F) Myoblasts fuse to form myotubes. (G) New myofilaments are synthesised to form myofibrils; nuclei remain centrally located. (H) Repaired fibre with peripherally displaced nuclei. *(From Hodgson DR, Rose RJ (1994) The athletic horse, with permission of WB Saunders, Philadelphia.)*

at risk of stretch-induced injury.[341] This 'weak sarcomere' theory provides an attractive explanation for why vigorous exercise can produce muscle pain and stiffness in untrained, but not trained, muscle.

BONE

Bone is a type of connective tissue with an abundant extracellular matrix specialised to provide a strong and rigid framework for the body. It has a rich blood supply. Nociceptive nerve endings capable of signalling pain are mostly located in the collagenous sheaths which surround bone.

Structure and composition

Bone tissue is found in solid blocks or sheets (cortical bone) or arranged as a lattice-work of slender struts (trabecular bone). In both cases, the adult tissue is composed of mature cells, osteocytes, trapped in small cavities (lacunae) within a rigid extracellular matrix. The extracellular matrix is approximately 5–8% water and 60–70% micro-crystalline solid, composed predominantly of hydroxyapatite. These plate-like crystals are 10–40 nm long and 2–5 nm thick. Their chemical composition is variable, but is similar to hydroxyapatite, $Ca_{10}(PO_4)_6OH_2$, where Ca is calcium, and PO_4 is phosphate. Individual crystals are very small, irregularly shaped, and contain impurities such as carbonate, sodium and magnesium. The remainder of the bone matrix is termed 'organic', and consists mostly of type I collagen (90%), other proteins such as osteocalcin and bone sialoprotein and the small proteoglycans biglycan and decorin. Collagen I fibres are bundles of fibrils, each made up of many collagen molecules lined up in a parallel array and held together by several types of cross-links (Fig. 7.8). Bone cells secrete individual collagen molecules which then lose their terminal regions so that they can self-assemble into fibrils within the matrix. Collagen cross-linking is a gradual chemical process which occurs in the test tube as well as in living tissue.[1463] Systematic gaps between collagen molecules (Fig. 7.8) form sites for the initiation and growth of the microcrystals.[1533]

The presence of crystals gives bone its rigidity and compressive strength, whereas collagen fibres confer tensile strength and toughness. The water-binding properties of proteoglycans enable them to 'capture space' in developing tissue, and then to regulate the diameter of collagen fibrils. Non-collagenous proteins appear to play a role in the mineralisation process.

The matrix is mostly arranged in concentric cylindrical lamellae with a central channel for blood vessels and nerve fibres, and with numerous osteocytes lying between adjacent lamellae (Fig. 7.9). The whole cylindrical structure is

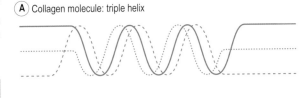

(A) Collagen molecule: triple helix

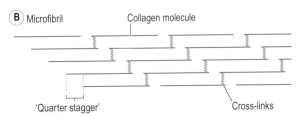

(B) Microfibril — Collagen molecule

'Quarter stagger'   Cross-links

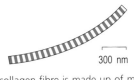

(C) Fibril (in electron micrograph)

300 nm

Figure 7.8 A collagen fibre is made up of many fibrils, (C) each of which is composed of a parallel array of collagen molecules, arranged end to end (B). An individual molecule of collagen type I or II comprises three polypeptide chains wound to form a triple helix, with short non-helical regions at either end (A). In bone, hydroxyapatite crystals are deposited initially in the gap regions between collagen type I molecules (B). For clarity, the helical region in (A) has been shortened.

termed an osteon, or haversian system. Irregular spaces between osteons and the slender struts of trabecular bone are filled with less-organised lamellae of similar composition (Fig. 7.10). The outer surface of a bone is covered with a fibrous membrane, the periosteum, and a similar membrane, the endosteum, lines the central medullary cavity of long bones. Each membrane consists of two layers, an outer protective layer containing many strong collagen fibres, which in the case of the periosteum blend in with the fibres from tendons, and an inner layer which contains two other types of bone cell, osteoblasts and osteoclasts.

Metabolism

Long bones, and vertebrae, develop from a 'model' of hyaline cartilage, which gradually turns into a bone as it grows and ossifies. Internal bone growth continues into adolescence at two growth plates by a process known as endochondral ossification, which involves an intermediate stage of calcium carbonate deposition and resorption. Growth plates enable a bone to increase in length while preserving the articular cartilage covering at each end. In addition, the width of a growing bone is increased by

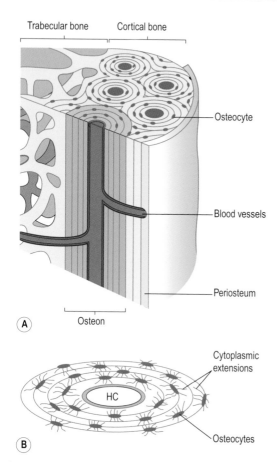

Trabecular bone   Cortical bone

— Osteocyte

— Blood vessels

— Periosteum

(A)   Osteon

Cytoplasmic
extensions

HC

(B)   Osteocytes

Figure 7.9 (A) Mature cortical bone is made of cylindrical osteons, comprising concentric layers (lamellae) of bone matrix surrounding a central blood vessel. (B) Bone maintenance cells, osteocytes, become trapped in small lacunae between the lamellae, but they can communicate with each other via long cytoplasmic extensions which extend radially outwards within small canaliculi (channels) in the solid matrix. HC, haversian canal. Compare with Figure 7.10.

direct deposition of bone from the inner layer of the periosteum. Active bone-forming cells, osteoblasts, secrete osteoid, which starts to mineralise into bone during the following few hours. Initially, the mineral structure and collagen alignment are disorganised, and the tissue is referred to as woven bone. This is then 'remodelled' by two types of bone cell which work in concert as a bone-forming unit to create haversian systems of mature bone: osteoclasts dissolve the old matrix, and osteoblasts then secrete new matrix in precisely oriented lamellae (Fig. 7.9). The mineralising process traps each bone-forming osteoblast in a rigid cell or lacuna, turning it into a less-active osteocyte. These bone maintenance cells communicate with each other by means of long cell processes which lie in

narrow channels (canaliculi) in the matrix. Remodelling occurs throughout adult life, so that bone matrix is turned over on a regular basis, and minor cracks are repaired before they can accumulate to cause major defects. The presence of microcracks in bone influences the tissue's mechanical properties, and may act as a stimulus to remodelling.[1632]

Bone cells can increase or decrease bone mass, or alter its shape and microarchitecture, in response to changes in external mechanical loading. This process is correctly termed 'modelling' to distinguish it from 'remodelling', in which bone mass stays the same. However, the mechanically adaptive response is often referred to loosely as 'adaptive remodelling' (Fig. 7.11), and the underlying principle that governs the bone's response to altered mechanical demands is known as 'Wolf's law'. In simple terms, Wolf's law states that bone architecture and mass adapt to best resist the forces applied to it, and there is plenty of experimental evidence to back it up.[512,805] Adaptation can involve optimising the entire shape of a bone to mechanical and metabolic demands,[1230] and this feat requires concerted action from many distant and apparently isolated cells. In fact, osteocytes are able to communicate directly with each other by means of gap junctions at the end of long extensions of their cell membranes which effectively create a 'nerve net' for the bone. They also communicate with osteoclasts and osteoblasts by means of chemical messengers (cytokines). Some cytokines, such as growth factors, stimulate a hypertrophic response, while others, including the interleukins, are associated with reductions in bone mass. Bone cells also respond to systemic signals (hormones) that are distributed through the blood to many bones. Mechanical and hormonal influences on bone metabolism are difficult to separate, because mechanical strain can stimulate osteoblast proliferation through the oestrogen receptor.[320]

The maximum speed at which whole bones can strengthen or weaken is not well characterised. It probably takes a year for newly deposited bone to be substantially mineralised.[454] The mineral content of a frequently loaded turkey bone can increase by 40% in just 6 weeks, or fall by 10–15% after 8 weeks of continuous unloading.[1226] The racquet arm of male professional tennis players contains 35% more cortical bone than the other arm.[698] Thirty years or more of vigorous physical activity increased various measures of bone size and strength by 8–18% compared to the relatively inactive identical twins who served as controls.[862] Bone adaptation can be quite extreme, as evidenced by the exceptionally high bone mineral content of vertebrae in elite weight lifters.[524] Bone mineral density is closely related to strength.[525]

Bone adaptations may not always be beneficial. Scalpel-induced disc degeneration in sheep[1081] leads to marked increases in sclerosis, and in the number of trabeculae in the adjacent vertebrae,[1001] presumably because the mechanically altered disc is less able to distribute stress evenly on

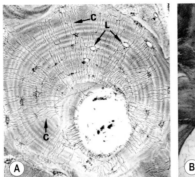 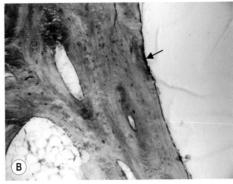

Figure 7.10 (A) Histological section of bone showing a large osteon. The contents of the central haversian canal are indistinct, but osteocytes in their lacunae (L) and their radiating cytoplasmic extensions which lie in canaliculi (C) are clearly visible. *(Reproduced from Young B, Heath JW 2000 Wheater's functional histology. Churchill Livingstone, Edinburgh, with permission.)* (B) Histological section of vertebral body cortex, showing flattened osteons. In the vertebral body, trabeculae (on the left) appear to condense to form the cortex.

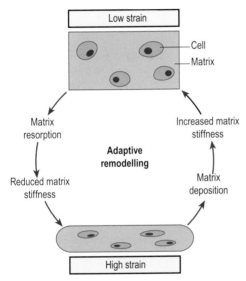

Figure 7.11 Most skeletal tissues are able to adapt their mechanical properties to match the mechanical environment. If mechanical loading increases so that tissue deformation (strain) is high, then more matrix is deposited by cells until the matrix stiffness increases sufficiently for strain to return to the normal range. Similarly, low loading will reduce strain and encourage matrix resorption until strain rises to normal levels again.

the bone (Fig. 11.8). Denser bone could then hinder the transport of metabolites into the adjacent disc.[1017] Osteophytes around the margins of the vertebral body, and in the apophyseal joints, may represent an attempt by bones to spread high loading over a greater area, and so to reduce stress and strain within the bone. Unfortunately, these adaptations can also lead to nerve root entrapment within the intervertebral foramen.[666]

The precise mechanical signal which controls adaptive remodelling in bone is probably the maximum dynamic deformation (strain) experienced locally by the tissue, and this is communicated to cells by the flow of fluid within the canaliculi.[895] Static loading has little effect,[805] whereas bone mass increases with increasing maximum strain.[1227] Only 36 cycles of dynamic loading per day are capable of producing a maximal response.[1226] According to the 'mechanostat theory',[453] bones strengthen when strains exceed a certain threshold value (approximately 2000 microstrains, or 0.2% change in length) and weaken when they fall below another threshold (approximately 200 microstrains). Strain thresholds can be altered by disease and by circulating hormones. Thresholds must also depend on genetic inheritance, because genes are reported to explain 40–66% of the variation in human bone density,[582,1309] depending on which bone is considered.[1437] For lumbar vertebrae, genes have been reported to explain 83% of the variation in bone density, with some of this influence being mediated through mechanical factors such as lean body mass and lifting strength.[1493] Genes similarly explain 27–75% of the variation in bone size, after the influences of age, gender and physical activity have been accounted for.[582]

Bones can be injured by gross fracture, or by the accumulation of microdamage leading eventually to a 'stress fracture'. Bone consists predominantly of the rigid crystalline matrix, so injury mechanisms probably resemble those found in engineering materials more closely than in any other bodily tissue. Fractures heal by the migration of cells from the periosteum and endosteum to the fracture site, where they link the broken bone ends with a deformable fibrous material ('fracture callus') which subsequently mineralises to form new bone. Once the new bone has been turned over by the continuous remodelling process, it is often difficult to detect the original break, and the healed bone can regain full strength. This remarkable ability of bone to repair itself makes it highly unlikely that an injured vertebra could be a direct source of chronic back pain (unless the bone became infected).

HYALINE (ARTICULAR) CARTILAGE

Hyaline cartilage is a connective tissue with an abundant extracellular matrix composed of proteoglycans and very fine collagen II fibrils. It combines the properties of toughness and compressive strength. It has a sparse population of cells (chondrocytes) but contains no blood vessels or nerve endings. The endplates of the intervertebral discs are composed of hyaline cartilage. Articular cartilage (Fig. 7.12) is a type of hyaline cartilage that covers the opposing surfaces of synovial joints, including the apophyseal joints in the spine. It provides a low-friction and low-wear bearing surface, and is able to distribute loading evenly on to the underlying bone.

Structure and composition

The matrix of hyaline cartilage consists mainly of water (70%), collagen (75% of dry weight) and proteoglycans (20% of dry weight). Proteoglycan molecules have a protein core, with side chains of the glycosaminoglycan (GAG) molecules chondroitin sulphate, keratan sulphate and dermatan sulphate. The most common proteoglycan (90% of the total) is a large molecule, aggrecan, which combines with hyaluronan to form huge aggregates up to 10 μm in length (Fig. 7.13). GAGs attract water electrostatically, and the main role of proteoglycans is to attract and retain water within the tissue. Their tendency to absorb water and swell is resisted by tension in the network of very fine type II collagen fibrils, which hold the cartilage together and anchor it to the subchondral bone[1383] (Fig. 7.14). The structure of collagen II fibrils is similar to that of collagen I (Fig. 7.8), but only the latter aggregate to form large fibres. Approximately 2% of articular cartilage collagen is type IX, a non-linear molecule with a projecting GAG side chain. Collagen IX binds to the surface of collagen II fibrils, with its projecting part possibly serving to interconnect fibrils into a three-dimensional network, or to anchor them in the proteoglycans.[1335] Mechanical interactions between collagen and proteoglycans help to resist cartilage deformation,[641,1268] but proteoglycan depletion does not reduce the tissue's tensile strength[200,1268] possibly because at very high strains, the collagen fibrils interact directly with each other, like tangled threads of cotton.[199] The high water content of articular cartilage enables it to distribute loads evenly between opposing bones,[34] and water loss during sustained loading allows the tissue to deform ('creep') so that the contact area increases, and the contact stress decreases (Fig. 7.15).

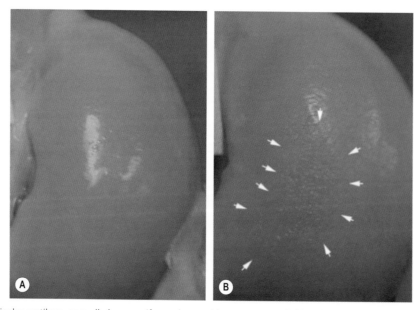

Figure 7.12 Articular cartilage normally has a uniform glossy white appearance (A) but becomes dulled and roughened following damage, or in the early stages of degeneration (B, arrowed). Images of sheep femoral condyle. *(Reproduced from Lu et al.[853] with permission.)*

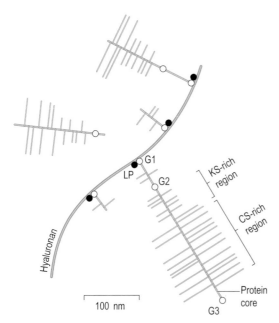

Figure 7.13 Diagram showing the structure of the proteoglycan molecule aggrecan. It has a linear protein core, with three globular regions (G1–G3). Side chains are of the glycoaminoglycans chondroitin sulphate (CS) and keratan sulphate (KS). Many individual aggrecan molecules aggregate together by binding on to hyaluronan by means of a link protein (LP).

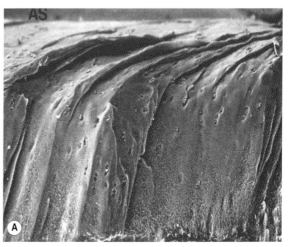

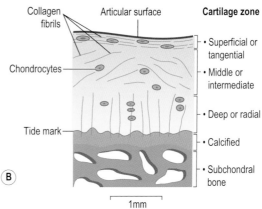

Figure 7.14 (A) The arcade structure of articular cartilage is suggested by this scanning electron micrograph of freeze-fractured bovine articular cartilage. AS, articular surface. (Reproduced from Jeffery et al.[685] with permission of the publishers.) (B) Diagrammatic interpretation of the structure of articular cartilage. Some collagen fibrils join the cartilage to bone, and others run parallel to the cartilage surface, but the length of individual fibrils is unknown. The various zones reflect differences in collagen alignment, chemical composition and cell morphology. Below the 'tide mark', the cartilage matrix is calcified, and its mechanical properties are intermediate between cartilage and bone.

The remainder of the cartilage matrix is composed of the small proteoglycans decorin, biglycan and fibromodulin, and non-collagenous proteins including cartilage oligomeric protein, fibronectin and anchorin. The function of these relatively small molecules is not fully understood, but they appear to regulate the formation of collagen fibrils, and help to bind the matrix components to each other, and to the cells.

Type II collagen fibrils in hyaline cartilage are so fine (10–100 nm in diameter) that they are difficult to visualise ('hyaline' means glassy). However, the gross structure of cartilage can be inferred from scanning electron micrographs of freeze-fractured tissue[283,685] as shown in Figure 7.14A. The surface (tangential) zone has a relatively high proportion of horizontal collagen fibrils which curve over in the proteoglycan-rich transitional zone, and become vertical in the radial zone, before entering a region of calcified cartilage below the 'tide mark', which forms a transition between relatively soft cartilage and stiff bone. The uppermost few microns of the tangential zone, the lamina splendens (Fig. 7.16), act like a tensile skin for the underlying cartilage, and probably play an important role in maintaining the internal fluid pressure within the tissue, which in turn assists lubrication.[237]

Metabolism

Chondrocytes (Fig. 7.16, left) manufacture and turn over the matrix constituents. In adult tissue, cells cease to divide and are normally isolated from each other, each being surrounded by a 'basket' of type II collagen to form a chondron.[685] Cell division, and consequent clustering, can occur when cartilage integrity is threatened, as in osteoarthritis (Ch. 15), but new cells do not appear to migrate to the location of any defect,[1412] and their metabolic rate is limited by the lack of a blood supply. Nutrients must reach the chondrocytes across long distances of matrix, either by diffusion, which is important for small molecules, or by bulk fluid flow, which is important for large molecules.[1057]

Matrix breakdown is controlled by enzymes which include the matrix metalloproteases (MMPs) and their tissue inhibitors, both of which are produced by chondrocytes. Some MMPs are called collagenases because they cleave individual collagen molecules at a specific site, causing the triple helix to unwind or denature. Other MMPs (gelatinases) further break down the denatured collagen. A third group of MMPs, the stromelysins, break down other matrix proteins, and also the proteoglycan molecules by cleaving their protein core. Another protease, aggrecanase, which is chemically distinct from the MMPs, is primarily responsible for the cleavage of aggrecan between the globular domains G1 and G2 (Fig. 7.13) and for the subsequent loss of proteoglycans from cartilage in osteoarthritis.[844]

Chondrocyte activity is controlled and coordinated by cytokines, which can be produced locally by the chondrocytes themselves, or by more distant cells such as those in the joint synovium. Cell activity is also influenced by mechanical loading applied to the tissue. The synthesis of matrix constituents is maximal at an applied pressure of 5–15 MPa, and decreases when the loading is greater or less than this.[555] Generally, cyclic loading at moderate load levels tends to stimulate synthesis, whereas prolonged static loading slows it down.[1454] The precise nature of the stimulus is unknown: it may be deformation of the cell membrane or cytoskeleton,[538] or changes in the fluid pressurisation within cartilage.[11] Matrix turnover in articular cartilage is much slower than in bone, with the half-life of proteoglycans being weeks or months, depending on distance to the nearest cell. The half-life of collagen could exceed 100 years.[1486] There is growing evidence that mechanical loading strengthens cartilage by blocking the action of catabolic cytokines that otherwise would encourage the chondrocytes to weaken their matrix.[1425]

Evidence that articular cartilage adapts to mechanical loading comes from studies showing that patients have a higher concentration of the water-binding GAG molecules in heavily loaded regions of their joints,[1216] and that vigorous physical activity in middle age protects against future cartilage thinning and damage.[1408] Animal experiments have confirmed that physical activity leads to thicker and stiffer cartilage, whereas inactivity or static loading has the opposite effect.[84] Results, however, depend on the size of the animal and the intensity of loading. For example,

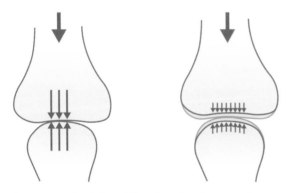

Figure 7.15 The deformability of cartilage increases the area of contact between articulating bones, reducing contact stress on the cartilage. Sustained 'creep' loading can increase this effect.

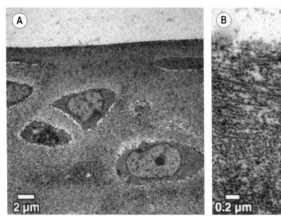

Figure 7.16 Transmission electron micrographs of articular cartilage from mice, showing the lamina splendens which forms a thin 'skin' on the surface, superficial to the chondrocytes (A). Under high magnification (B) it appears highly fibrous, with fine fibrils parallel to the surface. (*Reproduced from Jay et al.[683] with permission.*)

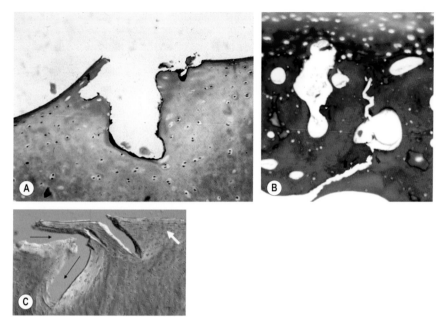

Figure 7.17 Compressive damage to articular cartilage. (A) Histological section of bovine cartilage: note the heavily stained cartilage 'skin' (lamina splendens) which appears to have recoiled backwards. (B) Histological section of the junction between articular cartilage (stained blue) and subchondral bone (red) in young bovine tissue. Note the marrow spaces in the subchondral bone, some of which are in direct contact with cartilage, and the two large cracks in the subchondral bone. (C) High-resolution micrograph of the surface of articular cartilage following compressive overload, showing typical oblique fissures which extend approximately 150 µm into the tissue. *(Reproduced from Thambyah and Brown[1414] with permission.)*

voluntary exercise protects cartilage from degenerative changes in hamsters,[1086] whereas in the horse, imposed high-intensity exercise thickens cartilage and subchondral bone[1430] and may cause cartilage deterioration in regions of highest loading.[1013] The difference may be attributable to the cube-square law (p. 7), which explains why heavy animals load their joints more severely than light ones.[44] Age may also play a part, because cells from old cartilage are less active[1429] and less responsive to mechanical stimuli[917] than cells from young tissue. It is difficult to estimate from these experiments just how much exercise is good for human cartilage, or how quickly, and to what extent, human cartilage can strengthen in response to exercise. It might be expected that strengthening would be slower in cartilage than in bone, because cartilage has no blood supply. Enzymatic breakdown of cartilage, however, could conceivably be rapid. Some degree of articular cartilage adaptation must occur in humans, because variations in its thickness and stiffness across a joint surface correspond to the varying mechanical demands placed upon it.[1606]

Excessive mechanical loading leads to cartilage damage rather than adaptation. A single impact can create oblique fissures in the cartilage surface[1414] (Fig. 7.17), allowing disruption of the underlying collagen network in a manner that resembles osteoarthritis.[1413] Impact can also cause cell death and proteoglycan loss,[646] and may injure the subchondral bone,[35] as shown in Figure 7.17B. More moderate but repetitive compressive loading can also kill a proportion of cartilage cells,[286] and cause fissures in the cartilage surface to increase in number and width (Fig. 15.17).[738] If an injury penetrates the cartilage to reach the subchondral bone, then fibrous tissue can grow from the bone to fill the defect, but this does not integrate well with surrounding articular cartilage: eventually it fails, and the joint becomes degenerated.[1297] Prior proteoglycan loss makes cartilage cells increasingly vulnerable to mechanical injury, especially in the cartilage surface zone.[1085]

TENDON AND LIGAMENT

These connective tissues contain a few cells embedded in a fibrous extracellular matrix which is specialised for tensile strength and energy absorption. They have blood supply, and contain a variety of nerve endings capable of monitoring tissue stress, strain and pain. The essential functional difference between tendons and ligaments is that tendons generally transmit tensile force in one direction only, from muscle to bone, whereas ligaments must resist the separation of bones in more than one direction. This difference is reflected in the orientation of their collagen fibres, which tend to be longer and more unidirectional in tendons. The chemical and biological properties of the two tissues are similar, although ligaments generally contain slightly less collagen.

Structure and composition

These tissues consist mostly of a fibrous extracellular matrix containing a few elongated cells, called fibroblasts (in growing tissue) or fibrocytes (in mature, less active tissue). The matrix is 60% water, with the solid component being composed mainly of collagen type I (80%), proteoglycans and elastin. Elastin is a fibrous protein rather like collagen, but elastin fibres can be stretched much further than collagen because individual elastin molecules straighten out. The original molecular shape is regained as soon as the tension is removed, so elastin fibres enhance elastic recoil in tendons and ligaments (and also in skin and the walls of blood vessels). Ligaments which have a high elastin content, such as the ligamentum flavum, have great extensibility. Small quantities of proteoglycans help to keep the tissues hydrated, and their presence may partly explain why injured tendons and ligaments can swell slightly. One of the small proteoglycans, decorin, probably acts to regulate the diameter of collagen fibres. Large proteoglycans are present in regions of tendon which are compressed against bone, where they probably serve to maintain tissue hydration, as in articular cartilage (see above).

Most of the collagen is organised in hierarchical fashion,[720] from the basic collagen molecule right up to large collagen fibre bundles which can be seen with the naked eye (Fig. 7.18). Increasing cross-linking between collagen molecules causes tendons and ligaments to become stronger and stiffer up until skeletal maturity. In both tissues, gross collagen fibres exhibit a zigzag planar waveform called 'crimp', which gradually straightens out when the tissue is subjected to high tensile forces.[1247,1285] Tension also causes a certain amount of sliding between collagen fibres, and some relative sliding of fibrils within each fibre.[1285] These mechanisms enable tendons and ligaments to be stretched by approximately 15% (with a stress of 100 MPa) before failure occurs.[1257] The main benefit of crimping is that considerable energy is required to straighten out crimps against the elastic resistance of other matrix constituents (Fig. 1.5), and this enables tendons, in particular, to function as giant elastic shock absorbers during locomotion.[59]

Metabolism

A sparse population of fibroblasts is responsible for the manufacture and turnover of the collagenous matrix. Their metabolic rate is low because tendons and ligaments are poorly vascularised, especially in their central regions, but there is evidence that these tissues can strengthen or weaken in response to changes in applied mechanical load. In humans, the strength of spinal longitudinal ligaments is related to the bone mineral content of the vertebrae to which they are attached,[1036] suggesting that they have adapted to the same mechanical demands. Spinal fixation, on the other hand, leads to softer and weaker spinal ligaments, presumably as a result of chronic underloading.[782] A tendon must surely adapt in line with any changes in strength of the muscle to which it is attached (see above) but it may not be capable of adapting as quickly, and this may explain why 'overtraining' injuries so often affect tendons or the musculotendinous junction. The beneficial effects of moderate exercise on tendon appear to be achieved in part by a proliferation of metabolically active stem cells within the tissue, and their differentiation into matrix-building tenocytes.[1625] The nature of mechanical loading, as well as its magnitude, influences the tendon matrix: compressive stresses arising from a tendon passing over a bone may cause the matrix to become more cartilaginous.[500] Quantitative evidence concerning tendon adaptation comes from a recent experiment on sheep, which showed that shielding the patellar tendon from all mechanical loading for 6 weeks reduced its stiffness by 79% and strength by 69%.[1229] These changes were almost fully reversed after loading had returned to normal. Slow overstretching of tendon can impair collagen stability and resistance to enzymatic degradation,[1568] possibly allowing accelerated adaptive remodelling under high static loading.

Tendon damage can occur as a result of injury or repetitive loading, and Achilles tendon ruptures are especially common in young to middle-aged men involved in sporting activities.[823] Fatigue injuries occur because tendon strength in vitro can fall by up to 90% if 1 million loading cycles are applied.[1257,1258] Injury often affects the musculotendinous junction, although collagen fibres can rupture at mid-length, or near their attachment to bone. Damaged fibres are degraded enzymatically as fibroblasts migrate to the injury site to lay down new collagen. Several stages in the healing process can be recognised:[834] (1) inflammation; (2) fibroplasia; and (3) maturation. Depending on tendon size, location and injury severity, healing can be predominantly intrinsic, or else extrinsic, in which the blood supply to neighbouring structures plays a major role.[834] New fibres are thinner than old, and have a disorganised crimp structure,[682] so their original mechanical properties are probably not regained, even after 14 months.[511,1570] Restoration of collagen fibril diameter is probably essential to restoration of ligament strength[1027] but it is not known if either can recover completely. Tendon repair can be frustrated by repeated minor injuries, resulting in a chronic degenerative condition or tendinosis.[1196,1409] Ligament injuries may affect only those fibres

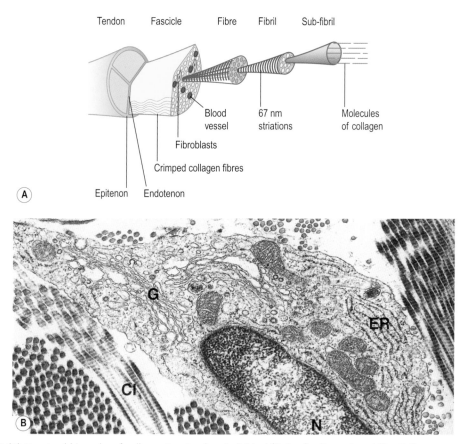

Figure 7.18 (A) Structural hierarchy of collagen in a tendon. Individual fibrils of collagen type I (Fig. 7.8) are grouped to form fibres that have a planer zigzag shape called 'crimp'. Many fibres are bundled together, along with fibroblasts and blood vessels, to form a fascicle. Each fascicle is surrounded by a sheath of more randomly arranged collagen, the endotenon, and the entire tendon is surrounded by the epitenon. (B) Electron micrograph of a tendon fibroblast secreting collagen into the extracellular matrix. Collagen molecules self-assemble into fibrils which appear striped in longitudinal section (Cl) and as dark spots in transverse section (bottom left). Active fibroblasts have a pale nucleus (N), and abundant rough endoplasmic reticulum (ER) and Golgi apparatus (G). *(Reproduced from Young B, Health JW (2000) Wheater's functional histology. Churchill Livingstone, Edinburgh.)*

which were oriented to resist the damaging movement. In the spine, interspinous ligament injuries are common,[1198] and are characterised by apparently non-functional fibres adjacent to a smooth hole filled with fatty deposits.[458,1198]

A different type of injury can affect large tendons during vigorous activity. So much heat is produced by the shock-absorbing mechanism that the temperature in the poorly vascularised centre of the tendon rises by more than 5°C.[1579] This is sufficient to denature collagen molecules by unwinding the triple helix (Fig. 7.8) and to interfere with fibroblast metabolism. However, tendon fibroblasts contain heat shock proteins, which makes them more heat-resistant than fibroblasts in other tissues such as skin.[144]

INTERVERTEBRAL DISCS

From a histological perspective, discs are classified as fibrocartilage, but they are really complex structures composed of several different tissues. Their gross structure, innervation and blood supply are considered in Chapters 2 and 4, and detailed functional anatomy is described in Chapter 10. It used to be assumed that intervertebral disc biochemistry and metabolism are similar to articular cartilage, which has been investigated more thoroughly (see above). However, such comparisons can be misleading, because cells of the annulus fibrosus and nucleus pulposus are now known to be phenotypically distinct (i.e. express slightly different genes) from the chondrocytes of articular cartilage, as well as from each other.[287]

Structure and composition

A disc varies from a highly hydrated gel in the centre of the nucleus to a tough ligamentous tissue in the outer annulus, while the cartilage component of the endplates resembles amorphous hyaline cartilage. The nucleus is composed of water (70–85%), proteoglycans (50% dry weight) and collagen (less than 20% dry weight). These proportions change gradually towards the outer annulus, which is approximately 50% water, proteoglycans (10% dry weight) and collagen (up to 70% dry weight).

The proportion of collagen type I (which is usually found in tensile structures such as ligaments) is highest in the outer annulus, and very low in the inner annulus and nucleus; conversely, collagen type II (which is normal in compressed tissues such as articular cartilage) is abundant in the nucleus, less common in the inner annulus and absent in the outer annulus.[406,1271] There is some evidence from work on tendons that the predominant collagen type can change from type I to type II if the habitual loading of the tissue changes from tension to compression,[500] so the varying collagen distribution in different parts of a disc probably reflects their different mechanical functions. The particularly coarse collagen fibre bundles in the annulus (Fig. 8.13) display the same crimp pattern seen in tendon and ligaments,[259,1124] and probably for the same reason: to enable them to stretch more, and to absorb more energy before failure (Fig. 1.5). Approximately 10–15% of disc collagen is type VI, which forms a network of short fibrils within the pericellular matrix. Small quantities of types III, V, IX, XI and XII are also present. Endplate cartilage contains collagen type X,[52] which is associated with hypertrophic chondrocytes involved in calcification.

An elaborate network of fine elastin fibres has been described within the disc[1620] and contributes 2% to its dry weight.[289] Elastin allows a tissue to recover its shape following large deformations, and its organisation (Fig. 7.19) suggests that it might help to resist radial expansion of the nucleus, and regulate shearing movements of the lamellae of the annulus.

Proteoglycan molecules in the nucleus tend to be smaller, and aggregate less, than in articular cartilage. This is presumably because they are in less danger of diffusing to the edge of the (comparatively large) disc and being lost from the tissue. Proteoglycan concentration is not uniform across the nucleus, and can exhibit localised variations in the annulus which suggest focal damage and swelling.[656]

Metabolism

Tissue mechanical function appears to determine cell type. The rounded cells in the nucleus are notochordal during development and early childhood,[1433] but then are replaced

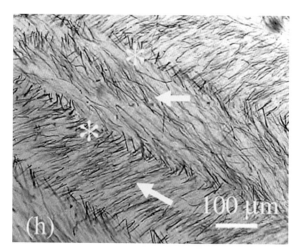

Figure 7.19 Elastin fibres (stained black) in the inner annulus fibrosus of a human intervertebral disc (female, aged 12 years, L3–4). Arrow, parallel fibres in adjacent lamellae show alternating orientation. *Interlamellar fibres with criss-cross pattern. (Reproduced from Yu et al.[1620] with permission.)

by cells which resemble articular cartilage chondrocytes (Fig. 7.20A).[743] The more elongated cells in the outer annulus (Fig. 7.20B) resemble fibroblasts, and have long processes which interconnect with each other[400] and which may form gap junctions.[378] Annulus cells are more deformable.[539] Each disc cell is surrounded by a collagenous 'basket' to form a chondron, with the matrix lying between the cell and basket being rich in collagen III and VI.[1204] As in the other skeletal tissues, disc cells manufacture and repair the matrix, but metabolic rates are comparatively very low because the avascular discs are so large: in fact they are the largest avascular structures in the body. A chronic lack of oxygen causes nucleus cells to become quiescent.[630] A chronic lack of glucose kills some disc cells so that the cell population decreases to a level that can be maintained by the availability of glucose.[701] Difficulties in metabolite transport probably explain why cell density is four times greater in the disc periphery compared to its centre.[581]

Metabolites of small molecular weight are transported mostly by diffusion, but the movement of large molecules is dominated by bulk fluid flow[424] which accompanies variations in physical activity (Fig. 7.21). These two processes can be distinguished by imagining a quantity of coloured dye thrown into a slow-moving stream: the spreading out of the dye into a large cloud is due to the random molecular movements which underlie diffusion, and the slow drift of the dye downstream illustrates the effects of bulk fluid flow. There are two transport routes: through the peripheral annulus, and through the perforated bone and hyaline cartilage of the central regions of

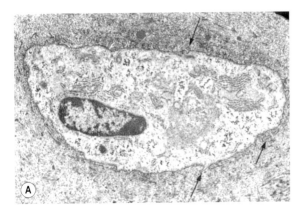

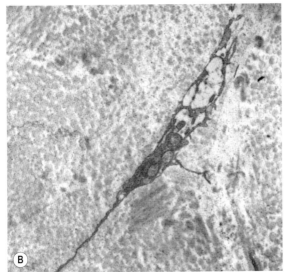

Figure 7.20 Intervertebral disc cells as visualised by transmission electron microscopy. (A) Nucleus pulposus cell (arrows indicate small extensions of the cell membrane). (B) Outer annulus cell, showing very long extensions. *(Reproduced from Errington et al.[400] with permission.)*

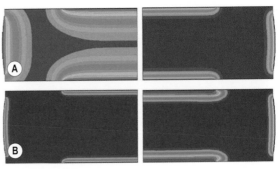

Figure 7.21 Penetration of nutrients into an intervertebral disc, as predicted by a finite element model. Each panel represents the anterior or posterior half of a disc in mid-sagittal section. Colours tending from blue to red indicate increasing penetration of molecules from the periphery. Top left: small solutes, diffusion; Top right: small solutes, fluid flow; Bottom left: large solutes, diffusion; Bottom right: large solutes, fluid flow. *(Reproduced from Ferguson et al.[424] with permission.)*

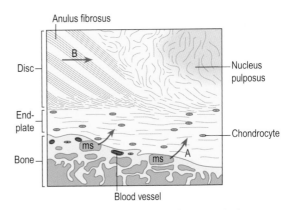

Figure 7.22 Diagram showing part of the vertebral endplate, which consists of a hyaline cartilage layer loosely bonded to a plate of perforated cortical bone. (Adapted from Roberts et al.[1205] with permission.) Note how the coarse collagen fibres of the annulus blend into the hyaline cartilage of the endplate. There are two routes for metabolite transport into the centre of the avascular disc: (A) through the marrow spaces (ms) of the endplate, and (B) through the annulus. Compare the lower half of this figure with Figure 7.23.

the endplates[1458] (Figs 7.22 and 7.23). The high negative fixed-charge density of the proteoglycans in the nucleus ensures that negatively charged ions mostly enter the disc by the annulus route, whereas neutral and positively charged molecules enter by the endplate route. Disc metabolite transport is hindered by sustained mechanical loading, which expels water from the disc,[957] reducing its permeability,[592] and hence reducing the rate of diffusion within it.[85] Sustained loading can also inhibit the fluid exchange that normally accompanies fluctuations in disc mechanical loading[585] and which assists metabolite transport.

Cells in the nucleus and inner annulus respond to changes in their mechanical environment in a similar manner to the chondrocytes of articular cartilage: very high and very low hydrostatic pressures both decrease proteoglycan synthesis, whereas loading within the normal physiological range (0.5–2 MPa) increases it.[667] Nucleus pressure rarely falls below 0.1 MPa in living people, even when they lie down,[1250] so maintaining disc tissue in culture at zero pressure would allow the tissue to swell,

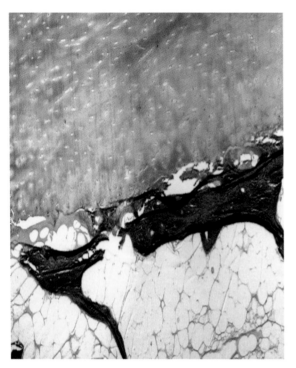

Figure 7.23 Histological section of a human vertebral endplate showing where a large marrow cavity in the vertebra (lower) meets the hyaline cartilage of the endplate (upper, stained orange). Some mechanical disruption is evident. Compare with Figure 7.22.

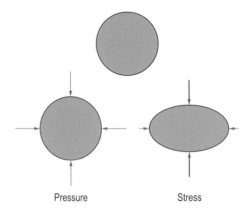

Pressure   Stress

Figure 7.24 A disc cell (upper) would not be deformed if it was subjected to a hydrostatic pressure (lower left) but it would be deformed if subjected to a directional stress (lower right). These mechanical considerations may partly explain the contrasting shapes of nucleus and annulus cells seen in Figure 7.20.

and may alter its metabolism compared to that found in vivo. Nucleus pressures in excess of 3 MPa (which would be equivalent to severe manual labour[1565]) increase the synthesis of the matrix-degrading enzyme MMP3.[559]. Static and cyclic loading of disc tissue tends to decrease and increase matrix synthesis, respectively,[1528] and there is growing evidence that excessive loading is most detrimental.[1592] Nucleus cells respond to cyclic stretching by proliferating and producing more collagen,[933] suggesting that these cells may be capable of behaving like chondrocytes or fibroblasts (see below), depending on whether the mechanical loading is in compression or tension.[181,703]

Cells of the outer annulus synthesise some proteoglycan, but these fibroblast-like cells are largely unaffected by hydrostatic pressure,[667] probably because they do not normally experience such pressures in life: they are embedded in a fibrous solid rather than a fluid, as indicated in Figure 7.24. Spinal compression causes the outer annulus to be stretched circumferentially by up to 3%,[600] and spinal bending stretches the outer annulus vertically by up to 18%,[600] and possibly by up to 50% (Fig. 12.9). However, some of this tissue strain involves sliding between collagen

fibrils, so that the outer annulus cells are probably stretched by only a few per cent at most.[378] Disc cell deformations and responses to loading ('mechanobiology') have been extensively reviewed.[1293]

Disc metabolism is too slow to study accurately in living humans. Follow-up magnetic resonance imaging studies indicate that changes in disc height and bulging progress extremely slowly in adults.[1490] Higher body mass and greater lifting strength are associated with reduced disc height and increased disc hydration,[1492] suggesting that habitual mechanical loading can have mixed effects on discs and their adjacent bones. A cadaveric study has shown that a disc's proteoglycan content is proportional to the thickness of the adjacent bony endplate,[1203] suggesting that both tissues can adapt to similar mechanical stimuli. Another cadaveric study showed that annulus strength is proportional to vertebral strength,[1326] but only in the outer annulus (where cell density is greatest[581])and in males (who may load their spines more vigorously). A third cadaveric study showed that men who were very physically active prior to death had stronger vertebrae and discs than less active men, although their discs were more likely to fail under extreme loading.[1153] Taken together, this evidence suggests that adult human discs can adapt to increased mechanical demands, but they adapt imperfectly, and more slowly than adjacent bones. Discs are therefore likely to be vulnerable to accumulating fatigue damage when the spine is subjected to a sudden increase in the level of mechanical loading.[15]

Intervertebral disc metabolism has been studied extensively in animals, although it is not easy to extrapolate from these experiments to the much larger and older discs of humans.[62,850] Static compressive loading of dog discs appears to stimulate synthesis of collagen type I and inhibit proteoglycan synthesis in the nucleus pulposus.[652] Requiring dogs to run on a treadmill for up to 40 km/day for 1 year showed several conflicting changes in the composition and metabolism of the discs: proteoglycan synthesis decreased at some spinal levels, but increased at others[1171] and collagen levels also were variably affected.[1170] A small group of these discs were found to creep more under load, suggesting that adaptive remodelling effects were being countered by the accumulation of fatigue damage during the severe exercise.[327] Experiments on rats and mice show that their intervertebral discs degenerate under prolonged immobilisation, and that degeneration is accelerated by static compressive loading.[657,851] Conversely, moderate running exercise increased matrix synthesis, and annulus cell numbers, in rat lumbar discs.[193]

Discs show only a limited ability to heal following injury, presumably because of difficulty in remodelling the large collagen fibre bundles of the annulus. In sheep, scalpel-induced peripheral annular tears lead to collagenous scar formation and granulation tissue in the outer annulus, and vascular ingrowth into the middle annulus.[558,703,1081] However, few inflammatory cells are found in the disc[711] and the inner regions of a tear do not heal: in fact they continue to progress inwards.[1081] Peripheral annular tears lead to reduced proteoglycan and collagen content within the nucleus, in both the affected and adjacent discs, but the annulus itself shows minimal biochemical changes.[968] Experimental enzymatic destruction of the nucleus leads to reduced proteoglycan synthesis,[1382] but this later recovers to a certain extent,[176] probably because proteoglycan turnover is faster than collagen turnover.[1222] Proteoglycan–collagen interactions within the annulus (p. 129) may partly explain why old radial fissures can 'heal' in the limited sense that they do not readily allow nucleus pulposus material to escape, even under severe loading.[30] In contrast, herniated tissue which escapes from the pressurised confines of the disc can undergo extensive biochemical changes, starting with rapid swelling (Fig. 11.29), leaching of proteoglycans[361] and final shrinkage or resorption.[90]

BIOLOGICAL COMPATIBILITY OF SPINAL TISSUES

Biological differences between spinal tissues could give rise to problems if the spine has to adapt to changing mechanical demands. The most metabolically active tissue, muscle, can change its size and force-generating capacity by a significant amount in just a few days, and it is muscle which applies most of the high forces to underlying tissues. Bone also has a rich blood supply, but it has

a much higher volume of extracellular matrix per cell than does muscle, so it requires several weeks to make substantial changes to its strength and internal architecture. Tendons and ligaments are poorly vascularised, and the high proportion of large collagen type I fibrils in their extracellular matrix ensures that it cannot be turned over rapidly. Adaptations in strength are possible, but they are slow, and repair following injury takes many months. The lack of a blood supply, and a low cell density, ensure that articular cartilage responds very slowly to changes in its mechanical environment. Nevertheless, significant adaptations can be measured after 1 year of exercise in young animals, and human cartilage thickness depends on the density of subchondral bone.[371] Finally comes the lumbar intervertebral discs, the largest avascular structures in the body, with such a low cell density that they are incapable of remodelling the collagen fibre bundles of the annulus within the working lifetime of an adult. Structural damage to a disc may be patched up with scar-like tissue, but is not fully repaired. Only in the outer annulus, which is close to the peripheral blood supply, is there any evidence that disc tissues can adapt to the strength of the adjacent bone.[1326]

Consider now some consequences of these marked differences in tissue biology. Suppose a young man starts his first manual job, with a back that has been mechanically conditioned to attending school and watching television. In the new job, his muscles will presumably strengthen quickly, and his vertebrae will soon catch up. But what will happen to his tendons, to his apophyseal joints and his lumbar discs? What if the man is not so young, or healthy, when he starts this manual job? The research summarised in this chapter indicates that the man's spinal tissues will be unable to adapt as quickly as his muscles, especially if he is middle-aged, and that the biggest problem will confront his intervertebral discs.

As another example, consider the future of an intervertebral disc that lies next to a damaged vertebral body endplate. (Minor damage to these endplates, or to the trabeculae which support them, is very common in life: see Ch. 15.) The vertebra will heal rapidly, perhaps with a few microcalluses to mark the site of injury.[1485] However, the nucleus of the disc adjacent to the damaged endplate will be decompressed (p. 145) and this may leave it incapable of manufacturing sufficient matrix to restore its normal volume and pressure. Accordingly, more of the force on the disc would be resisted by the annulus rather than the nucleus, creating long-term problems for the disc rather than the adjacent bone.

Potential problems arising from the different adaptive potential of adjacent tissues remain to be investigated. Two longitudinal epidemiological studies have produced evidence to suggest that strengthening muscles can pose a threat to the underlying spine during the first year of an arduous job,[36,756] but more work is required to rule out alternative explanations. In the mean time, the results of cross-sectional occupational surveys should be treated with some caution, because their study populations are likely to be self-selected to a certain extent: people with particularly weak backs are unlikely to survive long in the most arduous jobs, and those who do survive will include those whose backs have adapted successfully to the rigours of the job. Conversely, sedentary jobs will attract a proportion of those people who leave more arduous work because of back problems. In this way, cross-sectional surveys may systematically underestimate the adverse effects of mechanical loading on poorly vascularised spinal tissues.

Chapter | 8 |

Growth and ageing of the spine

INTRODUCTION

The spine undergoes changes during the course of a lifetime, from embryo to old age. Changes before birth show how specialised spinal structures emerge from relatively simple tissues according to the genetic 'recipe'. These early changes offer some insights into the advantages and limitations of the final structure. Changes after birth show how various spinal tissues cope with the challenges of increasing size during growth, and of upright posture. Changes which occur beyond skeletal maturity can broadly be separated into the more-or-less inevitable and continuous processes of ageing, and into the variable, discontinuous and harmful processes of degeneration. Spinal degeneration is considered in Chapter 15.

PRENATAL DEVELOPMENT AND GROWTH

Differentiation

After fertilisation, the human egg undergoes multiple cell divisions. Progressively, various cells become and stay different, giving rise to lines of cells that eventually produce specific types of tissues and particular organs. This process is called differentiation.

All cells in an individual have the same set of approximately 20 000 genes which code for the proteins that the cells make. No cell actually makes all those proteins. Early in embryonic life, cells are still capable of switching on ('expressing') any of these genes, and so these cells have the potential to become any cell in the future body. As development proceeds, however, each cell becomes more and more specialised by switching on more specialised genes, and by losing (permanently) the ability to express other specialised genes. For example, some cells in the 4-week embryo still have the ability to become cartilage or bone cells, but have lost the ability to form the endothelial cells which line blood vessels. Later, some of them will lose the ability to express the gene for collagen type I, and they may become 'terminally differentiated' as cartilage cells (chondrocytes) which are capable of producing only the matrix of articular cartilage.

Differentiation is important because it indicates the lineage of cells in adult tissues, and therefore indicates their inherent limitations and potential to adapt to changing circumstances, perhaps following an injury. Also, the great adaptive potential of certain undifferentiated cells means they could be extremely useful in helping to rebuild an injured tissue or organ, and that is why cell biologists and tissue engineers are currently making great efforts to isolate these cells and get them to reproduce under laboratory conditions.

Embryological development

The embryological phase is conventionally taken to represent weeks 2–8 of gestation (i.e. postfertilisation). At 2 weeks the human embryo is a small disc that consists of two layers: a ventral endoderm and a dorsal ectoderm. The ectoderm produces a third layer of cells, the mesoderm, which insinuate themselves between the original two layers. Within the mesoderm, a column of cells, called the notochord, develops from the future tail end of the embryonic disc, along its dorsal midline, towards the future head end. The notochord induces the formation around itself of all the axial structures of the body. Behind the notochord, the ectoderm folds into a tube, called the neural tube, which is the progenitor of the spinal cord and brain.

The early embryo elongates, and at about 3 weeks, the mesoderm changes its appearance from rows of regular epithelial-like cells to a less ordered structure, and the tissue is then referred to as mesenchyme. At about this time, transverse clefts appear on the surface of the embryo, dividing it up into 42–44 longitudinal segments or somites. This process of segmentation starts from the future head end of the embryo and progresses to the the future tail end. Most of the tissue in each segment or somite then differentiates into a cranial and caudal layer, as shown in Figure 8.1. The lighter cranial layer produces little more than the perineural tissues of the spinal nerve of the segment. The denser caudal layer of each somite produces two clusters of cells: a peripheral dermomyotome and a central somitic mesenchyme. The dermomyotome eventually forms the muscles and skin of the body. The somitic mesenchyme grows around the notochord and around the neural tube to form the vertebral column.

After 6 weeks, chondrification (cartilage formation) begins. This is a preliminary phase in the formation of bone. Cartilage is an appropriate tissue from which to produce bone, for it is sufficiently tough to maintain the shape of the bone, yet sufficiently pliable that cells can divide and push apart to allow the bone to grow in size. Chondrification is achieved by some of the cells of the somitic mesenchyme specialising in producing proteoglycans and type II collagen which form the matrix of the emerging cartilage. This process results in a rudimentary

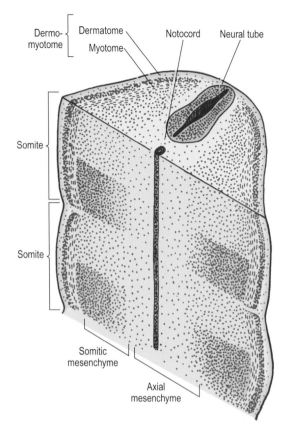

Figure 8.1 Segmental (somite) structure of an early embryo, in the combined coronal and transverse planes. Each somite has differentiated into a cranial and caudal layer. The latter will grow around the notochord to become the future vertebral column. *(Reproduced with permission from Bogduk N. Clinical anatomy of the lumbar spine and sacrum. Churchill Livingstone, Edinburgh, 1997.)*

cartilaginous vertebra being formed. The mesenchyme surrounding the notochord forms the centrum, which constitutes the core of the future vertebral body. The mesenchyme around the neural tube forms a cartilaginous neural arch and its processes. Above and below the developing cartilaginous vertebra, other cells in the somitic mesenchyme become arranged in concentric layers. These will eventually form the lamellae of the annulus fibrosus. Central to these concentric layers, cells of the notochord remain unaligned.

Fetal development

After 8 weeks of gestation, the embryo is referred to as a fetus, and this is marked by the beginnings of ossification, as many cartilage structures turn into hard bone. Cartilage is invaded by blood vessels from which cells emerge to

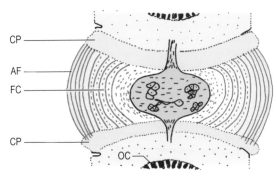

Figure 8.2 Sagittal section through a fetal intervertebral disc, showing the notochord expanding to fill the centre of the disc, and yet already almost entirely absent from the vertebral centrum. CP, cartilage plate; AF, annulus fibrosus; FC, fibrocartilage; OC, ossification centre of vertebral centrum. *(Reproduced from Bogduk N. Clinical anatomy of the lumbar spine and sacrum. Churchill Livingstone, Edinburgh, 1997.)*

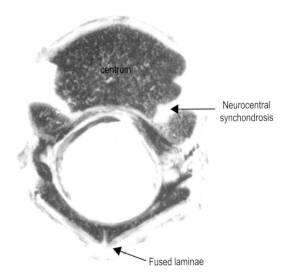

Figure 8.3 Transverse section through a lumbar vertebra of a young child (anterior on top). The laminae of the neural arch have just fused but the centrum is still separated from the neural arch by two cartilaginous neurocentral synchondroses. Note that regions of the neural arch, including the tips of the processes, remain cartilage.

remove cartilage and form small cavities. Other cells can then deposit calcium on to the free surfaces lining the growing cavities within the cartilage, and thereby form rigid bone. Ossification starts at the cranial end of the fetus and proceeds caudally. In each cartilaginous vertebra three primary ossification centres arise: one surrounding the notochord, and one on each side in the neural arch. Ossification of the centrum squeezes the notochordal cells out of the future vertebral body. Ossification of the vertebral body is largely complete by week 25. Not infrequently, remnants of the notochord can persist in the centre of an adult centrum, manifesting as a vertical fibrous canal. In the intervertebral disc, a reciprocal phenomenon occurs. The notochord actually expands outwards, to fill most of the area of the future nucleus pulposus with a semiliquid mucoid material (Fig. 8.2). The aligned cells in the annulus fibrosus deposit layers of collagen type I, and other regions of mesenchyme lay down the collagen type I of the future intervertebral ligaments.

Ossification in the neural arch proceeds dorsally and ventrally. Dorsally, the ossifying arches from each side approach each other in the midline. Ventrally, ossification extends towards the dorsolateral corners of the developing vertebral body.

Before birth, ossification of the vertebra is not complete (Fig. 8.3). Most of the vertebral body is ossified but its superior and inferior surfaces remain capped by a layer of cartilage. Its dorsolateral corners remain cartilaginous where they meet the ventral end of the ossifying neural arch on each side. The dorsal ends of the laminae remain cartilaginous, as does the spinous process, and the tips of the transverse and articular processes. These several, remnant islands of cartilage constitute growth plates. They allow the various parts of the vertebra to increase in length.

Those of the vertebral body allow growth in the height of the vertebral body. Those of the neural arches allow for growth in the length of the arch, and those of the processes allow for elongation of each process. Growth in the thickness of each part is achieved by apposition of bone on its surface.

In the disc, notochordal cells of the nucleus begin to degenerate and to be replaced by chondrocyte-like cells from the inner annulus. Discontinuous 'lamellar bundles' have been reported in the posterior annulus of fetal discs,[1438] but these persist into adulthood and must be considered normal.[913]

Occasionally, one or more of the emerging lumbar vertebrae becomes wholly or partially incorporated into the sacrum, a process known as sacralisation. Alternatively, lumbarisation can occur, in which a sacral vertebra develops with a full intervertebral disc between it and the next sacral vertebra. These developmental abnormalities lead to four or six lumbar vertebrae in the adult, rather than the usual five, but anomalous vertebrae are not particularly associated with future back pain or disability.

POSTNATAL GROWTH

Neonatal and infant growth

After birth, ossification of the vertebrae continues, and they increase in size. The rate of longitudinal growth is maximal at birth, but falls rapidly during the first 2 post-natal years. The annulus fibrosus retains its lamellar structure, but the nucleus pulposus becomes a translucent gel populated only by remnant notochordal cells, which are metabolically very active.[537]

Spinal curvatures begin to develop in response to functional requirements. The age of sitting up and looking about coincides with the emergence of a cervical lordosis (curvature with concave side-pointing posteriorly). Similarly, standing up and walking are accompanied by a growing lumbar lordosis which keeps the upper body vertical. A thoracic kyphosis is required to compensate for the other curves, and to increase the volume of the thoracic cavity to improve breathing. The emergence of spinal curves is accompanied by differential growth of anterior and posterior regions of vertebral bodies and intervertebral discs, so that both structures become slightly wedge-shaped at the apices of the curves.

Childhood and adolescence

In the growing vertebrae, the pedicles fuse with the centrum at the age of 6 to complete the vertebral body. Secondary ossification centres appear in the tips of the spinous, transverse and articular processes around puberty, and complete vertebral ossification is achieved by the age of 18–25 years, at which time these centres fuse with the rest of the vertebra. (Gymnasts and dancers who aspire to exceptional spinal mobility would need to start training before this happens!)

The apophyseal joints form initially in the coronal plane, such that their articular surfaces are directed anteriorly and posteriorly. By the age of 11 years, these joints adopt the oblique and variable orientation seen in the adult (Figs 10.8 and 10.9), presumably as a result of increased tension in the multifidus muscle, which attaches to the mamillary processes, and which becomes more active as the upright posture is more regularly assumed. In approximately 20% of lumbar vertebrae, the final orientation of the left and right apophyseal joints differs by 10° or more, a condition known as 'articular tropism' (Fig. 10.8). Tropism leads to asymmetrical resistance to shear forces and consequent axial rotation,[315] and is associated with posterolateral radial fissures in the annulus fibrosus.[414] However, tropism is not closely associated with back pain or disc degeneration,[1473] and is unlikely to play a major role in predisposing the intervertebral disc to injury.[379]

In the growing disc, the remaining notochordal cells in the nucleus are lost by 8 years, being replaced by chondrocytes from the inner annulus and cartilage endplate.[743] Chondrocytes are more resistant to nutritional stress in the growing disc[537] but are less active,[537] and the nucleus gradually becomes more fibrous. Notochordal cells persist into the adult in some species, forming clusters with interconnecting gap junctions,[644] and they are currently being investigated as a potential source of nucleus regeneration in adult humans. Disc cell density decreases throughout growth, but not thereafter (Fig. 8.4). During childhood, the vertebral endplates change from being convex facing the disc (Fig. 8.2) to flat, and then to concave, and their rounded corners gradually become more squared. Shape changes in vertebrae, and longitudinal growth of intervertebral discs, appear to require the stimulus of mechanical loading, because they are greatly impaired in non-ambulant spastic children who cannot subject their spines to high axial loading.[1405] The blood supply to the vertebral endplate decreases, and microstructural clefts and tears become common by the age of 15 years, especially in the nucleus and endplate.[170] Macroscopic defects in the endplate and annulus can occur before age 20 years[551] and have been reported on lumbar magnetic resonance imaging (MRI) scans in 3–8% of 13-year-olds.[755]

Most of the histological changes in discs resemble changes in other growing collagenous tissues, and their significance is unclear. Reductions in endplate vascularity could simply reflect necessary adaptations to increased mechanical loading at the onset of ambulation, because all structures made of hyaline cartilage lose their blood vessels when they become weight-bearing. Similarly, reduced cell density probably reflects increasing difficulties of metabolite transport in a growing disc, and may represent the maximum number of cells that can be maintained by the precarious supply. The appearance of microstructural clefts and tears roughly coincides with the adolescent growth spurt, which occurs between the ages of 11 and 13 years in girls, and 13 and 15 in boys. Microstructural defects affect all spinal levels to a similar extent,[170] and may possibly lead to more extensive disruption in later life, but while they remain small they appear to have little effect on the internal mechanical function of the disc.[40] In contrast, macroscopic changes in young discs occur mostly between L4 and S1, particularly in the posterior annulus,[551] and so cannot be considered a normal part of growth.

Vertebrae have a plentiful blood supply and so grow in height faster than the avascular intervertebral discs. Between 0 and 13 years, for example, the height of a typical lumbar vertebral body increases from 5 to 22 mm, whereas the height of the L45 disc nucleus increases from 3 to 10 mm.[1405] Discs show little, if any, growth beyond the age of 12 years, at least in patients with scoliosis.[1370] Growth in the disc is interstitial, which means that cells simply push out more matrix in all directions. Vertebrae, however, can grow in height only in the cartilage endplates which cover their superior and inferior surfaces (Fig. 8.2) and which blend with the discs on their other side. Vertebral growth stops between 18 and 25 years, when the cartilage endplates become calcified on the

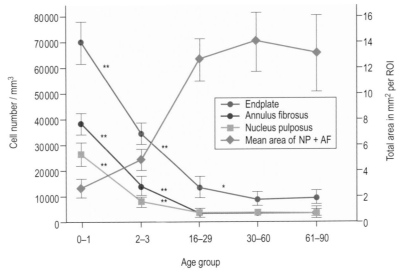

Figure 8.4 Cell density declines with age in all regions of the intervertebral disc, but only up until the cessation of growth (as indicated by disc area), after which it changes little. Note how cell density is greatest in the disc periphery (endplate and annulus) and least in the nucleus. NP, neural plate; AF, annulus fibrosis; ROI, Region of Interest. *(Reproduced from Liebscher et al.[830] with permission.)*

vertebral side to form the bony endplates. Blood vessels which supplied the growth plate are lost. The 'ring apophysis' is a hoop of bone that forms during childhood by ossification within the cartilage growth plate, opposite the outer margins of the vertebral body. It is complete by about 12 years, and then fuses with the outer rim of the vertebra at the end of the growth period, forming the raised rim around the vertebral margin in the adult. Its main functional significance is that the collagen fibres of the outer annulus fibrosus, which initially blended in with the cartilage endplate, later become firmly embedded in the bony ring, forming a very strong anchorage for the outer annulus.

Spinal curvatures continue to change during this period. Between the onset of walking and 7 years, the sacrum rotates forwards by approximately 3° and then remains constant during adult life.[863] Between 4 and 18 years, the pelvis rotates backwards and the 'pelvic incidence' (Fig. 8.5) increases by approximately 10°.[863] These changes may improve balance in the upright posture by ensuring that the sacral table stays slightly posterior to the hip joint to balance the abdomen which lies anterior to it. During the same period (4–18 years), lumbar lordosis increases by 6° and thoracic kyphosis by 10°.[863] Increased spinal curvatures may assist in shock absorbtion (p. 114), and complementary changes are required in different spinal regions in order to maintain upright balance and line of sight. An increasing thoracic kyphosis may also allow a greater thoracic cavity and enhanced respiratory performance.

Spinal mobility decreases during growth as the ratio of disc height to vertebral height decreases. Range of flexion motion decreases particularly between the ages of 10 and 14 years.[1497] Interestingly, spinal mobility falls more in western populations than in developing countries, possibly reflecting the tendency of western children to sit on chairs rather than in squatting postures which require considerable spinal flexion.[409]

AGE-RELATED CHANGES IN THE ADULT SPINE

Skeletal growth stops when the cartilage growth plates within bones fuse, generally around the age of 20 years. Subsequent changes in the adult spine cannot be interpreted as necessary adaptations to increasing size or changes in posture, but they need not be harmful either. Age gradually makes skeletal tissue cells less efficient, and some of them die, making it increasingly difficult for the remaining cells to repair and renew ('turn over') their extracellular matrix. Consequently, microscopic defects begin to accumulate in most tissues, weakening them slightly. In addition, some chemical reactions occur in the matrix which depend simply on chronological and time are not controlled by the cells at all. Above all, the tissues of the spine respond to the

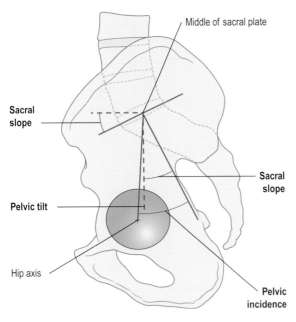

Pelvic incidence = sacral slope + pelvic tilt

Figure 8.5 Diagram of a pelvis in the sagittal plane (anterior on left), showing the relationship between several postural angles referred to in the text. *(From MacThiong et al.[863] with permission of Lippincott Williams & Wilkins, Philadelphia.)*

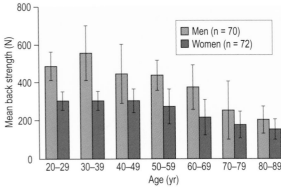

Figure 8.6 The isometric strength of back extensor muscles decreases greatly in old age, for men and women. Values refer to forces exerted by the back on a load cell and do not indicate the tensile force within the muscle. Error bars indicate the SD. *(Reproduced from Sinaki et al.[1314] with permission of Lippincott Williams & Wilkins, Philadelphia.)*

decreasing levels of physical activity commonly found in elderly people and which are probably related to decreasing muscle strength. So, this account of ageing must begin with the muscles, and explain why they become weaker with age.

Muscles

Muscle mass and strength both decrease with age,[295,532] a process known as sarcopenia. There is growing evidence that age-related sarcopenia is due not only to muscle fibre atrophy, which is greatest for the type II fibre population,[355,1219,1472] but also to a decrease in fibre number due to a loss of motor neurones.[355,938] Changes are greater in men than in women[467,468,679] and in people who are less physically active,[645] and they can be accelerated by chronic disease. Age-related changes vary between different muscles,[645,992,993] and in appendicular muscles they are also influenced by limb dominance.[645] Back extensor muscles usually attain maximum strength between the ages of 30 and 40 years, but 50–65% of this is lost in old age (Fig. 8.6), indicating a more severe age-related decline than is seen in limb muscles.[1314] This effect may have been

overestimated somewhat in the latter study because of a failure to account for the weight of the upper body.

Declining levels of physical activity no doubt contribute to age-related sarcopenia. However, the loss of muscle mass and strength occurs even in the active elderly, suggesting that other factors are important. Possible influences include: reduced levels of growth hormone, insulin-like growth factor, and sex steroids,[679] increased production of catabolic cytokines such as interleukin-6,[1221] insufficient dietary intake of calories and protein,[1005,1006] and reduced rates of protein turnover.[96,580,1550,1607] Sarcopenia can be reversed by high-intensity progressive resistance exercise,[427] although ageing human muscle is less responsive to exercise training than younger muscle,[807] and animal studies suggest that ageing muscle takes longer to regenerate following injury.[341] There is also evidence that testosterone administration can increase muscle mass and strength in elderly men,[425,1459] and that a combination of hormone replacement therapy and high-resistance training can increase muscle mass and power in younger postmenopausal women.[1318] Most intervention studies in the elderly have concentrated on the appendicular muscles, but one study has shown that back muscle strength could be improved in elderly men by administration of adrenal sex steroid precursors.[1002]

As well as becoming weaker, old muscle has a reduced oxidative capacity, which cannot be explained simply by reduced mass.[295,296] This may be due to an age-related increase in the number of fibres that are deficient in cytochrome c oxidase, a mitochondrial enzyme involved in aerobic energy metabolism.[776]

Ageing also affects the extracellular matrix of muscle. Collagen content increases, especially in the endomysium and perimysium,[506] and animal experiments indicate that

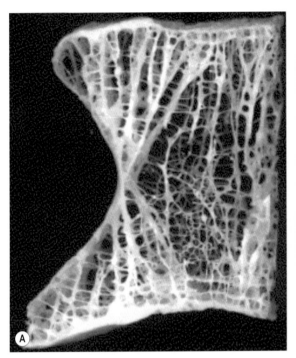 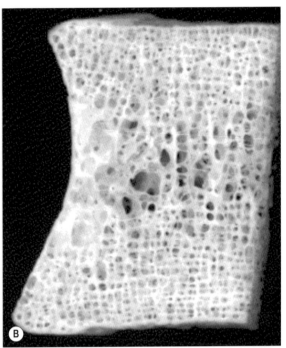

Figure 8.7 Anterior regions of macerated L2 vertebral bodies from a 97-year-old male (A) and a 27-year-old male (B). The old bone shows marked thinning and loss of trabeculae, and there is evidence of local buckling of vertical trabeculae, presumably following loss of support from horizontal trabeculae. *(Reproduced from Rajapakse et al.[1180] with permission of Elsevier, Amsterdam.)*

the epimysium becomes much stiffer with age,[471] presumably because of non-enzymatic glycation (p. 95). These changes increase passive muscle stiffness. Perhaps as a consequence of this, proprioceptive ability is impaired, contributing to slower reactions and poorer motor control.[1324]

The overall effect of all these changes is to make old muscles weaker, slower, more fatigable and stiffer, so that they become a major cause of disability and frailty in the elderly.

Vertebrae

Bone tissue deteriorates markedly with age (Fig. 8.7). Reduced levels of physical activity no doubt play a part, but so do changes in the levels of sex hormones such as oestrogen which reduce bone mass and strength, especially in women after the menopause.[1015] Age- and hormone-related weakening of bone is termed 'osteopenia'. The mineral component of bone matrix, hydroxyapatite, can readily be dissolved by acids secreted by osteoclasts. The collagenous component of bone also falls with age,[94] and when osteopenia is advanced, collagen is 'turned over' more rapidly so that thinner and less cross-linked fibres

are present.[911] However, the main determinant of the physical properties of ageing bone is its mineral content[94] and this is what is detected by dual-energy X-ray absorptiometry scans. These biochemical processes do not reduce bone mass uniformly: trabecular bone is affected more than the cortical shell[312] because it provides more surfaces on which the osteoclasts can operate. Horizontal trabeculae are lost in preference to vertical,[1404,1445] probably because they do not directly resist gravitational forces (although they prevent the vertical trabeculae from buckling). If trabeculae are thinned so much that they break, then they are not replaced, at least in adults. In this way, bone strength depends not only on bone mass, but also on aspects of bone architecture such as the orientation and connectivity of trabeculae.

Vertebral bodies are often severely affected by osteopenia because they contain so much trabecular bone. Cubes of vertebral trabecular bone lose more than 90% of their compressive strength between the ages of 30 and 80 years,[1538] whereas whole vertebral bodies, reinforced by the cortical shell, lose 50–75%.[1123] Microfracture of the vertically oriented trabeculae which support the vertebral body endplate are so common[1485] that they probably explain why endplates generally bulge into the vertebral body in old age,[609,1445] as shown in Figures 8.7 and 8.9. Localised

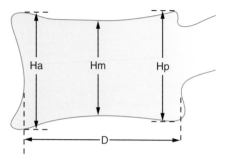

Figure 8.8 The shape of a vertebral body can be characterised by its anterior, middle and posterior heights (Ha, Hm and Hp) and its anteroposterior diameter (D). Types of vertebral deformity and fracture (see Fig. 11.7) are conventionally defined in terms of these parameters.

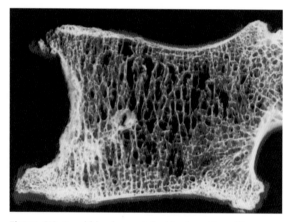

Figure 8.9 An old lumbar vertebral body sectioned in a parasagittal plane through a pedicle (anterior on left). Note the large anterior osteophytes, the smooth depression in the upper endplate which suggests previous repeated microtrauma and the trabeculae radiating from the pedicle to the lower endplate.

microfractures would be encouraged by the way old discs press unevenly on their vertebrae (Fig. 10.18).

Vertebral bodies tend to change their shape with increasing age even if they do not become fractured. Atraumatic deformation can occur by adaptive remodelling (Fig. 7.11), by the accumulation of microfractures which individually would be undetected, and also by creep (Fig. 1.6), which is much slower in bone than in soft tissue but can nevertheless be detected.[1141,1336,1596] It is conventional to define vertebral body height in three places: the anterior and posterior margins (Ha and Hp), and halfway in between (Hm), as shown in Figure 8.8. Three type of vertebral deformity can then be defined by comparing these

heights with each other and with the anteroposterior diameter (D) of the vertebral body. Thus, an anterior wedge deformity is characterised by a low Ha/Hp ratio; a biconcave deformity (Fig. 8.9) is characterised by a low Hm/Hp ratio, and a compression deformity is characterised by a low Hp/D ratio, as shown in Figure 8.8. There is a steady age-related increase in both anterior wedge and biconcave deformities in the thoracic spine, even in subjects with no evidence of traumatic fractures.[504] The Hp/D ratio increases during and beyond growth, peaking at 30–60 years and declining after age 65 years.[504] Similar trends have been observed in the lumbar spine, and they imply that ageing vertebral bodies normally lose height, especially from their anterior and central regions. Anterior vertebral height loss may arise following disc degeneration, for reasons explained on page 100, and central height loss is more likely if the disc is not degenerated so that the hydrostatic nucleus presses on the weak central part of the endplate.

Vertebral deformation is often exaggerated by the appearance of small outgrowths or osteophytes arising from the junction between the cartilage endplate, vertebral cortex and annulus fibrosus, usually on the anterolateral region of the vertebral body (Fig. 8.9). These outgrowths increase the effective cross-sectional area of the body by 25–30% from the age of 20–80 years,[1008] and so may be viewed as a purposeful adaptation to reduce compressive stress on the spine. However, vertebral body osteophytes typically resist only 10–20% of the compressive force on the spine[55] and their main purpose may be to resist bending (p. 208). Histologically they are mostly trabecular bone which appears to arise by the process of endochondral ossification from new cartilage laid down by cells originating in the annulus fibrosus.[843] Vertebral body osteophytes can be induced in animals by cutting into the disc so that it bulges anteriorly[843] and this may explain why, in humans, marginal osteophytes are associated with rim lesions in the adjacent annulus fibrosus.[608] The orientation of osteophyte trabeculae in human vertebrae[1404] suggests that bone formation may be driven by tensile forces in the fibres of the bulging outer annulus.

Thinning and loss of trabeculae are more common in the anterior part of the vertebral body,[1061] as shown in Figure 8.7. This could be related to the manner in which it is loaded by the intervertebral disc, as described on page 100. The central region of the vertebral body, midway between the two endplates, is also badly affected.[88]

To a certain extent, bone weakening can be countered by appropriate exercises, particularly those which involve impact loading of the bones,[108,109] and also by drug therapy (including hormone replacement therapy). However, the best advice is to exercise vigorously earlier in life to ensure that bone mass is sufficiently high that the normal age-related loss does not take it below the level at which the risk of fracture becomes high.

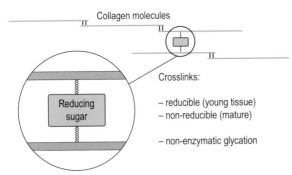

Figure 8.10 Diagram showing cross-linking between parallel collagen molecules in a fibril. Reducible and non-reducible cross-links are formed and broken by cellular activity, but non-enzymatic glycation involving sugar molecules is uncontrolled.

Some other causes of bone deterioration, including nutritional defects and rheumatological conditions, lie outside the scope of this book.

Hyaline cartilage

Hyaline cartilage forms the cartilaginous endplates, and articular cartilage (a type of hyaline cartilage) covers the articulating surfaces of the apophyseal joints. With increasing age, the number of live cells in hyaline cartilage falls, and the matrix shows a range of progressive biochemical changes. Enzyme-mediated cross-linking between adjacent collagen molecules proceeds steadily, with the links becoming increasingly mature (stable). Collagen cross-linking is a gradual chemical process which occurs in the test tube as well as in living tissue[1463] and it influences the mechanical properties of many connective tissues in the body, including skin.[1191] Another type of collagen cross-linking is non-enzymatic glycation. This process is not directly controlled by cells, and involves reducing sugars such as glucose forming cross-bridges between collagen molecules (Fig. 8.10). Non-enzymatic glycation is encouraged by low oxygen concentrations in the tissue combined with low matrix turnover. It results in advanced glycation end products which discolour the tissue (Fig. 10.19B), make it stiffer[100] and inhibit proteoglycan synthesis by chondrocytes.[334] Increased stiffness makes cartilage more brittle, and therefore more vulnerable to injury during impact loading.[335,1486] This line of research provides a biochemical explanation of why articular cartilage (and other collagenous tissues) weakens with age. Previously, it was supposed that the reduced strength of old cartilage[734,1543] was attributable to fatigue damage accumulating over many years, even though this explanation was never

entirely compatible with the known ability of cartilage to strengthen biologically in response to mechanical loading (Ch. 7).

Tendon and ligament

Tendons and ligaments become stronger and stiffer up until skeletal maturity, as collagen type I fibrils grow in diameter and are stabilised by more non-reducible cross-links.[93] Vigorous exercise can cause cross-sectional area to increase more rapidly during growth, at least in horses.[719] During subsequent ageing, tendons and ligaments become weaker[126] and less able to absorb strain energy (Fig. 1.5),[372] although these effects can probably be modified by physical exercise.[881] Age-related weakening may be related to focal microdamage, perhaps involving crimp mechanisms in the central core of the tendon.[1578] Impaired energy absorption may be due to excessive cross-linking involving tissue sugars (Fig. 8.10) making the tissue less extensible.

Intervertebral discs
Biochemical changes

Most age-related changes in the disc occur first, and to the greatest extent, in the nucleus and endplate. Proteoglycan fragmentation starts during childhood,[211] and with increasing age the overall proteoglycan and water content of the disc decreases, especially in the nucleus[28,78,1456] (Fig. 8.11). Loss of proteoglycan fragments from the disc is a slow process due to the entrapment of the nucleus by the fibrous annulus and the cartilage endplates of the vertebrae[1457]. As long as large proteoglycan fragments remain entrapped in the disc they can fulfil a functional role similar to that of the intact proteoglycan.[1222]

Reduced matrix turnover in older discs enables collagen molecules and fibrils to become increasingly cross-linked with each other, and existing cross-links become more stable,[375] and this in turn leads to further reductions in turnover. As a result, the half-life of disc collagens increases from 95 to 215 years between the age ranges 20–40 years and 50–80 years.[1322] The process of non-enzymatic glycation (Fig. 8.10) gives old discs their characteristic yellow-brown colour[1320] (Fig. 10.19) and makes the tissue stiffer[1519] and more easily damaged.[335] Despite increased cross-linking, the overall content of disc collagen decreases with age, independently of degeneration.[1316] Fine type II collagen fibrils in the inner annulus are replaced by type I fibres, as the annulus encroaches on the nucleus (Fig. 8.12). In the centre of large avascular discs, these reactions may be accelerated due to oxidative stress arising from harmful chemical reactions that can be likened to rusting, and which may be associated with nutritional compromise.[1035] Similar changes occur in the cartilage endplates,[146]

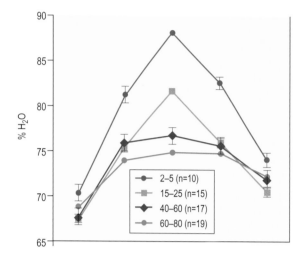

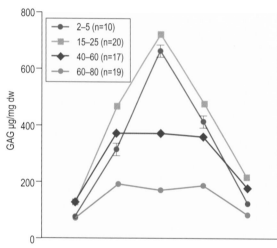

Figure 8.11 In human intervertebral discs, the concentration of water (H_2O) and glycosaminoglycan (GAG) decreases with advancing age (shown in years in the key). Each panel also indicates how concentration varies with location, from the anterior annulus (left edge of panel) through the nucleus to the posterior annulus (right of panel). *(Reproduced from Antoniou et al.[78] with permission.)*

and accompanying calcification of the endplate may compromise the nutrient supply to the adjacent nucleus (evidence reviewed by Moore[998]). Increased cross-linking inhibits matrix turnover and repair in old discs, encouraging the retention of damaged (denatured) collagen, and probably leading to reduced tissue strength. Some degraded matrix molecules such as fibronectin can impair disc cell metabolism.[68] In the annulus, more non-reducible cross-links are formed between adjacent collagen molecules[1035,1138] so that they aggregate into increasingly thick

fibrils and fibres (Fig. 8.13). These age-related biochemical changes (including water content) are largely responsible for the changing appearance of intervertebral discs when sectioned (Fig. 8.14) or imaged by MRI (Fig. 8.15).

Histological changes

Disc cell density does not generally decline after the cessation of growth (Fig. 8.4), although regional cell density can be modified adjacent to major pathological changes.[1035,1484] From skeletal maturity onwards there is a steadily increasing incidence of structural defects extending from the nucleus into the annulus.[1035] The nucleus pulposus tends to condense into several fibrous lumps (Fig. 8.14), separated from each other and from the cartilage endplate by softer material.[17] Annular lamellae become thicker[913] and gross defects in lamellar structure become more frequent after the age of 40 years.[134] Translamellar bridging elements (Fig. 10.14) become more numerous with age in sheep,[1272] but there are no equivalent human data. Sequential histological changes across nine decades have recently been classified.[170] Generally, these changes affect the endplate first, then the nucleus, and finally the annulus, and different spinal levels are affected to a similar extent.

Metabolic changes

Matrix synthesis decreases steadily after childhood, although it can increase again in some old and severely disrupted discs,[77,78] in which case it probably represents attempted healing. Reduced synthesis is partly attributable to decreased cell density, although proteoglycan synthesis rates per cell also fall.[880] Age-related changes in the types of collagens and MMPs synthesised suggest that cell phenotype can change in the vicinity of annulus fissures,[1544] possibly in response to altered matrix stress distributions (see next section).

Functional changes

Old but non-degenerated discs do not normally narrow with age: in fact the nucleus often becomes taller and the endplates more curved, as the nucleus pushes further into the adjacent vertebral bodies,[1126] which may be weakened by osteoporosis (Fig. 8.9). Annulus height does not increase and tends either to remain the same or to decrease as a result of increased bulging by the lamellae, either outwards or inwards. It is annulus height which determines the separation of adjacent pedicles and hence compressive load-bearing by the neural arch (see below). The region of inner annulus which exhibits hydrostatic pressure is reduced with age, and the pressure itself is reduced so that more of the compressive load-bearing is taken by the annulus, especially the posterior annulus[38] (Fig. 10.18). If disc cells are as adaptable as tendon cells, then

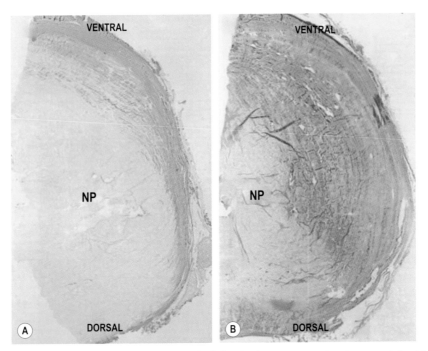

Figure 8.12 Large histological sections of human intervertebral discs in the transverse plane immuno-stained (brown) for collagen type 1. This increases in density and distribution with increasing age, as shown in (B). NP: nucleus pulposus. *(Reproduced from Schollmeier et al.[1271] with permission.)*

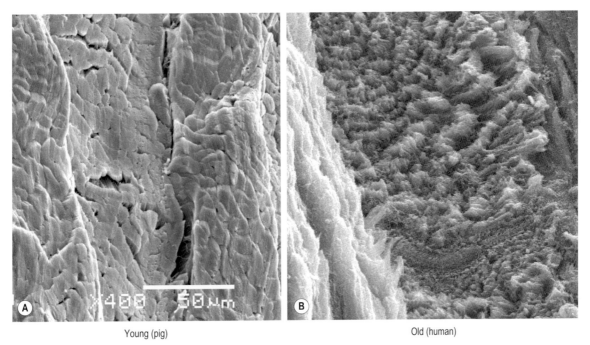

Young (pig)   Old (human)

Figure 8.13 Scanning electron micrographs of two pieces of annulus fibrosus. (A) This immature pig tissue shows three thin lamellae, each packed with small smooth-edged collagen fibres. (B) This old human tissue shows larger 'frayed' collagen fibres arranged in two thick lamellae. *(Courtesy of Dr Lee Neylon, Curtin University, Western Australia.)*

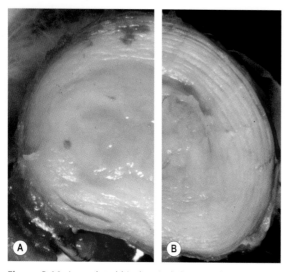

Figure 8.14 Age-related biochemical changes alter the gross appearance of intervertebral discs, sectioned in the transverse plane (anterior on top). (A) Young adult disc. (B) Middle-aged non-degenerated disc, showing the yellowing effects of non-enzymatic glycation, and how collagen changes thicken the lamellae of the annulus.

this profound age-related change in their mechanical environment may influence their appearance and function.[500]

With increasing age, the nucleus pulposus becomes dry, fibrous and physically stiff.[17,1453] The tensile properties of the annulus are only slightly impaired with age,[3,385,464] even though increased collagen cross-linking should improve them.[100] This apparent contradiction may be explained by the age-related accumulation of macroscopic defects,[551] which would weaken gross tissue samples. The outer annulus has the highest cell density[581] and most plentiful nutrient supply[424] and this region of the annulus does show some tendency to weaken with age, at least in male spines.[1326] Perhaps only the most metabolically active region of the disc is able to adapt to the reduced mechanical demands in old age?

Gross functional changes in the ageing spine

Spinal mobility decreases steadily during adult life, as shown in Table 8.1. Lumbar flexion and extension both decrease by about 20% between the ages of 20 and 55 years, with a tendency for extension to be lost more in the

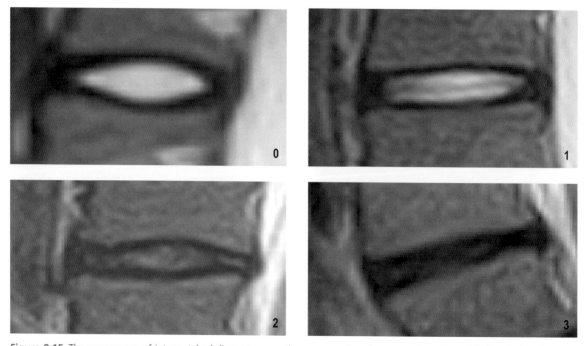

Figure 8.15 The appearance of intervertebral discs on magnetic resonance imaging scans depends on biochemical and structural changes in the tissue. Typical appearances can be graded 0 (young) to 3 (old, degenerated), as shown on these scans. *(Reproduced from Kjaer[752] with permission.)*

later years.[1381] Both genders are affected equally, but men of all ages appear to have more flexion but less extension than women, presumably reflecting a tendency for women to have slightly more lordotic spines. Data in Table 8.1 were obtained using inclinometers held next to the skin, and angles refer to the actual lumbar kyphosis or lordosis in full flexion and extension (i.e. they do not represent movements relative to any neutral position). Similar trends have been reported using a flexicurve technique,[223] which showed that mobility continues to decrease in old age, so that approximately 50% of the full lumbar range of motion is lost between 16 and 85 years of age. The flexicurve technique also showed that more mobility is lost in the upper compared to lower lumbar regions.[223] A radiographic study on patients with back pain found that the full sagittal range of movement fell by 3° per decade,[137] although some of this loss may be attributable to worsening disc degeneration. Declining mobility with age has been measured on excised cadaveric spines[33,610] and so must be due to altered properties of discs and ligaments, rather than to changes in muscle extensibility.

Movements of the cervical spine similarly decrease with age. A multivariate radiographic study[1310] found that the full range of flexion/extension between C2 and C7 decreased by 5° per decade, independently of degeneration (which caused additional reductions in mobility). Skin surface measurements[804] showed that lateral bending and axial rotation movements also decrease with age (Table 8.2), and suggested that proprioceptive ability decreases along with mobility.

Static postures are also affected by age. Older people tend to sit with an increased thoracic kyphosis, and with a forward head posture that involves increased flexion in the lower cervical spine, and increased extension in the upper cervical spine.[796] Similarly, they stand with a more anterior head position, an increased thoracic kyphosis, and with a pelvis that is displaced posteriorly relative to the feet and tilted so that the sacral table is more inclined to the horizontal.[1278]

Age affects load-sharing in the spine. Old intervertebral discs are more likely to be degenerated and narrowed, and this brings the adjacent neural arches closer together. As a result, the apophyseal joints resist an increasing proportion of the compressive force acting on the spine. Cadaver experiments have shown that, in the presence of severe disc narrowing, and when positioned in 2° of extension to simulate erect standing postures, the neural arch resists up to 90% of applied compression (Fig. 8.16). This can explain the severe osteoarthritic changes observed in the

Table 8.1 Angles of full lumbar flexion and extension for men and women of various ages. Data indicate mean values, obtained using hand-held inclinometers, from 686 men and 440 women with no history of back pain[1381]

	Flexion		Extension	
Age range (years)	Men	Women	Men	Women
16–24	33	26	54	63
25–34	31	24	52	60
35–44	28	22	49	53
45–65	26		45	

Table 8.2 Cervical spine range of motion declines with age. Averaged data refer to three-dimensional movements of the head relative to the thorax measured using a skin-surface infra-red tracking device on 140 asymptomatic volunteers (70 men and 70 women)

Age range (years)	Flexion/extension		Lateral bending		Axial rotation	
	M	F	M	F	M	F
20–29	119	128	86	87	140	152
30–39	110	115	70	82	137	146
40–49	118	122	77	80	136	138
50–59	114	100	70	65	128	122
60–69	99	110	67	61	124	115
70–79	97	107	44	68	99	123
>80	76	87	44	53	99	103

(From Lansade et al.[804])

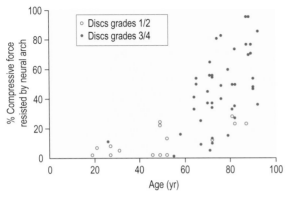

Figure 8.16 Compressive load-bearing by the neural arch increases greatly in old spines, especially if the discs are degenerated (dark symbols). Data refer to cadaveric lumbar 'motion segments' loaded to simulate the erect standing posture.[1142]

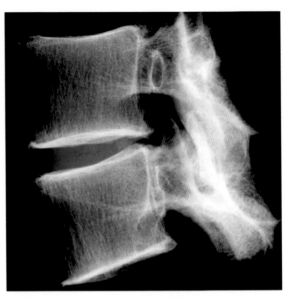

Figure 8.17 Radiograph of an old human lumbar motion segment, showing marked bone loss from the anterior vertebral body (left), and dense bone in the articular processes of the neural arches. Bone density is so low in the spinous processes that they are barely visible. These bone changes reflect altered load-sharing in the ageing spine.

Table 8.3 Altered load-sharing in degenerated spines, as measured in cadaver experiments.[16] Distribution of an applied compressive force of 1.5 kN between the neural arch (N arch), and the anterior (Ant) and posterior (Post) halves of the vertebral body (VB)

	Distribution (%) of applied compressive force					
	Upright posture			Flexed posture		
	Ant VB	Post VB	N arch	Ant VB	Post VB	N arch
Grade 2 (n = 4)	32 ± 27	49 ± 25	19 ± 8	62 ± 5	31 ± 7	7 ± 6
Grade 3 (n = 24)	21 ± 20	41 ± 20	38 ± 18	58 ± 17	36 ± 17	6 ± 6
Grade 4 (n = 13)	10 ± 8	12 ± 8	78 ± 9	51 ± 16	41 ± 16	8 ± 5

Mean values (± SD) are shown for each grade of disc degeneration (n is the number of specimens). Note that, in the presence of severe (grade 4) disc degeneration, upright postures concentrate loading on the neural arch, and flexed postures transfer it on to the anterior vertebral body. Few comparable data are available for young (grade 1) discs.

apophyseal joints of many old spines (Ch. 15). On the other hand, altered load-sharing causes the vertebral body (and especially its anterior regions) to resist less, so that it becomes 'stress-shielded' by the neural arch (Table 8.3). According to the principles of adaptive remodelling (Fig. 7.11), the anterior vertebral body then loses bone mineral and becomes vulnerable to anterior wedge fracture (Fig. 11.7). The overall effects of this profound age-related change in spinal load-sharing on bone mineral density are illustrated in Figure 8.17.

Chapter 9

Forces acting on the thoracolumbar spine

COMPRESSION, SHEAR, BENDING AND TORSION

All of the forces acting on a given part of the spine can be added up to form a single 'resultant' force (Fig. 1.2). For convenience, the resultant is usually divided into components, as shown in Figure 9.1. The component which acts perpendicular to the mid-plane of the disc is usually defined as the compressive force acting on that part of the spine, and the other component acting parallel to the disc is the shear force. In three dimensions, there would also be a lateral shear force acting perpendicular to the plane of the paper in Figure 9.1, but lateral forces are usually small, and will not be considered further.

The resultant force may cause the spine to bend or twist about its centres of rotation, which usually lie within the intervertebral discs (Fig. 10.5). The torque (force × lever arm) responsible for the bending and twisting can be divided up into components in a similar manner to forces. The components which cause the spine to bend in the sagittal and frontal planes are referred to as the bending moment and lateral bending moment respectively, and the component which causes the spine to twist about its long axis (Fig. 9.1) is defined as the axial torque on the spine. Bending moments and torque have the same units (Nm), and the words are sometimes used interchangeably. The word 'torsion' can refer to the axial torque (in Nm), or the axial rotation (in degrees) that it causes.

WHERE DO THE FORCES COME FROM?

Gravity and inertial effects

Gravity exerts a vertical force on each part of the body in direct proportion to its mass. This force is the 'weight' of the object (p. 4). When a person stands upright, the mass of the trunk, head and arms presses vertically on the lower lumbar spine with a force of approximately 55% of body weight,[1228] which is 385 N for a 70-kg man. Assuming the

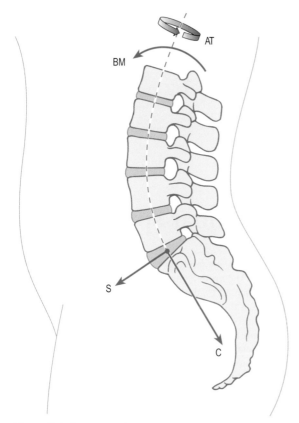

Figure 9.1 Component forces acting on the lumbar spine. C, compression; S, shear; BM, bending moment in the sagittal plane; AT, axial torque. In three dimensions, there could also be a lateral shear force and a lateral bending moment.

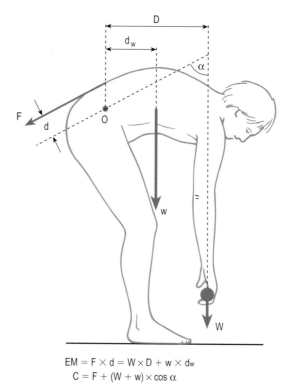

$$EM = F \times d = W \times D + w \times d_w$$
$$C = F + (W + w) \times \cos \alpha$$

Figure 9.2 During manual handling, the back muscles must generate an extensor moment (EM) to overcome the forward-bending moment due to upper body weight (w) and the weight being lifted (W). The average lever arm (d) of the extensor muscles in the lower lumbar spine is approximately 7.5 cm, whereas W and w act on much larger lever arms (D and dw). For this reason, the tensile force in the back muscles (F) is much greater than w or W, and the spine is subjected to a high compressive force (C).

lumbosacral disc is inclined at an angle of approximately 30° to the horizontal, the gravitational force will give rise to intervertebral compressive and shear force components of approximately 335 N and 190 N respectively.

The mass of body segments can give rise to much greater inertial forces when they are rapidly accelerated or decelerated. According to Newton's second law of motion (p. 4), the force rises in proportion to the acceleration (change of velocity divided by time). The high vertical acceleration experienced by a fighter pilot ejecting from a plane generates an impulsive compressive force on the spine that may be sufficient to crush a vertebra.[614] Similarly, rapid decelerations experienced during a fall on the buttocks can be sufficient to crush the spine.[440] The maximum velocity reached by a falling body just before impact depends on the distance of fall, whereas the time taken to stop depends on the amount of cushioning at impact. Therefore the peak deceleration (and peak force) generated during a fall from upright standing depends mainly on the length of a person's legs, and the softness of the landing.

Muscles

Muscles of the back and abdomen act to protect the spine, by stabilising it in upright postures[1368] and by preventing excessive bending and axial rotation movements. However, the muscle tension required to protect and to move the spine also subjects it to high compressive forces, because many of the strongest trunk muscles lie approximately parallel to the long axis of the spine. According to circumstances, the back muscles can be the spine's best friend, or worst enemy.

Even during relaxed standing and sitting, muscle tension increases the compressive force on the lumbar discs to approximately twice the superincumbent body weight.[1022,1250] During activities such as bending forwards and lifting weights, the back muscles need to generate much higher forces in order to overcome the effects of gravity acting on the upper body.[67,358] These forces can be estimated by using a moment arm analysis (Fig. 9.2). The simple analysis explained in this figure refers to a static equilibrium, where nothing is moving. In practice, manual handling activities require the upper body to be moved quickly, often from a stationary position, and so even higher muscle forces are required to generate high accelerations of the trunk.[363,946] Manual handling typically involves movements in several planes,[924] and these require additional lateral bending moments and axial torques which increase muscle tension further.[136,360,747,921]

The general principle illustrated by Figure 9.2 is that internal muscle forces must often be high because they act close to the centre of rotation of the body's joints, and yet they must attempt to move superincumbent body weight that may, in cetain postures, act far from the pivot. The same leverage principle can readily be applied to other joints such as the hip and knee: for example, adopting a squatting position can result in body weight acting a long way posterior to the knee, so that the quadriceps muscles, which act only a few centimetres anterior to the knee, must generate a tensile force of several times body weight. This is why your knees feel under pressure during deep squats, and why peak knee loading can exceed three times body weight when climbing or decending stairs.[798]

The force a muscle generates is due to a combination of active force, as a result of cross-bridge formation within muscle cells (Fig. 7.3), and passive tension in non-contractile structures. When muscles are lengthened beyond their optimum length, overlap between actin and myosin filaments decreases, and cross-bridge formation falls. Consequently, an increasing proportion of the force generated is due to tension in the stretched collagenous tissue sheaths of the muscle (Fig. 7.2), and to passive force transmission by large structural proteins such as titin.[1030,1162,1182] Titin connects the thick myosin filament to the Z-line of the sarcomere (Fig. 7.3) and is thought to transmit force longitudinally when the muscle is stretched.[1159,1427] It also helps to provide elastic recoil when the stretch is released.[984]

Fascia and ligaments

Fascia and ligaments are passive (non-contractile) structures that can sustain high tensile forces when stretched. This is demonstrated by the flexion–relaxation phenomenon (Fig. 9.3), in which the back muscles fall electrically silent when a person bends forwards to touch the toes.[431,543,749,1399] The effect extends to include the hamstring muscles and much of the thoracic erector spinae.[951] Evidently, the forward-bending moment generated by the upper body (Fig. 9.2) must be resisted by tension in passive tissues such as the ligaments of the neural arch, the erector spinae aponeurosis, lumbodorsal fascia and fibrous proteins in the muscle itself (see above).

The involvement of passive tissues in lifting is an important and controversial topic, because it can be both beneficial and harmful to the spine. Stretched passive tissues

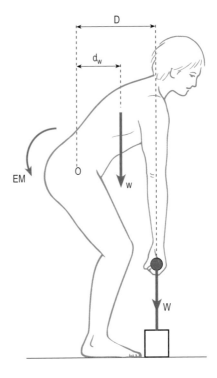

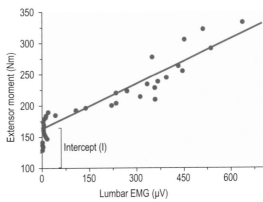

Figure 9.3 During an isometric contraction in the stooped position, the electromyographic (EMG) activity of the erector spinae muscles is linearly related to the extensor moment (EM) generated. (A) The subject pulled up on a load cell, reaching maximum force in approximately 3 seconds. Extensor moment was calculated from D, dw, w and W, as shown in Figure 9.2. (B) The intercept on the y-axis (I) indicates the moment generated when the erector spinae are electrically silent.

store elastic energy when the spine is flexed, and then release the energy when the person straightens up again, so that the back muscles do less work.[516,795] In addition, the supraspinous ligament and the strong posterior band of the lumbodorsal fascia both lie posterior to the back muscles,[163] and so act on longer lever arms relative to the centre of rotation in the discs than do the muscles.[948] Therefore, any extensor moment generated by these passive structures has a smaller compressive 'penalty' as far as the spine is concerned. (In other words, the ratio of extensor moment to tensile force is high.) On the other hand, most of the ligaments of the neural arch act on shorter lever arms than the back muscles, so any extensor moment generated by them is at the expense of a high compressive penalty. Also, too much flexion can leave the discs vulnerable to prolapse when the compressive force is high (Ch. 11). These considerations suggest that, during manual handling, the spine should be flexed sufficiently to tension the lumbodorsal fascia, but not so much that high forces are generated in the intervertebral ligaments and disc.

The feasibility of doing this was investigated in 149 healthy volunteers who lifted 10-kg weights from the ground, either with their knees flexed (squat lifts) or straight (stoop lifts).[366] On average, these volunteers flexed their lumbar spine by 83% and 96% in the squat and stoop lifts respectively, where 0% and 100% flexion refer to the erect standing and fully flexed positions (Fig. 13.3). Complementary static experiments investigating the relationship between lumbar flexion, electrical silence in the back muscles and extensor moment generation (Fig. 9.4) showed that 'passive' structures must have contributed 22% of the extensor moment in the squat lift, and 31% in the stoop lift. Furthermore, comparisons with the bending properties of cadaveric motion segments[13] showed that tension in the ligaments of the neural arch and in the posterior annulus fibrosus would have been low in both lifts, and contributed less than 25% of the total 'passive' extensor moment. Calculations suggest that the lumbodorsal fascia, and collagenous tissue within the back muscles themselves, are indeed strong enough to generate large extensor moments during lifting activities.[366] Previous estimates of the strength of the lumbodorsal fascia were based on testing excised samples of it,[1411] but the collagen fibre disruption caused by the excision of small samples can probably lead to the strength of the whole structure being underestimated.[23]

The experimental evidence therefore indicates that it is possible to make use of passive tension in the lumbodorsal fascia and stretched back muscles during lifting, without generating high stresses in the intervertebral ligaments and disc. This can be achieved simply by flexing the lumbar spine by 80–90% of the range between upright standing and touching the toes. It has been suggested that the lumbodorsal fascia can be tensioned in other ways, in particular by raising the intra-abdominal pressure (IAP), and by contracting the abdominal muscles so that they pull sideways on the fascia and generate a longitudinal tension within it.[517,518] However, attempts to demonstrate these mechanisms either directly in cadavers[1411] or using detailed anatomical data from cadaveric dissection[873] showed that the effects were small.

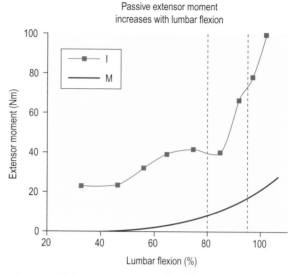

Figure 9.4 Extensor moments attributable to non-contractile tissues (I) can be calculated during isometric contractions, as shown in Figure 9.3. If the experiment is repeated with the subject in varying amounts of lumbar flexion, I increases markedly when flexion exceeds 80% of the in vivo range of movement. M represents the bending stiffness properties of cadaveric osteoligamentous spines (Fig. 9.11). A comparison of the two curves (I and M) suggests that, in the range 80–95% flexion, less than 25% of I is attributable to the osteoligamentous spine. *(Reproduced from Dolan et al.[366])*

Intra-abdominal pressure

Raising the IAP during lifting has been advocated by some as a means of transmitting load directly from the shoulders to the pelvis in order to reduce spinal compression[104] (Fig. 9.5). Pressures above 150 mmHg have been recorded during weight lifting,[388,925] which is sufficient to occlude the blood supply to the abdominal cavity and make the lifter go red in the face. However, a raised IAP is normally associated with increased abdominal muscle activity, which actually produces a flexion moment on the trunk.[122] This would act to increase spinal compression, so any benefit of the IAP mechanism is difficult to assess. An electromyographic (EMG) study (summarised in Fig. 9.4) showed that volunteers were able to generate an extensor moment of 20–25 Nm in the absence of any erector spinae muscle activity and without flexing forwards to stretch intervertebral ligaments and lumbodorsal fascia.[366] This extensor moment could possibly be due to a raised IAP, although there was no direct evidence to support this. However, a potential load-relieving effect of IAP was demonstrated in a study in which IAP was increased by electrical stimulation of the diaphragm via the phrenic nerve.[618] The resulting contraction of the diaphragm produced extensor moments in the absence of abdominal or back

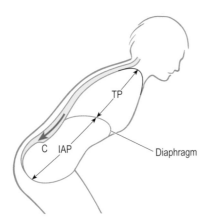

Figure 9.5 When a person lifts a heavy weight, a raised intra-abdominal pressure (IAP) and thoracic pressure (TP) have the potential to transmit force directly from shoulders to pelvis, bypassing the lumbar spine. In this manner, it is hypothesised that a high IAP can reduce the compressive force (C) acting on the lumbar spine.

extensor muscle activity, and the size of the moment was directly related to the increase in IAP.

In practice, any benefit of increasing IAP during lifting will depend to a large extent upon which muscles are employed to achieve the increased pressure. Transversus abdominis, which is composed of transversely oriented fibres, does not induce a flexor moment on the trunk when it contracts, so selective recruitment of this muscle (along with the diaphragm) could conceivably increase IAP and reduce compressive loading of the spine. During back extension movements, transversus abdominis shows the highest levels of abdominal muscle activity,[304] suggesting that, under these circumstances, it makes the greatest contribution to IAP. A mathematical model which considered transversus abdominis activation concluded that increases in IAP contributed about 10% to maximal voluntary extension moment during back extension efforts.[319] However, the exclusion of all other abdominal muscles from this model has been criticised on the grounds that the combined activation of these muscles, even at low levels of contraction, would be likely to produce flexor moments roughly equivalent to the estimated extensor moments generated by transversus abdominis,[278] so the debate continues. It is possible that the main benefit of increasing IAP is to stiffen the trunk and reduce spinal movement rather than to relieve compression.[617] Personal preferences may also be a factor, because holding the breath during trunk exertions increases IAP and gives a subjective feeling of spinal stability.[949]

Use of lifting belts

Wearing a wide abdominal belt helps to raise IAP, and could possibly reduce the compressive force on the spine during lifting by approximately 15%.[949] However, the effectiveness of lifting belts in reducing spinal loading is debatable, and depends on the type of belt.[522] There is some evidence from experiments on cadaveric human torsos that an increased IAP (simulating belt-wearing or breath-holding) has a greater effect on torso stiffness during lateral bending and axial rotation than in flexion and extension.[940] A raised IAP could therefore help stabilise the trunk in asymmetric manual handling tasks.[925] Some of this extra stability may be due to the belt increasing pressure within the muscles themselves.[986] It may be significant that abdominal belts are worn with their widest part next to the spine, rather than next to the abdominal wall they are supposed to be supporting. Perhaps weight lifters like to use a belt because it helps to keep the lumbar spine flat (i.e. moderately flexed) rather than in lordosis or kyphosis? There is some evidence that a belt can reduce sudden spinal bending movements during unexpected loading events.[809] The influence of back belts on low-back pain is considered on page 222.

COMPRESSIVE LOADING OF THE SPINE

For many years, spinal loading was equated with compressive loading, which is unfortunate because mechanisms of spinal injury depend greatly on the presence of bending and torsion. Nevertheless, the spine is compressed for most of the time, day and night, and compressive loading is undoubtedly an important contributor to the fatigue failure of spinal tissues. The following sections explain how the spinal compressive force can be measured, and what influences it.

Measuring spinal compression

Intradiscal pressure

The 'gold standard' measurements of spinal compression were made originally by Nachemson and Morris, who inserted a pressure-sensitive needle into the L3–4 disc of conscious volunteers.[1018] Measurements of pressure were later converted into compressive forces[1022] using the results of cadaver experiments to calibrate the pressure readings against force.[1020] Many of the results were later confirmed using better technology.[1250,1565] Intradiscal pressure techniques have limitations, however, because subjects are unlikely to move in a natural or vigorous manner with a long needle in their backs. Also, recorded pressures in vivo have been calibrated in terms of the compressive force applied to cadaveric discs that would have been swollen by postmortem storage, whereas the experiments on living people were performed after their discs had been dehydrated by hours of activity. In cadaveric experiments, load-induced fluid expulsion from intervertebral discs (Fig. 13.12), and this effectively transfers compressive loading from nucleus to annulus,[38] and from the disc to the neural arch.[39,1142] As a result, the ratio of nucleus pressure to spinal compressive force decreases by up to 36% following creep loading.[38] In vivo estimates of spinal loading which are based on intradiscal pressure measurements may therefore underestimate true spinal loading by a similar amount.

Spinal shrinkage

An indirect approach to quantifying the compressive force on the spine is to measure the amount of disc creep that it causes over a specified time period. Procedures have been developed to detect small time-dependent changes in the length of the spine, while minimising errors due to changes in posture.[64,224,350,586] Interindividual comparisons are difficult because the rate of disc creep depends on many factors, including age,[350] loading history,[38] the degree of disc degeneration,[28] disc area[64] and posture (which influences water expulsion from the discs[28] as well as load-bearing by the apophyseal joints: p 177). These variable factors may help explain why spinal shrinkage has been reported to be greater in standing postures than in sitting,[64,821] less when performing overhead work compared to standing,[224] and why a stature gain has been reported following dynamic hyperextension exercises.[883] Increased spinal shrinkage after sitting on a vibrating seat[1379] may be attributable to increased disc creep under oscillating loads, or increased muscle activity in the subjects being vibrated. However, another study showed that vibrations had no effect on stature over and above the effect due to sitting.[64]

Despite these variable factors, spinal shrinkage does provide a simple cumulative measure of spinal loading over time which may complement measurements of peak spinal loading in ergonomic studies.[328,433] The technique is most suitable when the spine is loaded predominantly in flexed postures (when all of the compressive load is resisted by the discs) and when comparisons are made between the same subjects performing different activities, so that individual factors such as disc area and degeneration are controlled for.

Accurate measurements of stature change do more than estimate cumulative spinal loading: they also indicate directly the speed and extent of fluid exchanges within the intervertebral discs. Water loss from discs leads to stress concentrations in the disc itself (Fig. 13.15) and apophyseal joints,[380] impairs disc cell metabolism,[118] and hinders metabolite transport within the disc. Stature changes are therefore of more than mechanical interest. They have the potential to give functional information concerning the biochemical and metabolic status of intervertebral discs, and it is not surprising to find that stature changes are different in people with back pain.[586]

Linked-segment and EMG-assisted models

Various mathematical models essentially elaborate the moment arm analysis approach (Fig. 9.2). Some are static[67] but most of them make allowance for the extra forces required to accelerate body segments.[119,746] Parts of the body such as the thigh, pelvis and lumbar spine are likened to a series of rigid segments which are linked by frictionless hinges (joints) and moved by the action of muscles which join the segments together. The position of each body segment is measured on living volunteers at frequent time intervals using a device such as a video camera. The change in position of each body segment per unit time gives the velocity of each segment, and the change in velocity per unit time indicates acceleration. Anthropometric data regarding the mass and centre of mass of each body segment can then be used to compute the net moments (force × distance) acting about each joint. Net moment is divided by the lever arm of the muscle mass responsible for the movement, yielding the muscle force acting on the joint. Detailed anatomical data required in these calculations, including the lever arms and cross-sectional areas of individual back muscles, are presented in Table 3.1 and in previously published work.[164,874,922] Force plate data can be incorporated to account for the effects of the ground reaction force during dynamic movements. Fully dynamic linked-segment models are able to measure accurately three-dimensional forces acting on each joint of the body[746] but they do have one drawback: they are unable to detect antagonistic muscle activity which can increase joint loading without affecting the movement of adjacent body segments.

The influence of muscle activity on spinal loading has been tackled by more complicated models which acknowledge that each joint is moved by several muscles, some of which could act antagonistically to each other. EMG measurements can be combined with data concerning muscle cross-sectional areas in order to determine the relative activity of each muscle, so that moments can be distributed between them.[519,927,943] Other models use optimising principles to divide up the overall moment between different muscles: for example, they may stipulate that spinal compression should be minimised, or that the square of muscle power should be minimised. Unfortunately, optimising principles can appear somewhat arbitrary, and the relationship between EMG activity and muscle tension is influenced by variable factors such as muscle length and speed of contraction. The importance of muscle length can be appreciated from Figure 9.6, which shows that the EMG signal can fall to near zero even when a high compressive force is acting on the spine, as verified by intradiscal pressure.

Direct EMG estimates of spinal loading

Because most of the compressive force acting on the lumbar spine arises from tension in the back muscles

Figure 9.6 Electromyographic (EMG) signals can fall to zero in stretched muscle, even when that muscle transmits a high tensile force. The graphs show simultaneous recordings from a healthy subject who flexed forwards to lift a weight from the floor, over a period of 6 seconds. Intradiscal pressure (which indicates spinal compression arising from muscle tension) is measured in kPa, trunk tilting angle (a rough measure of back muscle stretching) is measured in degrees (°) and skin surface EMG from the erector spinae is measured in μV. *(Data from Takahashi et al.[1399] with permission.)*

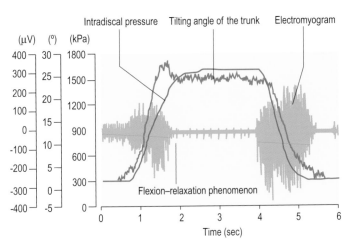

(Fig. 9.2), it is tempting to try to quantify spinal compression directly from the EMG activity of these muscles.[358] This approach does not attempt to predict forces or moments generated by individual muscles. Instead, it uses the EMG activity of the erector spinae to predict the extensor moment generated by them all, and then divides the moment by an effective lever arm[948] which refers to the whole muscle group in order to estimate the aggregate tensile force generated by the group.

Initially, the EMG activity from several sites overlying the erector spinae is calibrated against extensor moment when a volunteer pulls up with gradually increasing force on a chain attached to a load cell (Fig. 9.3). Linear regression is used to determine the gradient and the intercept of the relationship between EMG and extensor moment during isometric contractions. By repeating these calibrations in a range of postures which require different amounts of lumbar flexion, the effect of back muscle length on the EMG–extensor moment relationship can be determined.[358] In flexed postures, the intercept indicates the moment generated when there is no EMG activity in the back muscles, so the technique can be used to determine the extensor moment resisted by passive tissues such as the lumbodorsal fascia.[366] During concentric muscle contractions, the relationship between extensor moment and EMG activity is also influenced by the rate at which the muscles shorten.[141] This effect can be accounted for by repeating the EMG–extensor moment calibrations at a range of different contraction speeds, using an isokinetic dynamometer.[358] Forces associated with an upwards thrust by the legs on the spine, and acting in the direction of the long axis of the spine, must be measured separately using a force plate, but these 'hidden' inertial forces are generally only 2–4% of the maximum spinal compressive force.[365]

The main advantage of this EMG approach is that it requires no minimising principles, and it accounts directly for the variable effects of muscle length and contraction velocity on the EMG–moment relationship. It also measures antagonistic muscle activity, because any contractions

of the abdominal muscles cause a compensatory increase in erector spinae activity which is detected by the EMG electrodes.[365,899] The technique is portable and particularly well suited for measuring spinal compression in the workplace, especially when there are rapid movements of the trunk. It has been developed to include bilateral EMG recordings, which makes it suitable for investigating asymmetric lifting tasks,[364,1158] and it could be extended to record from the abdominal muscles also. The technique's main drawback is the inherent variability of EMG signals, which may be attributable to varying recruitment strategies for individual motor units within a large muscle.[745]

Comparison between direct EMG and linked-segment model techniques

In an attempt to validate the two main approaches for measuring spinal compression during dynamic lifting activities, a three-dimensional linked-segment model and the direct EMG technique were applied simultaneously to a group of volunteers.[365,745] Both techniques demonstrated similar increases in spinal loading in response to changes in the load lifted, the speed of lifting or the technique of lifting. However, the EMG model consistently predicted higher extensor moments than the linked-segment model. In the less arduous lifts (6.7 kg lifted slowly and without any trunk rotation), the EMG predictions were approximately 8% greater,[745] and this could be due to differences in the anthropometric assumptions of the two models.[364] However, in the most arduous lifts (15.7 kg lifted rapidly with 90° of trunk rotation), the EMG predictions were up to 40% higher. Some of this large difference may be due to varying amounts of electrical filtering applied in the two techniques, and some would have been due to antagonistic muscle activity.

Compressive loading in vivo

Nachemson's revised measurements of intradiscal pressure[1022] and subsequent experiments[1250] indicate that the

107

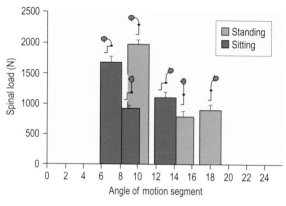

Figure 9.7 Intradiscal pressures measured in different standing and sitting postures in vivo. *(Reproduced from Sato et al.[1250] with permission.)*

compressive force on the lumbar spine rises from about 150 to 250 N when lying, to 500–800 N when standing erect, 700–1000 N when sitting erect and 1900 N when stooping to lift a 10-kg weight (Fig. 9.7). The higher compressive force during sitting (when the normal lumbar lordosis is flattened) can be explained in two ways: some back muscles are more highly activated in upright unsupported sitting postures than in standing,[362] and tension is increased in the stretched posterior ligaments of the spine whenever the spine is flexed (Table 13.1). A study on a single volunteer reported similar intradiscal pressures in standing and sitting, and suggested that the higher levels in sitting recorded by Nachemson may be an artefact caused by bending of the pressure-sensitive needle.[1565]

Results from EMG-assisted linked-segment models suggest that spinal compression at L4–5 rises to approximately 4 kN and 5.5 kN when healthy young men lift weights of 14 kg and 29 kg respectively[1155] and that about 20% of this is due to inertial forces.[946] These values are similar to those obtained using the direct EMG approach[363] but lower than those calculated by early moment-arm models which assumed that the lever arm of the back muscles was only 5 cm,[264] rather than the 6–8 cm currently accepted.[948] Complete time histories of spinal loading during dynamic lifting tasks are shown in Figure 9.8.

Antagonistic contraction of the abdominal muscles (sometimes called 'co-contraction') increases the stability of the trunk[472,521] but at the cost of increasing spinal compression by up to 45% during simulated lifting movements.[520] This high figure is applicable to semiupright postures which require considerable stabilising muscle activity. When the spine is more flexed and stabilised by a tensioned lumbodorsal fascia, antagonistic muscle activity in the abdominal muscles tends to be slight and have little influence on spinal compression.[1399] A vibrating environment increases spinal compression largely by increasing stabilising muscle tension, and effects can be large near the spine's resonant frequency of 4 Hz.[120]

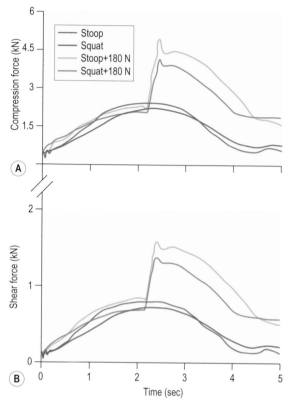

Figure 9.8 Dynamic forces acting on the L5–S1 disc during lifting. Graphs show the calculated compressive force (A) and the anterior shear force (B) for four trials: stoop and squat lifting actions with no weight, and stoop and squat lifts of a 180-N (40-lb) weight positioned 20 cm above the ground. Forces are normal and tangential to the disc mid-plane. *(Adapted from Bazrgari et al.[119] with permission.)*

During forward-bending and lifting tasks, compressive forces due to muscle tension are influenced by factors such as the mass and position of the load lifted, the amount of asymmetry and the technique and speed of lifting.[358,363,41 6,462,520,1291] The direct EMG approach was used to compare the effects of all these factors on a group of 21 young men who lifted various objects from the ground.[363] The peak compressive force on the lumbosacral disc increased from approximately 2.5 kN when lifting 10 kg to 5.0 kN when lifting 30 kg. Increasing the distance of a 10-kg weight from the feet, from 0 cm to 60 cm, increased the peak compressive force from 2.8 kN to 5.2 kN, and lifting 10 kg quickly (in 1 second) increased the peak compressive force to 5.3 kN compared to 3.2 kN when the lift was performed slowly over 4 seconds (Fig. 9.9). Lifting with the knees bent increased the compressive force slightly compared to straight-leg ('stoop') lifts, possibly because bent knees can prevent the lifter getting close to a bulky weight on the ground. More generally, however, dynamic analyses

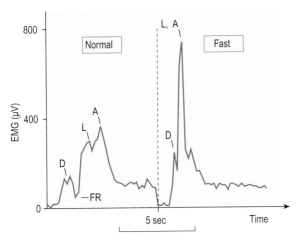

Figure 9.9 A subject bent forwards to lift a 10-kg weight from the ground at normal speed, and then as quickly as possible. Electromyographic (EMG) activity was averaged from electrodes overlying the erector spinae at T10 and L3. At normal speed, the first EMG peak (D), which represents deceleration of the upper body, is followed by a brief spell of flexion relaxation (FR). The following peaks represent lifting the weight off the ground (L), and accelerating the body and weight upwards (A). During the fast lift, L and A coincide, and the EMG peak is doubled After correcting the EMG signal for the effects of contraction velocity, this still indicates a 60% increase in spinal compression. *(Data from Dolan et al.[363])*

show that squat lifting reduces spinal compression and shear compared to stoop lifting,[119] as shown in Figure 9.8. In the workplace, manual handling tasks often combine several of the factors considered above, so that compressive loading would be particularly high when bulky objects are lifted rapidly from an awkward position relative to the lifter's feet.

Peak forces are not directly proportional to the weight lifted, because much of the muscle tension is generated to lift the weight of the upper body, which is usually much heavier than the weight being lifted. Similar trends were observed in 18 female subjects, but the overall forces were reduced by an amount which reflected their smaller upper body mass and shorter limbs.[363] Lifting with a rotated trunk (bending forwards and to one side) has little effect on the peak spinal compressive force as inferred from the 'total moment' generated by the back muscles.[747] However, this experimental approach neglects antagonistic activity from the abdominal muscles, and there is other evidence that lifting in a plane rotated by 45° or more increases antagonistic muscle forces[520,810] and therefore increases spinal compression.[360]

Values of peak compressive forces measured in these studies are approximately 50–70% of the ultimate compressive strength of cadaveric lumbar spines of similar age

and gender so they would not be expected to cause injury.[13] However, repetitive loading can damage cadaveric specimens at 40–50% of their ultimate compressive strength (Table 11.2), so compressive fatigue damage might be expected to accumulate at forces above 4 kN in a typical young man. It appears, therefore, that a change in just one variable factor (weight, distance or speed) can be enough to raise the estimated peak compressive force above the 4-kN threshold for fatigue damage during manual handling. Evidently, the risk of compressive back injury in the workplace depends on more factors than just the weight of the object lifted.

Many reported low-back symptoms are associated with sudden and alarming events[886] such as stumbling while carrying a heavy weight, or misjudging the weight of an object to be lifted. Under these circumstances, muscles can overreact and apply unnecessarily high forces to the spine.[121,351,882,1560] Typically, an experimental study showed that peak spinal compression during manual handling was increased by 30–70% when the subjects were alarmed.[899] It made little difference whether or not they were blindfolded, suggesting that the increased spinal loading was largely due to compensatory reflex contractions of the trunk muscles caused by stimulation of muscle spindles and Golgi tendon organs (Ch. 14). Even if an unknown load proves to be lighter than expected, it can lead to increased anticipatory muscle activity prior to lifting, and a faster, less-controlled movement during the lift.[351] Because of the risks to human volunteers, the experiments described above examined rather conservative loading regimes. However, a simulation study predicted spinal compressive forces up to 13 kN when an applied load of 40 kg or more was dropped into the hands.[65] Evidently, trying to catch a heavy falling object (such as a patient) could injure even a healthy back.

SHEAR

The shear force resisted by the osteoligamentous spine has never been measured in vivo. It is probably higher at the lowest lumbar levels where the discs are inclined at a steep angle to the horizontal so that a substantial component of the gravitational forces acts to shear the joint (Fig. 9.1). If the lumbosacral disc is inclined at 30° to the horizontal, the weight of the upper body will give rise to an intervertebral shear force of approximately 190 N. This increases in stooped postures, and when weights are carried, and is estimated to oscillate between 380 and 760 N when a man marches with a heavy backpack.[313] This is a 'worst-case' analysis, and other models based on detailed anatomical observations and EMG recordings suggest that shear is limited to 250 N by back muscle activity.[874,1157] Co-contraction of the abdominal muscles has been reported to increase shear by up to 70%.[520]

BENDING

Measuring spinal bending

The bending moment acting on the osteoligamentous lumbar spine plays a major role in damaging the intervertebral discs and ligaments (Ch. 11), yet few attempts have been made to measure it in vivo. Ligament forces have been calculated by some mathematical models, but the predictions are based on many assumptions[67,943] and the results can be inconsistent.[1155] A more straightforward approach is to compare lumbar flexion movements measured in vivo with the bending stiffness properties of the lumbar spine measured in vitro.[13]

In this technique, the bending moment acting on the spine in vivo is determined from dynamic measurements of lumbar flexion. Flexion can be measured using an electromagnetic tracking device, the 3-Space Isotrak (Polhemus, Vermont), which records lumbar curvature between L1 and S1 up to 60 times per second during dynamic activities (Fig. 9.10). Values of peak lumbar flexion are expressed as a percentage of the individual's in vivo range of flexion between the erect standing and fully flexed (toe-touching) positions (Fig. 13.3). These normalised flexion values are then compared with normalised bending–stiffness curves for cadaveric osteoligamentous lumbar spines[13] (Fig. 9.11). The normalised bending–stiffness curve takes into account the different flexibilities and strengths of different spines, and allows the bending moment in vivo to be quantified with an accuracy of ±8% of the bending moment required to cause the first signs of damage to a motion segment (i.e. ± 5 Nm for a typical young man). The technique can be summarised by the equation:

$$M = 0.1 \times (0.093V - 2.25)^3$$

where M is the bending moment expressed as a percentage of that required to bend a motion segment right up to the elastic limit, and V is the flexion angle measured in vivo, expressed as a percentage of the full range from erect standing to full flexion. M can be converted into absolute units by multiplying by 60 Nm, which is the approximate strength in bending of an average cadaver lumbar spine.

Spinal bending in vivo

Bending moments on the spine during manual handling

Results obtained using the above technique indicate that peak bending moments are about 10 Nm when lifting a 10-kg weight with the knees bent, and 19 Nm when lifting with the knees straight.[363] Bending forwards and to one

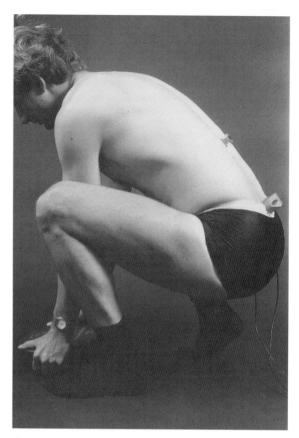

Figure 9.10 It is normal to flex the lumbar spine substantially when lifting weights from the ground, even if the knees are bent. Here, lumbar flexion is measured using the 3-Space Isotrak device mounted over the spinous processes of L1 and S1/S2. Comparison with Figure 13.3C indicates that the lumbar lordosis has been eliminated, so that the lower back is flat.

side increases the bending moment on the lumbar spine by up to 30% compared to lifting in the sagittal plane,[363] probably because a smaller proportion of the movement can be accommodated by the pelvis. In bent-knee squat lifts, increasing the mass of the load from '0 kg' (a pen) to 20 kg increased the bending moment from 7.5 Nm to 13 Nm, whereas increasing the distance of a 10-kg load from the body increased peak bending moment up to 20 Nm (calculated from Dolan et al.[363]). Preliminary data indicate that lifting style also influences bending moments on the thoracic spine.[498]

When do bending moments rise to high levels?

Evidently, spinal bending during lifting depends on several variable factors, but it is noteworthy that none of these

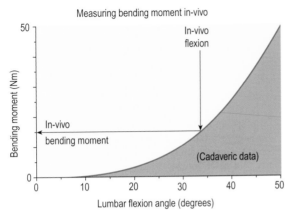

Measuring bending moment in-vivo

Figure 9.11 Composite bending stiffness curve for a cadaveric lumbar spine L1–S1. Values of lumbar flexion measured in vivo can be compared to this curve in order to estimate the bending moment acting on the spine in vivo. Note that the bending moment doubles over the last 10° of flexion. *(After Adams and Dolan.[13])*

factors caused the peak bending moment to exceed 25 Nm, which is 40% of its value at the elastic limit. It seems that the back muscles adequately protect the spine from excessive bending during moderate lifting tasks, at least in the group of young, healthy subjects who took part in the aforementioned experiments.[363] However, average values can conceal valuable information: several of the volunteers consistently flexed so far that the estimated peak bending stresses exceeded 50% of the value at the elastic limit. These subjects actually flexed further forwards during the dynamic lifting tasks than when attempting to reach full flexion in a static posture, so that peak flexion values were up to 115% of their normal range. It would be expected that these individuals, who possibly had impaired proprioceptive or motor function (Ch. 14), would be more likely to sustain fatigue damage to spinal tissues during repetitive bending and lifting tasks. A prospective epidemiological study showed that people who applied most bending to their spine during arduous laboratory lifting tasks were indeed more likely to develop back pain in the follow-up period.[898]

Peak bending moments acting on the lumbar spine rise to higher levels in people with poor spinal mobility, and are lower than normal in those who are particularly supple.[357] This could explain why limited lumbar mobility predicted future back pain in a prospective study of nurses and other healthcare professionals.[36] The peak bending moment can also increase when particularly heavy or large objects are lifted, or when the bending movement is forwards and to one side.[357,363] Rapid flexion movements are resisted more strongly by the spine so peak bending moments in vitro increase by 10–15%.[14] Sudden and

alarming incidents can increase spinal bending, especially when the trunk muscles are not preactivated.[789,899]

High lumbar flexion during lifting means that non-contractile tissues contribute to the total extensor moment. When a 10-kg weight is lifted from the floor using the stoop (straight-leg) and squat (bent-leg) techniques, the 'passive' contribution is approximately 20% and 30% respectively.[366] This can be reduced if the weight is lifted from a convenient height off the ground.[276] Only a small proportion of the 'passive' extensor moment can be attributed to the intervertebral discs and ligaments (Fig. 9.4) so most of it must be due to tension in the lumbodorsal fascia,[1411] the supraspinous ligament,[1016] and non-contractile tissue in the muscles themselves.[721]

Dangers of sustained and repeated bending

During repetitive lifting, fatigue of the quadriceps muscles and/or back muscles is associated with increased lumbar flexion[359,1156,1428] and increased bending moments on the lumbar spine.[359] Prolonged sitting or standing in flexed postures causes creep in spinal ligaments and fascia,[944] and just 5 minutes of this creep (simulated in vitro) is enough to reduce by 40% the ability of intervertebral ligaments to protect the discs in bending.[14]

Sustained and repetitive flexion can also compromise the protective action of the back muscles, which normally contract automatically in response to signals from mechanoreceptor afferents in spinal ligaments, fascia and muscles (Ch. 14). So, when a person bend forwards to lift an object from the ground, a sudden burst of back muscle activity decelerates the upper body (Fig. 9.9) and prevents excessive lumbar flexion.[358] However, experiments on anaesthetised cats have shown that repeated stretching of the supraspinous ligament over a period of 10 minutes almost eliminates reflex contraction of the back muscles.[1344] A similar effect was noted after just 3 minutes of simulated sustained flexion.[1572] Full recovery of the protective muscle reflex can take several hours[485] and full creep recovery takes even longer.[1342] This loss of reflexive muscle activity can probably be explained in terms of time-dependent changes in the viscoelastic tissues of the spine as a result of creep. Creep allows strain to increase progressively as a function of time. As a result, the close correspondence between tissue stress and strain is removed and this may impair the sensitivity of mechanoreceptors to stretch.

In humans, trunk flexion following creep would also activate muscle spindles, and their afferent signals could possibly compensate for any loss of sensitivity in ligamentous mechanoreceptors. However, another study in cats showed that afferent output from muscle spindles was similarly reduced in response to sustained stretches of the paraspinal muscles, provided that the muscles were in a lengthened position.[482] This could explain why prolonged sitting in a flexed posture impairs spinal proprioception in humans, and delays the activation of the erector spinae muscles during subsequent forward-bending tasks (Ch. 14). It appears that prolonged flexion can reduce the ability of the back muscles to protect the lumbar spine from excessive bending, thereby increasing the risk of bending injury to the intervertebral discs and ligaments.

Diurnal variations in bending moment

Although prolonged spinal flexion can increase the risk of bending injury, prolonged compressive loading has the opposite effect. Compressive loading expels water from the discs, reducing their height, and also their resistance to bending (Fig. 13.18). Muscles appear not to compensate for this by allowing proportionally more spinal flexion,[18] so peak bending moments acting on the osteoligamentous spine fall considerably. This can be viewed in reverse: in the first few hours of each day, the discs are swollen with water and peak bending moments acting on the spine are approximately 100% higher than later in the day.[360] This phenomenon is described in more detail in Chapter 13.

TORSION

The lumbar spine is subjected to torsion during activities such as golf and discus throwing, and small coupled axial rotation movements generally accompany lateral bending movements.[1116] However, very little is known about the torsional stresses acting on the spine in vivo. Trunk muscles can exert torsional moments of 50–80 Nm about the long axis of the spine[942] with the back muscles contributing approximately 5 Nm.[875] These same muscles would be expected to protect the underlying spine from any externally applied torque (perhaps applied to an outstretched arm), but the extent to which they do this is difficult to quantify.

In theory, it should be possible to measure torsional stresses in vivo by measuring axial rotation movements and comparing them with the torque rotation properties of cadaveric spines. However, in practice this approach has considerable difficulties. The full range of axial rotation in vivo is only about 1° to each side for each lumbar level (Fig. 10.2), and in this range, torsional stresses acting on the posterior annulus of the disc are minimal (p. 147). However, contact stresses in the apophyseal joints, and hence the axial torque on the spine, rise rapidly with increasing angle of rotation,[26] so a small experimental error in the measurement of angular rotation would lead to a large error in the prediction of torque. Because skin movements lead to gross overestimates of axial rotation when measured by skin surface techniques,[1112] this makes any attempt to predict torque from skin surface measurements unfeasible. More accurate measurements of axial rotation can be obtained by inserting pins into the spinous processes (p. 118), but this invasive procedure could inhibit normal movement patterns.

In cadaveric specimens, torsional damage is first detectable at a torque of 15–30 Nm,[26] so this is probably the upper bound of torque acting in vivo. The normal in vivo range of bending moment appears to be approximately 40% of the bending moment required to cause damage[363], so if a similar safety margin is applicable to torsion, that would suggest maximal torques of approximately 6–12 Nm acting on the lumbar spine in life.

Evidently, the precise torque acting on the osteoligamentous spine during vigorous activities remains elusive, and is likely to remain so. Nevertheless, non-invasive measurements of axial rotation[423,1112] do give some comparative measure of torque on the spine, which may be sufficient for occupational studies attempting to assess the risks for low-back pain.[924]

Chapter | **10**

Mechanical function of the thoracolumbar spine

INTRODUCTION

This chapter describes how the spine 'works' during normal daily life, and explains the mechanical function of each component part. Mechanical damage is considered separately in Chapter 11, and a discussion of how posture affects spine mechanical function is included in Chapter 13. Most of the data refers to the lumbar spine, but many details can be extrapolated to thoracic levels if due allowance is made for their smaller size (which makes them weaker) and narrower discs (which makes them less mobile). This generalisation is consistent with a recent matched comparison of four-vertebra specimens, from T1–4, T5–8, T9–12 and L1–4 spinal levels, that were all subjected to the same small bending moments and torques.[233] Cervical spine mechanics are considered separately in Chapter 12.

To a certain extent, spinal function can be inferred from a careful consideration of anatomy, and this is why form and function were described together in Chapters 2 and 3. However, this is not always good enough, because some 'common-sense' inferences regarding mechanical function can be misleading, and often it is difficult to decide between two equally plausible explanations of how something works (or fails to work) without detailed quantitative information. For example, to appreciate the relative role of the lumbar discs and ligaments in resisting torsional stresses, it is necessary to compare the amplitude of axial rotation movements measured in vivo with torsional stiffness data obtained from cadaveric spines in vitro. Only then is it possible to infer the relative loading of certain structures, or to specify at what angle of rotation a given structure begins to resist strongly.

WHY IS THE SPINE CURVED?

The purpose of the S-shaped curvature of the spine in the sagittal plane (Fig. 10.1) is not straightforward. The cervical lordosis develops when an infant first lifts its head to move around, and the lumbar lordosis follows when the child starts to walk upright. A lumbar lordosis can be induced artificially in growing monkeys and rats by forcing them to walk on their hind legs.[258,1160] It appears therefore that spinal curves have 'something to do' with locomotion in upright posture. But what?

Spinal curves are not required to give a level line of sight during upright walking, because a straight spine would do that just as well. To a certain extent, the curves provide rotational stability in the sagittal plane by distributing body mass away from the straight line between skull and pelvis. This mechanism can be likened to a tight-rope walker extending his arms out sideways to reduce side-to-side wobble. In both cases, distributing body mass away

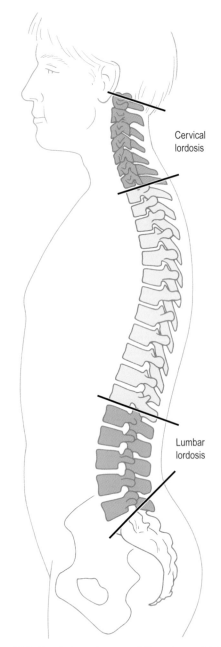

Figure 10.1 The S-shaped curves of the spine assist in shock absorption during locomotion. See text for details.

from a central axis of rotation increases the moment of inertia about that axis, and therefore makes it easier to maintain balance. In addition, a lumbar lordosis increases motion coupling in the lumbar spine (for example, linking lateral bending with axial rotation[275]) and this has been proposed as a fundamental mechanism to facilitate pelvic movements during locomotion.[516] However, the soldier's habit of swinging the arms backwards and forwards when marching can achieve pelvic rotation just as well.

The most important function of the spinal curves is revealed by the manner in which they vary during the walking cycle. Sagittal-plane curves increase and decrease during every stride, with an amplitude of approximately 1–2° per lumbar level.[1392] This suggests that the curved spine can absorb and release energy during each stride, somewhat in the manner of a bed spring. Generally, a curved shape allows a compressed structure to be deformed in bending, rather than pure compression, and this in turn enables it to act as a shock absorber.

But this is still not the whole story, because flexion–extension movements of only 1–2° per lumbar level are resisted very little by the spine, so spinal tissues themselves are unable to absorb much strain energy.[60] This is perhaps just as well, because a proportion of absorbed strain energy is always lost as heat (this is hysteresis energy: Fig. 1.5), and the avascular discs would find it difficult to dissipate much heat during vigorous exercise. Very large and poorly vascularised tendons in the legs of race horses have a similar problem, so that exercise-induced temperature rises may cause degenerative changes within them.[1579] The usefulness of the spinal curvature during locomotion becomes apparent when it is realised that large muscles of the back and abdomen must be working vigorously to oppose gross changes in spinal curvature, in much the same way that the quadriceps and calf muscles oppose knee and ankle flexion.[59] Substantial antagonistic activity of the trunk muscles in supporting the upright spine has been measured using electomyography[520] and can be inferred from measurements of intradiscal pressure.[1022] The stretched tendons of these trunk muscles are the real spinal shock absorbers. The importance of musculotendinous shock absorption can be appreciated by jumping off a chair and landing with straight legs and back: the elasticity of discs, bones and articular cartilage could do little to protect from a damaging impact unless the body's joints were allowed to flex, against the resistance of their muscles. The experiment is better imagined than performed!

Spinal curves, therefore, allow some of the energy associated with up-and-down movements of locomotion to be absorbed by the tendons of trunk muscles and, to a lesser extent, by the ligaments and discs of the spine itself. In this way, they reduce the vertical accelerations which would otherwise be transmitted from the pelvis to the skull. These mechanisms could also operate when a person sits on a vibrating surface such as a tractor seat, although most sitting postures involve some reduction of the spinal curves (Ch. 13), so the shock absorption would be less. During static postures, either sitting or standing, there is no obvious benefit to be gained from the spinal curvature. It has been suggested that a lumbar lordosis strengthens the spine by allowing it to behave as an arch,[87] but the conclusions of this paper have been questioned.[5]

There has been considerable recent interest in the sagittal alignment of the whole spine and pelvis during upright standing. Associations have been demonstrated between thoracic kyphosis, lumbar lordosis, inclination of the sacral table, pelvic tilt, sagittal offset and 'pelvic incidence', which is an anatomical characteristic of the pelvis (Fig. 8.5).[863,173,864] Some of these angles change slightly with growth and ageing,[863,864] as described in Chapter 8. They can also differ in patients with disc degeneration[568] and osteogenesis imperfecta,[2] although it is difficult to discern cause from effect. Obviously, surgical disturbance to one or more of these angles is likely to cause compensatory changes in other angles if the spine is to maintain its overall upright balance, with muscle activity minimised.

MOVEMENTS OF THE LUMBAR SPINE

Range of movement: radiographs, CT, MRI and implanted pins

The range of spinal movements can be measured in vivo accurately using stereo radiographs[1110,1369] and three-dimensional magnetic resonance imaging (MRI),[455] and average values for young men are given in Figure 10.2. Broadly similar in vivo results have been reported for T11–L1.[488] The overall range of sagittal-plane movement is approximately 14° at most lumbar levels, although the changing proportions of flexion and extension indicate that the reference position (erect standing) involves more extension at L3–4 and L4–5 than at other lumbar levels.

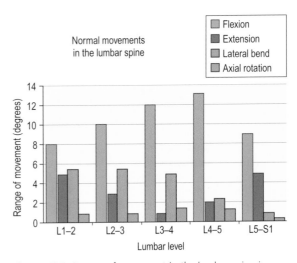

Figure 10.2 Ranges of movement in the lumbar spine in healthy young men: data from bilateral X-rays.[1110,1116] Values for lateral bending and axial rotation are averaged for movements to the left and right of the neutral position (relaxed standing).

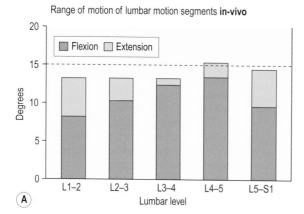

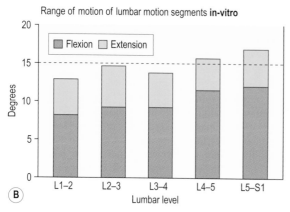

Figure 10.3 (A) Ranges of sagittal-plane movement in young men as measured by bilateral X-rays.[1110] The reduced range of extension at L3–4 and L4–5 suggests that these levels were already extended in the reference position, which was erect standing. (B) Ranges of movement for cadaveric spines of similar age. Overall mobility is similar to that in (A), but there is rather more extension in the cadaveric spines, presumably because their reference position (unloaded) involves some flexion compared to the reference position for living people (erect standing).

Figure 10.3 compares flexion-extension in vivo with values obtained from cadaveric spines which have been flexed and extended right up to the elastic limit of their ligaments. The similarity between in vivo and in vitro ranges of movement suggests that healthy people can flex and extend their lumbar spine close to their ligamentous limits, although the back muscles normally provide a small margin of safety in full flexion.[13,32]

Lateral bending movements are slightly less than in the sagittal plane, especially at L5–S1 (Fig. 10.2). Axial rotation movements of the lumbar spine are barely larger than the errors in the techniques used to measure them, but their small size (approximately 1–2° to each side at each spinal level[455,1116]) has been confirmed by a variety of techniques.[488,1060,1358]

Range of movement: skin surface techniques

Assessment of techniques

Invasive techniques can be used on small groups of subjects, but other methods must be devised to characterise the effects of age, gender, pathology and physical training on spinal range of movement. Most of these methods use devices attached to the surface of the back. Devices such as inclinometers and flexicurves which measure spinal curvature directly agree well with radiographic measurements of vertebral rotations, with small systematic errors, and correlation coefficients greater than 0.9.[20,1251] Accuracy is better for flexion than for extension.[1251] Reported disagreements between skin surface measurements and radiographs in one particular study can be attributed to the measurements being taken at different times in different postures.[1365] It is important to realise that it is difficult for a supple person to flex the lumbar spine fully while sitting in a chair with the knees flexed.[1169] Skin-stretching as measured by the Schober test does not correlate well with radiographic measurements of mobility.[368,1150] Schober measurements are unreliable[982,1150] and are affected by body weight, lumbar lordosis and trunk length.[36,967] The electromagnetic 3-Space Isotrak device can give accurate values of lumbar flexion if it is mounted on the back with its electrical cables running horizontally,[357,368] but if the cables run over the shoulders then flexion movements tend to be exaggerated,[612] possibly because the cable tilts the sensor. Isotrak measurements of lateral bending appear reasonable, but measurements of axial rotation must include large movements of the skin and thorax because they greatly overestimate the movements measured by radiographs.[1112] Optical movement analysis devices can track the position of skin-mounted markers with considerable accuracy, but the computed values of spine angular movement do not agree closely with radiographs.[1114]

Variations in lumbar mobility with age and gender

Skin surface measurements[223,384,1381] and radiographs[137] indicate that sagittal mobility decreases with age, especially in the upper lumbar spine (Ch. 8). Mobility in the frontal plane also decreases with age, but axial rotation appears to be unaffected.[950] Gender differences in the full range of sagittal movement are generally small,[384] although women extend more from the standing position, whereas men flex more.[223,383,1381]

Other influences on lumbar mobility

African-American women appear to have an increased range of lumbar extension (but not flexion) compared to white American women.[1435] More generally, genetic inheritance influences the range of flexion and extension, probably because genes influence body weight and disc degeneration which then impact on mobility.[112] Increasing body mass index (an indicator of obesity) tends to reduce lumbar mobility.[137] Mobility measurements must be taken according to a strict time protocol, because during sustained or repeated flexion, the restraining ligaments 'creep', allowing in vivo flexion angles to increase by 5–10% in just a few minutes.[359,944] Attention must also be paid to the time of day, because fluid expulsion from the discs increases the range of spinal flexion (Fig. 13.18). For the whole lumbar spine, the diurnal increase in flexion is 5–6.5° in healthy subjects[18,384] and 11° in back pain patients.[398] The range of lateral bending also tends to increase as the day progresses,[384] but the range of extension is unaffected.[398]

The range of axial rotation is decreased in stooped postures because the increased forward shear force presses the apophyseal joint surfaces firmly together.[541] It has been suggested that flexion could increase the range of axial rotation by allowing more 'free play' to the tapered inferior articular processes,[1112] but the Isotrak measurements in support of this theory contain large artefacts.

Appropriate physical training can increase the range of lumbar flexion and lateral bending in adults by 5% and 9% respectively,[1588] but it seems unlikely that lumbar extension can be increased much.[794] The evident suppleness of certain athletes and dancers is mostly attributable to increased flexibility of their hamstring muscles.[794]

Patterns of movement

Centre of rotation

During spinal flexion, extension and lateral bending, adjacent vertebrae do not simply rotate about the centre of the nucleus pulposus as if it were a rigid pivot or ball bearing. Instead, the annulus fibrosus and intervertebral ligaments undergo complex deformations which cause the vertebrae to glide past each other as they angulate. Such complex movements can be described as rotations only if the instantaneous centre of rotation (CoR), or notional pivot, is itself allowed to move around. For a small incremental movement, the location of this CoR can be calculated as shown in Figure 10.4. During a more substantial movement, the proportions of compression and bending acting on the spine will vary continuously, and so will the proportions of sliding and rotational movement. This causes the position of the CoR to vary also, so it is usual to speak of the locus or path taken by the CoR during the movement. It is difficult to locate this moving centre accurately, and experimental errors may partly explain the long and tortuous locus reported for the CoR in some spines.[489] For practical purposes, it is best to define an ellipse (or three-dimensional ellipsoid) which contains the entire path of the CoR, and then average the data over a group of healthy people (Fig. 10.5). According to experimental

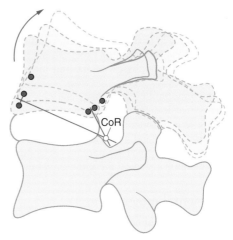

Figure 10.4 The position of the centre of rotation (CoR) during an intervertebral movement can be calculated by drawing straight lines between the initial and final positions of two anatomical landmarks on adjacent vertebrae. Then perpendicular bisectors of these lines are drawn, and where these two bisectors meet is the CoR.[1113] In life, the position of the CoR varies continuously during most movements, and the above procedure must be repeated for each increment of movement.

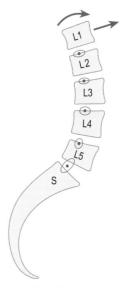

Figure 10.5 During sagittal-plane movements, the centre of rotation (CoR: see Fig. 10.4) moves around the intervertebral disc, normally within the limits shown by the ellipses, and with average positions shown by the blue dots. Each vertebra effectively moves by a combination of pure rotation and translation (or sliding) as indicated for L1. *(Data from Pearcy and Bogduk.[1113])*

data[489] and mathematical models,[1264] lumbar CoRs lie below the centre of the disc during small movements, and migrate anteriorly in flexion, and posteriorly in extension. In degenerated cadaveric spines, CoRs can migrate posteriorly towards the apophyseal joints, and inferiorly into the vertebral body.[1627]

CoRs are important because they determine how compressive and tensile deformations vary across the disc, and between various ligaments. However, they cannot be measured accurately, and are inherently variable because they depend on the relative amounts of compression, shear and bending acting on the spine at any moment.

Intersegmental movements

The time course of lumbar flexion or extension movements during simple bending and lifting tasks has been measured using a variety of techniques. The best is videofluoroscopy, which is effectively a continuous X-ray image recorded by a video camera. It is invasive, and the image enhancement techniques required to obtain sharp pictures reduce sampling frequency to 2.5–5 Hz.[708,1066] This technique has shown that, when healthy subjects bend forwards slowly from the upright position, the initial and final movement must take place in the hips, and that lumbar flexion usually either starts in the upper lumbar spine and spreads smoothly to the lower levels,[708] or else all levels flex at the same time. No particular pattern predominates in the lumbar spine when subjects straighten up again,[1066] and no contrary or 'paradoxical' movements at individual lumbar levels were observed.[708] Translational (gliding) movements between adjacent vertebrae were 1.1–3.3 mm in flexion, and 0.3–1.3 mm in extension.[708] Videofluoroscopy has also shown that expert weight lifters flex their lumbar spine when lifting a bar bell from the ground, sometimes by a considerable amount.[276]

Patterns of intersegmental movement have also been studied using skin-mounted devices or markers, but errors arising from skin movement artifact may explain why movements of individual vertebrae appear inconsistent.[480] Oscillating intervertebral movements during treadmill walking have an amplitude of 1–2° per lumbar level in both the sagittal and frontal planes, and a similar movement appears to occur at the hips.[1392]

Coupled movements

Any primary movement of the spine deforms the intervertebral discs and ligaments, and may cause the neural arches to make contact with each other. Because the materials properties of spinal structures vary from place to place, and because the geometry of the neural arch is so irregular, the primary movement usually creates small coupled movements in other planes, as the spine bends and twists in order to minimise resistance to the primary movement. For example, a primary movement in lateral

bending may cause the bony surfaces in one of the apophyseal joints to meet at an oblique angle, and this would cause one vertebra to move in the direction of this contact force. Generally, coupled movements measured in vitro are small, inconsistent and depend on posture.[275,1096] In living people they are small and probably modified by muscle action.[455,1116] However, consistent motion coupling has been measured in living people by inserting steel pins into the L3 and L4 spinous processes of healthy volunteers: primary movements in lateral bending were consistently coupled with small twisting movements to the opposite side, and with some flexion.[488,1358]

Movements of the whole lumbar spine

Skin surface measurements of overall movement between L1 and S1 made with the Isotrak show that, when people lift weights from the floor, they flex their lumbar spine by 85–105% of the range between upright standing and full flexion.[13,363,366] Subjects with poor spinal mobility often exceed 100% of their static range of flexion[357] and this is not a contradiction in terms, because static limits can be exceeded during dynamic lungeing movements. Even if they bend their knees, normal subjects find it impossible to lift a 10-kg weight without flexing the lumbar spine by more than 50%.[366] When bending forwards from a standing position, with legs straight, the initial angular movement probably starts in the hips[708] but this is soon followed by a phase of motion dominated by lumbar flexion. The contribution from hip flexion then increases and dominates the final phase of movement.[401] Straightening up again with a weight in the hands involves hip extension at first, and then the lumbar spine extends.[1033] When asked to lift a heavy weight while keeping the knees bent, young men tend to raise their hips and straighten their legs first, and then extend the lumbar spine only when the main effort of lifting is over.[325] The thoracic spine does not move much during such activities.[325]

Spinal movements and spinal disorders

Attempts have been made to distinguish between 'normal' and 'back pain' populations on the basis of spinal movements. In general, patients with back pain move more slowly[953] and through a smaller range of movement[227,935,1111,1151] presumably because full-range movements exacerbate their pain. Patients sometimes show abnormal coupling of movements[1369] or show 'steps' in an otherwise smooth movement.[953] Patients with degenerative spondylolisthesis tend to move the slipped level first when bending forwards, sometimes in a disordered way, and when returning to the upright position again the affected level can be slow to extend.[1066] Differences can be demonstrated between different groups of patients as regards their spinal movement patterns[1115,1397] or torque-generating capacity[1043,1044] and those with back pain can be predicted accurately.[145] However, the large variability in mobility and movement patterns found in normal pain-free people makes it difficult to assign an individual patient to a specific diagnostic group on the basis of these measurements.[953]

Movement analysis techniques can also be used to monitor patient progress during rehabilitation.[884,935] Again, the natural variability of spinal movements hinders the identification of significant progress in specific individuals or patient groups. The use of large isoinertial machines to monitor the mobility and strength of patients' backs has been extensively and critically reviewed.[1044]

A restricted range of sagittal-plane movement causes the lumbar spine to be subjected to increased bending stresses,[357] and reduced lumbar mobility increases the risk of future low-back pain.[36] A similar increase in risk is associated with a tendency to bend the lumbar spine more than average when performing standardised lifting tasks in the laboratory.[898] This association could be interpreted in terms of impaired coordination or motor control, and is analogous to the increased risk of knee pain in those people ('microklutzes') who walk heavily.[1178]

TECHNIQUES USED TO INVESTIGATE SPINAL FUNCTION

Our knowledge of spine mechanics is derived mainly from experiments on animals and cadaveric spines, and from mathematical models, so it is appropriate to consider the limitations of these techniques before dealing with the information they produce. The following account is based on a previously published methodological review.[9]

Mechanical testing of cadaveric tissues

Load and loading rate

Most biological tissues are stiffer when high forces are applied to them (i.e. they are non-linear), and they are also stiffer when forces are applied rapidly[14,560] (i.e. they are viscoelastic). It follows that the spine's response to loading depends on the magnitude and rate of loading, so both of these should be as realistic as possible. As described in Chapter 9, the spine is subjected to 3–6 kN of compression and 10 Nm of bending during routine manual handling tasks, and these forces are applied rapidly, typically between 0.2 and 5 seconds. Cadaveric specimens should be loaded with similar severity. Also, the spine's resistance to one form of loading depends on other forces which are applied at the same time (for example, a compressive

preload increases resistance to bending[473,677]) so cadaveric experiments should aim to reproduce the combined complex loading encountered in life. It is not normally necessary to apply separate forces to simulate the action of each individual muscle, because any number of forces acting in the same plane can be represented by a single resultant force (Fig. 10.4), provided that the vertebrae can be assumed to be rigid, which is usually a reasonable approximation. Finally, cadaveric tissues must be protected from dehydration during prolonged testing, but on the other hand, intervertebral disc tissue must not be allowed to come into contact with water unless the disc is under load, because unloaded disc tissue can absorb water and swell to an unphysiological extent.

Centre of rotation

If natural movements of the spine are to be reproduced in cadaver experiments, it is necessary to apply physiologically reasonable complex loading to the specimen and then allow it to deform freely in response to these forces. The apparatus should not seek to impose a fixed CoR (p. 117) about any one position because this would impose abnormal forces on some parts of the specimen. One solution is to apply a pure 'couple' (twisting effect) to a specimen. Another is to apply offset loading, as shown in Figure 10.6. This has the additional benefit of applying compression and shear as well as bending.

Effect of death on the spine's mechanical properties

In this materialistic age, there is no reason to suppose that the moment of death changes the mechanical properties of the spine. Certain changes have been noted when creep tests were performed on pig spines, just before and after death,[728] but similar changes were noted in repeated tests even when the animals did not die in between,[726] so the changes are due, at least in part, to poor reproducibility of the experimental measurements.[8] Respiration may possibly influence the spine's mechanical properties,[728] but this would constitute a very small mechanical perturbation which could be simulated on cadaveric material if considered worthwhile.

Changes in the hours following death

The loss of muscle tension after death reduces loading of the intervertebral discs, allowing them to imbibe water from surrounding tissues. The same physicochemical process causes discs to swell up every night when individuals relax their muscles during sleep, and it is reversed during the following day's activity. It is misleading to talk of a 'normal' or 'physiological' disc hydration because hydration depends on many factors, including loading history and age. Preliminary creep tests can be used to

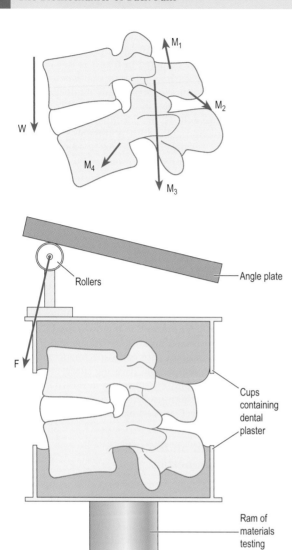

Figure 10.6 (A) The many muscle forces (M), and body weight (W), that act on a lumbar vertebra. In cadaveric experiments, it is convenient to sum all of these forces into a single resultant force (F) which has a specified magnitude, direction and point of application.

bring cadaveric discs into the physiological range before other tests are performed on them.[18,957,1129] The water content of cadaveric discs differs slightly from that of discs removed during anterior fusion operations[694] but it is not clear just how much of the difference is due to postmortem changes, and how much to degenerative changes in the surgically removed discs.[957] Apparent postmortem changes in disc hydration and swelling pressure[694] may be an experimental artifact caused by storing discs for several hours after they have been cut away from the vertebral body: this would cause the nucleus to lose its intrinsic

prestressing by the annulus and ligamentum flavum, and allow a redistribution of water and swelling pressure throughout the disc.[957]

The cooling-down of cadaveric tissues after death influences their mechanical properties. Spinal ligaments shrink slightly at 21 °C so that they are less extensible,[576] and laboratory temperatures reduce the rate of creep in intervertebral discs and tendons by approximately 10–15%.[291,766] Bones are 6% less extensible at 21 °C[1286] and the fatigue life of vertebrae is probably higher at laboratory temperature.[184] Currently we do not know if differential thermal contraction in different spinal tissues leads to a measurable change in load-sharing between them.

Effect of frozen storage on mechanical properties

Frozen storage has a variable effect, generally being greater when freezing is at −20 °C than at −80 °C, and affecting time-dependent creep properties more than elastic. Freeze-thawing at −80 °C has a negligible effect on tensile properties of the annulus,[464] ligaments[1421] or bone.[1286] Freeze-thawing at −20 °C has little effect on ligament[995] or bone.[1029] Nor does it change the compressive stiffness of motion segments[1329] or intradiscal pressure.[1020] Only minor changes in the gross elastic mechanical properties of motion segments occur during subsequent prolonged laboratory testing.[1102] Freeze–thaw cycles at −20 °C lead to faster creep in the highly hydrated discs of young pigs, possibly as a result of minor cracking of the vertebral body endplate[106] or because of increased proteoglycan loss from cartilage after a freeze–thaw cycle,[1629] but this does not happen with mature human discs.[347] Freeze–thawing has been reported to increase the compressive strength of young pig spines by 24%,[238] but this odd result may not be applicable to human discs.

The combined effects of death, cooling and postmortem storage can change certain mechanical properties of cadaveric spines, but these changes are small compared to the differences in mechanical properties between individual spines. Their effects can be minimised in cadaveric experiments by appropriate experimental design: for example, by comparing mechanical properties in the same specimens before and after some planned intervention.

'Motion segment' experiments

Additional problems arise when spines are dissected into 'motion segments' consisting of two vertebrae and the intervening disc and ligaments. The longitudinal and supraspinous ligaments are weakened during dissection because they contain fibres which span several vertebrae and this reduces slightly their resistance to bending.[349] Also, the inferior and superior surfaces of the vertebral bodies of a motion segment must be loaded by rigid plaster or metal plates, rather than by an intervertebral disc. However, this is unlikely to have much effect because compressive failure always occurs in the inner endplates, which are loaded naturally.[186] Testing whole lumbar spine specimens, from L1 to S1, avoids these problems, but it creates others, because a curved lumbar spine buckles when compressed in vitro without any support from living muscles. Buckling can be avoided by using steel cables to simulate the action of individual muscles[1564,1566] or by using cables to follow the line of action of the resultant force from numerous muscles,[1108] but neither of these techniques is suitable for applying high forces in a rapid manner.

Mathematical models

Analytical models

These models are essentially analogies, in which complicated biological structures are likened to simple mechanical devices in order to gain insight into how the biological structure works. For example, an intervertebral disc might be likened to a car tyre in order to explain how disc bulging and height depend on pressure in the nucleus (p. 130).[189] Analytical models usually involve gross simplifications, and this can create problems if the model is used to make quantitative predictions (for example, the angle at which annulus fibres become damaged in torsion[640]).

Finite element models

Finite element (FE) models are quite different. They accurately represent the anatomy of a biological structure by recreating it from large numbers of small blocks of material (Fig. 11.25), each of which is assigned simple materials properties such as 'linear elastic' or 'fluid-like'. Forces are then applied to the outer surfaces of the model and the deformation of each little block (or element) is calculated, and then summed. Because the elements interact with each other, it is necessary to solve a large number of simultaneous equations in order to determine the mechanical response of each element, and hence of the whole structure, and this requires a fast computer. Finally, forces and deformations of particular groups of elements are calculated in order to infer the loading on some substructure of interest. For example, an FE model of a human vertebral column could be used to determine the compressive force acting on a particular apophyseal joint surface. All FE models must be validated by comparing their predictions with known mechanical behaviour, preferably using the same biological specimens in the experiments and when capturing the three-dimensional anatomy for the model. Only then can the predictions of the model be trusted.

The strength of FE models is that they can be used repeatedly to examine the influence of variable factors such as applied load, displacement or angular rotation on the specimen's responses. The variable influences of age, disc height and disc degeneration can be investigated

systematically by repeating the simulations with different materials or geometric properties.[465,854] FE models are therefore ideal for iterative 'what if' studies. Also, they can quantify stress distributions and internal deformations that would be very difficult to measure experimentally.[800,1306]

The main weakness of FE models is that they can predict almost anything. Depending on the rigour of the validation experiments, the modeller can choose between a variety of assumptions, material properties and shapes, until the output of the model appears reasonable. FE models therefore have little true predictive power, and rarely predict anything strikingly new. If they did, they would not be believed! Also, FE models depend on materials properties that must be obtained from cadaver experiments, and so incorporate the same postmortem artefacts. A practical problem is that limited computing power generally compels the modeller to make simplifying assumptions regarding the mechanical behaviour of complex fibre-reinforced composite materials such as the annulus fibrosus. Another practical problem with FE models of the neural arch is that the precise shapes and spacing of the opposing apophyseal joint surfaces have a critical effect on the predicted contact stresses, and reliable input data cannot easily be obtained from cadaveric material.[1304,1307] A more general limitation with some FE models is that they are constructed around the three-dimensional anatomy of a single motion segment, so that their predictions cannot be generalised to other spinal levels, or other spines. Often it is the diversity of mechanical behaviour that explains phenomena of clinical interest.[37] However, it is possible to capture the geometry of several spine specimens in order to model diversity of behaviour as well as typical behaviour.[1208,1384]

Animal models

Some mechanical properties of spinal structures can be assessed in living animals[726,728] but these experiments present severe technical problems, including poor reproducibility.[8] Experiments on animals can be used to demonstrate underlying biological principles within living spinal tissues.[657,851,1081] However, there are problems when interpreting results from small animals to humans,[62,850] including: the easier transportation of metabolites into small animal discs; the cube-square law (p. 7), which explains why structures cannot simply be scaled up unless the materials used to make them also increase in strength; and small interspecies differences in morphology, which affect the magnitude and location of maximum stresses within the structure.[854] The age of experimental animals must also be taken into account, because age greatly affects the distribution of compressive stress within the intervertebral discs (p. 132), and the ability of cartilage cells to respond to mechanical stimuli falls with age.[917]

The above discussion highlights one of the underlying problems with spinal research: only very limited interventions can be contemplated with the spines of living people, so is it often necessary to turn to some cadaveric, mathematical or animal model in order to make progress, and each of these types of model has its strengths, weaknesses and areas of applicability.

VERTEBRAE

Vertebral body

Lumbar vertebral bodies (and the intervening discs) resist most of the compressive force acting down the long axis of the spine, although the proportion decreases with age (Fig. 8.6), and depends on posture and loading history (Ch. 13). Most of the compressive load must be resisted by the dense network of trabeculae, because removal of the outer shell of cortical bone weakens the structure by between 10%[936] and 35–44%.[1615] FE models suggest that the load-bearing role of the vertebral cortex increases in old vertebrae (which lose trabeculae preferentially) and at mid-vertebral body height: typically, in old and osteoporotic vertebrae, the cortex resists 15% of the compressive load close to the endplates, and 45% at mid-body height.[402]

The endplates which mark the boundary with the intervertebral discs are thin plates of cortical bone, perforated by many small holes (Fig. 7.22) which allow the passage of metabolites from bone to the central regions of the avascular discs.[1205,1206] These holes doubtless weaken the endplate, and may explain why it is the most easily damaged structure in the lumbar spine (Ch. 11). Endplate thickness is least in the centre of the endplate, opposite the disc nucleus (Fig. 10.7). Mechanical loading is greatest

in this region (if the disc is non-degenerated), so endplate thickness clearly reflects a trade-off between strength and permeability to nutrients passing from the vertebral body into the disc nucleus.[1628] The superior (cranial) endplate is consistently thinner than the inferior (caudal) endplate of the same vertebral body[642,1203,1628] (Fig. 10.7) and it is supported by less dense trabecular bone.[1628] This assymmery could be explained by the additional loading applied to the lower half of the vertebral body by muscles attached to the neural arch (Fig. 10.6) Not surprisingly, compressive overload usually fractures the cranial endplate, both in vivo and in cadaveric experiments.[1628] Age-related deterioration in vertebral bodies is described on page 93.

Vertebral bodies may possibly be hydraulically strengthened during rapid loading by the blood and marrow trapped inside them, but this theory has not been supported by experimental evidence.[648]

Neural arch

The neural arch is mostly cortical bone, with only a small volume of trabecular bone inside, so it does not weaken as much with age as the vertebral body. Numerous processes serve as attachment points for muscles and for ligaments. If muscle and ligament forces become unbalanced, then the entire neural arch can bend upwards or downwards relative to the body. For example, touching the toes generates high forces in the erector spinae, which pull down on the neural arches of lumbar vertebrae and bend them downwards (in vivo) by 2–3° on average.[529] When full flexion is simulated on cadaveric motion segments, tension in the intervertebral ligaments causes the inferior articular processes to bend forwards and downwards by 1–6° relative to the vertebral body, pivoting about the pars interarticularis.[529] Similarly, in full extension, bony contact between the neural arches bends the inferior articular processes backwards and upwards. The relevance of this to spondylolysis is considered on page 162. The spinous processes can make firm contact in full extension, or following pathological disc narrowing, so that a proportion of the compressive force acting on the spine can be resisted by these 'kissing spines'.[19]

ZYGAPOPHYSEAL JOINTS

Articular surfaces

These small synovial joints have gently curved articulating surfaces (Fig. 10.8A) with an average area of 1.6 cm[2,1387] They stabilise the lumbar spine in compression, and prevent excessive bending and translation (gliding movements) between adjacent vertebrae. Articular cartilage removed from these joints will swell up if it is immersed in saline, suggesting that the joint surfaces are

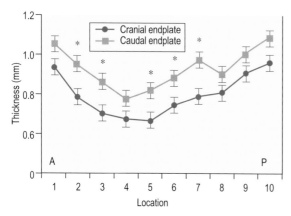

Figure 10.7 Average endplate thickness for caudal and cranial endplates of human thoracolumbar vertebral bodies, aged 48–92 years, measured in the mid-sagittal plane. Both endplates were thinnest in the middle, and at locations marked * caudal endplates were thicker than cranial. Error bars represent the SEM. (Reproduced from Zhao et al.[1628] with permission.)

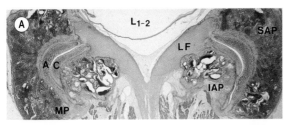

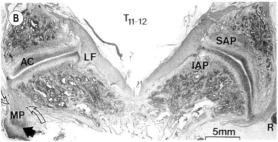

Figure 10.8 Histological sections of zygapophyseal joints, sectioned in the transverse plane (anterior on top). (A) Note the curving joint surfaces covered in articular cartilage (AC) and the thick amorphous ligamentum flavum (LF) which blends in with the anterior margin of the joint capsule. IAP/SAP, inferior/superior articular process. (B) T11–12 joints showing marked asymmetry (tropism) between right and left joints. (Reproduced from Singer KP 1994 Anatomy and biomechanics of the thoracolumbar junction. In: Boyling JD, Palastanga N (eds) Grieve's modern manual therapy, 2nd edn, with permission of Churchill Livingstone, Edinburgh.)

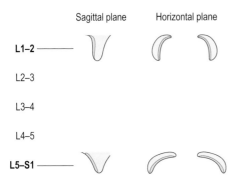

Figure 10.9 The orientation of the apophyseal joints varies with lumbar level, in both the sagittal and horizontal planes. Changes are gradual between L1–2 and L5–S1. Cartilage-covered articular surfaces are shaded.

permanently prestressed in situ,[1422] presumably by the ligamentum flavum. In this manner, they are able to protect the intervertebral discs. The articular surfaces are approximately vertical in the upper lumbar spine, but are more oblique at L4–5 and L5–S1 (Fig. 10.9). This explains why the lower lumbar apophyseal joints resist approximately 20% of the compressive force acting perpendicular to the mid-plane of the discs, while at the upper levels they resist only half as much.[25] Most of the resistance to axial compression comes from the lower margins of the articular surfaces,[380,1304] but with increasing backwards bending, direct extra-articular contact with the inferior lamina can occur.[380,1262] In lordotic (extended) postures, and following pathological disc narrowing, the apophyseal joints can transmit more than 50% of the spinal compressive force from one vertebra to the next (Fig. 8.6). Flexion movements, on the other hand, reduce load-bearing by the neural arches (Table 8.2) and probably cause contact to occur in the superior anteromedial regions of the joint surfaces.[1304]

Lumbar apophyseal joints are best able to resist forces acting perpendicular to their broad articular surfaces, approximately in the plane of the disc. Cadaver experiments[1254] and mathematical models[1264] suggest that these forces vary between 40 and 105 N during simulated postures and movements in vitro. Interfacet forces severely limit the range of axial rotation in the lumbar spine,[26,50,379] with the greatest contact stresses probably occurring in the superior–posterior margins of the joint surfaces,[1304] and they are capable of resisting forward shearing forces of 1 kN each.[318] If the apophyseal joints are asymmetrical in the transverse plane (Fig. 10.8B), then shear induces a small axial rotation.[315] Muscle forces pulling down on the spinous processes may serve to increase the intervertebral shear force resisted by the apophyseal joints according to a 'door knocker' mechanism.[651] This would help to 'lock' the apophyseal joints and enhance their stabilising action in flexed postures.[541]

Joint capsule

The joint capsule consists of a strong outer layer of collagen fibres, 13–20 mm long, and an extensible inner layer containing elastic fibres which are 6–16 mm long.[1602] It is thickest in the inferior margins of the joint, where the fibres are longer and run in a superior-medial to inferior lateral direction. Thickenings of the capsule are often referred to as the 'capsular ligaments' (see below). Full extension can stretch the joint capsule as it resists the backwards rotation of the inferior articular processes about the pars interarticularis[529,1605] and there is some evidence that this can cause back pain.[262] The joint capsule is lined by a thin cellular layer, the synovium, which is responsible for creating and maintaining the synovial fluid that lubricates the joint.

Lubrication

All synovial joints are lubricated by synovial fluid, which ensures that there is little friction or energy loss when the articular surfaces rub against each other. The most

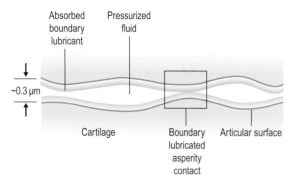

Figure 10.10 Lubrication between opposing cartilage surfaces in a synovial joint: fluid film lubrication is provided by small pockets of pressurised synovial fluid, and boundary lubrication is provided by a lubricant adhering to the asperities of the cartilage surfaces.

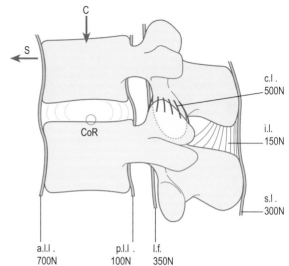

Figure 10.11 Lumbar motion segment, showing typical values (in newtons) for the strengths of intervertebral ligaments (9.81 N = 1 kg). Data compiled from various sourses. CoR, centre of rotation; C, Compression; S, Shear; a.l.l., anterior longitudinal ligament; p.l.l., posterior longitudinal ligament; l.f., ligamentum flavum; c.l., capsular ligaments of the apophyseal joints; i.l., interspinous ligament; s.l., supraspinous ligament.

active ingredient in synovial fluid is hyaluronan,[1586] a long glycoasaminoglycan molecule which attracts water and gives the fluid a thick, slimy consistency which is not easily squeezed out from between the articular surfaces when the joint is loaded. Microscopic undulations in the cartilage surface (Fig. 10.10) help to create pools of synovial fluid which then allow the cartilage surfaces to slide past each other on a thin film of fluid, an effect which is similar to a car tyre aquaplaning on a wet road. This mode of lubrication is referred to as 'fluid film' lubrication, and is very effective at reducing friction if the joint is loaded lightly, and for just a few seconds. Severe and chronic loading, however, squeezes out most of the synovial fluid, so that the opposing asperities of the cartilage surfaces come into direct contact with each other (Fig. 10.10). Lubrication is then provided by another glycoprotein, lubricin, which has one end bonded to the cartilage surfaces, and the other end free to attract water.[683] The free hydrated regions of lubricin separate the cartilage surfaces and act as a boundary lubricant in the manner of a thick grease.

Most synovial joints combine fluid film and boundary lubrication mechanisms to ensure that friction is low,[607] and consequently that the articular surfaces are not damaged by high shear stresses (Fig. 1.1D). The apophyseal joints, however, are somewhat unusual in that static spinal postures press their articular surfaces forcibly together for long periods, with little movement. Under these circumstances, fluid film lubrication would be minimal, and boundary lubrication would predominate. This may partly explain why the apophyseal joints are so often affected by cartilage damage, leading to osteoarthritis (p. 208). Lubricin and hyaluronan must be continually synthesised by cells in articular cartilage and in the joint synovium, and any deficiencies in this synthesis can lead to joint damage.[683]

SPINAL LIGAMENTS

Most of the intervertebral ligaments lie posterior to the centre of sagittal-plane rotation (Fig. 10.11), which lies within the intervertebral discs.[1113] Therefore their primary action is to protect the spine by preventing excessive lumbar flexion. This protective action is not entirely beneficial, because ligament tension acts to compress the intervertebral discs, so that nucleus pressure increases by 100% or more in full flexion, even for the same applied compressive force.[39]

For ease of reference, typical strengths of the intervertebral ligaments are compared in Figure 10.11. Average lengths and cross-sectional areas (measured in sagittal and transverse sections, respectively) have also been reported from eight cadavers with an average age of 63 years.[1134] Strength values are from various studies described below. Data of this sort should be viewed with caution, because some ligaments vary markedly with spinal level, and some are oriented at an angle to the horizontal and sagittal planes. Other ligaments consist of several bundles of fibres with slightly different lines of action, so their overall strength is underestimated by simply pulling them apart in a given direction and noting the force at which the first fibres fail. Experimental details given below characterise the mechanical function of individual ligaments when tested to simulate specific functions in life, such as resisting flexion. The large comparative study of spinal ligament strength by Myklebust et al.[1016] was performed on old cadaveric material (average age 67 years) and so its results are supplemented by those of smaller studies performed on younger specimens.

Interspinous and supraspinous ligaments

The fibres of these two ligaments merge in with each other, so that a scalpel cut along their common boundary reduces their combined tensile stiffness by 40%.[376] Mechanically, therefore, they should be treated as a single unit.[499] Together they have a tensile strength of 160 N and fail at a nominal 39% strain when resisting flexion.[33] This very high value of strain for a ligament reflects their position far behind the CoR. Collagen fibres cannot be stretched much more than 10%, so it appears that these two ligaments must either be slack in the neutral position (when the motion segment is neither flexed nor extended) or else their fibres must reorient during flexion movements. The gross anatomy of the interspinous ligament (Fig. 10.11) suggests that its fibres do reorient in the initial stages of flexion.[602] This probably explains why the lumbar interspinous and supraspinous ligaments provide minimal resistance at small angles of flexion, but resist 19% of the applied bending moment in full flexion, and are the first structures to be damaged beyond the normal range of movement.[18,33] In the thoracic spine, for comparison, the interspinous and supraspinous ligaments together contribute approximately 13% of flexion stiffness when motion segments are moderately flexed.[66]

When considered in isolation, the supraspinous ligament is weak or absent in the lower lumbar spine[639,1198] and its tensile strength has been reported as 77 N at L1–3, falling to 49 N at L3–5.[376] In the upper lumbar spine, its fibres are difficult to distinguish from those of the lumbodorsal fascia (p. 38), which may explain why some studies accord it a much greater tensile strength.[1016] The isolated interspinous ligament has been reported to have a tensile strength of 100 N.[376,1016] Another study suggested that it could resist 100 N without damage.[611]

Intertransverse ligament

This is stretched by up to 20% during lateral bending movements, which is more than any other ligament, and it may play a major role in resisting lateral bending.[1100] However, its strength has not been assessed, and it could possibly be weak, and slack in the neutral position. In the thoracic spine, it was not considered to be a true ligament by Jiang et al.,[690] who found it to be inseparable from interweaving muscle tendons in the region between transverse processes.

Ligamentum flavum

This unusual ligament contains a network of uncrimped collagen fibres loosely arranged about its long axis together with a high proportion of elastin, a fibrous protein which is more extensible than collagen. Elastin gives the ligament its yellow colour, and enables it to be stretched by 80% without failure.[1024] At 100% strain (which would be difficult to achieve in life) the ligament fails by pulling away from the bone.[639] In an unloaded motion segment, the ligamentum flavum is prestretched by 11–17%, and therefore prestresses the disc in the normal upright posture.[639,1024] It also provides much of the spine's resistance to small flexion movements.[33] Its primary mechanical function may be to provide a smooth posterior lining to the vertebral foramen, a lining which does not become slack or buckle when the spine is bent backwards.[1274] This would be a considerable advantage, because anterior buckling of a ligament in this critical position could compromise the spinal cord, and this is now known to be a major factor in spinal stenosis.[563] The ligamentum flavum provides 13% of the spine's resistance to full flexion[33] and its tensile strength is approximately 250–350 N.[1016,1024]

Zygapophyseal joint capsular ligaments

These localised thickenings of the joint capsule are sometimes considered as distinct ligaments. They are short but very strong, and appear to be deployed to provide maximum resistance to spinal flexion. Fibres at the anterolateral margins of the joint capsule are shorter than those at the posterior margin, but because they lie closer to the CoR, they become taut at the same angle of flexion.[7] However, if the vertebrae are simply pulled apart in the vertical direction, the two fibre bundles fail separately, the shorter ones first,[317] and the peak recorded tensile force (for left and right joints combined) is then typically 350–1100 N.[317,1016] In full flexion, these ligaments provide 39% of a motion segment's resistance to bending, and transmit an average tensile force of 591 N.[33] The capsular ligaments lie lateral to the mid-sagittal plane, so are able to resist lateral bending as well as forward bending, and they could possibly be the first spinal structures to suffer injury during an excessive movement in anterolateral bending. They also resist hyperextension,[19,588,1605] but offer little resistance to axial rotation, at least in the lumbar spine.[26,1100] Equivalent data for the thoracic spine suggest that facet joints, including their associated capsules and ligaments, contribute approximately 45% of a motion segment's resistance to moderate flexion.[66]

Posterior longitudinal ligament

This thin band adheres to the posterior surface of the discs, but is only weakly attached to the vertebral bodies in between. It contains crimped collagen fibres which straighten out when the ligament is stretched by 7–8%,[639] and it applies a small pre-tension to the disc of approximately 3 N.[1421] Its tensile strength has been variably reported as 100 N[1016] and 180 N,[1421] which may reflect some difficulty in determining the precise boundary between disc and ligament. It lies close to the CoR, so can play only a negligible role in protecting the disc from excessive flexion. On the other hand, it is capable of protecting the spinal cord from herniated disc material: when cadaveric discs are induced to prolapse in the laboratory, the displaced fragment of nucleus pulposus can be contained, or even deflected upwards, by this ligament (Fig. 11.19). Because it is so much weaker than the posterior annulus, the ligament could perform this function only by yielding to the posteriorly displaced disc material until it is sufficiently far from the nucleus that it is depressurised. The posterior longitudinal ligament is innervated by a plexus of nerves from the sinuvertebral nerve (p. 44), with capsulated and unencapsulated nerve endings,[613,780] so it may possibly function as a 'nerve net' to detect abnormal posterior deformations of the underlying disc.

Anterior longitudinal ligament

This is thicker and stronger than its posterior counterpart, and adheres to the anterior margins of the vertebrae rather than to the discs. Its crimped collagen fibres straighten out at a stretch of 8–10%.[639] Its strength increases with the speed at which it is stretched[1037] and is typically 600 N when tested in situ[1016] and 330 N when stripped from the underlying bones.[1421] The anterior longitudinal ligament helps to resist spinal extension movements, but its proximity to the CoR, and to the much stronger anterior annulus, suggests that this is not an important function. Excessive extension would be resisted more effectively (but perhaps, more painfully) by impaction of the neural arches. The anterior longitudinal ligament is very broad, so it could conceivably protect the inferior vena cava and dorsal aorta from rubbing against anterolateral vertebral body osteophytes.

Iliolumbar ligaments

Like the intervertebral ligaments, the iliolumbar ligaments resist bending and axial rotation of the L5 vertebra relative to the pelvis.[280,822,1598] Lateral bending is particularly restricted.[1598] The extra stability conferred by the iliolumbar ligaments may explain why L5–S1 is less mobile than L4–5 in living people, but not in cadaveric motion segments, in which this ligament is cut through (Figs 10.2 and 10.3).

INTERVERTEBRAL DISCS

These complex structures lie between the vertebral bodies, and their primary function is to transfer compressive

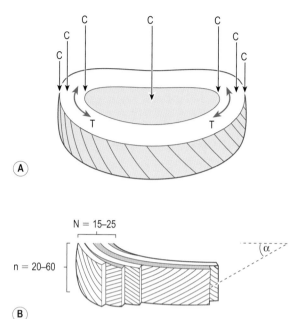

Figure 10.12 (A) When an intervertebral disc is loaded in compression (C), a hydrostatic pressure is generated in the nucleus (shaded), and this creates a restraining tensile stress (T) within the annulus. (B) Detail showing individual lamellae of the annulus: note the discontinuities in lamellar structure. The alternating fibre angle (α) is approximately 30°, but varies locally. N = number of lamellae in a typical region of annulus; n = number of collagen fibre bundles visible in a vertical section of a typical lamella. *(Data from Marchand and Ahmed.[913])*

forces evenly from one vertebral body to the next, while allowing small intervertebral movements. They are too stiff to be good shock absorbers, and are not well suited to resist high bending, shearing or twisting forces acting on the spine. The soft nucleus pulposus ensures that an even distribution of compressive stress acts on the vertebral bodies, with the encircling lamellae of the annulus holding the nucleus in place. Hydrostatic pressure within the nucleus generates a tensile 'hoop stress' in the surrounding annulus, as indicated in Figure 10.12. The hyaline cartilage endplate (Fig. 7.22) acts as a buffer between the nucleus and the adjacent vertebral endplate, hindering the expulsion of water and proteoglycan fragments from the nucleus.[1207]

The tendency of the proteoglycan-rich nucleus to swell up in tissue fluid is resisted by tension in the collagen fibres of the annulus and longitudinal ligaments, so that the nucleus exhibits a pressure of approximately 0.05 MPa in a cadaveric vertebral body–disc vertebral body unit, even when it is unloaded. Pre-tension in the ligamentum flavum[1024] raises the intrinsic nucleus pressure in an intact, but unloaded, cadaver motion segment to 0.05–0.12 MPa,

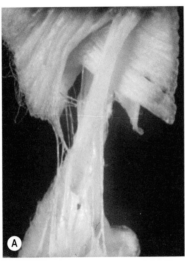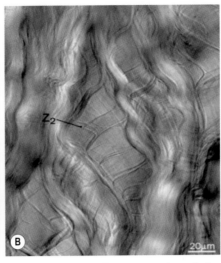

Figure 10.13 Collagen fibres of the annulus fibrosus. (A) Photograph of a piece of human annulus pulled apart in the vertical direction. Note the large collagen fibre bundles oriented in two directions in adjacent lamellae, and a few fine collagen fibres, coated in proteoglycans, that have been pulled out of the matrix. (B) Crimped collagen fibres in bovine annulus fibrosus, visualised by differential interference contrast microscopy. The tissue has been stretched laterally to emphasise how the fibres have a branching structure. *(Reproduced from Pezowicz et al.[1124] with permission.)*

with degenerated discs being at the low end of this range.[40,1095] Low-level muscle activity in living subjects lying prone raises the nucleus pressure to 0.08–0.15 MPa.[1250,1565] However, small tensile forces in the annulus, ligaments and muscles are not sufficient to prevent the disc from swelling. Consequently, human stature increases by 2 cm overnight (p. 184), and astronauts exposed to zero gravity for long periods of time are reputed to return to Earth up to 5 cm (2 inches) taller. Under normal gravity, everyday loading of the spine is sufficient to expel water from the interverte-bral discs, leading to a diurnal cycle of nocturnal swelling and daytime height loss.

Annulus fibrosus

The annulus consists of approximately 15–25 concentric lamellae[259,913] which contain a high proportion of large branching collagen fibre bundles arranged in alternate directions, as shown in Figures 10.12 and 10.13. The structure shown in Figure 10.12 is an idealisation, because individual fibre bundles often take a curved course from bone to bone, and irregularities in the lamellar structure are common, especially in the posterolateral annulus.[913] Note that the alternating dark and light banded appearance of the annulus (Fig. 8.14) is due to the way incident light is reflected by collagen fibres reaching the surface at different angles in successive lamellae; it is not due to bands of collagen alternating with bands of softer matrix. Annulus lamellae are held together in the radial direction

by a network of cross-ties or 'bridging elements' (Fig. 10.14). These structures appear to be comprised of crimped collagen type I fibres that branch off from collagen fibre bundles within the lamellae,[1272] but they also contain aggrecan and other collagens.[970] They can span many lamellae, and their twisting morphology probably allows some interlamellar movement while preventing gross delaminations. The possibility of small interlamellar movements is suggested by the presence within the disc of lubricin,[1301] a glycoprotein which plays a major role in boundary lubrication of cartilage surfaces in a synovial joint. The interface between adjacent lamellae is also rich in elastin fibres and associated microfibrils,[1621] which would aid recovery from large deformations.

Different regions of the annulus have different functions. The outer lamellae have a high proportion of crimped type I collagen fibres, and they function as strong ligaments which resist excessive bending and twisting of adjacent vertebrae.[24,189] The middle lamellae are sufficiently deformable that the tissue can behave like a fluid in young non-degenerated disc (p. 132), although after the age of 35 years they usually behave like a fibrous solid and directly resist high compressive loading, even when unsupported by the nucleus.[189,916] The vertical compressive stiffness of annulus tissue is greatest anteriorly, and decreases with age and degeneration.[1453] The innermost lamellae are sufficiently deformable that the tissue normally behaves like a pressurised fluid, even though the collagen fibres form distinct lamellae.

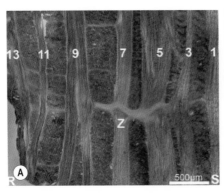
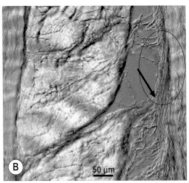

Figure 10.14 Annulus bridging elements. (A) Low-magnification view of 13 lamellae bridged by a single element (Z). (Reproduced from Schollum et al.[1272] with permission.) (B) High-magnification view of individual collagen fibrils passing between adjacent lamellae that have been pulled radially apart. Note that the lamella in the centre shows two large collagen fibre bundles in cross-section, whereas the lamellae on either side show crimped collagen fibres in longitudinal section. *(Reproduced from Pezowicz et al.[1124] with permission.)*

Tensile properties of the annulus

Tensile tests performed on small samples of annulus show that adjacent lamellae are only weakly bound together and can be pulled apart with a tensile stress of 0.2–0.3 MPa at a strain of 100–250%.[456,912] This stress probably represents an upper bound on the strength of the proteoglycan matrix, though it must include the strength of bridging elements and elastin fibres which hold the lamellae together. The annulus is much stronger in the plane of individual lamellae, especially when stretched in the horizontal direction or parallel to one of the two predominant fibre directions.[464] If small horizontal samples of outer annulus are stretched very slowly (0.01% per second) then failure occurs at a stress of 1–3 MPa and a strain of 10–25%, with the anterior annulus being stronger than the posterolateral, and the outer annulus stronger than the inner.[3,385] These variations may be due to structural differences within the collagen network[913] because they cannot be explained by differences in chemical composition.[1323] At faster strain rates, the stress at failure rises to approximately 3.5 MPa in the horizontal direction[464,1590] and 10 MPa in the direction of the collagen fibres.[464,912] When large samples of outer annulus are stretched in the vertical direction, in order to simulate spinal bending, then failure occurs at a stress of 2–4 MPa, and a strain of 30–70%.[528] The anterior annulus is softer and weaker in tension than the posterior annulus, and the inner annulus is much weaker again.[528] Comparisons between studies are difficult, because small specimens appear to be disproportionately weak, especially when stretched vertically, on account of the extra disruption to their collagen fibres (see below). Because of this effect, the vertical tensile strength of the outer annulus in situ may be 4–9 MPa.[528] Regional variations in the tensile properties of the annulus are summarised in Table 10.1.

These properties suggest that the disc's primary role is to resist compressive force (which generates approximately horizontal tensile stresses in the annulus) rather than bending (which stretches the annulus vertically) and that stretching of the posterior annulus needs to be resisted more vigorously (or more often) than stretching of the anterior annulus. The reduced strength of the inner annulus might be expected from its collagen composition, and from the fact that tensile stresses in the walls of thick pressure vessels are lowest near their inner surface.

As with most skeletal tissues, the tensile strength and stiffness of the annulus fall with age and degeneration.[3,456,464] They also fall during cyclic loading, presumably because microdamage accumulates within the tissue: if 10 000 loading cycles are applied, then annulus tissue fails at approximately 40% of the tensile stress required to damage it in a single loading cycle.[528]

How does collagen reinforce the annulus?

The marked effect that specimen size has on annulus stiffness and strength[23] is typical of chopped-fibre composite materials,[638] and suggests that the tensile properties of the annulus depend on collagen–proteoglycan interactions rather than the strength of intact fibres passing from bone to bone. In effect, the collagen fibres may provide tensile reinforcement of the annulus in the manner of a material like fibreglass, and the degree of reinforcement is proportional to the average length of fibre fragments within the tissue[23] (Fig. 10.15). This important property means that local damage to the collagen network does not lead rapidly to widespread failure (as it would do if the fibres provided all of the tensile strength, as in a nylon stocking, for example) and it explains how the annulus is able to grow without lengthening existing collagen fibres.

Table 10.1 Tensile properties of the annulus fibrosus vary between inner, middle and outer regions. Data for human specimens aged 48–91 years are presented as the mean (sd)[1326]

	Inner annulus	Middle annulus	Outer annulus
Number of specimens	39	46	47
Length (mm)	6.8 (1.7)	6.8 (1.6)	6.3 (1.7)
Cross-sectional area (mm²)	5.2 (1.6)	4.9 (1.2)	4.8 (0.9)
Failure load (N)	9.9 (7.6)	20.0 (11.0)	34.8 (19.0)
Ultimate strength (MPa)	2.0 (1.5)	4.1 (2.3)	7.4 (4.3)
Elongation (%)	64 (36)	44 (15)	40 (11)
Stiffness (N mm)	5.7 (5.3)	13.3 (7.6)	26.5 (14.8)
Normalised stiffness	1.20 (1.11)	2.77 (1.62)	5.67 (3.38)
Failure energy (N/mm)	15.5 (13.7)	21.6 (15.4)	33.2 (23.9)

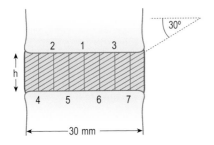

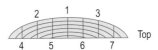

Figure 10.15 If a vertical slice of annulus and bone is taken from the lateral margin of a motion segment, as illustrated, then its tensile properties do not depend greatly on the number of collagen fibres which pass directly from bone to bone. The tensile stiffness of the annulus in the vertical direction is reduced by only 33% when vertical cut 1 is made, even though this cut would be expected to sever all collagen fibres linking the two bones.[23] This suggests that fibre–matrix interactions make an important contribution to annulus integrity, just as in a fibre–composite material such as fibreglass.

The fibre-composite behaviour of the annulus also ensures that a great deal of energy is required to pull it apart completely.[23,528] This property is termed 'toughness' (p. 6), and the annulus is one of the toughest materials in the body. Lateral cohesion within each annulus lamella probably depends on the manner in which collagen fibres split and branch (Fig. 10.13B), so that they resist deformations in

all directions. Discrete bridging elements (described above) also contribute to holding annulus lamellae together.

Nucleus pulposus

The high water content and loose collagen network of the nucleus give the tissue unusual mechanical properties. The water ensures that the tissue has very low rigidity, so it deforms easily in any direction and equalises any stresses applied to it.[40] In this respect, it resembles a fluid, and so it is correct to speak of a fluid 'pressure' within the nucleus, rather than a compressive 'stress' (Fig. 7.24). When loaded rapidly, however, small samples of nucleus can withstand considerable shear stresses and behave more like a viscoelastic solid.[658] Certainly, the collagen network limits the amount of deformation that the nucleus will undergo: if two soft regions of nucleus are gripped with forceps and pulled apart, there is negligible resistance up to the point where the collagen fibres become taut, but then considerable force is required to separate the two regions entirely. The tensile strength of the nucleus has never been measured, but may be comparable to that of the annulus when it is stretched in the radial direction. In effect, the nucleus behaves like a 'tethered fluid', and these peculiar properties blend in gradually with more conventional solid behaviour in the middle of the annulus. In old and mildly degenerated discs, the nucleus contains firm fibrous regions surrounded by a softer gel which ruptures easily when fluid is injected into it. The typical positions of fibrous and gel-like regions within the nucleus explain the 'hamburger' discograms characteristic of mature and non-degenerated discs.[17] A reduction in the proteoglycan content of the nucleus compared to the annulus could result in the latter attracting water from the former, so that

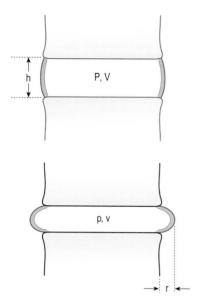

Figure 10.16 The height (h) and radial bulge (r) of an intervertebral disc depend on the pressure (P) and volume (V) of the nucleus pulposus. If the volume is reduced (Lower diagram), either by water expulsion or by surgical intervention, then the nucleus pressure falls, and the annulus bulges more.[189] This is rather like letting air out of a car tyre.

clefts open up in the nucleus.[1585] This mechanism could also explain how circumferential (but not radial) fissures form in the annulus.[12] The ease with which injected fluid can separate the fibrous nucleus from the hyaline cartilage endplates in discography argues against the theory that the creation of loose 'fragments' within the nucleus of a middle-aged disc is an important step in the process of disc protrusion.[191] In severely degenerated discs, the nucleus is a fibrous solid, often likened to 'crab meat'.[17]

The large proteoglycan molecules which attract and hold water in the nucleus also act to hinder the movements of other molecules through the matrix, even small ones such as glucose, and water itself. There are no empty 'pores' within the matrix for fluid to pass through quickly, so fluid flow in response to a change in mechanical loading takes place slowly over a number of hours. The precise water content of the nucleus depends on a number of factors, including age and loading history,[28,957] and it has a profound effect on internal mechanics of the disc. Any increase in water content (by unopposed swelling, or by injection) increases the pressure within the nucleus[73,1183] and this in turn reduces disc bulging,[190] increases disc height[190] and increases the disc's resistance to bending.[18] This is rather like pumping air into a tyre (Fig. 10.16). Conversely, a disc becomes decompressed and bulges like a flat tyre if the water content and volume of the nucleus are reduced, whether by creep loading, by degenerative changes or by injury.[190,1300]

Cartilage endplates

These thin layers of hyaline cartilage cover the central region of the vertebral body endplates, on the disc side (Figs 7.22 and 7.23). Physically, this tissue is similar to articular cartilage near its junction with bone, but, unlike articular cartilage, it is only loosely bonded to the underlying bone,[24,528] presumably because it is always pressed up against it by the hydrostatic pressure of the nucleus. Its function appears to be to help equalise loading of the vertebral body,[1294] while preventing the migration of the much softer nucleus material into the pores in the vertebral endplate. The hyaline cartilage may also act as a chemical and biological filter between the nucleus pulposus and the blood vessels in the vertebral body. It will also prevent rapid fluid loss from the nucleus into the vertebral body during sustained loading, and so will assist in maintaining the water content and internal pressurisation of the disc.

Stress distributions within intervertebral discs

This technique has revealed the internal mechanical functioning of the disc to an unprecedented extent, both in vitro[22,40,959] and in vivo.[962] Because of its importance, it is appropriate to consider briefly how it is performed, and what is actually being measured.

A static compressive load, sufficient to simulate light manual labour, is applied to a motion segment for a period of 20 seconds, and during this time, the distribution of compressive stress within the disc is measured at a frequency of 25 Hz by pulling a miniature pressure transducer through it, along its sagittal midline (Fig. 10.17). The transducer is a small 2 mm-long strain-gauged membrane, mounted in the side of a 1.3 mm diameter needle.[959,960] The annulus has excellent self-sealing properties[916] and no disc material is expressed through the needle hole during the experiments. Rotating the needle about its long axis enables the vertical and horizontal components of compressive stress to be measured in successive tests, using the same needle track.

Validation tests have shown that the output of the transducer is approximately equal to the average compressive stress acting perpendicular to its membrane,[958] even in a degenerated annulus fibrosus.[281] This implies that there is negligible resistance to the matrix deforming into the slight recess in the needle to press on the transducer membrane. The outer 2–4 mm of annulus is a fibrous solid in which there is unlikely to be sufficient coupling between matrix and transducer membrane for reliable recordings to be made. Note that there may be high tensile forces in the collagen fibres in this region of disc, but these are not detected by the transducer. The transducer output represents an average stress acting on the 2-mm-long membrane, and this may help to explain why measured

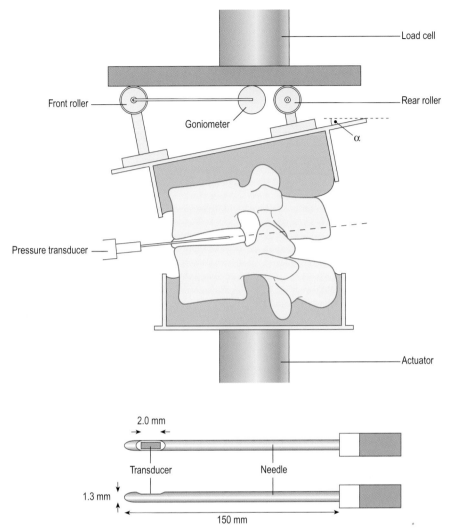

Figure 10.17 Measuring stress distributions inside cadaveric intervertebral discs. A cadaveric lumbar motion segment is secured in cups of dental plaster (shaded) and subjected to constant compressive loading by means of a hydraulic actuator. During this time, a needle-mounted pressure transducer (lower) is pulled through the disc along its mid-sagittal diameter in order to measure a stress profile. Two rollers are used to load the specimen in various angles of flexion or extension, as measured by the goniometer.

compressive stress usually falls steadily to zero near the disc periphery.

Typical stress profiles are shown in Figure 10.18 for discs of all grades of degeneration, as defined by ourselves[17] and by others.[1416] The visual appearance of similar discs is shown in Figure 10.19. In the young grade 1 disc, the measured vertical and horizontal compressive stresses are approximately equal to each other, and do not vary with position across most of the disc. Evidently, the whole interior region of the disc behaves like a bag of fluid, with an outer 'skin' of annulus only 2–4 mm thick. The extension of fluid-like behaviour into the annulus may explain why

capillaries and nerve fibres do not grow more than a few millimetres into the annulus of healthy discs: fluid pressures would press on hollow blood vessels from all sides, and collapse them if the disc were heavily loaded. In the mature grade 2 disc, which is typical of non-degenerated spines aged over 35 years, the size of the hydrostatic central region shrinks to that of the histological nucleus, and small stress concentrations can be seen in the annulus, usually posterior to the nucleus. Grade 3 discs are moderately degenerated, and this is reflected by an irregular stress profile indicating variable resistance to compression from a disrupted fibrous matrix in which the central hydrostatic

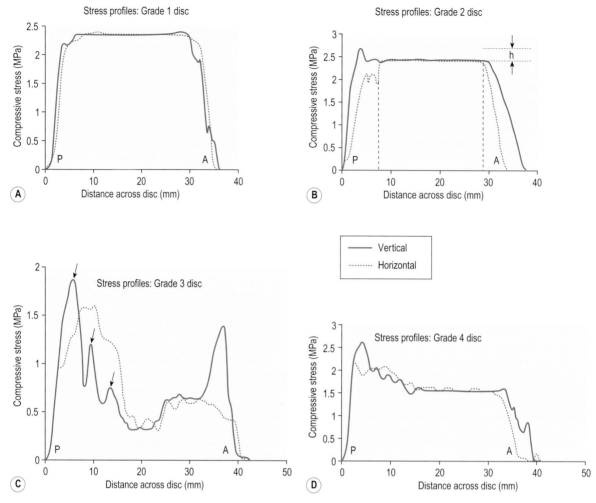

Figure 10.18 Typical stress profiles for lumbar intervertebral discs subjected to a compressive force of 2 kN. Vertical and horizontal compressive stress is plotted against position along the mid-sagittal diameter (P, posterior). (A) In a young, non-degenerated disc, there is a large functional nucleus in which the horizontal and vertical stresses are equal, suggesting hydrostatic conditions. (B) With increasing age, stress concentration (peaks) appears within the annulus, and the size of the hydrostatic nucleus is reduced. (C) and (D) refer to young discs showing moderate and severe degenerative changes respectively. Note the greatly reduced hydrostatic nucleus, and the high stress concentrations within the annulus.

region is small or absent. Severely degenerated grade 4 discs are characterised by highly irregular and variable stress profiles, and by an overall reduction in compressive stress. This suggests that such discs, which are often severely narrowed, are being shielded from compressive loading by adjacent structures such as the neural arch, or by bridging vertebral body osteophytes.[37,40]

Compression of an intervertebral disc

When a disc is compressed, the hydrostatic pressure in the nucleus rises and generates a tensile hoop stress in the restraining annulus (Fig. 10.12). According to the theory of thick-walled pressure cylinders, the hoop stress increases from the inner lamellae to the outer. The annulus also resists compression directly, causing it to bulge radially outwards, and therefore to lose height. This forces the vertebral body endplates closer together, but the central regions of the endplates cannot come much closer together because the nucleus lies between them, and its high water content makes it virtually incompressible. Therefore, the central region of the endplates bulges into the vertebral bodies.

Some of these effects have been quantified in cadaveric experiments. Compressive forces of 0.5–2 kN stretch the collagen fibres on the disc surface by 1–3%[600,1362] and cause the disc to bulge radially by 0.4–1.0 mm. Bulging

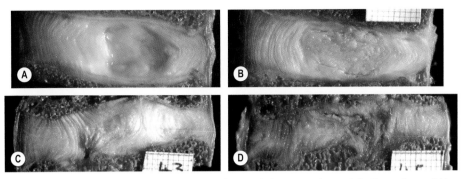

Figure 10.19 Lumbar intervertebral discs sectioned in the mid-sagittal plane, anterior on left. These discs, which were not subjected to any postmortem loading, represent the first four stages of disc degeneration. (A) Grade 1 disc, typical of ages 15–40 years. (Male, 35 years.) (B) Grade 2 disc, typical of ages 35–70 years. The nucleus is fibrous, and there is brown pigmentation typical of ageing. However, the disc's structure is intact, and the disc is not degenerated. (Male, 47 years, L2–3.) (C) Grade 3 disc, showing moderate degenerative changes. Note the annulus bulging into the nucleus, damage to the inferior endplate and the lack of pigmentation in some regions of the disc. (Male, 31 years, L2–3.) (D) Grade 4 disc, showing severe degeneration. Note the brown pigmentation, the disruption to both endplates and internal collapse of the annulus, with corresponding reduction in disc height. (Male, 31 years, L4–5.)

varies around the disc periphery, being greatest in the anterior annulus[1363] or posterolateral annulus,[1551] with the difference possibly being due to the age and lumbar level of specimens tested. Outwards bulging is also greater in the peripheral annulus (0.36 mm for a 1 kN compressive load) compared to the inner annulus (0.16 mm).[1056] Compared to a preload of 250 N, a compressive force of 4.5 kN reduces the height of a motion segment by 0.9 mm, but the height loss in the nucleus is only half of this, so each endplate must bulge into its vertebral body by approximately 0.25 mm.[188,624] Endplate bulging can reach 0.8 mm before failure.[188] A disc's response to compression depends very much on its precise shape and size: for example, discs which have a high ratio of height/area will exhibit higher tensile stresses in the outer annulus, and more radial bulging, for the same applied compressive force.[854] This makes it difficult to extrapolate mechanisms of disc structural mechanical failure from one spinal level to another, or from animal to human discs.

Bending of an intervertebral disc

Flexion movements cause the lumbar discs to pivot about a CoR close to the nucleus pulposus (p. 117). The anterior annulus becomes compressed and thickened, while the posterior annulus is stretched and thinned. Tension in the posterior annulus acts to increase the hydrostatic pressure in the nucleus.

Experiments have shown that flexion reduces the height of the anterior annulus by 25–35%[27,709] and causes it to bulge radially outwards by approximately 0.1 mm/degree of movement.[599,1363] Concentrations of compressive stress can appear, or grow, in the matrix of the anterior annulus.[39] The posterior annulus flattens its radial bulging[1363] and stretches by 50–90% in full flexion.[27,709,1117] Crimped

collagen fibres can be stretched by 10–15% before failure, and direct measurements of disc surface strain indicate fibre strains of only 0.7% per degree of flexion,[1362] so these high vertical deformations of the annulus can only be achieved by removal of radial bulge, and by interfibre sliding.[204] Some fibre reorientation has been suggested by the results of X-ray diffraction experiments,[758] although this may be influenced by changes in radial bulging. The elastin network of the disc (Fig. 7.19) may help return collagen fibres to their original orientation.[1620] During flexion movements of short duration, the fluid content and volume of the posterior annulus must remain constant, so vertical stretching is accompanied by a corresponding thinning in the radial direction,[31,1290] as shown in Figure 13.9. This may have important consequences for disc nutrition (p. 180). However it can be misleading to refer to a 'migration' of the nucleus in certain postures[58]: the nucleus merely fills the space made available to it by the annulus, and annulus deformations are reversible. True nucleus migration requires the prior formation of radial fissures in the annulus.

The reduced water content and increased stiffness of old and degenerated discs impair their ability to spread load evenly on to their adjacent vertebrae during flexion and extension movements. Consequently, high concentrations of compressive stress can appear in the annulus, anteriorly during flexion, and posteriorly during extension (Fig. 10.20). These concentrations of compressive stress imply high tensile forces within the disc's collagen network; indeed, it is only the collagen tension which prevents disc matrix from moving to equalise loading across the disc.

Equivalent mechanisms must operate when the disc is bent backwards and laterally. The ratio of disc height to width is so small that angular movements of the vertebrae of only a few degrees entail large vertical deformations in

Figure 10.20 Degenerated discs are unable to distribute loading evenly on to the adjacent vertebral bodies, especially when the vertebrae are oriented at an angle to each other. Stress concentrations in this severely degenerated disc appear in the anterior annulus (in flexion) and posterior annulus (in extension). Stress profiles are explained in Figure 10.17. A, anterior; P, posterior.

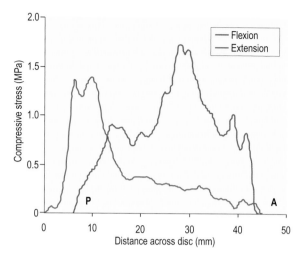

the annulus (Fig. 13.9). This will lead to particularly high tensile and compressive stresses in the annulus of thin discs with a large side-to-side diameter, especially when they are laterally flexed about their shorter diameter. Shear strains in a disc, which probably contribute to delamination, rise to their maximum values in the peripheral posterior and lateral annulus during lateral bending movements.[300]

Axial rotation of an intervertebral disc

Torsional movements of the spine generate most tension in half of the collagen fibres in the annulus, with the other fibres tending to become slack,[793] as indicated in Figure 2.6. It has been suggested that only 3° of axial rotation is permitted by the lumbar discs,[640] but this theoretical analysis neglected the natural radial bulge of the annulus, and the crimp in its collagen fibres. When cadaveric discs are rotated to 6° by a torque of 15 Nm, collagen fibres on the disc surface are stretched by up to 7%[1362] and annulus bulge is reduced by 0.2 mm.[1363] Torsion raises the pressure within the nucleus of the disc, presumably because tension in the oblique collagen fibres which resist torsion acts to compress the disc at the same time. A torque of 10 Nm applied to a vertebral body–disc–vertebral body unit raises intradiscal pressure in the nucleus by 0.16 MPa, whereas a bending moment of 10Nm raises it by approximately twice that amount.[1277]

SACRUM AND SACROILIAC JOINTS

Sacrum

This large wedge-shaped bone comprises five fused sacral vertebrae. Several of its features are derived from its

component vertebrae, and some are more or less redundant. The sacrum transfers mechanical loading between the lumbar spine and pelvis by means of the sacroiliac joints, and it anchors the insertions of several back muscles (Ch. 3). In addition, the sacral canal and sacral foramina provide a particularly safe passage for the cauda equina and sacral nerve roots in what would otherwise be an exposed and vulnerable location.

Sacroiliac joints

Movements in vivo

Stereo radiography has been used to visualise the position of implanted metal markers in patients with suspected sacroiliac joint problems.[386,1377,1378] These studies have shown that sacroiliac joint movements are small in all planes. The greatest movements occur when patients move from the upright standing position to lie prone with one leg hyperextended: in the latter position, the sacrum rotates backwards relative to the pelvis by approximately 2°, the iliac crests rotate inwards (towards each other) by up to 0.2° and translational (gliding) movements of 0.5–0.7 mm occur between the sacrum and ilium.[1377] Most rotations are approximately symmetrical in the sagittal plane, and differ little in symptomatic and painfree joints, although small differences were observed between patients with unilateral and bilateral symptoms. Movements were 30–40% smaller in men, and tended to increase slightly with age.[1377] Implanted metal wires in the sacrum and ilia have been used to demonstrate a similar small range of movement in healthy volunteers, but no significant variations with sex, age or parturition were found.[751] Interestingly, angular rotations of 6–8° and translations of 2.5 mm were observed in a single subject who reported recurrent sacroiliac joint problems.[751] However, manipulation of patients with sacroiliac joint problems failed to cause any angular or translational movement of the joint that could be detected by subsequent stereo radiography, even though there was clinical improvement.[1440] Skin surface measurements made on healthy subjects and on gymnasts[1332] indicate sacroiliac joint rotations of up to 18°, but this probably includes skin movement artifacts, because the accuracy of the measurements (as opposed to their reproducibility) was not assessed.

Movements in vitro

Large sacroiliac joint movements have been observed in five cadavers (four male, one female) aged 52–68 years, which were placed in extreme striding positions with the legs straight, one stretched out in front, and one stretched out behind.[1333] Joint movement was measured to an accuracy of 1.3 mm or 1.0° by detecting embedded lead spheres using computed tomography (CT) scans. The total range of sacroiliac joint movement in the sagittal plane averaged 5° for the left joint and 8° for the right, with extreme values ranging from 3° to 17°.[1333] Movements in other planes were 4° or less. Maximum linear displacements of the posterior superior iliac spines relative to the sacrum were 5–8 mm. The authors suggest that similar movements would be observed in living people during vigorous activities such as running or jumping. When eccentric forces of up to 60% body weight were applied to the sacrum of cadaveric pelvises, rotations and translations of approximately 1° and 1 mm were observed.[980,1529] Rotations increased by 10% when either the posterior or anterior ligaments were cut, and by 30% when both were cut.[1529]

Mechanical function

These joints allow small movements between the base of the spinal column (the sacrum) and the pelvis (ilia). Corresponding movements at the pubic symphysis allow relative motion between left and right hip bones, which is

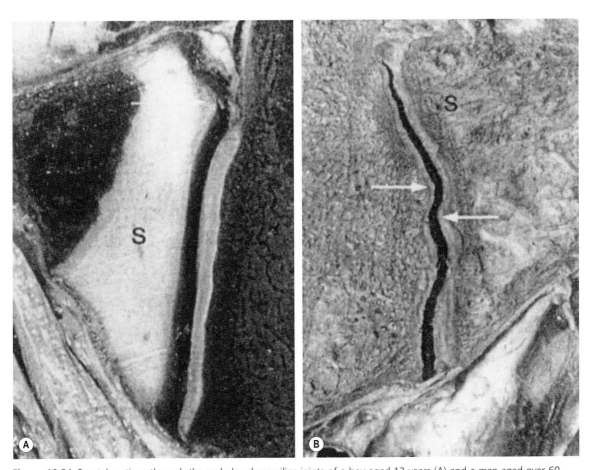

Figure 10.21 Frontal sections through the embalmed sacroiliac joints of a boy aged 12 years (A) and a man aged over 60 years (B). S indicates the sacral side. Note that the flat surfaces and abundant cartilage of the young joint are replaced with undulating surfaces (arrows) and thinner cartilage in the old joint. *(Reproduced from Vleeming et al.[1502] with permission of J B Lippincott, Philadelphia.)*

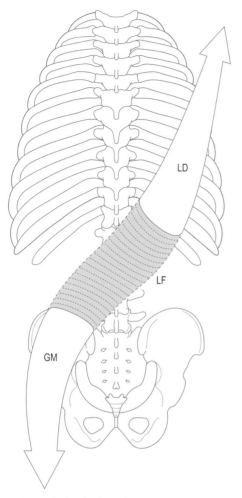

Figure 10.22 The lumbodorsal fascia (LF) forms a mechanical link between the gluteus maximus muscle (GM) on one side of the body, and the latissimus dorsi muscle (LD) on the other. The force transferred across the pelvis will act to press the surfaces of the left-hand side sacroiliac joint closer together. In this way, the bilateral effects of this linkage may be to stabilise the sacroiliac joints, by the mechanism of force closure.[1501]

increased during (and after) childbirth as a result of ligament laxity.[478] Apart from this, it is not obvious just what mechanical purpose the sacroiliac joints serve, although this uncertainty has led to various theories. Sacroiliac joints could play some role in shock absorption[60] but they are too stiff to absorb much strain energy, and during locomotion most shock absorption would come from the tendons of the leg and foot.[60] However, even a small amount of shock absorption may serve a useful function in protecting the integrity of the pelvic ring if it is subjected to a direct blow, perhaps during a fall on the buttocks or hip (p. 22). Another possibility is that small movements of the sacroiliac joints somehow facilitate locomotion, but it is difficult to imagine how a few degrees of extra movement would be of much mechanical benefit to bones whose other ends are attached to mobile joints such as the hip and lumbosacral joints.

In a young person the joint surfaces are approximately flat, but with increasing age they develop a series of undulating peaks and troughs which interdigitate with each other (Fig. 10.21). These anatomical changes greatly increase the joint's resistance to shearing movements,[1503] by a mechanism which has since been termed 'form closure'.[1501] The undulations suggest that a small relative displacement of the opposing surfaces might become 'locked' if two peaks were to oppose one another. Sacroiliac joint locking and slipping have not been demonstrated experimentally, although there is an extensive clinical literature on the subject.

Sacroiliac joint stability could possibly be increased by muscle action. Tension generated in the gluteal muscles on one side of the body can be transmitted diagonally across the back to the contralateral latissimus dorsi by means of the lumbodorsal fascia,[102,1500] as shown in Figure 10.22. These diagonal forces will act to press the surfaces of the sacroiliac joints closer together, and may increase their stability by a mechanism termed 'force closure'.[1501] This is an attractive hypothesis which seeks to explain how the lumbodorsal fascia can coordinate the function of some of the largest muscles in the body, whilst increasing pelvic stability. However, the size of the forces acting on the passive link – the lumbodorsal fascia – is not yet known.

Chapter | 11 |

Mechanical damage to the thoracolumbar spine

INTRODUCTION

This chapter considers how the thoracolumbar spine can be damaged during the activities of daily living. Mechanisms of violent trauma are dealt with only briefly because they are not of widespread interest, and there is little scientific work to support the classifications of injury that are currently accepted. On the other hand, a great deal of effort has been spent on trying to understand the origins of limited structural failure in spinal tissues, because such failure is extremely common, is linked to back pain and tissue degeneration and may be both preventable and treatable. Mechanisms of sacroiliac joint damage are not discussed because of a lack of relevant experimental data. As in Chapter 10, most of the data is reported for the lumbar spine, but much of it can be extrapolated to thoracic levels also. Damage to the cervical spine is considered in Chapter 12.

Not everyone with back pain has a damaged back, and many patients have no detectable spinal pathology of any kind. Evidence is mounting that mechanical back pain can arise directly from high (but non-damaging) stress concentrations within innervated tissues. This is the underlying concept of a 'functional pathology', and is considered separately in Chapter 13.

DAMAGE, INJURY AND FATIGUE FAILURE

Damage can be defined in terms of an acquired defect to, or disruption of, a given structure. In practice, damage manifests itself as a permanent impairment of that structure's ability to withstand applied mechanical loading. An injury refers to damage to a living tissue, either by mechanical loading or by a chemical or electromagnetic influence (such as a burn). In cadaver experiments, gross damage can be detected directly by sight or sound, but the threshold of clinically relevant (painful) damage is probably the 'elastic limit' at which non-reversible deformation first occurs.[33,1174,1617] Beyond this limit, the gradient of a force deformation graph decreases, as shown in Figure 1.4. Strains of this magnitude can have other biological consequences as well as pain: they impair collagen stability throughout the matrix, and render the collagen more vulnerable to matrix-degrading enzymes.[1568]

If forces are applied slowly to a cadaveric specimen, then water is expelled from it and a certain amount of 'creep' in soft tissues occurs (Fig. 1.6). Creep is reversible and is entirely physiological, but creep deformation is not easy to distinguish from non-reversible residual deformation attributable to mechanical damage. For this reason, investigations of failure mechanisms in biological tissues require that mechanical loading be applied rapidly, in a physiologically reasonable time scale, rather than slowly or incrementally. Quasistatic 'weights in pans' tests are unsuitable for this purpose.

'Fatigue' failure occurs by the accumulation of micro-damage caused by the repetitive application of forces which are too small to cause detectable damage if applied only once (Fig. 1.7). There is only a tenuous connection with the quite distinct metabolic process of muscle fatigue, or with 'fatigue' used to mean 'tiredness'. Note however, that fatigue failure is an engineering concept which must be interpreted with caution when applied to living tissues. Repetitive mechanical loading, and the microscopic damage resulting from it, can initiate a beneficial adaptive remodelling response within a living tissue, so that it becomes stronger rather than weaker (Fig. 7.11). For fatigue failure to occur in a living tissue, microscopic damage must accumulate faster than the adaptive remodelling response can cope with, and this critical rate will depend upon the metabolic rate of the tissue in question, and on the age and health of the individual.[15] Clearly it would be meaningless to perform very long low-intensity fatigue tests on cadaveric tissues, because the lack of a normal biological response would ensure that the outcome could not be applied to living tissues. It would be acceptable, however, to use cadaver testing to study a tissue's response to short-term high-intensity fatigue, because this would be modified less in living tissues. For example, in a tissue with a low metabolic rate such as the annulus fibrosus, in vitro fatigue testing of a few thousand cycles could be used to study the effect of spinal flexion occurring in vivo over a period of hours or weeks; but the application of millions of cycles to simulate several years' activity would be inappropriate.

COMPRESSION

As far as the vertebral column is concerned, it is conventional to speak of the 'compressive force' as being that force which acts down the long axis of the spine, at 90° to the mid-plane of the intervertebral discs (Fig. 11.1). As discussed in Chapter 9, this force arises mostly from tension in the paraspinal muscles, and from gravity acting on the mass of the upper body.

Resistance to compression

Compressive loading is resisted mostly by the anterior column consisting of the vertebral bodies and intervertebral discs, but a variable proportion falls on the apophyseal joints. In the simulated erect standing posture, these joints resist 16% of a typical 1 kN spinal compressive force[25] and much of this is concentrated on the inferior margins of the joint surfaces.[380] Intervertebral disc

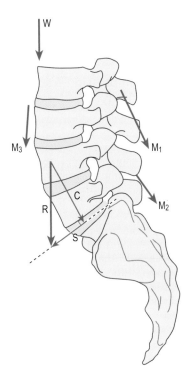

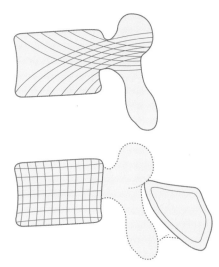

Figure 11.2 Drawing of sagittal sections through a lumbar vertebra showing the orientation of trabeculae (anterior on left). **(A)** The plane of this section passes through one of the pedicles, and it suggests how trabeculae from the pedicles can reinforce the vertebral endplates, especially the lower endplate. (Compare with Figure 8.9.) **(B)** In the mid-sagittal plane the trabecular architecture is more symmetric.

Figure 11.1 The lumbar spine is subjected to various muscle forces (M₁, M₂ etc.) and to the weight of the upper body (W). All of the forces acting on a particular intervertebral disc can be represented by a single resultant force (R), and this in turn can be represented by two components (C and S) which act at 90° to each other in anatomically meaningful directions. The component (C) which acts perpendicular to the mid-plane of the intervertebral disc is referred to as the compressive force, and the component (S) which acts in the mid-plane of the disc is referred to as the shear force. Approximately, the compressive force acts down the long axis of the spine, but it is not necessarily vertical: indeed, it could act horizontally in someone in a stooped position.

narrowing of 1–3 mm causes increased loading of the articular surfaces, and may also cause extra-articular impingement of the tip of the inferior facet on the lamina below.[380] If the disc height is severely reduced by degenerative change, then up to 90% of the compressive force can act on the apophyseal joints in lordotic postures (Fig. 8.16). Under these circumstances, severe compressive loading may possibly damage them.

The disc is well designed to resist high compressive forces and has a higher compressive strength than the adjacent vertebrae. Even if the annulus is cut into with a scalpel blade, there is no herniation of nucleus pulposus material through the fissure in response to pure compressive loading.[183,1498] This type of loading is much more likely to affect the vertebral body.

Vertebral compression fracture

The endplate is usually the spine's 'weak link' in compression

The vertebral body endplate is the 'weak link' of the lumbar spine, and when the compressive force rises to high levels, the first unequivocal signs of damage usually occur in the endplate, or in the trabeculae which support it.[186,647,1123,1614] This happens even if the posterolateral annulus of the adjacent disc is weakened prior to loading, by cutting into it from the nucleus so that a full-depth radial fissure is formed, passing from the nucleus to within 1 mm of the disc periphery.[183] The relative weakness of the endplate may be a consequence of the need for it to be as thin as possible to facilitate nutrient transport into the intervertebral disc (p. 83). Compressive overload usually fractures the cranial endplate, both in vivo and in cadaveric experiments.[185,1628] This is because the cranial endplate is thinner and weaker than the caudal endplate of the same vertebral body (Fig. 10.7), and it is less well supported by the trabecular arcades from the pedicles (Figs 8.9 and 11.2). (Confusion can arise by referring to the superior and inferior endplates of a disc, and the latter would constitute the superior endplate of the vertebra below.)

Failure is caused by the nucleus pulposus of the adjacent disc causing the endplate to bulge into the vertebra.[188,561,624,1614] The various types of vertebral compressive

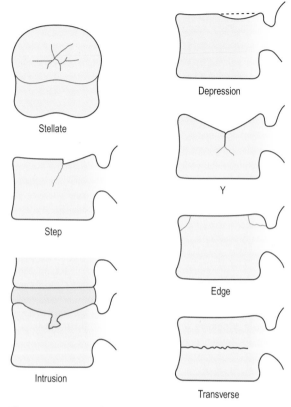

Figure 11.3 Types of vertebral compressive failure, as classified by Brinckmann et al.[185]

damage have been classified by Brinckmann et al.[185] (Fig. 11.3) and a typical example is shown in Figure 11.4. Damage can be difficult to visualise and it is sometimes necessary to press on the bone in order to detect the fine line of fracture running through the endplate or trabecular bone. Endplate disturbance caused by compressive overload tends to be more irregular in older cadaveric specimens with reduced bone mineral density.[561] In some cadaveric experiments, small quantities of nucleus pulposus are expressed vertically through the damaged endplate to form an intraosseous herniation (Fig. 11.5), which in life can lead to a calcified defect known as a Schmorl's node (p. 206). Vertical movement of disc material probably explains why the intraosseous pressure can increase rapidly to 100 mmHg (0.013 MPa) in the damaged vertebra.[1614]

Adolescent vertebrae may fail in a slightly different manner: compression tests on young pig spines show that they fail by a posterior edge fracture (Fig. 11.3) running from the endplate down to the cartilage growth plate, which appears to be a zone of weakness before skeletal maturity.[857]

It is important to realise that typical endplate fractures are difficult to detect on plain X-rays[188,689,857,1614] (Fig. 11.6). However, magnetic resonance imaging (MRI) can help by revealing any vertical displacement of nucleus pulposus,[857] and biological reactions to endplate fracture known as Modic changes (p. 206).[988]

'Osteoporotic' compression fractures of the vertebral body

Osteoporosis is a condition which involves marked systemic bone loss in elderly people (p. 93) and osteoporotic vertebrae can fail by several mechanisms which are unusual in younger spines. Anterior wedge fractures (Fig. 11.7 and 15.21) involve the collapse of the anterior vertebral body cortex together with a wedge-shaped region of trabecular bone behind it. Wedge fractures are probably caused by anteriorly located trabeculae losing thickness and connectivity more than posteriorly located trabeculae[42,642,1311] (Figs 8.7 and 8.17) so that this region of the vertebra is weakened. The vertebral endplate also is weakest anteriorly.[634] The underlying cause of anterior weakening appears to be 'stress shielding' of the anterior vertebral body by the neural arch, following intervertebral disc narrowing.[42] Subsequently, spinal flexion unloads the neural arch, even when the disc is degenerated (Table 8.2), and concentrates the applied compressive force on to the weakened anterior vertebral body. This explanation of anterior wedge fracture assumes that vertebral bone mineral density adapts to forces acting in habitual upright postures, rather than in occasional flexion movements, but this is a reasonable assumption because animal experiments show that between 4 and 36 loading cycles per day are required to induce an adaptive remodelling response.[1226] This, in combination with the reduced responsiveness to mechanical stimuli of old compared with younger bone,[110,1441] suggests that many elderly people will not bend forwards far enough, or often enough, to protect against bone loss from the anterior vertebral body. The importance of stress shielding in osteoporotic fractures of old vertebrae is emphasised by the finding that these fractures are more closely linked to reduced body weight and muscle strength than are fractures of other bones.[428] Young vertebrae can also sustain anterior wedge fractures, but the underlying cause is different: full flexion or hyperflexion concentrates so much of the loading on to the anterior region of bone that it fails first, even though it has normal strength.

A second type of fracture common in elderly spines is the biconcave fracture in which both endplates are collapsed inwards (Fig. 11.7B). The smooth curvature often exhibited by affected endplates (Fig. 8.9) suggests that the underlying cause is repeated microfractures of the weakened trabeculae which support them.[1447,1485] Traumatic compression fracture of younger vertebrae generally creates more discontinuous endplate damage (Fig. 11.5). Intervertebral discs which lie between vertebrae with biconcave fractures often have a high nucleus, because the nucleus has met little resistance in pushing into the

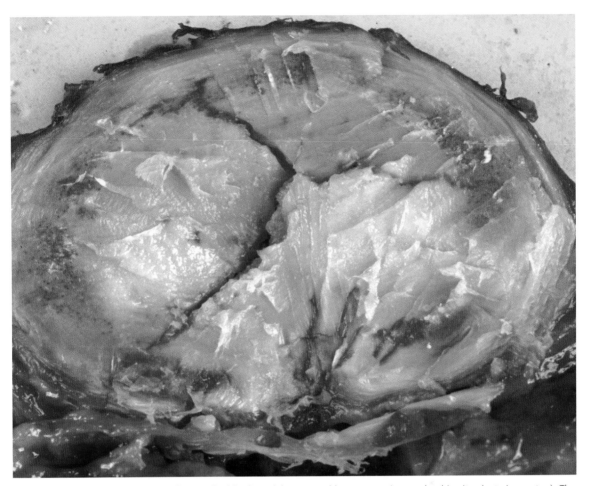

Figure 11.4 Large stellate fracture of a vertebral body endplate caused by compressive overload in vitro (anterior on top). The disc has been cut away to reveal the underlying bone, covered centrally by the hyaline cartilage endplate.

weakened vertebrae. However, this does not necessarily mean that the disc is not degenerated: the annulus may be collapsed, and the height of the annulus is a better indicator of disc integrity and (dys)function than nucleus height.

'Crush' fractures (Fig. 11.7C) in elderly spines may represent the effects of sudden compressive loading collapsing both the anterior and posterior vertebral cortices together. Cadaveric experiments suggests that this is more likely to occur if the spine is flexed slightly, so that the apophyseal joints do not resist most of the loading. The relatively flat endplates sometimes seen in such fractures suggests that the adjacent nucleus pulposus is decompressed when fracture occurs, so that it has little effect on deforming the central region of the vertebral endplates. In young spines, compressive trauma can sometimes cause 'burst fractures', which have a similar appearance to crush fractures.

Gradual creep deformation of old vertebrae is considered on p. 183.

Compressive strength of thoracolumbar vertebrae

The compressive strength of the lumbar spine ranges between 2 and 14 kN, depending on the sex, age and body mass of the individual, with a typical value for a young man being 6–10 kN. The high and low extremes refer to male athletes, and old women with osteoporosis, respectively. The strength of human lumbar motion segments in different forms of loading is summarised in Table 11.1.

Vertebral compressive strength can be predicted to an accuracy of about 1 kN using quantitative computed tomography (QCT) and endplate area[185,186] or from measurements of bone mineral content obtained using dual X-ray absorptiometry.[562] QCT is better at predicting vertebral fractures in elderly people,[189] presumably because it measures volumetric density of trabecular bone, and is little influenced by cortical bone and osteophytes. Endplate area, and presumably spinal compressive strength, can be

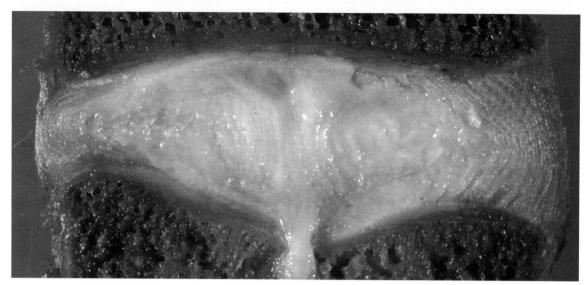

Figure 11.5 Lumbar disc sectioned in the mid-sagittal plane following mechanical loading in vitro (anterior on right). The disc was subjected to a minor compressive overload injury (which damaged the upper endplate of the lower vertebra and decompressed the nucleus) followed by cyclic loading in compression. Some nucleus pulposus has herniated down into the vertebral body, and the inner lamellae appear to be collapsing into the nucleus. Note the concavity of the damaged endplate. (Male, 42 years, L4–5.)

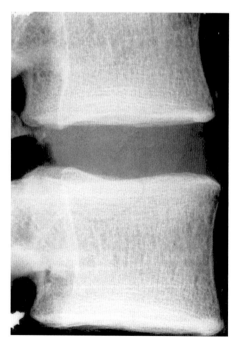

Figure 11.6 Radiograph of a cadaveric lumbar motion segment following endplate fracture. At subsequent dissection, one of the endplates adjacent to the disc was found to be damaged, but this is not apparent from the radiograph.

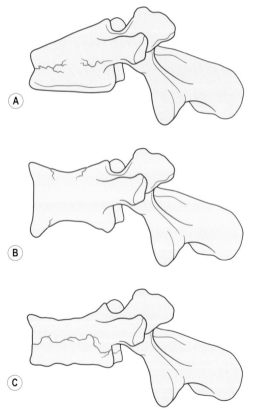

Figure 11.7 Three types of vertebral deformity commonly seen in elderly osteoporotic vertebrae. **(A)** Anterior wedge fracture; **(B)** biconcave fracture; **(C)** crush fracture.
(Reproduced from Rao and Singrakhia[1184] with permission.)

Table 11.1 Strength of lumbar motion segments and intervertebral discs. Sources of data are given in the text. Values in parentheses indicate the standard deviation, and a dash indicates a range of values. B refers to specimens tested without a neural arch

	Site of failure	Average strength	Comments
A. Motion segments			
Compression	Vertebral endplate	5.2 (± 1.8) kN (all specimens)	Depends on endplate area and bone mineral density
		6.1 (± 1.8) kN (male, 20–50 years)	
		10.2* (± 1.7) kN (male, 22–46 years)	
Shear	Neural arch?	2.0 kN?	Strength of disc uncertain
Flexion	Posterior ligaments	73 (± 18) Nm	0.5–1.0 kN compressive preload
Backwards bending	Neural arch	26–45 Nm	Disc can be damaged
Torsion	Neural arch	25–88 Nm	Strength depends on criterion of failure
Flexion + compression	Disc or vertebra	5.4 (±2.4 kN)	Disc can prolapse
B. Disc + vertebral bodies			
Shear	Annulus?	0.5 kN?	Uncertain
Flexion	Posterior annulus	33 (± 13) Nm	Strength unrelated to disc pressure
Torsion	Annulus?	10–31 Nm	Depends on criterion of failure

*Tested in moderate flexion.

estimated from certain anthropometric factors.[294] Body weight is a good predictor of vertebral strength in men, but not women,[647] and this may be because in men body weight is influenced more by muscle mass than body fat. Strength increases down the lumbar spine by approximately 0.3 kN per lumbar level.[184] Reported average strengths of motion segments from young men aged approximately 20–50 years range between 10.2 kN[647] and 6.1 kN.[184,186] The difference between these values may be attributable to several factors: unlike Hutton and Adams,[647] Brinckmann et al.[184] tested all specimens 'fresh' without prior frozen storage; they applied the compressive force only to the vertebral bodies so that the neural arches probably resisted less than if the force had been applied to the entire vertebrae; they used a sensitive definition of the first signs of failure; and many of their specimens were from patients who had prolonged bed rest prior to death. There are no systematic studies of spinal strength in powerful male athletes, but measurements of bone mineral density suggest that it may approach 20 kN.[524] The strongest

motion segments so far tested were from an athletic young coal miner (13.0 kN[1153]) and from a 21-year-old male (14.1 kN[1614]).

Additional information on vertebral strength comes from experiments on animal spines. The strength of pig cervical spines increased if they were compressed rapidly (1 kN/s compared to slowly (0.1 kN/s), but very rapid loading (16 kN/s) had no further strengthening effect.[1613] Frozen storage has been reported to increase the compressive strength of young pig spines by 24%[238] but it is not apparent why this should be so, or if this result can be extrapolated to mature human spines.

Variations in posture (angle of flexion or extension) do not exert a large influence on lumbar motion segment compressive strength.[39,525] This is probably attributable to two opposing effects: in neutral and lordotic postures, the apophyseal joints share in the load-bearing, as described above, and this would be expected to increase strength; but these postures also generate concentrations of compressive stress within the posterior annulus of the disc (Fig. 13.10),

Table 11.2 Cyclic loading reduces the compressive strength of the lumbar spine

Relative load (%)	Number of loading cycles				
	10	100	500	1000	5000
60–70	10%	55%	80%	95%	100%
50–60	0%	40%	65%	80%	90%
40–50	0%	25%	45%	60%	70%
30–40	0%	0%	10%	20%	25%
20–30	0%	0%	0%	0%	10%

Values in Table 11.2 indicate the probability of compressive failure if a motion segment is loaded for the specified number of cycles at the specified relative load. Relative load is the actual compressive load expressed as a percentage of the load required to cause compressive failure in a single loading cycle.
(Data from Brinckmann et al.[184])

and this would act to reduce strength. Isolated thoracic vertebrae were reported to be substantially weaker if compressed to failure with the addition of a forward-bending moment[210] but this could be because the vertebrae were very old and would have lost bone mineral preferentially from their anterior regions.[42]

Fatigue failure of the vertebral body

Compressive failure occurs at lower loads during cyclic loading,[184,565,846] as shown in Table 11.2. Typically, compressive strength is reduced by 30% if 10 loading cycles are applied, and by 50% if 5000 cycles are applied. Damage is reported to be similar to that which occurs during a single loading cycle (Fig. 11.3). However, some slight differences might be expected, because sustained or cyclic loading expels water from the central region of the intervertebral discs,[957] causing them to concentrate more of the loading on to the periphery of the endplate (Fig. 13.15). Compressive fatigue damage is probably a common event in life, because microfractures and healing trabeculae are found in most cadaveric vertebral bodies.[1485]

Vibrations

Fatigue damage can accumulate rapidly if the spine is exposed to mechanical vibrations, for example by sitting on a tractor seat. Vibration frequencies close to the natural resonant frequency of the seated human spine (4–5 Hz) cause the largest vertical accelerations[1098,1561] and the largest intervertebral movements.[1146] Considerable muscle tension is then required to hold the upper body steady.[1292,1379] In erect standing, the resonant frequency can rise to 5.5–7 Hz, depending on posture, but a distinct resonance is lost when the knees are flexed,[1145] presumably because this allow the quadriceps tendons to act as shock

absorbers (Fig. 1.5). Increased muscle tension associated with vibrations would increase disc creep, and cause back muscle fatigue, as discussed in Chapter 14.

Internal disc disruption

The idea that compressive overload can directly damage lumbar discs has been disproved by the experiments described above, but compression may lead indirectly to intervertebral disc failure. Compressive damage to the vertebra allows the endplate to bulge into the vertebral body to a greater extent.[190] This effectively increases the volume available for the nucleus, and causes a large and immediate drop in nucleus pressure.[22,41,1165] (A similar pressure drop would occur in any closed hydraulic system if its volume were suddenly increased.) The decompressed nucleus resists less of the applied compressive force, so more of it falls upon the annulus fibrosus, where it generates large peaks of compressive stress within the tissue, particularly posterior to the nucleus (Fig. 11.8). This makes the annulus unstable: the approximately vertical lamellae are more severely compressed than before, and yet receive less lateral support from the decompressed nucleus. It might be expected that the inner lamellae would buckle and collapse into the nucleus, as shown in Figures 11.5 and 11.9, and there is recent evidence from cadaver[22] and animal[621] experiments that this does in fact happen. The inner lamellae also bulge inwards when the nucleus is decompressed by experimental removal of nucleus material.[1290] Internal derangements of intervertebral discs are more common than disc prolapse,[307] and reverse bulging of the inner lamellae is found in approximately 35% of severely degenerated discs[542,1403] Inwards-bulging lamellae are often found in conjunction with endplate fracture in cadaveric spines (Fig. 11.5).

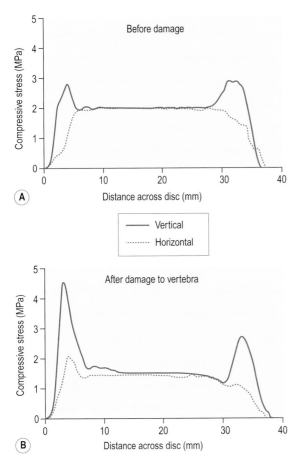

(A)

Vertical
Horizontal

(B)

Figure 11.8 The distribution of compressive stress along the sagittal mid-plane of a cadaveric intervertebral disc is greatly affected by damage to an adjacent vertebral endplate. **(A)** A normal distribution of horizontal and vertical stress for a 46-year-old disc (anterior on right). **(B)** Endplate damage, caused by overloading the motion segment in compression, reduces the pressure in the nucleus, and generates high stress peaks in the annulus. *(Stress profiles are explained in Figure 10.17.)*

The effect of endplate damage on internal disc function depends greatly on age,[22,41] with young discs being less affected than those aged 50–70 years. This is probably because the inner annulus of a young disc behaves like a fluid which can deform readily to accommodate the altered shape of the endplates. Hence, the pressure in the nucleus does not fall, and no stress gradients can be sustained within the annulus. Old and severely degenerated discs may also be less affected by endplate damage than middle-aged discs, but for a quite different reason: they may be narrowed and therefore stress-shielded by the apophyseal joints, so that decompression of the nucleus leads to extra compressive loading of the neural arch rather than the annulus.[1142]

Cadaveric experiments can indicate only the short-term effects of endplate damage on disc function. Longer-term effects would be dominated by the reaction of disc cells to changes in their mechanical environment. Paradoxically, this could make matters worse, because disc cell metabolism is impaired by very high and very low matrix compressive stresses.[667] Therefore, the irregular stress distributions created by endplate damage (Fig. 11.8) would probably inhibit metabolism throughout the disc. Reduced proteoglycan synthesis in the nucleus would serve only to reduce nuclear volume and pressure further, so that a vicious circle of decompression and cell inactivity could be initiated. Stress peaks in the annulus greater than 3 MPa, such as those in Figure 11.8, would stimulate the production of matrix-degrading enzymes[559] so the annulus might suffer progressive mechanical and enzymatic disruption.

The mechanism just outlined shows how an initial compressive injury to a vertebral body endplate could lead to internal collapse of the annulus, followed by cell-mediated enzymatic degradation of the matrix. It is not necessary to invoke more elaborate biological events, such as inflammatory or autoimmune reactions of the nucleus cells to blood from the vertebral body,[156] although these could occur nonetheless.

Endplate disruption may threaten the adjacent discs in yet another way: healing of the damaged bone may block

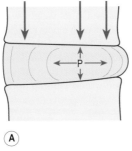

(A)

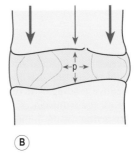

(B)

Figure 11.9 Diagrams of a mid-sagittal section through an intervertebral disc (anterior on left). **(A)** In a normal disc, the pressure (P) in the nucleus pulposus prevents the lamellae of the annulus from collapsing inwards in response to high compressive loading. **(B)** Endplate damage decompresses the nucleus and increases the direct compressive loading on the annulus. Under these circumstances, the inner lamellae can collapse into the nucleus.

the nutrient pathways which appear to be essential for normal cell function in the nucleus.[918] Endplate impermeability has been associated with degeneration of the adjacent disc[1017] although there is recent strong evidence to the contrary.[1210]

Activities which could injure the spine in compression

During normal living, most of the compressive force acting on the spine is generated by tension in the muscles of the back and trunk (Ch. 9), and any activity which requires maximal contraction of these muscles can threaten the spine with compressive overload. Vertebrae are frequently crushed during grand epileptic seizures, when normal neurological inhibition of muscle contraction force is lacking.[1475] (Many of these injuries occur with the subject lying in bed, so they cannot be attributed to falls.) Alarming events, or emergencies during manual handling, could have a similar effect on muscle action and spinal loading. Lifting heavy or bulky objects in a rapid or awkward manner can generate compressive forces higher than the fatigue limit (Fig. 1.7) so fatigue failure would occur if such activities were performed sufficiently often that microdamage accumulated at a faster rate than the body's adaptive remodelling response could cope with. Accidents involving falls and collisions could also injure the lumbar spine in compression.

SHEAR

It is convenient to define a 'shear' force on the vertebral column as that force which acts parallel to the mid-plane of the intervertebral disc, at 90° to the compressive force discussed above. (This is not quite what engineers usually mean by shear when discussing stress analysis, but there is little scope for confusion.) The shear force arises mostly from gravity acting on the upper body, and so is greater in the lower lumbar spine where the discs are inclined at a steep angle to the horizontal (Fig. 11.1), and in forward-stooping postures.

Resistance to shear

Collagen fibres in the disc and intervertebral ligaments are poorly oriented to resist shear, and indeed the disc just 'creeps away' from it during repetitive loading.[316] It can therefore be assumed that, under most circumstances in life, most or all of the shear force acting on the lumbar spine is resisted by the neural arch. If the apophyseal joints are asymmetrical in the horizontal plane (articular tropism: Fig. 10.8) then the intervertebral shear force tends to cause the upper vertebra to rotate towards the side of the facet which is oriented more in the frontal plane.[315] Even if the apophyseal joints are symmetrical, an eccentric

shear force acting lateral to the mid-sagittal plane can cause axial rotation, and may contribute to rotational deformity in the thoracic spine.[783] The erector spinae muscles have many fascicles which pass in an inferior posterior direction from the transverse processes to the sacrum and ilium (Ch. 3), and these are capable of resisting most of the intervertebral shear force.[1157] However, it is not certain whether or not they do this in practice, and in the upright posture, the muscles of the trunk exert a net anterior shear force on the lumbar spine.[164]

Damage in shear

The orientation of the lumbar apophyseal joints suits them well for resisting shear, and when loaded perpendicular to the pars interarticularis, the inferior articular processes can resist approximately 2 kN (range 0.6–2.8 kN) before fracture occurs in the pars, or pedicle.[318] Fracture of the pars can also occur in response to cyclic forces oscillating between 380 N and 760 N.[313] Fractures resemble the pars defects seen in spondylolysis, and this may indeed be one cause of spondylolysis. (Other causes probably include repeated flexion and extension movements, as discussed on page 162.) Shear damage would be more likely to occur if the apophyseal joint surfaces were oriented more medially (Fig. 2.14), or if they were so asymmetrical that one or other of them was called upon to resist most of the shear force by itself. If the apophyseal joints are removed, then repetitive loading in compression and shear causes the disc to slip forwards by several millimetres, with a greater slip occurring when the disc is degenerated.[316] More than 20 mm of forward slip can occur if the loading is severe.[316] This may explain why spondylolisthesis (Fig. 19.3) often follows bilateral spondylolysis.

Activities which could injure the spine in shear

Vertical gravitational loading creates a forwards shear force on the L4 and L5 vertebrae, because these tend to be inclined forwards to the horizontal (Fig. 11.1). The forward shear force would increase if the trunk was inclined forwards and if its weight was increased, so marching long distances with a heavy backpack could be a common cause of shear failure of the neural arch.[651] Standing in a very lordotic posture would increase the inclination of the sacrum and increase the shear force acting on L5 and S1. So too would landing upright from a jump.

TORSION

Centre of rotation

The lumbar spine does not have a clearly defined axis for axial rotation (torsion) movements. It probably lies

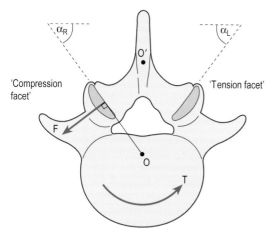

Figure 11.10 Superior view of a lumbar vertebra, showing how the orientation of the apophyseal joint surfaces restricts axial rotation (torsion) movements. An applied torque (T) causes a superior vertebra to rotate about an axis (O) within the posterior annulus fibrosus, rather than about a posterior axis representing the centre of curvature of the joint surfaces (O'). This brings the articulating surfaces of the compression facet into firm contact and generates a high compressive force (F) on those surfaces. The capsule and ligaments of the opposite tension facet provide little resistance. Note that the orientation of the apophyseal joints, represented by the angles α_L and α_R, is often asymmetrical, a condition referred to as facet tropism.

somewhere in the posterior annulus fibrosus, because this is where the axis of minimal torsional stiffness lies[26] and where a motion segment appears to rotate around if it is subjected to a pure torque.[299] However, small rotational movements bring one of the apophyseal joints into firm contact (Fig. 11.10) and this probably causes the axis to migrate towards that joint as the applied torque increases. Note that the axis does not lie near the centre of curvature of the apophyseal joint surfaces (Fig. 11.10). Such a location would minimise the resistance to torsion from these joints, but their function is to limit and guide movement, not merely facilitate it.

Resistance to torsion

Lumbar motion segments offer little resistance to very small angles of axial rotation. Collagen fibres in the annulus simply straighten out their 'crimp' waveform. Further movement then brings the articular surfaces firmly together in one of the two apophyseal joints (the 'compression joint') and this restricts movement to 1–2° in young and healthy spines.[26,1089] A similarly restricted range of movement (RoM) has been measured in vivo (Fig. 10.2). The range of axial rotation increases with increasing disc degeneration,[1089] and old lumbar motion segments

can be axially rotated up to 8° without apparent damage.[26] This could be because age-related degenerative changes reduce the thickness of articular cartilage in the apophyseal joints, allowing more 'free play'. If a torque of 8.5 Nm is applied to a motion segment, without any compressive loading, then the anterior and lateral annulus resist torsion more strongly than the apophyseal joints.[793] However, the resistance from the latter increases at higher torques, and when high compressive preloads press the vertebrae closer together: typically, at the limit of the physiological RoM, 30–70% of the applied torque is resisted by the apophyseal joint in compression, 20–50% by the disc and only 0–5% by all of the intervertebral ligaments combined.[26] Of the ligaments, only those associated with the apophyseal joint capsule are stretched more than 5% when the applied torque reaches 15 Nm.[1100]

The fact that torsion is resisted more by bony surfaces than by ligaments or annulus fibrosus may explain why torsion has less effect than bending on intradiscal pressure: the measured increase in pressure in response to an applied torque is less than 15% of that which occurs when an equivalent bending moment is applied.[1277]

Torsional damage

Damage is initiated when the applied torque rises to approximately 10–30 Nm, which is equivalent to a force of 250–500 N acting on the compressed apophyseal joint.[26] The precise nature of the initial torsional damage is uncertain, but probably involves the articular cartilage or subchondral bone of the compressed apophyseal joint.

The effects of torsional loading on the disc have long been controversial, but the experimental evidence appears simple enough: in the small RoM permitted by the lumbar apophyseal joints, no disc damage has been demonstrated, and none would be expected. Several authors have repeated the suggestion of Farfan et al.[413] that a change in torsional stiffness which occurs at approximately 3° of rotation represents microdamage to the disc. However, similar changes in stiffness with increasing displacement are seen in all other disc movements, and is attributable to the opening-out of the 'crimp' structure of the disc's collagen fibres (Fig. 7.18). This is not evidence of damage. Collagen fibres in discs, ligaments and tendons all show this initial region of low stiffness before entering a linear region, up to approximately 10% strain, at which damage really does occur. No evidence of torsional damage to the disc can be detected in the RoM 1–9°.[29] It would be difficult to reconcile the suggestion that lumbar discs suffer microscopic damage at 3° of rotation with the fact that thoracic discs, which receive less torsional protection from the apophyseal joints, can be rotated by an average of 3° to each side in vivo, and by up to 10° at T12–L1, without apparent harm.[531] If motion segments are subjected to cyclic torsional loading, then the only demonstrable damage occurs in the apophyseal joints rather than the disc.[845] Finite

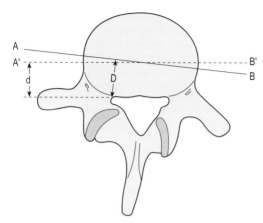

Figure 11.11 Asymmetrical apophyseal joints (here exaggerated) could possibly contribute to disc degeneration by causing the disc to flex about an oblique axis (solid line, AB) rather than about a symmetrical axis (dashed line, A'B'). In this example, the left posterolateral corner of the disc lies further from the oblique axis (D) than from the symmetric axis (d) and so would be stretched more during bending movements.

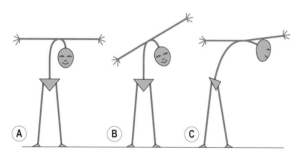

Figure 11.12 (A) Bending directly forwards flexes the lumbar spine. **(B)** If the lumbar spine is axially rotated at the same time as it is flexed, then the upper body will be rotated as shown. This is not a common movement in life. **(C)** Adding lateral bending to the forward flexion produces the asymmetrical bending which is common in manual handling. This asymmetrical bending may also involve some coupled axial rotation, but axial rotation is not a primary movement.

element modelling of the lumbar spine also suggests that disc failure in pure axial rotation is unlikely.[1307]

It has been proposed that the range of axial rotation, and the consequent risk of disc injury, depends on the obliquity of the apophyseal joint surfaces, or on asymmetry in the obliquity of the two joints at a given level ('facet tropism'), as shown in Figures 10.8 and 11.11. However, the experimental evidence does not support this theory,[50,541] not even when coupled movements are taken into account.[379] Associations between facet tropism and disc degeneration[153,415,1052] can be explained by a mechanism involving bending rather than torsion (Fig. 11.12), because

tropism could lead to asymmetrical bending and increased stretching of the posterolateral annulus (Fig. 11.11).

The precise range of torsional movement, and the risk of disc injury, will also be influenced by other components of spinal loading. For example, in a forward 'stooped' posture, the intervertebral shear force rises[651] and presses the apophyseal joint surfaces closely together, reducing the small range of axial rotation even more.[541] It has been proposed that the tapered shape of the articular facets allows them more free play in certain flexed postures, and this may explain why sitting with the lumbar spine flexed and the legs stretched out in front appears to increase the range of axial rotation.[1112] However, the skin surface measurements offered in support of this mechanism greatly overestimate the true axial rotation movements of the vertebral column; they may also be influenced by the posteriorly directed shear force which acts on the lumbar spine in this peculiar sitting posture, and which may 'open up' the space between the articular surfaces.

If the apophyseal joints are cut away, then forced axial rotation damages the disc at approximately 10–20° of rotation, with ultimate failure occurring at 11–32°.[413] Circumferential tears appear in the outer annulus, but there is no formation of radial fissures or displacement of nucleus pulposus.[413] Torsional stresses would be greatest in that region of the disc which lies furthest from the centre of rotation, and this region is always the anterolateral annulus, even when the centre of rotation moves towards the apophyseal joint in compression. In life, this mechanism might explain the 'rim tears' which commonly affect the anterolateral annulus[542,1483] and its attachments to bone.[608] It appears that severe torsional damage must be inflicted on the apophyseal joints, causing a 'crumpled neural arch'[1380] before lumbar discs are adversely affected.

The role of torsion in causing damage to thoracic motion segments has not yet been investigated.

Activities which could injure the spine in torsion

The lumbar spine would be subjected to a large torque if a force were exerted on an outstretched arm, perhaps during a fall, or during some contact sport such as rugby. Activities such as hurling a discus would generate substantial angular momentum in the upper body, and this would have to be resisted by the spine and trunk muscles in order to bring the body to rest. Serving in tennis, fast bowling in cricket and driving in golf similarly twist the lumbar spine, but the effects of torsion are difficult to distinguish from accompanying movements in backwards and lateral bending. The back muscles are poorly positioned to oppose any dynamically applied torque, but axial torques of up to 100 Nm can be generated by a combination of other muscles, particularly the external obliques and latissimus dorsi.[941] A certain amount of torque would be generated on the lumbar spine when someone bends forwards and twists round to one side. Such awkward twisting movements are closely related to disc prolapse and back pain,[732,924] but it is likely that the main movements of the lumbar spine are forward and lateral bending, rather than torsion (Fig. 11.12).

BACKWARDS BENDING

Centre of rotation

During flexion and extension movements in the sagittal plane, the axis of rotation is not fixed, but moves slightly within the nucleus pulposus of the intervertebral disc (p. 117). In effect, the superior vertebra glides anteriorly and posteriorly, respectively, as it flexes and extends about the nucleus. However, when discs become degenerated the centre of rotation can change markedly and inconsistently.[489] Cadaver experiments show that it can migrate towards the apophyseal joints during backwards-bending movements.[1627]

Resistance to backwards bending

The neural arch resists 60–70% of the applied bending moment when a motion segment is extended right up to its elastic limit. On average, damage can be detected after 3–8° of movement (mean 5°) with a bending moment of 28 Nm[19] or 45 Nm,[529] depending on the criterion of damage and the accompanying compressive force. Typically, an extension moment of 10 Nm combined with a compressive load of 190 N creates an apophyseal joint force of 200 N.[1262] Forces on the neural arch increase further if compressive loading is high, as would often be the case in vivo. For example, if a normal motion segment were subjected to 3 kN of compression while positioned in 4° of extension, the neural arches would resist approximately 570 N (calculated from Adams et al.[39]). Such a high force would generate very high stress concentrations in the lower margins of these joints, or adjacent laminae.[380]

The rest of the resistance to backwards bending must come from the intervertebral disc, and from the anterior longitudinal ligament.[1100,1262] Concentrations of compressive stress appear in the posterior annulus after just 2° of extension and increase considerably at 4° of extension (p. 179).[37,39] The posterior annulus bulges into the vertebral canal, reducing its diameter by 2 mm.[1274][Schonstrom, 1989 #1128] Stress concentrations within the neural arch and disc may explain why so many people find it uncomfortable to extend their lumbar spine fully while in the erect standing position. Although backward bending usually develops high stress concentrations within the posterior annulus, there are exceptions to this 'rule'. In one study, several motion segments showed a reduction in peak compressive stress within the posterior annulus

in 2° and 4° of extension, compared to the neutral posture.[37]

Damage in backwards bending

It is not easy to identify the first structure to be damaged in hyperextension, and it may depend on anatomical details such as the height of the disc, and the spacing and shape of adjacent spinous processes.[19] Most likely, the apophyseal joints would be damaged first, but the interspinous ligament may be squashed between opposing spinous processes, and primary disc damage cannot be ruled out. A combination of full backwards bending and 1 kN of compressive loading can cause the inferior articular processes to be deflected posteriorly by approximately 2° (Fig. 11.13), presumably because they make contact with the lamina below, and pivot about the pars interarticularis.[529] The deformation is not entirely elastic,[39,529] so it could involve damage to the joint capsule, as suggested in Figure 11.13. This was first proposed as a mechanism for back pain by Yang and King.[1605] Rapid lumbar extension movements, which occur in sports such as gymnastics, athletics, tennis and cricket, could conceivably force the neural arches together with sufficient violence to fracture the pars interarticularis, and cause spondylolysis.

If a motion segment is positioned in hyperextension and compressed rapidly to failure, then in certain cases the nucleus pulposus of the intervertebral disc can herniate through the anterior annulus.[19] The mechanism is probably similar to that for posterior disc herniation (see Fig. 11.18, below) but anterior prolapse is harder to achieve (at least in the laboratory) because the anterior annulus is usually thicker than the posterior. If the neural arches are removed from cadaveric motion segments, then severe repetitive loading in backwards bending and compression leads to posterior bulging of the posterior annulus. Extreme 'hairpin bending' of individual lamellae can persist after cessation of loading (Fig. 11.14). This mechanism probably explains why backwards bending leads to posterior disc protrusion in the tails of experimental rats[836,837] and mice.[851] In living humans, prior or accompanying damage to the neural arch may be necessary in order to deform the disc sufficiently. If a complete radial fissure exists already in the posterior annulus, then repeated extension movements can force injected radiographic contrast fluid down the fissure and into the vertebral canal.[497] It is unclear if nucleus pulposus material can migrate as easily as contrast fluid.

Activities which could injure the spine in backwards bending

Full backwards-bending movements of the lumbar spine can occur during overhead manual work, such as painting a ceiling. It is difficult to measure lumbar extension

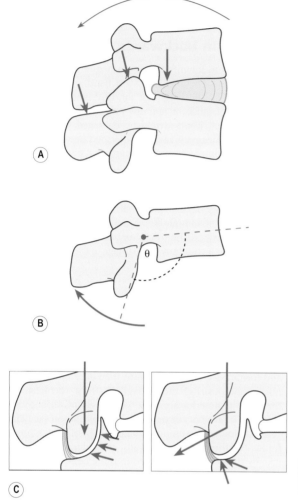

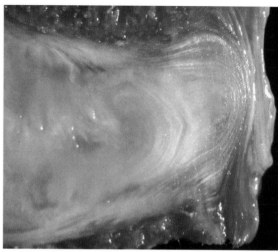

Figure 11.14 Disc protrusion reproduced in the laboratory. Photograph of a cadaveric lumbar disc, sectioned in the mid-sagittal plane, following cyclic mechanical loading in compression and backwards bending. Note the hairpin bending of the outermost lamellae, causing the posterior annulus to protrude beyond the posterior margin of the adjacent vertebral bodies.

Figure 11.13 The effects of backwards bending on a lumbar motion segment. **(A)** Concentrations of compressive stress appear in the posterior annulus, the apophyseal joints and between the spinous processes. **(B)** The inferior articular facets bend backwards about the pars interarticularis by several degrees. **(C)** Hyperextension can generate high contact forces in the lower margins of the articular surfaces, causing backwards rotation of the inferior facet and stretching of the joint capsule.

accurately using skin surface techniques, because skin wrinkling interferes with the measurements,[20] but approximate measures of thoracolumbar extension obtained from large electromechanical devices do indicate that lumbar extension movements are not uncommon in industry, and that they are closely associated with back pain.[924] Exertions in the upright or extended postures are also likely to generate substantial antagonistic activity of the trunk muscles, and lead to high compressive loading of the spine.[520]

Sporting activities such as serving in tennis, and fast bowling at cricket, subject the lumbar spine to combinations of backwards bending, lateral bending and torsion, and could cause a variety of injuries to the neural arch, including spondylolysis (see Fig. 11.33, below).

FORWARD BENDING

Centre of rotation

The centre of rotation for sagittal-plane flexion and extension movements is not static: it moves around as the vertebrae rotate and slide past each other. It normally lies in the inferior posterior region of the nucleus pulposus (Fig. 10.5).

Resistance to forward bending

When motion segments are subjected to complex loading in bending, compression and shear in order to simulate flexion of the lumbar spine in vivo, the intervertebral ligaments provide most of the resistance to movement.

During the first few degrees of flexion, there is slight resistance from the intervertebral disc and ligamentum flavum.[13,33] Reference is sometimes made to a 'neutral zone'(NZ) in which the motion segment has zero resistance to bending,[1100] but this is an artefact caused by applying discrete weights to cadaveric spines and then allowing

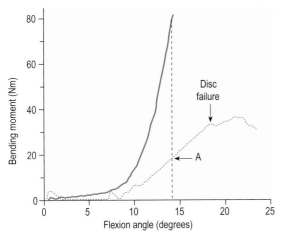

Figure 11.15 When a lumbar motion segment is subjected to a combination of bending and compression, to simulate forward flexion in life, its resistance to bending is initially slight, but increases rapidly as the limit of movement is approached (solid curve). This particular specimen (male, 28 years, L4–5), has a neutral zone of 7° and a full range of flexion of 14°. When the neural arch and ligaments were removed, then the remaining disc could be flexed to 18° before damage (dashed curve). The bending moment resisted by the disc at the limit of flexion **(A)** is usually much less than that required to injure the disc, indicating that the ligaments protect the disc in flexion. *(Adapted from Adams et al.[24])*

creep to occur before measuring the flexion angle. During dynamic activities, the lumbar vertebral column provides some resistance even to small movements.

Halfway to full flexion, the disc resists more strongly than the posterior intervertebral ligaments, and this is attributable to tension in the outer posterior annulus, and compression of the anterior annulus, which bulges anteriorly by approximately 0.1 mm per degree of flexion.[1363] Ligament tension rises rapidly over the last few degrees of movement, so that in full flexion, 39% of the resistance comes from the capsular ligaments of the apophyseal joint, 29% from the disc, 19% from the interspinous and supraspinous ligaments and 13% from the ligamentum flavum.[33] The bending moment resisted by the spine is almost doubled during the final 2–3° of movement (Fig. 11.15). Tension in the intervertebral ligaments can be sufficient to bend the inferior articular processes forwards by several degrees about the pars interarticularis[529] and it increases pressure in the nucleus by up to 110% in full flexion,[24] even if the applied compressive load stays the same. It has been suggested that the articular surfaces of the apophyseal joints resist flexion,[1446] but this is based on experiments which measured the joints' resistance to combined bending and shear, and it is shear that is resisted by the apophyseal joints. There is experimental and theoretical evidence that the smooth articular surfaces play a negligible role in resisting lumbar flexion.[33,1306]

There is an interesting diurnal variation in the spine's resistance to flexion. Prolonged loading expels water from the disc, reducing its height and allowing some slack to the short collagen fibres of the annulus and intervertebral ligaments. This has the effect of increasing the range of flexion, and reducing the proportion of bending moment resisted by the disc (Fig. 13.18). On the other hand, a high compressive preload removes any slack from collagen fibres in the annulus, and therefore increases the disc's resistance to bending.[13,473,677,1566]

Comparisons between in vivo and in vitro measurements show that the back muscles do not normally permit the vertebral column to be flexed right up to its elastic limit.[32] However, the margin of safety for the lumbar spine decreases in the early morning[18] and can be eliminated entirely by mechanisms described in Chapter 14.

Damage in forward bending

Rapid bending

Injury in flexion typically occurs when the bending moment rises to 50–80 Nm, but the spine's strength in bending can be as high as 124 Nm in strong young men.[13,24,33] The flexion angle at which injury occurs is usually between 5 and 9° per motion segment for the upper lumbar spine, and 10 and 16° for the lower lumbar spine. The similarity in mobility between cadaveric motion segments and living joints (Fig. 10.3) suggests that the RoM in life is influenced strongly by the mechanical properties of discs and ligaments, rather than by the length of the back muscles. This makes it feasible to estimate the bending moment acting on the lumbar spine of living subjects by comparing spinal movements with the bending stiffness properties of cadaveric spines.

The first structure to sustain damage beyond the elastic limit (50–80 Nm) is the interspinous–supraspinous ligament complex.[33] If forwards bending is combined with lateral bending, then the capsular ligaments of the contralateral apophyseal joint are put to an additional stretch because they lie at some distance from the sagittal midline.[1039] They could then sustain damage before the interspinous ligament (Fig. 11.16). In normal forward bending, however, a further 2° of hyperflexion is required to overstretch the capsular ligaments.[7]

In more violent flexion injuries, overt damage has been reported when the bending moment exceeds 70 Nm.[981] Gross damage is evident at 120 Nm[1039] and complete failure of the tissues occurs at 140–185 Nm, with a flexion angle of approximately 20°.[1083,1084] The last structure to fail is the outer posterior annulus fibrosus. Its strong fibres either pull a fragment of the vertebra away from the rest of the bone,[27] or else pull out of their vertebral anchorages, or rupture and pull out of the disc matrix at mid-disc

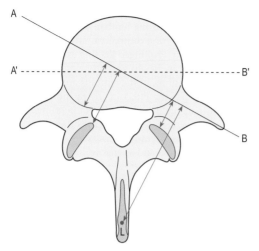

Figure 11.16 Superior view of a lumbar vertebra, illustrating the dangers of bending forwards and to one side. The oblique axis of bending (AB) then lies close to one apophyseal joint, but far from one posterolateral corner of the disc. Stretching of ligaments and annulus is proportional to their distance from the axis, so in this example, the left posterolateral annulus will be stretched more than in normal flexion about A'B'. This region of annulus must also resist a higher proportion of the applied bending moment, because the right apophyseal joint lies so close to the bending axis (AB) that its resistance to bending will be negligible. Furthermore, stretching of the interspinous/supraspinous ligament (L) will be reduced, so its apparent function as the check on forward bending would be jeopardised.

height (Fig 10.13A). These latter two mechanisms, which require a great deal of energy, indicate how well the collagen 'cross-weave' of the annulus is able to reinforce the matrix in the manner of a fibre-composite material, and prevent the propagation of tensile damage throughout the annulus. Once the outer ligamentous portion of the annulus has failed in hyperflexion, it is easy for the inner annulus to pull the cartilaginous endplate away from subchondral bone.[24] Discs tested to destruction in forward bending, without any ligamentous protection, resist 15–50 Nm before failing in this manner, at a typical flexion angle of 18°.[24] Strength in bending appears to be independent of nucleus pressure,[24] suggesting that, in extreme flexion, the posterior annulus behaves like a ligament in tension. The role of intervertebral ligaments in protecting the disc in flexion is illustrated in Figure 11.15.

Slow and sustained bending

The spine's strength and stiffness in bending depend on the speed of movement.[14,1084,1595] The viscoelastic properties of ligaments and discs cause their resistance to flexion to increase by 12% if the duration of the movement is reduced from 10 to 1 second; conversely, sustained flexion reduces motion segment resistance to bending by 42% in just 5 minutes, and 67% in 1 hour.[14] Most of the 5-minute effect is probably due to rapid stress relaxation in stretched spinal ligaments[1595] and this effect would probably be even quicker in living tissues at 37°C. Viscoelastic deformations of the disc are slower because they involve fluid movements over long distances. Because of these effects, rapid flexion movements are more likely to injure the discs and ligaments than slow movements to the same end position, and sustained flexion may reduce ligamentous protection of the discs during dynamic movements. Sustained bending also reduces the protective action of the back muscles (Fig. 14.2).

Interactions between bending and compression

Bending stiffness also increases in the presence of a substantial compressive preload,[13,677] presumably because a prestressed annulus resists deformation more strongly. Typically, raising the preload from 400 N to 1300 N increases motion segment resistance to flexion by 30%,[13] emphasising the importance of a realistic compressive preload in cadaveric experiments.

Activities which could injure the spine in forward bending

Healthy people flex their lumbar spine by 80–100% whenever they bend forwards to lift objects up from the floor (p. 110). Awkward bending movements (forwards and to one side) require some lateral flexion of the lumbar spine,[747] and this would increase stretching of the contralateral apophyseal joint capsule. Full flexion right up to or beyond the normal static limit can occur in simple tasks such as putting on a sock or shoe, especially in people with a low range of sagittal-plane movement in the lumbar spine and hips, who tend to lunge forwards in order to accomplish the task.[357] Risks would increase following a long period of flexed posture (for example, driving a car) because stress relaxation will occur in ligaments and other collagenous tissues which have been stretched for a long time. This presents a double risk to the spine: firstly, it allows the spine to creep into more and more flexion[944] so that conditions are then more favourable for disc prolapse (see next section). Secondly, stress relaxation of ligaments and tendons desensitises their mechanoreceptors, and greatly diminishes reflex muscular protection of the spine (Fig. 14.2). During repetitive bending and lifting activities, this loss of reflex muscular protection is exacerbated by muscle fatigue,[359] which reduces the muscles' ability to generate maximum force in an emergency.[902] Gross ruptures of the interspinous ligament have been reported in

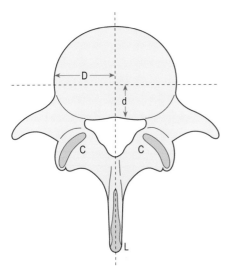

Figure 11.17 Superior view of a lumbar vertebra, showing that lateral bending stretches the peripheral annulus fibrosus more than the same angular movement in flexion. Stretching of a region of annulus is proportional to its distance from the axis of bending, and this can be much higher in lateral bending (D) compared to forward bending (d). The effect is greatest in lower lumbar discs where the ratio D/d is highest. The interspinous/supraspinous ligament (L) and apophyseal joint capsular ligaments (C) lie close to the axis of lateral bending and so do not offer much resistance to movement.

20% of cadaveric spines,[1198] suggesting that hyperflexion injuries to the lumbar spine are not uncommon in life.

LATERAL BENDING

Lateral bending movements of the thoracolumbar spine have not been studied in much detail. By itself it is an uncommon movement, but a component of lateral flexion frequently accompanies forwards flexion when people bend to reach objects which are not directly in from of them (Fig. 11.12). Small lateral bending movements can also accompany axial rotation, although this effect is variable, and may be under muscular control.[1116] Symmetry suggests that the axis of lateral bending lies along the midsagittal plane of the disc, so that most of the spine's resistance to lateral bending probably comes from compression of the apophyseal joint on the side towards which the spine is bent,[1262] and from stretching of the contralateral annulus fibrosus and capsular ligaments (Fig. 11.17). The intertransverse ligaments are stretched most by lateral bending,[1100] but they are weak and would be unable to protect the disc mechanically.

A lateral bending moment of 10 Nm causes 4–6° of lateral bending, with most of the resistance coming from

the disc.[1089,1277] Particularly high shear strains are then generated in the lateral and posterior annulus[300] and may contribute to delamination. If the disc is degenerated, then the RoM falls to 3–4°, and the NZ (see Fig. 11.31, below) is almost eliminated,[1089] suggesting that apophyseal joints are becoming impacted. The rise in nucleus pressure generated by a lateral bending moment is greater than when the same moment is applied in forward bending.[1277] This is probably because much of the resistance to lateral bending comes from collagen fibres in the lateral annulus, which lie further from the axis of bending than do the posterior intervertebral ligaments when resisting flexion, and so are stretched more by a given angular movement. When a lateral bending moment of 60 Nm was applied to three young motion segments, 12–15° of angular movement was observed, and two of the specimens were damaged.[981] Unfortunately, the method of gripping the specimen contributed to the damage, and may have influenced the mode of failure (the superior endplate was pulled away from the vertebral body).

BENDING AND COMPRESSION: DISC PROLAPSE

Direct compressive loading of a lumbar motion segment never causes direct damage to the disc.[186,387,647] The disc has a higher compressive strength than the vertebral bodies on either side of it, regardless of whether the disc is healthy or degenerated, or if the compression is applied rapidly or slowly[1123] or repetitively.[184,846] Even if the disc is deliberately weakened before testing, by cutting into the posterolateral annulus from the outside[1498] or from the nucleus,[183] the disc is not injured when the spine is loaded in compression. Usually, the thin plate of perforated cortical bone which constitutes the vertebral body endplate is the 'weak link' of the lumbar spine in compression (p. 139). Torsional loading also does not generate radial fissures, or cause discs to prolapse, not even if the apophyseal joints are first destroyed, and the disc twisted to angles 10 times greater than its normal range in life (p. 147).

The only proven method of injuring a disc without damaging its adjacent vertebrae is to bend the disc so much that the stretched and thinned annulus becomes weaker than the vertebral endplate (Fig. 11.18) and then to compress the disc in this vulnerable position. Two cadaveric experiments initially provided detailed evidence that discs can then prolapse in response to severe or repetitive loading, without artificial interference to the annulus.[27,30]

Disc prolapse by sudden loading

When lumbar motion segments are positioned in anterolateral flexion or hyperflexion, and then compressed rapidly to failure, approximately half of them fail by

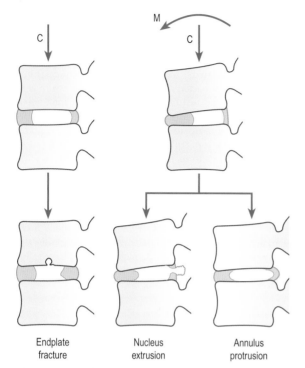

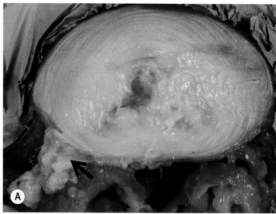

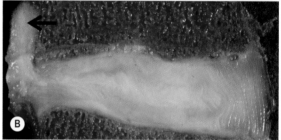

Figure 11.18 Left: compressive loading (C) damages the vertebral endplate before the intervertebral disc. Right: a bending moment (M) acting on the spine stretches and thins the annulus on the contralateral side, reducing its strength compared to the endplate. The simultaneous application of a high compressive force (C) raises the pressure in the nucleus pulposus, and the disc can then prolapse: either nucleus pulposus herniates through the weakened annulus (nucleus extrusion) or else it causes the annulus to collapse outwards (annulus protrusion).

Figure 11.19 (A) Lumbar intervertebral disc following mechanical loading in vitro (anterior on top). Note the large posterolateral herniation of nucleus pulposus (bottom left) which occurred suddenly following severe loading in bending and compression. (Male, 43 years, L4–5.) **(B)** Lumbar disc sectioned in the mid-sagittal plane following mechanical loading in vitro. The disc was compressed to failure (9.8 kN) while positioned in 6° of flexion. Note the radial fissure and the herniated nucleus pulposus trapped behind the posterior longitudinal ligament. (Male, 40 years, L2–3.)

posterior prolapse of the intervertebral disc (Fig. 11.19). In the original experiment,[27] discs which prolapsed most readily were non-degenerated discs from cadavers aged 40–50 years.[469] Severely degenerated discs (grade 4 on a scale of 1–4: Fig. 10.19) could not be made to prolapse.

The applied compressive force required to cause prolapse was 5.4 kN on average (range 2.8–13.0 kN) and the average flexion angle was 15.8° (range 9–21°). (Flexion angles reported in the original paper were 3° too low, because of a calibration error in the goniometer used to measure them.) Each motion segment would have been flexed several degrees beyond its normal range of motion defined by the interspinous ligament (p. 151), but this could not be verified because the neural arches were removed before testing in order to reveal the posterior annulus more clearly. This interference could have had little influence on whether the discs prolapsed or not, because in several subsequent experiments, the same

technique has been used as a matter of routine to cause disc prolapse in intact motion segments.[22,361,961,1153] These later experiments clarified one important detail: it is not absolutely necessary for the flexion angle to be high, provided that either the flexion angle or the compressive force exceeds normal everyday limits. The large prolapse shown in Figure 11.19B occurred in an intact motion segment flexed only 6°, which was well within the elastic range of its ligaments.

Some details of these experimental prolapses may be of clinical interest. Prolapse occurred in approximately 1 second, sometimes with an audible 'pop', and in one specimen the displaced nucleus material was projected through the air for a considerable distance! In each case, a complete radial fissure was created to allow posterior migration of nuclear material, but the excellent self-sealing properties of the annulus[183,916] make these fissures difficult to visualise when the disc is sectioned horizontally

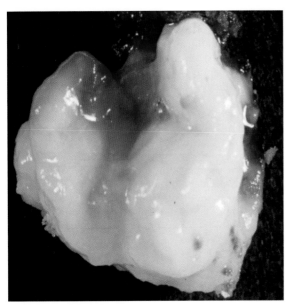

Figure 11.20 Close-up view of herniated nucleus pulposus obtained as in Figure 11.19. Note that there is some attached bone tissue, presumably from the vertebral endplate.

show age-related weakening of the annulus, and yet still retain the large pressurised nucleus of youth.[1266] Severely degenerated discs do not prolapse in the laboratory,[27,961] presumably because the nucleus is too fibrous and dehydrated to exert a hydrostatic pressure on the annulus.[40] Similarly, cadaveric discs which have been dehydrated by several hours of creep loading exhibit a reduced nuclear pressure[38] and a greatly reduced propensity to prolapse when loaded severely.[18] Mathematical models[855,1357] and experiments on animal discs[1312] also indicate that prolapse is more likely to occur when the loading is applied rapidly to a fully hydrated disc.

In another experiment on mostly non-degenerated motion segments aged 20–52 years, posterior disc prolapse was simulated using up to 8° of flexion, and between 1 kN and 6 kN of compression.[191] However, it was necessary to weaken these discs before testing began by cutting a 10 × 10-mm channel into the posterior annulus from the nucleus, so that only the outermost 1 mm of annulus was intact. Also, the nucleus was replaced by chopped pieces of annulus taken from another disc. This experiment explains how a severely degenerated disc could prolapse at low flexion angles after a large radial fissure and fragmented nucleus have been created by other means.

(Fig. 11.19A). In the sagittal plane, however, they are quite obvious (Fig. 11.19B). In a minority of specimens, prolapse appeared as a localised outwards collapse of the posterior annulus, but usually it involved the extrusion, or sequestration, of nucleus pulposus material, sometimes with harder material attached to it (Fig. 11.20). The displaced material either emerged from the posterolateral corner of the disc which was stretched most by the component of lateral bending (Fig. 11.19A), or else it was more midline and trapped behind, or displaced by, the posterior longitudinal ligament. Manual pulling of the vertebrae apart into flexion caused some of the nucleus material to be sucked back into the disc, but it was always expelled again as soon as the manipulation stopped. In contrast, it was a simple matter to push the material sideways away from the site of extrusion.

A later experiment showed that discs which prolapsed were more likely to exhibit peaks of compressive stress in the matrix of the posterior annulus when loaded in bending and compression.[961] The origin of these stress concentrations is unclear: they may indicate focal damage to the collagen network, causing a localised loss of proteoglycans and water, and resulting in a loss of hydrostatic properties in that region of the disc. Alternatively, they may reflect normal ageing processes in discs aged between 30 and 50 years.[40]

Mathematical models also predict that posterolateral disc prolapse should occur most easily in discs which

Disc prolapse by repetitive loading

The same combination of compression, bending and lateral bending can create disc prolapse at lower load levels during cyclic 'fatigue' loading.[30] This type of injury has been produced in vitro only in young non-degenerated discs, and it is typified by a large posterolateral radial fissure (Fig. 11.21) which allows extrusion of small quantities of soft nuclear pulp.

Motion segments with an intact neural arch were positioned in full flexion, with an additional component of lateral flexion, and subjected to 40 cycles of compressive loading per minute for up to 6 hours. An initial injection of radiopaque fluid (including blue dye) into the nucleus enabled a discogram to be taken to demonstrate the absence of radial fissures prior to testing. Cyclic loading was gentle at first, in order to expel the extra fluid associated with discography, but the peak compressive force increased gradually to a maximum value which depended on specimen age and body mass. As the experiment progressed, water expulsion from the disc increased its range of flexion (Fig. 13.18), and the flexion angle was increased accordingly, without exceeding the elastic limit of the ligaments. Of 29 specimens tested in this manner, six developed a complete radial fissure, and these were all grade 1 discs (Fig. 10.19), aged under 44 years, from the L4–5 and L5–S1 levels. Fissures were confirmed after testing by a second discogram, and the expulsion of small quantities of blue-stained nucleus pulp was plain to see (Fig. 11.22). For the six discs which prolapsed, peak cyclic compressive force was 3.5 kN on average (range 2.5–4.5 kN) and peak flexion angle was 14° (range 8–16°). The other 23 specimens either sustained vertebral fractures or remained undamaged, but many showed bell-shaped distortions of the annulus which resembled incomplete radial fissures (Fig. 11.21). Other young discs tested without the injected

blue dye also showed radial fissures at the end of the experiment (Fig. 11.23), although some of these may have been present in the disc before mechanical loading.

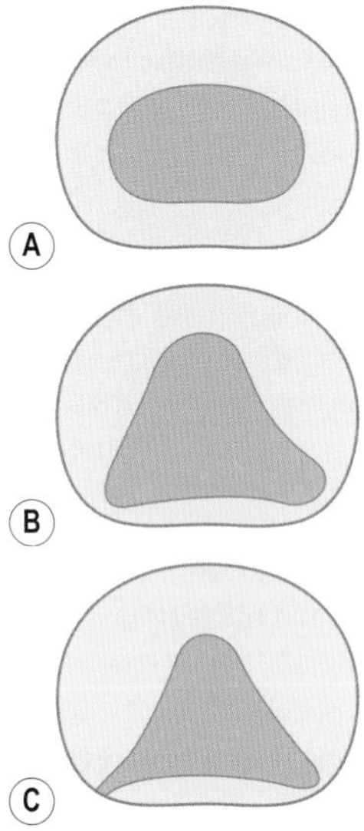

Again, some details may be of clinical interest. In several discs, the outermost lamellae of the annulus appeared to halt fissure progression by bulging outwards, and allowing nucleus pulp to accumulate behind them rather than penetrate them (Fig. 11.24). If this outermost 1–2 mm of annulus was removed with a scalpel during the period of cyclic loading, an immediate herniation of nuclear pulp occurred. (These were not included among the six 'prolapses'.) The pretest discogram revealed pre-existing radial fissures in 13 older discs, but none of these allowed posterior herniation of nucleus pulposus material during cyclic loading. Either old fissures heal efficiently, or else the nucleus becomes too fibrous to be expelled down the fissure, in the absence of severe bending or compression. One 33-year-old L5–S1 disc was cyclically loaded for 3 hours before being compressed rapidly to failure, at 17° of flexion and 5.9 kN of compression. The disc prolapsed suddenly, as described above, but it was probably weakened already by the cyclic loading.

Adding torsion to bending, lateral bending and compression increases compressive stresses in the inner posterolateral annulus[1357] and enables prolapse to occur at lower flexion angles during repetitive loading,[513] although the evidence that prolapse occurred during the course of the latter experiment is not compelling. Of 14 discs that prolapsed during cyclic loading, four involved extrusion of nucleus pulposus and 10 failed by annular protrusion. The relative importance of bending, lateral bending, torsion and compression in causing disc prolapse during repetitive loading has been analysed in finite element models.[1303,1266] They show that collagen fibre strains are greatest in the posterolateral annulus, and are greater in healthy discs than in severely degenerated discs (Fig. 11.25).

Figure 11.21 Superior view of intervertebral discs showing how posterolateral radial fissures develop. **(A)** Normal disc, with nucleus (shaded) having a similar shape to the peripheral annulus. **(B)** Repetitive loading in bending and compression can cause the annulus to be deformed into a typical bell shape. **(C)** Lamellae of the annulus eventually rupture in one or both posterolateral corners.

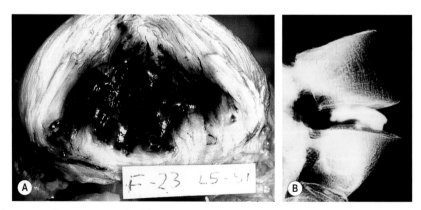

Figure 11.22 (A) Young cadaveric intervertebral disc showing a complete posterolateral radial fissure following cyclic loading in bending and compression. (B) Radiopaque blue dye was injected into the nucleus before loading in order to demonstrate that the annulus was initially intact and to show the path of the nucleus tissue through the annulus. *(Reproduced from Adams and Hutton[30] with permission.)*

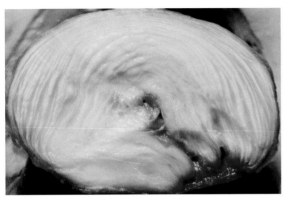

Figure 11.23 Cadaveric lumbar disc following cyclic mechanical loading in bending and compression (anterior on top). Note the deformation of the annular lamellae, and the complete posterolateral radial fissure. The endplate was fractured, allowing blood to pass down the fissure.

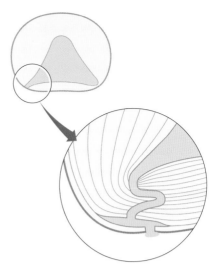

Figure 11.24 Radial fissure formation in young lumbar intervertebral discs, as inferred from cadaveric experiments. Upper: diagram of a disc in the transverse plane, showing nucleus pulposus tissue (shaded) tracking down a posterolateral radial fissure in response to cyclic loading. Lower: inset shows how nucleus tissue breaks through the peripheral annulus, and accumulates behind the outermost lamella, which is reinforced on the outside by the posterior longitudinal ligament. Finally, nucleus tissue leaks from the disc.

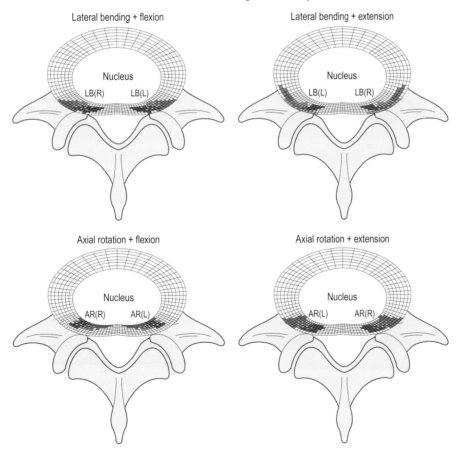

Figure 11.25 Output from a finite element (FE) mathematical model, suggesting how various combinations of complex loading influence deformations of the annulus fibrosus. There is a consistent tendency for maximum shear strains (shown red) to be concentrated in the posterolateral annulus in response to flexion or extension combined with lateral bending (LB) and axial rotation (AR). L/R indicate left and right. *(Reproduced from Schmidt et al.[1266] with permission.)*

The precise mechanism by which pressurised nucleus pulposus can create a radial fissure in the annulus has been further investigated in sheep discs.[1479] In these experiments, nucleus pressure was raised to very high levels by injecting a viscous radiopaque gel into the nucleus via a valve in the endplate until catastrophic disc failure occured. No flexion was used. Annular disruption was investigated using microcomputed tomography and differential interference contrast microscopy. As shown in Figure 11.26, the thin posterior annulus was the most common site of failure. The pressurised gel and nucleus forced itself into and between the annulus lamellae, usually at mid-disc height, with interlamellar disruption (i.e. delamination) predominating in the outer annulus (Fig. 11.27). Delamination in this region of annulus probably reflects pre-existing circumferential tears, or reduced interlamellar cohesion, and it led to contained disc prolapses or protrusions. However, some complete radial fissures were also formed. Subsequent work[1480] showed that the addition of

flexion to the loading regime encouraged more direct radial ruptures of the central posterior annulus, with the path of the growing fissure moving between one endplate and the mid-height of the disc. Flexion appeared to facilitate nucleus flow, and created additional tension in the posterior annulus that limited circumferential flow in favour of radial flow.

Another animal experiment showed that radial fissures and disc herniation can be created by repeatedly flexing and extending porcine cervical motion segments, while subjecting them to a compressive force of 1.4 kN.[1402] This loading regime is another approximation to the simulation of repeated heavy lifting, and it shows how (natural) nucleus pulposus can insinuate itself into and between the lamellae of the annulus until complete herniation occurs, without rupturing any collagen fibres. The extent of posterior radial fissure formation depends on (porcine) disc shape[1611] and can be increased by the addition of compressive vibrations at a frequency (4 Hz) that is close to the spine's natural frequency.[1612]

Consequences of disc prolapse

Mechanical consequences

When disc prolapse is simulated on cadaveric specimens, it causes an immediate drop in nuclear pressure (Fig. 11.28), which probably explains why only a small quantity of nuclear material is extruded during subsequent cyclic loading.[30] This decompression must persist in living patients, because the average resting pressure in the nucleus of herniated discs in vivo is 45% lower than that of healthy control discs (calculated from Sato et al.[1250]). A decompressed disc has a reduced resistance to bending, and the affected motion segment may well exhibit instability (p. 160). Radial fissures in the annulus following disc prolapse have good self-sealing properties[30] but they impair the disc's resistance to bending and torsion[1269] and increase shear stresses between adjacent lamellae,[502] so they probably predispose the disc to further mechanical disruption.

Once released from the pressurised confines of a (cadaveric) disc, any displaced nucleus material can swell up in saline to approximately 2–3 times its size in just a few hours.[361] During the following 96 hours, gradual leaching of proteoglycans from the swollen tissue causes it to shrink again to its original size (Fig. 11.29). If similar processes occur in vivo (and it would be difficult to imagine why they would not), then they could explain why some patients report a worsening of symptoms several hours after an incident during which they felt their back 'give way'.

Biological consequences

Inflammatory-like responses within nerve roots are probably more important in the aetiology of sciatica than mechanical compression,[725,1070] although the contribution of the mechanical compression should not be

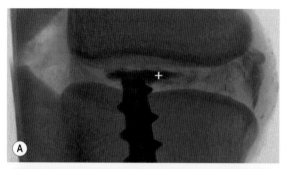

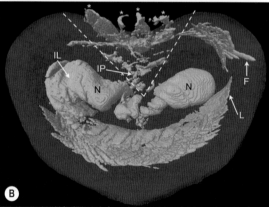

Figure 11.26 Radiographs of a sheep disc showing **(A)** how a radiopaque gel was injected into the nucleus under high pressure at the location marked +, and **(B)** how the pressurised gel created complete radial fissures in the posterior annulus. * gel extrusion. IL: inner lateral annulus. IP: inner posterior annulus. IA: inner anterior annulus. N: gel within the nucleus, F: gel contained within a fiber bundle. (Reproduced from Veres et al.[1479] with permission.)

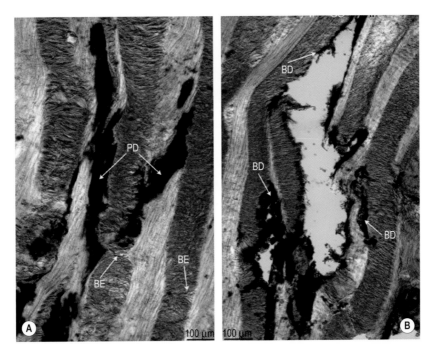

Figure 11.27 Phase-contrast microscopy showing how the (sheep) annulus can be disrupted by injecting a gel under high pressure into the nucleus (as in Fig. 11.26). **(A)** Intralamellar damage in the middle annulus. **(B)** Interlamellar disruption of outer annulus. Arrows indicate injected gel. PD: intralamellar disruption BD: interlamellar disruption BE: bridging elements. *(Reproduced from Veres et al.[1479] with permission.)*

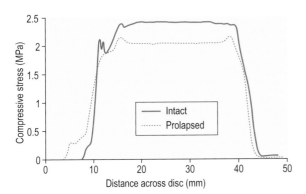

Figure 11.28 Distribution of vertical compressive stress along the sagittal midline of a cadaveric intervertebral disc, before and after the disc was induced to prolapse by loading in bending and compression. (Anterior on right. Specimen: male, 40 years, L23.) Prolapse reduces the pressure in the nucleus, and in some discs can generate stress peaks in the annulus. Note the increased diameter of the disc after prolapse, which can be attributed to increased posterior bulging. *(Stress profiles are explained in Figure 10.17.)*

disregarded.[1584] Inflammation could be triggered by proteoglycans leaching from herniated disc tissue, together with the matrix-degrading enzymes and cytokines which are produced in quantity in this tissue.[713] Animal experiments have shown that nucleus pulposus tissue can alter nerve root morphology after only 3 hours' contact[235] and subsequently can cause pain sensitisation of adjacent nerve tissue (p. 205). If an extruded fragment of nucleus pulposus is not removed surgically, it can shrink markedly over 2 years,[305] and may disappear entirely from the MRI image.[772]

Longer-term consequences of disc prolapse will be dominated by cell-mediated biological changes. In young animals, the nucleus pulposus is able to regenerate itself to a limited extent following chymopapain-induced injury,[176,1382] and this could help restore nucleus pressure and function. It could also lead to repeated prolapse down the same fissure, and explain the recurrent sciatica which can be such a problem in young humans. In older individuals, nucleus regeneration it not so apparent[1107] and the initial decompression following prolapse is likely to be more severe.[22] Disc prolapse is likely to set up a vicious circle of nucleus decompression, structural disruption, cell-mediated weakening of the matrix and further decompression, as described on page 196. In this way, disc prolapse may cause disc degeneration (rather than the other way round).

Activities which could cause disc prolapse

Most intervertebral disc herniations removed at surgery are composed primarily of nucleus pulposus tissue, as in the

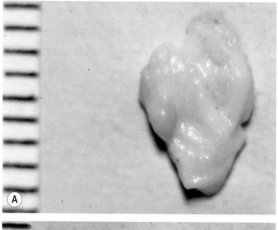

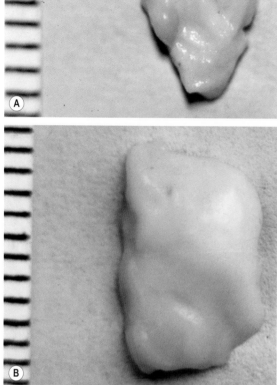

Figure 11.29 Herniated nucleus pulposus collected from cadaveric experiments, as in Figure 11.19. **(A)** Tissue as it herniated. **(B)** Same tissue following 4 hours of swelling in physiological saline at 37°C. The tissue has increased its weight by approximately 150%.

high bending. Excessive bending with high compression could occur when lunging to catch or retain a falling object, or when attempting a heavy lift after the spine has been allowed to creep into excessive flexion (p. 192). Any event involving the trunk being dragged forwards into a flexed posture is likely to be particularly dangerous because forces in the back muscles are highest when the muscles are stretched, and when contracting eccentrically (resisting further stretching). A great deal of biomechanical evidence suggests that disc prolapse is more likely to occur in the early morning, when the discs are swollen with water (p. 185), although there is currently no epidemiological evidence to confirm this.

Many repetitive manual handling tasks generate peak compressive forces on the spine greater than the 2.5–4.5 kN used in the fatigue experiments described above, and at the same time, these tasks frequently involve full lumbar flexion.[363] It appears therefore that discs could prolapse in vivo whenever the number of loading cycles per day is sufficiently high that fatigue damage accumulates faster than the discs' adaptive remodelling response can deal with (Fig. 7.11). It is difficult to predict when this might occur, because it depends on the age, health and work experience of the individual, as well as the work environment.

SEGMENTAL 'INSTABILITY'

Mechanical instability

In engineering terminology, a system is stable, unstable or neutral according to criteria depicted in Figure 11.30. This usage of the term 'instability' bears some relation to its clinical usage to describe a condition in which a motion segment exhibits an abnormal magnitude or direction of movement when subject to a normal load. There are three main possibilities: firstly, the range of motion (RoM) is excessive; secondly, the RoM is normal, but the motion segment exhibits a qualitatively abnormal resistance to movement within this normal range; and thirdly, the motion segment has an abnormally low resistance to movement within a normal RoM.

Excessive intersegmental movement

Excessive RoM can be caused by injury to the structure or structures which normally limit that movement. Mechanisms of injury to restraining structures such as ligaments and the neural arch have been described above. Any of them could lead to spinal instability, at least in theory. However, there are good reasons to prefer the term 'hypermobility' for excessive movements caused by injury to restraining structures,[86] leaving 'instability' to refer to abnormal movements within a normal range.

above experiments, and none contains only annulus fibrosus,[1000] so 'real-life' disc prolapses are probably similar to those shown in Figures 11.19 and 11.20. Many manual handling activities load the lumbar spine simultaneously in compression, bending and lateral bending, and so might be expected to cause disc prolapse if the severity of just one of these components rose to damaging levels.

Circumstances which could lead to excessive bending or excessive compression in vivo have been discussed above. Disc prolapse is most likely to occur when these circumstances are combined. For example, falling on the buttocks with the legs stretched out in front, or stumbling while carrying a heavy weight, or lifting a heavy object in an emergency, could combine excessive compression with

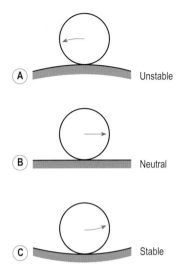

Figure 11.30 Mechanical criteria of stability as illustrated by a sphere on a surface. **(A)** In this unstable system, any displacement of the sphere will progress to further displacements, and the system will collapse. **(B)** In this neutral system, any displacement of the sphere will neither progress nor be reversed. **(C)** In this stable system, any displacement will be reversed as soon as the perturbing force is removed.

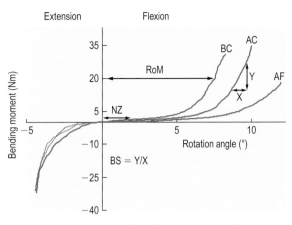

Figure 11.31 Typical set of bending moment–rotation curves for combined flexion and extension movements. Neutral zone (NZ) and range of motion (RoM) were defined as the angles when the applied bending moment reached 1.5 and 20 Nm respectively. Bending stiffness (BS) was measured as the slope of the bending moment–rotation curve at 20 Nm. BC, before creep; AC, after creep; AF, after failure.

Qualitatively abnormal intersegmental movement

Abnormal intervertebral movements within a normal range could conceivably be caused by a structure such as an osteophyte causing a temporary block or 'catch' at a particular point during an otherwise smooth movement. This concept is supported by the subjective experiences of some people with back pain, and by small flexion/extension oscillations which can be measured in cadaveric motion segments when they are moved rapidly in the sagittal plane.[1063] However, there is little other experimental work to throw light on this concept.

Abnormally low intersegmental resistance to small movements

Instability may simply reflect a negligible resistance to small movements, so that the motion segment 'wobbles'.[10] In effect, the specimen has an enlarged neutral zone (NZ), which is the range of angular or translational movement within which the spine has minimal internal resistance to movement.[1097] The upper boundary of the NZ is the angle (or displacement) at which the resistance to movement is first detected, and this threshold has been variously defined. The NZ increases with age,[983] is a sensitive indicator of minor injury[1090] and is hypothesised to be closely related to clinical instability.[1097] The ratio NZ:RoM is

sometimes considered an index of instability,[983] because it expresses the range of joint laxity as a percentage of the full RoM.

Discogenic causes of segmental instability

Intervertebral discs provide most of the spine's intrinsic resistance to small movements[19,33] and so are likely causes of instability. With increasing age and degeneration, the size of the hydrostatic nucleus decreases,[40] and water content and pressure within it fall.[40, 1250] This allows the annulus to bulge more, both externally and internally, and the disc loses height. Height loss is exaggerated if the disc is disrupted, or the vertebral endplate is fractured.[41] Annulus height loss gives slack to the collagen fibres of the annulus fibrosus and intervertebral ligaments, reducing their resistance to bending[18] and giving rise to instability.

In a cadaveric experiment, two important physical aspects of early disc degeneration – nucleus dehydration and endplate disruption – were shown to generate segmental instability. The two interventions decompressed the nucleus, and reduced disc height by an average of 1.0 and 1.7 mm respectively, so that total disc height loss (2.7 mm) was similar to that seen in moderately degenerated discs in vivo. The effects on motion segment stability are shown in Figure 11.31. Both interventions increased the RoM, NZ and instability index in flexion, but not in extension. Averaged results, summarised in Figure 11.32, show that endplate damage had a particularly large destabilising effect, and that the resulting instability was most evident in lateral bending and flexion.[1627] The strength of

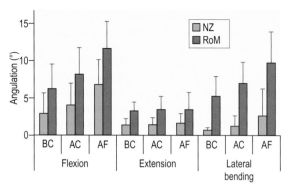

Figure 11.32 Average values of range of motion (RoM) and neutral zone (NZ) for 21 cadaveric thoracolumbar motion segments. In flexion and lateral bending, both NZ and RoM increased following the two disc degeneration treatments, but no such effects were apparent in extension. BC, before creep; AC, after creep; AF, after endplate failure. Error bars indicate the SEM.

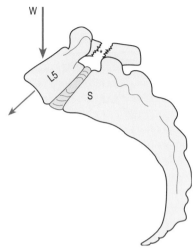

Figure 11.33 Spondylolysis is a defect of the pars interarticularis (*), which occurs either unilaterally or bilaterally. L5 is most commonly affected. Gravitational forces (W) sometimes cause a forward slipping of the upper (damaged) vertebra upon the one below, a condition known as spondylolisthesis.

this experiment is that structural and physical aspects of early disc degeneration were entirely separated from the biochemical changes of ageing, which tend to make discs more fibrous and less mobile (Table 8.1). The combined influences of ageing and degeneration were assessed in a previous cadaveric study, which showed that segmental mobility increases with increasing (pre-existing) disc degeneration, as assessed from MRI scans.[457] However, the most degenerated specimens were less mobile,[457] perhaps reflecting the stabilising influences of fibrosis and osteophytosis in severely degenerated spines. Certainly, vertebral body osteophytes play a major role in resisting and limiting spinal bending.[55] Restabilisation may explain why another cadaveric study, which graded disc degeneration radiographically in terms of osteophytosis, sclerosis and disc narrowing, reported that segmental mobility decreases uniformly with increasing disc degeneration.[740] A similar pattern has been observed in animal experiments, with injuries to the disc increasing the spine's RoM and NZ over a period of several weeks, until healing processes reduce them again.[49]

SPONDYLOLYSIS AND SPONDYLOLISTHESIS

Spondylolysis is a defect of the pars interarticularis which resembles both a fracture and a degenerative condition. Therefore, mechanical influences will be considered here, whereas certain clinical aspects are described in Chapter 19.

Fracture of the pars can be reproduced by applying a posteriorly directed shear force to the inferior articular processes of cadaveric lumbar vertebrae (Fig. 11.33). A single loading cycle causes fracture at a force of approximately 2 kN,[318] and cyclic loading oscillating between 380 and 760 N can cause fatigue failure.[313] In life, the shearing forces required for fatigue failure could arise when marching with a heavy backpack.[651] Alternating flexion and extension movements of the lumbar spine may also cause spondylolysis, by bending the inferior articular processes about the pars. In cadaver experiments, angular movements of 2–3° have been measured in the anteroinferior direction (in flexion) and posterosuperior direction (in extension), as shown in Figure 11.13. Alternating movements would therefore cause large and potentially damaging stress reversals in the pars, and pose the greatest threat of spondylolysis.[529] This may explain the high incidence of spondylolysis in gymnasts[672] and cricket fast bowlers.[567] The finding that the risk of spondylolysis does not depend on facet orientation or tropism[707] and yet is associated with facet osteoarthritis[707] suggests that intervertebral shear forces play a smaller role than spinal bending (especially hyperextension) in the aetiology of spondylolysis.

Genetic predisposition must also be important, because 26% of the close relatives of those with spondylolysis have a similar problem themselves.[1580] Inherited factor may simply be a small cross-sectional area of bone in the pars interarticularis.[314] Higher incidences of spondylolysis in Alaskan natives[1361] may depend partly upon (inherited) differences in lifestyle.[389]

Spondylolysis usually affects the lower lumbar vertebrae, which are normally inclined at a steep angle to the vertical (Fig. 11.1). The spondyolytic defect is filled with fibrocartilage with varying degrees of calcification,[171] which would be prone to time-dependent creep. Not surprisingly, loss of the resistance to shear of the apophyseal joints often results in a forwards slip of L4 or L5 relative to the vertebra below, under the influence of gravity. This forwards slip, spondylolisthesis, can in theory be opposed by the action of the erector spinae muscles resisting the forward shear force[1157] but only in stooped postures, and not in standing. Spondylolisthesis (Fig. 19.3) is associated with more sagittally oriented apophyseal joints rather than with asymmetrical facets, and this probably represents a predisposing weakness rather than secondary remodelling.[153]

SPINAL TRAUMA

Several classifications of spinal trauma have been published for the benefit of orthopaedic surgeons.[338,620] Much of the information appears to be based upon experience and conjecture rather than experiment, but nevertheless is consistent with the principles outlined in this chapter. Two particular types of injury have been investigated more methodically.

Flexion distraction ('seat belt') injuries

When a car occupant is thrown forwards on to a lap-type seat belt, the lumbar spine is loaded in combined flexion, forward shear and compression. Gross damage is evident at 120 Nm and complete failure of the tissues occurs at 140–185 Nm, with a flexion angle of 20°.[1083,1084] Interpreting these and other experiments, Neumann et al. suggested that total instability occurs when flexion exceeds 19° and spinous process separation increases by more than 33 mm.[1038]

Burst fractures of the vertebral body

These can be defined as comminuted vertebral body fractures with disruption of the anterior and posterior walls of the vertebral body,[338] and they are characterised by an increased interpedicular distance.[1302] They can cause severe neurological problems from the retropulsion of bone into the spinal canal. The name 'burst fracture' suggests some involvement from tissue fluid trapped within a rapidly loaded vertebra, and there is some evidence that rapid loading is more likely to damage the vertebral body cortex rather than the endplates.[1613] However, the involvement of trapped fluid may not be great, because the compressive strength of cadaveric lumbar vertebrae is little affected by preventing fluid outflow using paraffin wax.[648] Burst fractures can be simulated in the laboratory by dropping a heavy weight on to a section of thoracolumbar spine.[440,1103] The resulting severe compression injuries resemble the transverse fractures described by Brinckmann et al. (Fig. 11.3), but also involve damage to both of the adjacent intervertebral discs[440] with disc material being forced into the vertebral bodies. The loss of vertebral height creates severe rotational instability in the affected motion segment,[1103] presumably because of the consequent loss of tension in the intervertebral ligaments and annulus. Burst fractures are more common in the thoracic spine than in the lumbar, and they are less likely to occur if the intervertebral discs are degenerated.[1302]

Chapter | **12** |

Cervical spine biomechanics

INTRODUCTION

The cervical spine will not be described in as much detail as the lumbar spine. There is insufficient research on the cervical spine to make the attempt worthwhile, and the purpose of this short chapter is merely to point out some similarites and differences between the thoracolumbar and cervical spine in order to increase our understanding of the latter.

GROSS ANATOMY

Cervical vertebrae are distinguished by small bodies, long spinous processes which often are bifid and by the uncinate processes of the uncovertebral joints (Fig. 12.1). Cervical apophyseal joints are relatively large compared to elsewhere in the spine. Cervical intervertebral discs are relatively thick in comparison to vertebral body height,

and the resulting high ratio of cartilage to bone explains the high mobility of the cervical spine. The posterior annulus is often thin and rudimentary in cervical discs (Fig. 12.2) and the nucleus often appears rather fibrous for its age.[975]

MOVEMENTS OF THE CERVICAL SPINE

During flexion and extension of the cervical spine, the centres of rotation between adjacent vertebrae tend to be slightly lower (more caudal) than those in the lumbar spine (Fig. 10.5) so that they lie in the vertebral body, below the endplate (evidence summarised by Bogduk and Mercer[165]). This indicates a considerable degree of anterior–posterior translational movements, as the cervical vertebrae slide over the curved surfaces of the vertebral bodies (Fig. 12.1) and apophyseal joints.

Typical ranges of movement for the whole cervical spine in vivo are shown as a function of age in Figure 12.3. Movements between the head and thorax are greatest in axial rotation, followed by flexion/extension and then lateral bending, and all movements decrease with age. Much of the large range of axial rotation occurs between the axis (C1 vertebra) and the odontoid process of the atlas (C1), enabling the head to be turned freely to look over one shoulder.

Ranges of segmental movement in cadaveric cervical spines are shown in Figures 12.4 and 12.5. The segmental flexion/extension movements (Fig. 12.4) are comparable to those measured in vivo by radiographs,[1310] suggesting that the maximum bending moments applied in the cadaveric experiments (2 Nm) were sufficient to induce full-range movement.

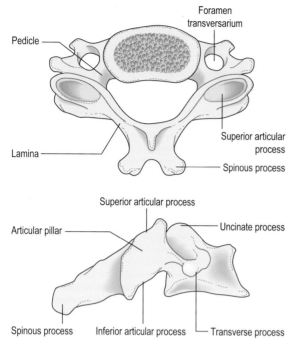

Figure 12.1 Typical cervical vertebra in the **(A)** transverse and **(B)** sagittal planes. *(Adapted from Bogduk N. In: Hochberg MC, Silman AJ, Smolen JS (eds) Rheumatology, 4th edn. Philadelphia, PA, U.S.A., 2008.)*

DISC MECHANICS

The internal mechanical functioning of cervical intervertebral discs can be appreciated from Figures 12.6–12.8. These pressure profiles[1327] are broadly similar to those shown in Chapters 10 and 13 for lumbar discs, but with two exceptions. Most notably, the cervical nucleus often exhibits a stress gradient, from anterior to posterior, even though the vertical and horizontal stresses are approximately the same at each location, as would be expected for a tissue that exhibits fluid-like behaviour. The gradient (Fig. 12.7) persists even if the needle is pulled through the disc in the opposite direction, so cannot be attributed to a needle volume artifact. One possible explanation is that the rather fibrous cervical nucleus behaves like a 'tethered fluid' which freely allows small displacements of tissue, but not large displacements, so that stress is equalised over small distances, but not large ones.[1327]

A second major difference is that cervical discs rarely exhibit large concentrations of compressive stress in the posterior annulus, not even when they are compressed while positioned in extension (Fig. 12.8). This could possibly be because the cervical posterior annulus is

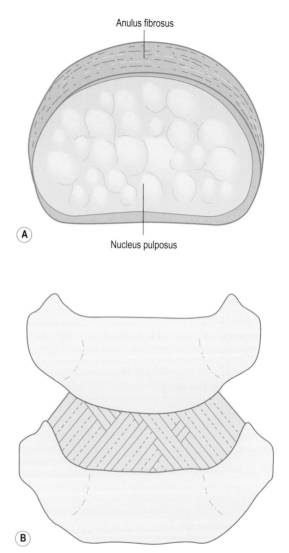

Figure 12.2 Cervical intervertebral disc **(A)** in transverse section (anterior on top) and **(B)** anterior view. *(From Bogduk N. In: Hochberg MC, Silman AJ, Smolen JS (eds) Rheumatology, 4th edn. Philadelphia, PA, U.S.A., 2008.)*

relatively thin, from interior to exterior (Fig. 12.2), so that it would buckle under a high compressive stress rather than sustain it.

STRENGTH OF THE CERVICAL SPINE

Cadaver experiments have assessed the strength of cervical motion segments in compression and bending.[1047,1166] Averaged results for specimens aged 64–89 years[1166] showed that the elastic limit in flexion was reached at 8.5°

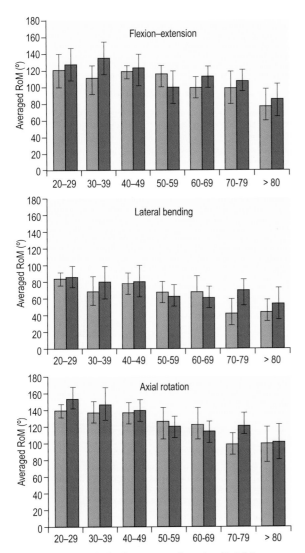

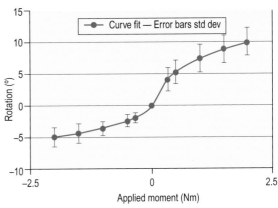

Figure 12.4 Bending moment–rotation curves for typical (C5–6) cervical motion segments tested in flexion and extension. Seven large cadaveric specimens from C2–T1, average age 33 years, were subjected to pure moments, with no compressive preload. Similar results were obtained for all levels C2–7, although C7–T1 was less mobile. Error bars indicate the SD. (*Reproduced from Wheeldon et al.[1555] with permission.*)

Figure 12.3 Cervical spine ranges of motion (RoM) in bending and axial rotation, plotted as a function of age and gender. Averaged data refer to three-dimensional movements of the head relative to the thorax measured using a skin surface infrared device on 140 asymptomatic volunteers (70 men (red bars) and 70 women (blue bars)). (*Reproduced from Lansade et al.[804]*)

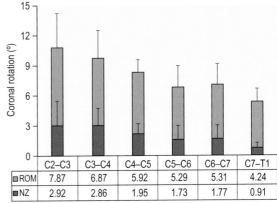

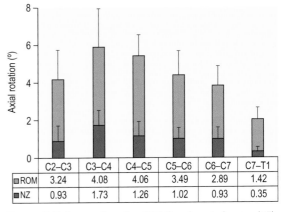

Figure 12.5 Range of motion (ROM) and neutral zones (NZ) for cervical motion segments tested in lateral bending (coronal rotation) and axial rotation. Values are for movement from one side to the other. Nine cadaveric specimens from C2–T1, average age 34 years, were subjected to pure moments of up to 2 Nm, with no compressive preload. The NZ refers to zero moment. Error bars indicate the SD. (*Reproduced from Yoganandan et al.[1616] with permission.*)

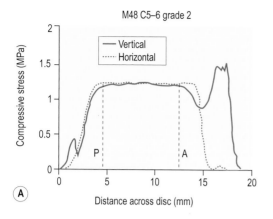

M48 C5–6 grade 2

(A)

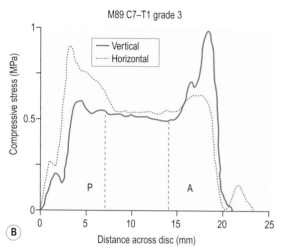

M89 C7–T1 grade 3

(B)

Figure 12.6 Anterior-posterior (A-P) stress profiles in cervical intervertebral discs, subjected to a compressive force of 200 N. The non-degenerated (grade 2) disc shows a large nucleus, exhibiting hydrostatic properties, between the vertical broken lines. The old and degenerated (grade 3) disc has a narrowed hydrostatic region, and increased stress concentrations in the annulus. Much of the compressive force acting on this old specimen was resisted by the neural arch. *(Stress profilometry is explained in Figure 10.17. A smaller transducer, mounted in a 0.9 mm-diameter needle, was used for cervical discs.)*

with a bending moment of 6.7 Nm. In extension, values were 9.5° and 8.4 Nm respectively. In compression, disc–vertebral body units from the same specimens reached the elastic limit at an average 1.23 kN and their ultimate compressive strength was 2.40 kN. Strength was greater in male specimens, depended on spinal level and tended to decrease with age.

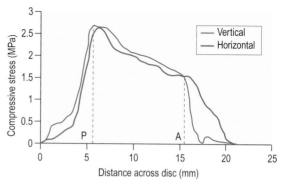

Figure 12.7 Stress profiles obtained from a non-degenerated cervical disc, showing unusual material properties. Measurements were repeated with the transducer oriented vertically and horizontally. In the functional nucleus pulposus (between the broken vertical lines) these two components were equal, suggesting hydrostatic fluid conditions, and yet a distinct stress gradient was apparent. *(Stress profilometry is explained in Figure 10.17.)*

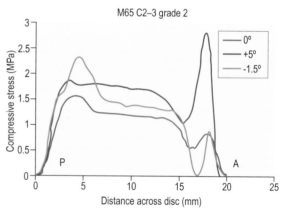

M65 C2–3 grade 2

Figure 12.8 Stress profiles obtained from a non-degenerated cervical disc, showing the influence of posture. Flexed posture (+5°) concentrated stress anteriorly, and extended posture (–1.5°) tended to concentrate it posteriorly, but not to the same extent, even if extension angles were increased. *(Stress profilometry is explained in Figure 10.17.)*

Rough comparisons can be made with the lumbar spine. The compressive strength of cervical motion segments (2.4 kN) is approximately 45% of the average strength of lumbar specimens of equivalent age (calculated from Brinckmann et al.[185]). However, the strength in bending of the cervical motion segments (6–8 Nm) is only 20% of the equivalent strength of lumbar motion segments of similar age (calculated from Adams and Dolan[13] and Adams et al.[19]). Evidently, the slender cervical spine (Fig. 12.9) is vulnerable to bending injuries and requires extra protection from the neck muscles.

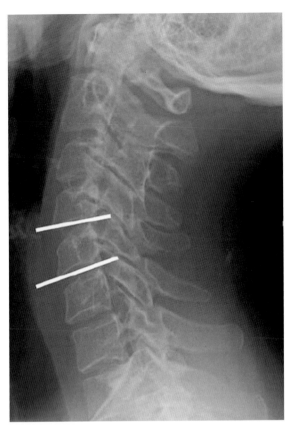

Figure 12.9 Sagittal-plane radiograph of the cervical spine with the head in an upright position. Note the overall slenderness of the cervical spine, and how the anterior column of vertebral bodies is less substantial than the posterior column of neural arches. *(Reproduced from Simpson et al.[1310] with permission.)*

Table 12.1 Resistance to bending of cervical specimens was reduced: (1) following surgical removal of the spinous processes and associated ligaments; (2) following removal of the apophyseal joints; and (3) following compressive failure of the remaining disc–vertebral body specimen

	Resistance to bending	
	Flexion (%)	Extension (%)
Intact motion segment	100	100
Spinous process removed	52 (17)	77 (14)
Apophyseal joints removed	24 (17)	30 (16)
After compressive failure	14 (11)	22 (12)

Results are expressed as a percentage of the resistance of the intact motion segment (row 1). Values indicate the mean (SD). Changes in moment resisted after each intervention can be attributed to the structure removed: for example, the spinous process and associated ligaments provide 48% (100 − 52) of the motion segment's resistance to flexion.
(Data from Przybyla et al.[1166])

RESISTANCE TO BENDING

The cervical spine structures that provide most resistance to bending were investigated in a cadaveric experiment, by measuring changes in resistance to bending after various structures were surgically removed. Results, summarised in Table 12.1, showed that ligaments lying between the spinous processes play a dominant role in resisting flexion, whereas the apophyseal joints provide most resistance to extension.

CERVICAL SPINE TRAUMA CLASSIFICATION

An injury classification system has been proposed and validated for the subaxial cervical spine.[1462] A weighted sum of scores is calculated for: (1) injury morphology; (2) discoligamentous complex; and (3) neurologic status to create a single severity score, which then informs treatment.

WHIPLASH

What is whiplash?

Whiplash is typified by low-velocity car crashes in which the upper body is thrown forwards and then back, or vice versa (Fig. 12.10). Whiplash injuries are commonly associated with the neck, but similar events can probably injure the lumbar spine, even if a seat belt is worn, because sitting down causes the lower lumbar spine to be almost fully flexed[72] so only a modest forward movement is required to throw the lumbar spine into hyperflexion.

What is injured in whiplash?

Practically every tissue and structure in the neck can be injured in cervical whiplash,[1187] although increasing evidence points towards the apophyseal joints as being the major source of chronic pain.[103] Magnetic resonance imaging (MRI) scans taken 2 weeks after a whiplash

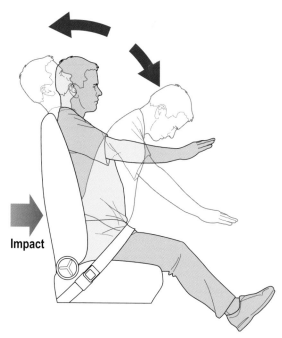

Figure 12.10 In a typical whiplash injury, a rear impact causes the driver's shoulders to be thrust forwards relative to his or her head, which is thrown backwards and upwards. Depending on the presence and location of the headrest, the head can bounce off, throwing the neck into hyperflexion.

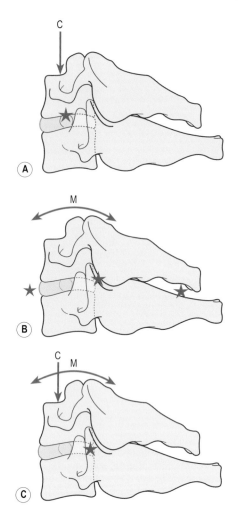

Figure 12.11 Diagrams illustrating the likely sites of injury (*) when the cervical spine is loaded in bending (M) and/or compression (C). **(A)** Excessive compression damages the vertebral endplate. **(B)** Bending damages peripheral structures, including intervertebral ligaments. **(C)** Combined bending and compression can cause disc prolapse.

incident reveal signs of gross trauma in fewer than 0.5% of patients.[774] Such gross MRI signs are unrelated to clinical outcome,[774] possibly because they are not reliably related to surgical findings.[892] The following sections therefore apply some biomechanical insights to the problem of what is injured in patients reporting whiplash.

Firstly, the site and severity of injury must depend on how much warning (and alarm) the victim received just prior to impact. Any screech of brakes or flashing image in the driver's mirror would allow time for the back or neck muscles to contract in a reflex manner to protect the spine, and there is evidence that a sudden loud noise increases neck muscle contractions.[149] In mechanical terms, reflex muscle contractions may be sufficient to reduce the peak bending moment acting on the spine (provided that the impact was not extremely violent) but only at the expense of increasing greatly the spinal compressive force.[899] The resulting injury would more likely be compressive in nature and involve the discs and vertebral bodies (as well as the muscles themselves) rather than intervertebral ligaments or the neural arch (Fig. 12.11). This may explain why a high proportion of intervertebral disc cells have been reported to be dead or dying shortly after cervical spine trauma.[1319] Cadaveric experiments have shown that cervical intervertebral discs can prolapse in a

similar manner to lumbar discs if they are loaded severely in bending and compression (Fig. 12.12).

On the other hand, if an impact occurred without warning, then the neck muscles would have insufficient time to prevent the spine from being injured in bending, although stretch reflexes[710] may cause them to generate enough force to influence the outcome to a certain extent.[885] Bending injuries would probably involve the posterior intervertebral ligaments (in the hyperflexion stage of whiplash) or the neural arch (in the hyperextension phase). Clearly, to assume that the forces acting on the spine during whiplash are small just because the vehicle impacts are usually of low velocity would be a

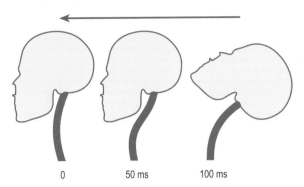

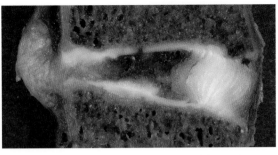

Figure 12.12 Diagrammatic representation of the changing curvature of the cervical spine during whiplash. The arrow indicates the direction of the impacting force. Approximately 50–75 ms after impact, the cervical spine develops an exaggerated S-shaped curvature, and maximal extension at all cervical levels occurs after 100 ms. *Data from experiments on cadaveric cervical spines.*[1099]

Figure 12.13 Cervical disc prolapse in a middle-aged cadaveric disc. This mid-sagittal section shows a large posterior herniation of nucleus pulposus (left) caused by loading the specimen in hyperflexion and compression (p. 154). There is blood in the nucleus from an endplate defect, and internal bulging of the inner anterior annulus.

serious mistake. Muscle forces can be magnified in alarming situations, and if the muscles do not have time to react, then the underlying cervical spine is extremely vulnerable to bending.

A second aspect of whiplash may also be applicable to both the cervical and lumbar spines: the site of injury will be affected by any axial rotation of the head or torso. If the victim was turning round at the moment of impact, then the spine could suffer a bending injury about an oblique axis (Fig. 11.16). This increases the risk of injury to structures which lie away from the mid-sagittal plane,[1101] and in particular the apophyseal joint capsule.[1308]

Whiplash injury mechanisms have been investigated in a variety of models. When whole human cadaveric cervical spines were subjected to a simulated rear-end collision,[1099] a biphasic response was noted. In the first phase (50–75 ms after impact), the cervical spine formed an exaggerated S-shaped curve as the lower cervical levels extended, and the upper ones flexed. In the second phase (>75 ms), all levels were extended, with overall maximum extension of the head occurring after 100 ms (Fig. 12.13). Injuries were most likely to occur by hyperextension in the C5–7 region during the first phase of neck movement, and involved both anterior and posterior structures. These experiments neglected the effects of muscle activation, as did several earlier 'crash test dummy' tests, and so they reproduced only the bending-type injuries which represent one end of a spectrum of injuries involving varying amounts of bending and compression. When living volunteers were subjected to mild rear-end collisions,[710] or direct blows to the face,[460] they also showed early S-shaped deformations of the cervical spine associated with abnormal and large extension movements of the lower cervical vertebrae, and flexion at upper levels. Radiographic movement data suggested particularly high stretching of the anterior annulus, and compression of the apophyseal joints, at C5–6. However, very different types of injury can result from rapid extension of the neck: an experiment on anaesthetised pigs showed that a 'shock wave' can develop within the cerebrospinal fluid which could possibly damage nerve cell membranes.[1385]

Chapter | **13** |

Posture, creep and 'functional pathology'

INTRODUCTION

Mechanical loading need not be severe to cause pain. Small forces can give rise to pain if they are concentrated into a small area of innervated tissue, and if you doubt this, try walking with a stone in your shoe! This is an example of a 'functional pathology' where pain arises directly from stress concentrations, in the absence of injury or degenerative change. In the spine, the distribution of loading across and between spinal structures depends on how the spine is used: in particular it depends on posture, and how long each posture is held for. This chapter on 'functional pathology' considers how different postures can generate high stress concentrations in undamaged but innervated spinal tissues.

Posture can be interpreted in terms of the orientation of adjacent vertebrae. If vertebrae are pressed together at an unusual angle, then high stress concentrations can arise in the intervertebral discs, ligaments and apophyseal joints. If the posture is held for a long time, some heavily loaded tissues will gradually 'creep' away from the load, while others will lose water, and with it their ability to distribute loading. Both effects will influence stress concentrations in spinal tissues. The final section summarises the evidence concerning stress concentrations in the lumbar spine, and suggests a rational basis for the concept of 'good' posture.

POSTURE AND THE LUMBAR SPINE

Spinal 'posture' can be characterised in various ways, depending on the shape or curvature of the spinal column and the orientation of the entire column to the vertical. Moment arm analysis (Fig. 9.2) explains why inclining the spinal column to the vertical requires trunk muscle activity to balance the external moment generated by gravity acting on the mass of the upper body. Any tendency to lean forwards or backwards therefore increases the spinal compressive force arising from muscle tension (Fig. 13.1), and spinal loading is minimised when the vertebral column is balanced vertically on the pelvis and/or supported by a chair. Quite separate from the effects of trunk inclination, and the presence or absence of support, is the effect of lumbar curvature itself. It is this which largely determines how the compressive force is distributed between the various structures of the spine.

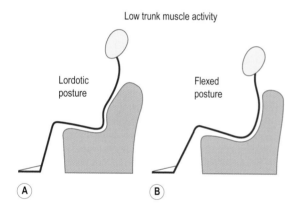

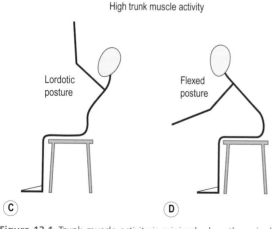

Figure 13.1 Trunk muscle activity is minimal when the spinal column is supported (**A** and **B**), and high when it is inclined to the vertical (**C** and **D**). The actual shape of the lumbar spine, either lordotic or flexed, has much less effect on muscle activity.

Posture and lumbar curvature in the sagittal plane

It is convenient to define spinal posture in terms of the angle subtended in the sagittal plane between the upper surface of the L1 vertebral body and the top of the sacrum (Fig. 13.2). This angle is referred to as the 'lumbar curvature' or 'lumbar lordosis', and typical values are 49–61° in erect standing, and 22–34° in unsupported sitting.[72,675,849] In full flexion, the angle is reversed and can be denoted by a negative value. For cadaveric lumbar spines, cut free from all muscle attachments and therefore entirely unloaded, the lumbar curvature is typically 41–45°.[19,414] This can be considered the 'neutral' configuration of the lumbar spine. Evidently, upright standing increases lumbar curvature by 8–16° compared to the neutral configuration (approximately 2° for each motion segment), whereas upright sitting decreases it by about 10–21°. Neither standing nor sitting corresponds to the neutral configuration, so neither should be considered a more 'natural' or 'normal' posture than the other.

The precise amount of lumbar flexion or extension in a given posture can be quantified from changes in lumbar curvature (Fig. 13.3). Lumbar curvature as defined above should really be measured from X-rays, but it can be estimated by measuring the angle between the tangents to the surface of the back at L1 and S2. There is no fundamental reason why these two measures of lumbar curvature should be the same, but they are similar because the skin surface lies at approximately 90° to the top surface of the lumbar vertebral bodies and sacrum. Changes in lumbar curvature defined in Figure 13.2 should correspond precisely to changes measured at the skin surface (Fig. 13.3), although skin movement artefacts can lead to small differences, especially in lordotic postures.[20]

When referring to living subjects, it is convenient to consider the upright standing position to represent zero flexion, and the fully flexed toe-touching posture is then 100% flexion. Typical values of lumbar flexion obtained with skin-mounted inclinometers are shown in Figure 13.4 for a wide range of postures. Note that common postural habits such as crossing the legs while sitting, or standing with one foot slightly raised, serve to reduce lumbar curvature by a small amount.[362] Nearly all sitting postures flex the lumbar spine, often substantially, and the L4–5 and L5–S1 levels are almost fully flexed.[72] Indeed, lumbar flexion is one of the defining characteristics of sitting, together with weight transfer through the ischial tuberosities.[54] Walking appears to involve a slight flattening of the lumbar lordosis compared to standing still,[1392] as does standing with a weight on the shoulders (for most people).[965] Lordosis increases during the early stages of pregnancy,[377] presumably to re-establish sagittal balance, and this postural adaptation is facilitated by the fact that women tend to have a relatively greater interspinous space, and less kyphotic vertebral bodies, at several

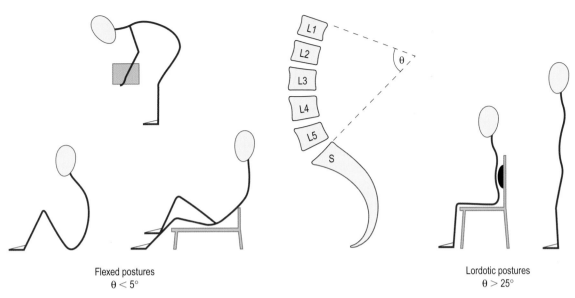

Figure 13.2 Lumbar posture can be categorised as lordotic or flexed depending on the size of the lumbar curvature (θ), as defined in the figure. The neutral configuration refers to the shape of an unloaded cadaveric lumbar spine (centre).

Flexed postures
$\theta < 5°$

Lordotic postures
$\theta > 25°$

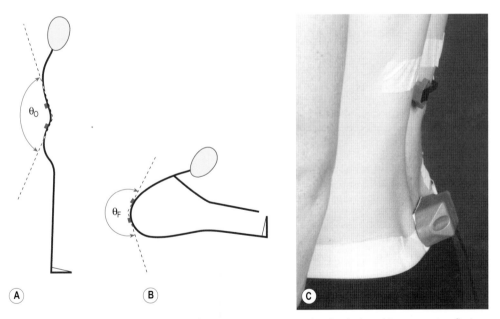

Figure 13.3 (A) If the lumbar curvature in a particular posture was measured to be θ, then this represents a flexion angle of $(\theta-\theta_O)$ degrees. This can be expressed as a percentage of the full range of movement between the erect standing position **(A)** and full flexion **(B)** using the formula: % flexion = $100 \times (\theta-\theta_O)/(\theta_F-\theta_O)$. **(C)** The Isotrak device which can be used to measure lumbar curvature.

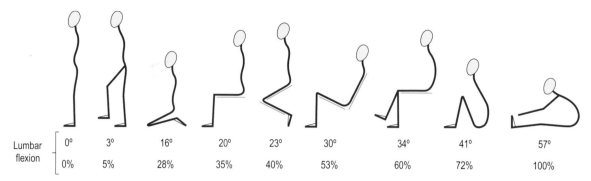

Lumbar flexion	0°	3°	16°	20°	23°	30°	34°	41°	57°
	0%	5%	28%	35%	40%	53%	60%	72%	100%

Figure 13.4 Many commonly adopted postures flex the lumbar spine to a greater or lesser extent. Percentage flexion is defined in Figure 13.3. *(Adapted from Dolan et al.[362] with permission.)*

thoracolumbar levels.[931] The overall standing lordosis is unrelated to (adult) age or gender, although lordosis in the lower lumbar spine is reduced slightly in older people.[487] Recent evidence suggests that the spinous processes increase in height with age, causing bony contact between them[92] and reducing lumbar lordosis in older people. Patients with back pain show reduced lordosis, especially in the lower lumbar spine,[675] and a particularly flat back is a risk factor for future low-back pain.[36]

Posture and load-sharing in the lumbar spine

Flexed postures stretch the posterior intervertebral ligaments, and tension in these ligaments increases the compressive force acting on the intervertebral disc. Lordotic postures cause these ligaments to become slack, and increase loading of the neural arch, so that compressive loading of the disc is reduced. These effects are demonstrated by experimental data for an individual motion segment in Figure 13.5, and are discussed in more detail below. The combined influences of posture and disc degeneration on load-sharing are summarised in Table 8.3.

Posture and the neural arch

The bony neural arches of adjacent vertebrae make sliding contact with each other in the apophyseal joints, and their spinous processes are separated by only a few millimetres of interspinous ligament. Not surprisingly, small changes in postural angle can lead to high stress concentrations at these points of contact.

The proportion of the compressive force acting on the spine which is transmitted through the apophyseal joints rises from 1% in the neutral posture to 16% in 2° of lordosis.[25] Furthermore, lordosis causes this increased force to be concentrated on the inferior margins of the articular surfaces, and on the very tips of the inferior processes as

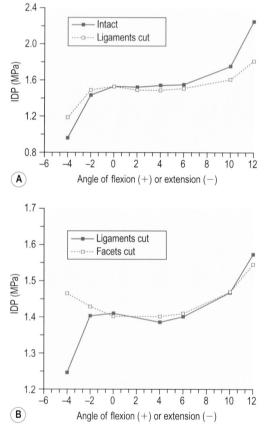

Figure 13.5 Intradiscal pressure (IDP), which is the hydrostatic pressure within the nucleus pulposus, is a good indicator of the overall compressive force acting on an intervertebral disc. **(A)** IDP increases in flexion, because of ligament tension. **(B)** IDP is reduced in extension because of load-bearing by the apophyseal joint surfaces (facets). Data for a cadaveric motion segment (male, 49 years, L23) which was subjected to a constant compressive force of 2 kN in each posture.

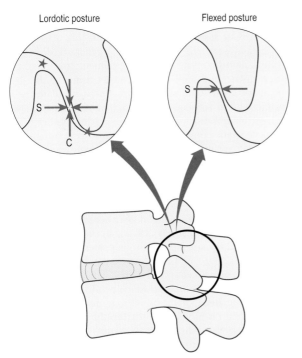

Figure 13.6 Lordotic postures (left) increase the compressive force (C) acting on the apophyseal joints, and concentrate stresses in the inferior margins of the articular surfaces. Direct bone–bone contact (indicated by stars) can also occur. Flexed postures (right) remove the compressive loading from these joints, and cause the shear force (S) to be resisted by the middle and upper margins of the articular surfaces.

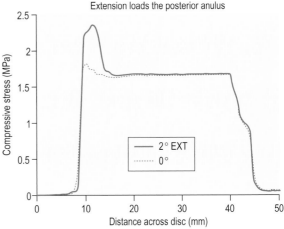

Figure 13.7 The distribution of vertical compressive stress along the sagittal mid-plane of a cadaveric intervertebral disc, compressed in the neutral configuration (0°) and in a lordotic posture (2° EXT). (Specimen: male, 19 years, L45, anterior on right. Compressive force = 2 kN.) Lordotic postures tend to increase the peak compressive stress in the posterior annulus. (Stress profiles are explained in Figure 10.17.)

they impinge on the lamina below[380,1304] (Fig. 13.6). There is no articular cartilage to soften this extra-articular impingement, so it could give rise to particularly high stress concentrations. Moderately flexed postures, on the other hand, cause the articular surfaces to be oriented parallel to each other, and contact stresses are low and evenly distributed. Extra-articular impingement does not then occur. 'Kissing' spinous processes can also transmit considerable compressive forces down the spine if the vertebrae are oriented in several degrees of extension.[19] However, the resulting stress concentrations have not been measured.

Disc degeneration and narrowing can cause up to 90% of the compressive force to be resisted by the neural arch in lordotic posture (Fig. 8.16).

Posture and intervertebral disc mechanics

Small changes in posture can have large effects on the distribution of compressive stress inside the annulus fibrosus of intervertebral discs. When discs are subjected to compressive loading in the neutral posture' (i.e. without any bending being applied) they generally exhibit a small 'peak' of compressive stress in the posterior annulus, and a fairly even compressive stress throughout the nucleus and anterior annulus (Fig. 10.18B). In a simulated lordotic posture such as erect standing (i.e. in 2° of backwards bending for a motion segment) the size of this stress peak usually increases (Fig. 13.7), whereas moderately flexed postures usually distribute stresses evenly across the disc (Fig. 13.8). In full flexion, stress peaks can appear in the anterior annulus, but they are rarely as high as those in the posterior annulus in full extension[39] unless the disc is severely degenerated and narrowed (Fig. 10.20). These stress concentrations can be explained in terms of the elastic properties of the annulus fibrosus which is deformed vertically during flexion/extension movements (Fig. 13.9).

Posture also affects the hydrostatic pressure in the nucleus pulposus. For an applied compressive force of 500 N, the nucleus pressure is 40% less in 4° of extension than in the neutral configuration because the neural arches of adjacent vertebrae are pressed more firmly together and resist more of the compressive force.[39] On the other hand, nucleus pressure rises by 100% in full flexion because flexion stretches the ligaments of the neural arch, and ligament tension acts to compress the disc. If the neural arch is removed from a motion segment, then lumbar extension and flexion both increase nucleus pressure, by 8% and 38% respectively.[39] This shows that a stretched annulus can act like a ligament to compress the adjacent nucleus. High compressive forces (up to 3 kN) increase the compressive stiffness of the disc, and these postural effects on nucleus pressure are then diminished (Table 13.1).

A young highly hydrated disc behaves more like a 'bag of fluid' (p. 131) so that stresses within it are affected less by changes in posture. Conversely, as discs become older and/or more degenerated, their water content falls and they become less able to distribute compressive stress evenly (Fig. 10.18). The effects of posture are then

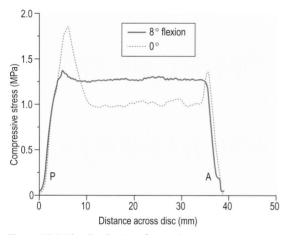

Figure 13.8 The distribution of vertical compressive stress along the sagittal mid-plane of a cadaveric intervertebral disc, compressed in the neutral configuration (0°) and in moderate flexion (8° flexion). (Specimen: male, 55 years, L45, P = posterior, A = anterior. Compressive force = 1 kN.) Moderate flexion tends to distribute compressive stress evenly across the disc, although it usually increases the pressure in the nucleus pulposus. P, A. *(Stress profiles are explained in Figure 10.17.)*

magnified (Fig. 10.20) and just 2° of bending can substantially increase stress peaks in the annulus (Fig. 13.10).

Increased sensitivity to posture in degenerated discs has been demonstrated in cadaveric specimens by damaging the endplate, and then expelling water from the disc by means of cyclic loading.[37] This treatment simulates two biomechanical consequences of advanced disc degeneration (structural disruption and dehydration) rather than the degenerative process itself, and it results in intradiscal stress profiles similar to those seen in severely degenerated discs in vivo.[962] On average such degenerated cadaveric discs showed stress peaks (over and above the nucleus pressure) of 1.9 MPa in the posterior annulus in 2° of extension. This was reduced to 0.6 MPa in moderate flexion. However, a minority of discs behaved quite differently from the average (Fig. 13.11): in these discs, extension reduced the stress peaks in the posterior annulus, by as much as 40%, and the hydrostatic pressure in the nucleus was also reduced.[37] Discs which appeared to benefit in this way from backwards bending tended to be more degenerated than the others in terms of the irregularity of their stress profiles recorded in the neutral posture. This suggests that when a disc is narrowed, it is possible for the neural arch to 'stress-shield' the posterior annulus in full extension, so that much of the compressive force on the spine is transmitted through the neural arch and anterior annulus (see below). The detailed results also illustrate two dangers of in vitro experimentation: the tendency to assume average results are generally true of all spines, and the tendency to extrapolate results on essentially 'normal' cadaveric material to the often-degenerated spines of patients with back pain.

The above discussion has considered only the compressive stress within the disc matrix, but it should be

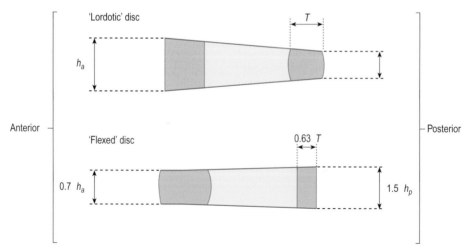

Figure 13.9 Diagram showing how an intervertebral disc deforms in the sagittal plane when the lumbar spine is in a flexed posture (lower) and a lordotic posture (upper). Changes in annulus height can be measured directly from radiographs.

Table 13.1 The effect of flexion and extension on intradiscal (nucleus) pressure (IDP), for isolated discs (below) and intact motion segments (above). Average data for 5–8 specimens[39]

Compression (N)	% Increase (+) Or Decrease (–) In IDP					
	–4°	–2°	0°	50% flexion	75% flexion	100% flexion
Motion segments						
500	–40	–10	0	+12	+45	+110
1000	–30	–6	0	+4	+23	+79
3000	–15	–4	0	+1	+6	+30
Disc vertebral body						
500	+8	+3	0	+3	+12	+38
1000	+3	+4	0	0	+5	+12
3000	0	+2	0	–1	+1	+4

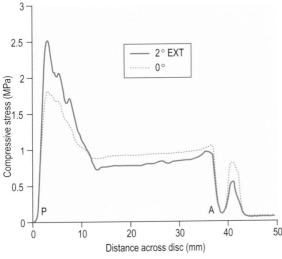

Figure 13.10 The distribution of vertical compressive stress along the sagittal mid-plane of a cadaveric intervertebral disc, compressed in the neutral configuration (0°) and in a lordotic posture (2° EXT). (Specimen: male, 54 years, L34, P = posterior, A = anterior. Compressive force = 2 kN.) This disc was damaged by compressive overload prior to testing, and structural failure makes the stress distribution very sensitive to small changes in posture. P, A. *(Stress profiles are explained in Figure 10.17.)*

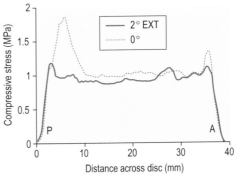

Figure 13.11 The distribution of vertical compressive stress along the sagittal mid-plane of a cadaveric intervertebral disc, compressed in the neutral configuration (0°) and in a lordotic posture (2° EXT). (Specimen: 55-year-old male, L45, P = posterior, A = anterior. Compressive force = 2 kN.) In some discs tested, lordotic posture reduced the stress peak in the posterior annulus, presumably because of stress-shielding by the neural arch. P, A. *(Stress profiles are explained in Figure 10.17.)*

remembered that the outer annulus behaves like a ligamentous structure in tension. Tensile stresses in the outer annulus are not detected by the pressure transducer used to record stress profiles. However, the presence of tension in the outer annulus can be inferred from its effect of increasing the pressure within the nucleus. Tension in the outer posterior annulus rises rapidly as the limit of flexion is approached, but the data in Table 13.1 suggest that they are unlikely to exceed 190 N (i.e. 38% of 500 N).

Posture and intervertebral disc nutrition

The supply of metabolites to cells within the intervertebral disc is barely adequate for normal requirements[918,1354,1455] and impaired metabolite transport is associated with disc degeneration.[623,1017] Cell culture experiments suggest that nucleus pulposus cells are tolerant of low oxygen concentrations, but die if the extracellular concentration of glucose falls below a critical level for a period of several days.[630] Any influence of posture on disc metabolism may therefore be important, and, in fact, posture appears to have large effects on both of the two transport mechanisms, diffusion and fluid flow.

The amount of a metabolite that can diffuse into a given region of the disc depends critically on the diffusion path length, which is the distance to the nearest blood vessel on the disc's surface or in the vertebral body. Compared to erect standing, flexed postures stretch the posterior annulus by 60%, and compress the anterior annulus by 35%.[27,1117] In order to maintain constant tissue volume, the thickness (and hence diffusion path length) of the anterior and posterior annulus must be correspondingly increased and decreased respectively (Fig. 13.9). Flexion therefore reduces the diffusion path length into the posterior annulus. In cadaveric experiments, flexion enhances metabolite diffusion into the inner posterior annulus[31] which is the region of the disc with the most precarious nutrient supply.[918] Similar events would occur in living discs because diffusion is a physical process, and measurements of diffusion into living discs agree with calculations based on cadaveric experiments.[1455] The beneficial effects of flexion would be compounded by the fact that the stretched posterior annulus has an increased surface area, so that a greater flux of metabolites could be 'funnelled' into the inner posterior annulus.[31] Flexion causes a corresponding decrease of metabolite diffusion into the thickened anterior annulus[31] but this is the last region of the disc to show degenerative changes.

Posture also affects fluid flow within discs, and this is particularly important for the transport of high-molecular-weight metabolites which diffuse very slowly,[424] as shown in Figure 7.21. Flexion increases intradiscal stresses, while at the same time thinning the posterior annulus and increasing its surface area, so fluid expulsion from the loaded disc is increased.[28] Fluid expelled under high load returns when loading is reduced, bringing metabolites with it. Flexion and extension tend to generate the highest compressive stresses in the anterior and posterior annulus, respectively (p. 177), so changes in posture will move the position of maximum compressive stress within the disc, and therefore enhance intradiscal fluid flow. These cadaveric experiments suggest that metabolite transport by fluid flow, both into and within the disc, is enhanced when flexed postures are alternated with lordotic postures.

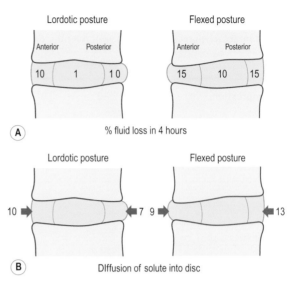

Figure 13.12 The influence of posture on metabolite transport into lumbar intervertebral discs. **(A)** Numbers indicate the percentage water loss from the anterior annulus, nucleus and posterior annulus of a cadaveric disc loaded at body weight during a 4-hour experiment.[28] **(B)** Numbers represent the average concentration of a small solute that has diffused into the anterior and posterior half of cadaveric intervertebral discs during a 4-hour experiment.[31]

Figure 13.12 summarises the evidence concerning posture and disc metabolite transport.

Posture and spinal nerve roots

Compared to the neutral (unloaded) position of a cadaveric lumbar spine, moderate flexion increases the cross-sectional area of the vertebral foramen by 12%, and extension reduces it by 15%.[666] In the same specimens, nerve root compression was judged to occur in the intervertebral foramen in 15%, 21% and 33% of specimens which were sectioned in the flexed, neutral and lordotic postures respectively. Extension decreases the volume and sagittal diameter of the neural sac when it is visualised by myelograms in cadaveric spines.[847]

Compressive loading also can decrease the cross-sectional area of the intervertebral foramen and contribute to foraminal stenosis. Compressive creep deformations of discs and vertebrae (see below) combine to reduce the height of the intervertebral foramen, and this loss in height causes a secondary reduction in foraminal width, as the outer annulus[601] and ligamentum flavum[563] both bulge horizontally into the foramen.

Although lumbar flexion would reduce the effects of nerve root compression, it would increase any effects of nerve root tension, especially if the nerve root were tethered to underlying structures by scar tissue.

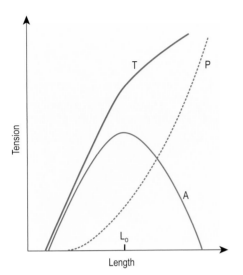

Figure 13.13 The length of a muscle affects the maximum active tension it can produce (A), as well as the passive tension (P) in stretched collagenous tissue within the muscle. Overall tension in the muscle (T) is greatest when the muscle is stretched compared to its resting length (L_o). *(After Wilke.[1563])*

Posture and muscle action

Posture affects three properties of the back and abdominal muscles: their length, the angles at which they pull on vertebrae, and their lever arms relative to centres of rotation. The most important of these influences is on muscle length. Muscles generate maximum active tension when they operate at their optimal length for cross-bridge formation, which is approximately 100–110% of resting muscle length. Cross-bridge formation and active tension both fall when the muscle is shortened or lengthened relative to this optimal length. Muscles can also generate passive tension in their non-contractile collagenous components, and this passive tension increases greatly as the muscle is stretched[1168] (Fig. 13.13). Trunk muscles are probably at their resting length when the spine is in the neutral configuration (Fig. 13.2). Therefore, erect standing, which extends the lumbar spine by approximately $12°$[19] will shorten the back muscles slightly, whereas flexed postures will stretch them. Not surprisingly, overall back muscle strength is substantially higher in flexed postures[363,366] compared to the erect standing posture,[964] and maximum strength increases by approximately 18% between 30% lumbar flexion and 60% flexion.[901] Although back muscle strength in more flexed postures has not been investigated thoroughly, it appears that strength is not diminished at 70% flexion.[366]

Above 80% lumbar flexion, the back muscles receive substantial help from the lumbodorsal fascia. This has been demonstrated in a large study which measured the maximum extensor moment that could be generated across the lumbosacral joint while the lumbar and thoracic back muscles remained electrically silent (Fig. 9.4). Extensor moment must therefore have been generated by more distant muscles, perhaps the gluteals and latissimus dorsi, and transmitted across the lumbar spine by the lumbodorsal fascia.[102] Stretched supraspinous and intervertebral ligaments would also have generated some passive extensor moment, but their contribution becomes substantial only when full flexion is approached (Fig. 9.4). The hypothesis that tension in the lumbodorsal fascia can be elevated substantially by the action of the abdominal muscles has been disproved by anatomically precise calculations,[873] so it appears that flexing the lumbar spine is the most effective way of employing the fascia to assist in heavy lifting. This assistance is beneficial in three ways: (1) the stored strain energy in the stretched fascia reduces the metabolic cost of lifting; (2) tension in the fascia increases the maximum load that can be lifted; and (3) because the fascia has a long lever arm relative to the centre of rotation in the disc, it also reduces the 'compressive penalty' of lifting, as discussed on page 104. The mechanics of weight lifting is considered in more detail in Chapter 9.

Lordotic postures enable the erector spinae to pull backwards at an increasing angle on the lower lumbar vertebrae and help them to limit the gravitational forward shearing force acting on these vertebrae to approximately 200 N.[1157] This may be of some benefit, although the apophyseal joints are able to resist 2 kN of shear without this assistance.[318] Full flexion reduces the posteriorly directed shear force exerted by muscles on the upper lumbar vertebrae, and changes the net shear force acting on L5/S1 from an anteriorly directed force to a posteriorly directed one.[874]

Lumbar curvature has little effect on the lever arms of the back muscles relative to the flexion–extension axis of rotation, and so does not greatly influence the compressive force acting on the lower lumbar spine. This has been demonstrated using bilateral X-rays to compare the attachment points of the back muscles (including multifidus) in the erect standing and fully flexed postures.[874] This study concluded that flexion increased the lever arms of some muscles, but reduced them in others, so that there was no overall difference in the muscles' ability to generate extensor moment. A magnetic resonance imaging (MRI) study has claimed that flexed postures reduce the lever arm of the erector spinae,[1442] but this may be an artefact caused by subjects squashing their back muscles against the confining walls of the MRI scanner whilst attempting to flex in a confined space.

Postures involving lateral bending of the lumbar spine

Lateral bending has received little attention from biomechanists, presumably because it is not a common movement in life. However, lateral bending is often combined with forward bending during asymmetrical manual handling tasks, and in awkward postures, so it is important to understand the significance of the component of lateral bending. The side-to-side diameter of a lumbar disc is approximately 50% greater than its anteroposterior diameter, so a given angular movement between two vertebrae in the frontal plane will cause 50% greater vertical deformations of the peripheral annulus than the same movement in the sagittal plane (Fig. 11.17). Intradiscal stress distributions should therefore be more sensitive to lateral bending than to flexion or extension, and the stress peaks shown in Figures 13.7 and 13.10 would probably be larger if the 2° angulation was in the frontal plane rather than the sagittal plane. Similarly, small angles of spinal bending in the frontal plane could possibly generate high compressive stresses in the ipsilateral apophyseal joint, and high tensile stresses in the capsule of the contralateral joint. By implication, postures which involve angular movements in both the sagittal and frontal planes will be capable of generating particularly high stress concentrations in the disc, apophyseal joints and intervertebral ligaments.

These possibilities have not been tested by experiment, but anterolateral bending does indeed create large concentrations of compressive stress in the lateral and posterior annulus fibrosus, and these stress concentrations are linked with the disc's susceptibility to prolapse under the influence of combined bending and compression.[961] Lateral bending is usually coupled with axial rotation (p. 118) and a combination of compression, bending and axial rotation generates particularly high intradiscal stresses in the inner posterolateral annulus.[1357] Finite element modelling suggests that shear and fibre strains in the annulus both increase when a component of lateral bending is added to primary loading in flexion or axial rotation.[1265]

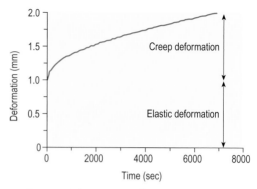

Figure 13.14 Typical creep curve for a cadaveric intervertebral disc (male, 55 years, L23). When a compressive force of 1.7 kN is first applied, the disc deforms immediately. This elastic deformation is followed by a slow creep deformation over a period of hours as water is expelled from the disc.

'CREEP' IN SPINAL TISSUES

Compressive 'creep' deformation of intervertebral discs

Sustained loading of intervertebral discs causes them to lose height gradually, a process known as 'creep' (Fig. 13.14). Most disc creep is due to the expulsion of water.[28,786,957] Approximately 25% of the height loss has been attributed to viscoelastic deformation of the annulus[195] but this may simply be a structural effect arising from the annulus bulging more when the volume and pressure of the nucleus are reduced (Fig. 10.16). As water is expelled from the disc, the notional 'pore pressure' within the tissue falls, so that more compressive load-bearing is resisted by the solid components of the matrix, and tension in the collagen network decreases.[1267] Annulus

tissue becomes more elastic (and less viscous) as a result.[765,1328] After 6 hours of creep loading at 1.5 kN, creep slows down markedly. The volume and hydration of the nucleus and inner annulus are then reduced by approximately 20%,[957] an increasing proportion of the inner annulus loses its ability to behave as a hydrostatic fluid (Fig. 13.15) and concentrations of compressive stress appear within the annulus, usually posterior to the nucleus.[38,81] Pressure in the nucleus is usually reduced by 30–40%, and this allows the annulus to bulge radially outwards, rather like a 'flat tyre',[189] and may cause the inner lamellae to bulge into the nucleus.[1305] The disc's resistance to shear is reduced.[316] Eventually, water expulsion causes the swelling pressure of the disc's proteoglycan-rich matrix to increase until it approaches a balance with the external mechanical pressure, and then water expulsion stops, or is greatly reduced.[1456]

When external loading is removed, the disc recovers from creep by sucking the expelled water back in again, until the original disc height is regained. Recovery from creep is rather slower than the creep process itself, but complete recovery is eventually achieved.[1466] Earlier cadaveric experiments reported incomplete recovery from creep, giving rise to speculation that postmortem blood clotting in the endplate might prevent the disc's swelling pressure from operating properly. However, the earlier results probably represent an artifact arising from postmortem superhydration of the disc, following several days of unloading in the wet environment of the cadaver. This interpretation is supported by more recent experimental results which show that repeated creep and recovery tests on goat discs soon reach a steady state of creep, followed by 100% recovery.[1466] The extremes of hydration in the repeatable tests probably reflect hydration in vivo at the start and end of every day. In these tests, attempting to block the disc

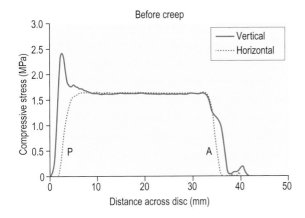

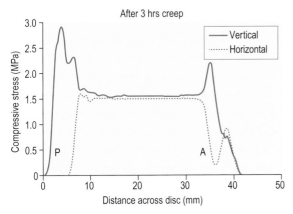

Figure 13.15 Distribution of vertical and horizontal compressive stress along the sagittal mid-plane of a cadaveric intervertebral disc, before and after a 3-hour period of compressive creep loading in a lordotic posture (2° of extension). (Specimen: male, 59 years, L34, P = posterior, A = anterior. Compressive force = 2 kN.) Creep increases stress concentrations in the annulus, and reduces the size of the region that exhibits a hydrostatic pressure. *(Stress profiles are explained in Figure 10.17.)*

endplate with silicone paste had little effect on creep recovery, suggesting that postmortem blood clotting is not a major factor.[1466]

Compressive 'creep' deformation of vertebrae

Many elderly people diagnosed with 'fractured' vertebrae do not recall any preceding trauma, and their radiographs may reveal no clear fracture plane.[689] This suggests that old vertebrae can deform gradually by some 'creep' mechanism in a similar manner to intervertebral discs. It has been known for many years that bone is a viscoelastic material,[311] and that repeated loading of small bone

samples leads to a residual deformation that recovers slowly, if at all.[1597] Recently, studies on whole human vertebrae have confirmed that they can creep under physiological load levels, provided that the bone mineral density is low.[1141] Interestingly, the less-dense anterior region of the vertebral body creeps faster than the posterior, so that the entire vertebral body develops a slight but measurable anterior wedge shape. Typically, a 2-hour creep test (at 21°C) results in an anterior wedge deformity of 0.1°. Recovery from creep takes approximately 20 times as long as the period of loading,[1597] and in whole vertebrae full recovery may not be possible.[1141] It is not easy to extrapolate from cadaver experiments to living humans, because the rate of creep decreases with time (Fig. 13.16) and may eventually approach an equilibrium. Also, creep would probably be faster at body temperature[1197] and may then recover more. The underlying mechanisms of bone creep are unknown, but could involve fluid flow within canaliculi, slipping at the cement lines which separate adjacent osteons (Fig. 7.9), or proliferation of microcracks. The last mechanism is known to be enhanced when bone is deformed slowly.[1633]

Creep mechanisms are accelerated if the vertebra suffers minor damage.[858] If elderly vertebrae are subjected to high compressive loading in vitro, then it is possible to create only focal damage to a single endplate and to its supporting trabeculae, without the injury being apparent on radiographs (Fig. 11.6).[689] It is difficult to assess the clinical impact of such minor injuries: they may or may not cause pain that is severe enough to lead to a medical consultation. However, even minor injuries can accelerate creep deformation of the affected vertebral body, typically by a factor of 700%.[858] This research is in its early stages, but it appears that focal damage to trabecular bone leads to increased loading on adjacent tissue, which then undergoes plastic deformation (i.e. permanent deformation beyond the elastic limit (Fig. 1.4)) if its bone mineral density is sufficiently low. This in turn throws increased loading on to adjacent bone, so that a progressive deformity develops. Prospective studies on patients are required to determine the influence of creep, and accelerated creep, on vertebral deformity in later life.

Total time-dependent compressive deformations of the elderly spine

The cadaveric studies described above show that, in elderly people with low bone mineral density, creep deformations are of similar magnitude in the intervertebral discs and vertebral bodies, and that elastic deformations can actually be greater in the bone than in the discs.[1143] Plainly, many old spines do not behave like segmented columns of rigid bones separated by soft discs. Figure 13.17 suggests an alternative model. The anterior column is much more deformable than in youth, and is represented by a dashpot

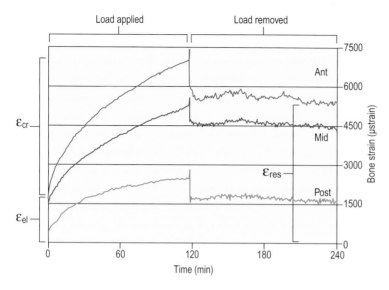

Load applied   Load removed

Ant

Mid

ε_{res}

Post

ε_{cr}

ε_{el}

Bone strain (µstrain)

Time (min)

Figure 13.16 Creep deformation and recovery curves for a 2-hour creep test on a lumbar vertebral body. (Male, aged 80 years, L2.) The three graphs show deformation (strains) in the posterior, middle and anterior vertebral body of one of the specimen's two vertebrae. Elastic (ε_{el}), creep (ε_{cr}) and residual strains (ε_{res}) are labelled for the anterior vertebral body. *(Reproduced from Pollintine et al.[1141] with permission.)*

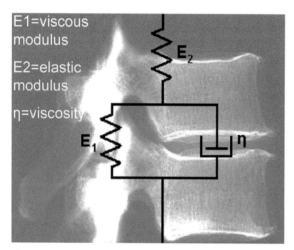

E1=viscous modulus

E2=elastic modulus

η=viscosity

E_2

E_1

η

Figure 13.17 The response of the elderly vertebral column to sustained compressive loading can be understood in terms of a three-parameter model, as shown. A dashpot or syringe (η) represents a propensity to time-dependent creep deformation in the anterior column, whereas the spring E_1 represents stiff resistance to compression from the increasingly compacted posterior column. Note the radiographically dense bone in the neural arches, indicative of their major load-bearing role in elderly spines. *(Reproduced from Pollintine et al.[1143] with permission.)*

(or syringe) to emphasise that both degenerated discs and osteoporotic vertebral bodies can creep markedly in response to sustained loading. This creep process is resisted, and may become limited, by bone-on-bone contact in the neural arches, which become heavily load-bearing and may develop relatively dense bone. The posterior column is therefore represented by a stiff spring.

Diurnal changes in human stature

Unfortunately, almost nothing is known about bone creep in vivo, or how it might be recovered during rest, so the following discussion is based on what we know about disc creep only. It will be relevant to those people who are too young to have developed severe spinal osteoporosis.

During the course of each day, physical activity reduces the height and volume of intervertebral discs by about 20%.[172] There is a corresponding reduction in human stature of 15–25 mm,[329,788,1449] much of which occurs during the first hour after rising. During the night, when the spine is relatively unloaded, the disc's elevated swelling pressure sucks in water from surrounding tissues, causing tissue hydration to increase and swelling pressure to fall, until it approaches equilibrium once more with external mechanical load. In this way, the disc's water content exhibits a cyclic diurnal variation, which is modified by periods of hard work or rest. Three hours of carrying a backpack weighing 20 kg, for example, reduces disc volume by 4.5%.[894] There is no evidence that the disc's water content ever achieves an equilibrium with applied load – only that it approaches equilibrium after several hours of constant loading – so there is no such thing as a precise physiological disc hydration, just a physiological range which depends on loading history. Measurements of spinal shrinkage during discrete time intervals can be used to infer the approximate magnitude of spinal loading (p. 106).

Diurnal changes in spinal mechanics

Any loss of disc height brings adjacent vertebrae closer together and increases loading of the apophyseal joints: approximately, a 1-mm height loss can increase their

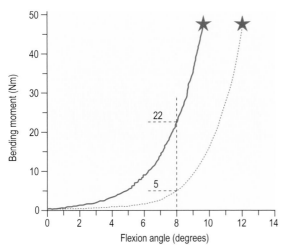

Figure 13.18 The resistance to flexion of a cadaveric lumbar motion segment before (solid line) and after (broken line) 2 hours of compressive creep loading at 1.5 kN. (Specimen: male, 52 years, L23, creep height loss =1.0 mm.) Creep reduced this specimen's resistance at 8° of flexion by 77%, and increased its range of flexion by 2°. Stars indicate the elastic limit of flexion.

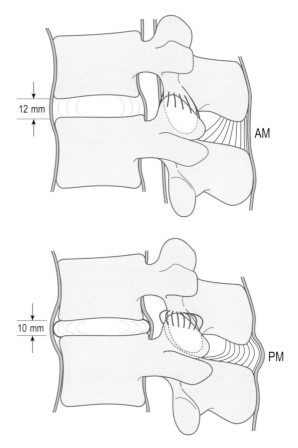

Figure 13.19 Representation of diurnal changes in spinal mechanics. In the early morning (AM), the discs are swollen with fluid, and collagen fibres in the discs and ligaments have no slack. Later in the day (PM), fluid expulsion from the discs causes them to lose height and bulge radially, giving slack to the intervertebral ligaments and increasing the load-bearing function of the apophyseal joints.

load-bearing from 4% to 16% of an applied compressive force of 1 kN.[25] As disc height is lost, compressive stresses become concentrated in the inferior margins of the apophyseal joints, especially in lordotic postures, and extra-articular (bone–bone) impingement of the inferior facets on the subjacent lamina can occur.[380] The height of the intervertebral foramen is reduced directly by disc creep, and its anteroposterior diameter is reduced also by the concomitant increase in disc radial bulging, so the space available for the spinal nerve roots is reduced considerably as the day progresses.

Loss of disc height slackens the intervertebral ligaments and fibres of the annulus fibrosus, so that they resist bending movements less.[18,1627] On average, 2 hours of compressive creep loading at 1.5 kN reduces disc height by 1.1 mm, reduces the bending moment resisted at full flexion by 41% and increase the range of flexion by 12%,[14] as shown in Figure 13.18. The effect of disc creep is relatively greater for the short fibres of the annulus than for the longer fibres of most intervertebral ligaments, so the disc becomes better protected in bending.[18] After creep, it becomes more difficult to cause discs to prolapse posteriorly, presumably because creep loading decompresses the nucleus and reduces tension in the posterior annulus in flexion (p. 155). Increasing the volume of the nucleus by injecting water into it has the opposite effect: the pressure increases[73,1183] and so does the motion segment's resistance to bending.[73]

Some of these changes have been measured in living people. The range of lumbar flexion increases by approximately 5° during the course of a day,[18] with 77% of the increase occurring during the first hour after rising.[360] When the peak bending moments acting on the osteoligamentous lumbar spine are quantified (p. 110), they are found to increase by more than 100% in the early morning compared to later in the day.[360] This supports the common experience that it is easier to touch your toes in the evening, when all of the intervertebral ligaments (and the spinal cord!) have more slack. Similarly, the range of straight-leg raising increases as the day progresses.[1154] Diurnal loss of disc height and approximation of the neural arches should make spinal extension movements more difficult in the evening, although this has not been quantified. Diurnal changes in spinal mechanics are summarised in Figure 13.19.

Spinal 'creep' in flexion and extension

Sitting in a slumped position causes the lumbar spine to 'creep' into more and more flexion.[944] This is not simply due to changes in the back muscles, because flexion creep has been measured in cadaveric spines subjected to sustained or repetitive bending.[14,1444] Typically, 5 minutes in full flexion reduces a motion segment's resistance to flexion by 42%, whereas 100 full flexion movements during the same period reduces it by 17%.[14] Experiments on isolated ligaments[1595] show that they creep substantially in a few minutes, whereas disc creep involves fluid redistribution over long distances and takes hours to approach equilibrium.[957] Therefore, sustained or repetitive lumbar flexion will have a relatively greater effect on the posterior intervertebral ligaments than on the disc, so that ligamentous protection of the discs will be reduced. Sustained backwards bending also causes creep in cadaveric specimens, but extension creep during 20 minutes amounts to less than 10% of the normal full range of movement, presumably because of bony impaction between the neural arches.[1068]

'GOOD' AND 'BAD' POSTURE FOR THE LUMBAR SPINE

Sitting and standing

Recommendations concerning 'good' or 'bad' posture should not be based on experimental data concerning only one or two structures: the whole lumbar spine must be considered, including muscles and fascia. Unfortunately, early investigations of the biomechanical effects of spinal posture concerned only the hydrostatic pressure in the nucleus pulposus of the intervertebral disc, which was measured in cadaveric specimens,[1021] and subsequently in living people.[69,1018] These studies found that lordotic postures reduce the pressure in the nucleus pulposus compared to flexed postures, and they concluded that lordotic postures reduce spinal loading. We now know that lordotic postures reduce nucleus pressure only because they transfer load-bearing to the posterior annulus fibrosus and apophyseal joints (p. 100). These latter structures are frequent sources of back pain,[797] whereas the nucleus is not, so the concept of 'good' posture needs to be re-evaluated.

The relative merits of a flexed and lordotic lumbar spine are summarised in Box 13.1. These statements suggest that moderate flexion is preferable in static postures, whereas a slight lordosis has certain advantages during locomotion. Too much lumbar flexion is worse than too little, because prolonged full flexion severely compromises the ability of the back muscles to protect the lumbar spine, as described in Chapter 14 (p. 192). The evident dangers of

excessive flexion may have been apparent before the benefits of moderate flexion were understood, and this could explain why the advocacy of lordotic postures was so readily accepted. But now that a more complete picture is emerging, it is time to recognise the benefits of moderation: not too much flexion, and not too much lordosis either.

On a practical level, it is reassuring that the biomechanical and nutritional benefits of moderate flexion are matched by a perception that a flattened lumbar spine is also more comfortable. Common postural habits such as standing with one foot raised on a bar rail, or sitting with the legs crossed, all tend to move the lumbar spine from lordosis to slight flexion (Fig. 13.4). However, there is no ideal sitting or standing posture, because no single posture can be comfortably maintained for a long period of time, presumably because of blood flow restrictions in compressed or contracted tissues. Therefore, any recommendations on 'good' sitting or standing postures must incorporate the need for intermittent postural adjustments. Recommendations should also pay attention to the additional stress concentrations which arise from lateral bending of the lumbar spine (p. 182), and to the benefits of minimising muscle activity. According to these criteria, the ideal posture would be the fetal position! Realistically, it would be better to advocate a straight (moderately flexed) back, with the head and vertebral column finely balanced so as to allow the supporting muscles to relax.

Box 13.1 **Relative advantages of moderately flexed and lordotic postures**

Advantages of moderately flexed postures

1. Even distribution of stress in the intervertebral discs
2. Increased supply of metabolites to vulnerable regions of discs
3. Reduced loading of the apophyseal joints
4. Increased volume of intervertebral foramen and spinal canal
5. Lumbodorsal fascia is able to resist lumbar flexion

Advantages of lordotic postures

1. Reduced pressure in the nucleus pulposus
2. Reduced compressive stresses in the anterior annulus
3. Apophyseal joints contribute to spinal compressive strength
4. Improved shock absorption during locomotion
5. Spinal stretch reflexes preserved

Manual handling

The benefits of moderate lumbar flexion can also be realised during vigorous activities such as lifting heavy weights. In fact, when spinal compressive loading rises to high levels, the only clear advantage of lordotic postures (reduced nucleus pressure) becomes insignificant (Table 13.1). The compressive strength of cadaveric lumbar motion segments appears to vary little in the range between the neutral position and moderate (4–10°) flexion,[39] presumably because two opposing effects cancel each other: flexed postures probably strengthen the disc–vertebral body unit by equalising the distribution of compressive stress within the disc, whereas lordotic postures will strengthen motion segments by sharing load-bearing between the disc and neural arch. In full flexion, tensile forces in the posterior intervertebral ligaments act to compress the disc, but this effect becomes smaller when the compressive force rises to high levels (Table 13.1). There is some slight evidence that motion segments are weaker when flexed to 15°, which is beyond the physiological limit of many specimens, and failure is then more likely to involve the anterior vertebral body rather than the endplate.[525] Also, in full flexion and hyperflexion, stretching of the posterior annulus fibrosus increases the risk of posterior disc prolapse (p. 154).

When heavy lifting is viewed in a wider perspective, it can be seen that a flat, moderately flexed lumbar spine has the additional advantage of stretching passive tissues, including the lumbodorsal fascia, so that the 'compressive penalty' of lifting is reduced (p. 104). Flexion also reduces the metabolic cost of lifting by causing elastic energy to be stored in stretched tissues (Fig. 1.5). It is not surprising, therefore, that healthy people flex their lumbar spine by approximately 80% when lifting weights from the ground, regardless of whether they adopt a 'bent-knees' style,[363] or lift in a manner of their own choosing.[366] Even when they attempted to maintain a lordosis throughout the lift, a group of experienced lifters found it impossible to avoid flexing their lumbar spine by less than 57% on average.[366] The widely held belief that weight lifters should, or even can, maintain a normal (standing?) lumbar lordosis is evidently mistaken, and may arise from a quite proper appreciation of the dangers of too much flexion during lifting. It may be of practical benefit to instruct novices to 'lift with a lordosis' in order to reduce the risk of them lifting with a fully flexed or hyperflexed back, but the instructor should know that the lumbar spine will in fact be moderately flexed, and that this is beneficial to the spine.

POSTURAL ADVICE FOR THOSE WITH BACK PAIN

The above discussion has considered how 'good' posture should be interpreted for people with a healthy back, but these arguments cannot necessarily be extended to those with an injured or painful back. Obviously, the need to avoid pain and to minimise loading of damaged tissues would take precedence. Maintaining an exaggerated lordosis may help some patients, but this is an expedient for particular individuals which should not be applied to healthy people.

The final word on 'good' posture should be reserved for evidence from living people, rather than the interpretation of laboratory experiments. Intervertebral disc degeneration is less common in populations who habitually adopt squatting postures which flex the lumbar spine than it is in industrialised populations who generally prefer chairs[408,409] and who have a reduced range of lumbar flexion.[127,695] Although several factors may contribute to the relative health of the 'squatters'' discs, this evidence makes it difficult to argue that flexed postures are harmful to the back.

Sensorimotor control

INTRODUCTION

Most spinal loading arises from muscle tension, as discussed in Chapter 9, and muscles are required to protect the spine from injury. Plainly, if the muscles of the trunk act in an unusual or uncontrolled manner, then there may be adverse consequences for the underlyng spine. This chapter considers how patterns of trunk muscle activity depend on sensory feedback information from spinal tissues, and how motor control patterns can be disturbed by factors such as creep, muscle fatigue and pain.

So many muscles are capable of moving the human torso that any particular task can be achieved by many different combinations of activated muscles. This inherent 'redundancy' in the problem of trunk muscle activation means that mathematical models of muscle function are unable to predict which is the optimum muscle strategy for a particular task, unless they introduce minimising principles in order to obtain a unique solution.[277,501] The somewhat arbitrary nature of these principles is considered on page 106, and they lead to uncertainty over the whole concept of optimal motor control patterns. A variety of patterns could be explained simply in terms of anatomical diversity, combined with personal preferences, or perhaps even a preference for variety because experienced workers show more variability in spinal loading when repeating a lifting task than do novice workers.[523] This argues against the physical importance of optimum muscle strategies during manual handling.

There have been attempts to explain back pain in terms of faulty motor (feedback) control leading to a lack of spinal stability.[1188] However, stability can be defined in such a manner that any injury necessarily represents a failure of stability, and of motor control, so the argument is somewhat circular.[6]

ASYMMETRICAL MUSCLE ACTIVITY

Large asymmetries have been detected in the electromyographic (EMG) signals from the back muscles of patients with back pain,[260] as shown in Figure 14.1, but there is currently no evidence to suggest that these asymmetries cause the pain. The spine is essentially symmetrical about the mid-sagittal plane, so gross left–right asymmetries in the activity of back muscles may represent an attempt by muscles on one side of the back to 'splint' a painful spinal segment. Or, they could represent reflex inhibition (p. 194). Alternatively, asymmetrical muscle activity could reflect selective muscle atrophy, possibly in response to injury, or asymmetrical muscle growth. In a similar manner, inferred imbalances in flexor/extensor muscle strength may be causes or consequences of back pain.

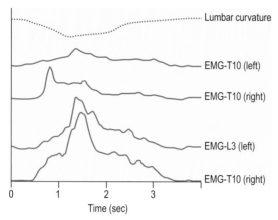

Figure 14.1 Evidence of asymmetrical back muscle activity in a patient with acute back pain, who flexed forwards to lift a 10-kg weight from the ground. The top curve shows that peak lumbar flexion occurred after 1.2 seconds. The other curves indicate the electromyographic (EMG) signal recorded from four sites on the surface of the back, at the levels of T10 and L3. Note the early activation of the muscle at T10 on the right-hand side of the back. *(Dolan 2000, unpublished data.)*

ANTAGONISTIC MUSCLE ACTIVITY

Muscles which flex the spine normally work antagonistically with those that extend it. Antagonistic muscle activity stabilises the vertebral column in the sense that it reduces the need to recruit additional muscles to deal with some unexpected event.[1368] However, antagonistic muscle tension increases the compressive force acting on the spine (p. 108). For each posture or activity, there must be an optimum level of antagonistic muscle activity which achieves adequate spinal stability, while minimising spinal loading and metabolic cost. When stability is a major concern, as in upright and rotated postures, then antagonistic muscle activity is relatively high, and can increase spinal compressive loading by up to 45%[277,520,810,941] Vibrations also induce stabilising muscle activity, increasing in proportion to the amplitude and frequency of vibration,[1144] and becoming especially large near the spine's natural frequency of 4.5 Hz.[1147] Conversely, when high compressive loading of the spine is more of a problem, as when lifting heavy objects from the ground, then antagonistic muscle activity is low, accounting for approximately 10% of spinal compressive loading.[745,947]

Antagonistic muscle activity is often increased in people with back pain,[47,586] although this is not necessarily the case in chronic sufferers.[260] Evidently, trunk muscles can increase their activity in order to 'splint' a painful spinal segment, and so reduce the risk of sudden movements deforming injured tissues. Alternatively, high antagonistic muscle forces could possibly cause pain by subjecting the underlying spine to high chronic loading, leading to accelerated creep and high stress concentrations. To the authors' knowledge, this possibility remains unsupported by experimental evidence.

Muscle spasm represents an extreme form of muscle splinting, in which a vigorous reflex contraction of a muscle is induced by stimulated nociceptors in adjacent tissue.[1344] Muscle spasm ensures that a painful spinal segment is effectively splinted, but muscle tension imposes high compressive forces on that segment, and the affected muscle can possibly become a source of pain in its own right.

FLEXION–RELAXATION

A similar problem is the loss of the normal flexion–relaxation phenomenon. When someone bends forwards, it is normal for the back muscles to fall electrically silent and allow the forward-bending moment of the inclined trunk to be supported by stretched non-contractile tissue within the muscles (Fig. 7.2) and by adjacent structures such as the lumbodorsal fascia and intervertebral ligaments.[431,945,1276] If the spine is sufficiently flexed, then the thoracic erector spinae fall silent as well.[366] Skin surface electrodes used in these investigations are capable of picking up signals from the deep muscles of the trunk as well as from superficial muscles.[939] The flexion–relaxation response is often lost in people with back pain,[48,1535] but there is no evidence that the response is lost before the pain starts. The simplest explanation is that the back muscles are attempting to 'splint' a painful spinal segment during a potentially threatening movement into full flexion.

REFLEX CONTROL OF SPINAL MOVEMENTS

Under most circumstances, muscles of the trunk act to protect the underlying spinal tissues from injury (Fig. 14.2). To do this effectively, muscles must be capable of generating rapid and forceful contractions in order to prevent excessive movements and maintain spinal stability. This protective action has been demonstrated when subjects bend forwards to lift an object from the ground[358]: a sudden burst of back muscle activity decelerates the upper body and prevents excessive lumbar flexion (Fig. 14.3). This muscle protection is achieved via both reflex and voluntary muscle activation that is dependent upon input from a wide variety of mechanoreceptor afferents found in spinal tissues.[956,1193,1201,1594,1601]

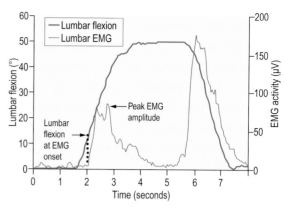

Figure 14.3 Recordings of lumbar flexion and electromyographic (EMG) activity at L3 while a subject bends forwards from a standing position, and then straightens up again after 2 seconds. Horizontal arrows indicate lumbar flexion at the onset of EMG activation, and peak EMG activity during the flexion. Experiments showed that, after sitting for 1 hour in a flexed posture, EMG onset would occur at higher angles of lumbar flexion. (*Data from Dolan et al. 2005.*[369])

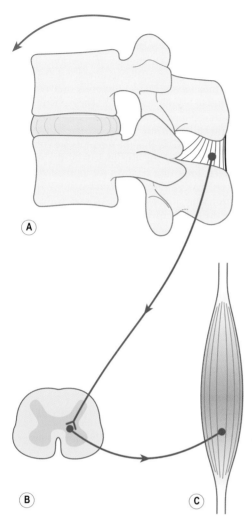

Figure 14.2 In a stretch reflex, stimulation of receptors in a stretched ligament or muscle **(A)** sends a signal to the spinal cord **(B)**, which sends a signal to the muscle **(C)**, causing it to contract in order to counter the initial stimulus. (If the receptor is in a ligament, one or more interneurones – not shown – may be involved within the spinal cord, which will slow the reflex slightly.) In a 'long-loop' or long-latency reflex, the incoming signal from the stimulated tissue reaches the spinal cord in the same manner, but is then reflected from the brainstem, before a modulated response is sent to the muscle.

The most rapid muscle response is achieved via monosynaptic reflexes initiated by muscle spindles that lie within skeletal muscle. The spindles are innervated by primary (IA) and secondary (II) muscle afferents that synapse directly with the alpha motor neurone of the muscle in which they lie. Primary afferents, which are sensitive to both strain and strain rate, initiate a rapid contraction of the muscle (typically within 30–50 ms) in response to a sudden increase in muscle length,[352,1317] thereby protecting the muscle from sudden strain injury. Secondary afferents, in contrast, are sensitive to slow or sustained stretch of the muscle, so they are responsible for providing continuous feedback to the central nervous system that contributes to proprioception.

In the back muscles, spindles in longissimus and multifidus show greater sensitivity to movement compared to spindles in the limb muscles,[245,246] which may reflect their important protective role in limiting spinal bending. Small intervertebral muscles contain a high density of spindles[1049] which may contribute to spinal proprioception and explain why a high degree of proprioceptive acuity is maintained throughout a range of motion.[1391] During spinal movements, spindles in these short muscles may be more highly activated than in the longer paraspinal muscles because of the higher relative strains in their fibres. These findings suggest that the intervertebral muscles, which are mechanically weak, may nevertheless play an important role in controlling intervertebral motion. There is also evidence that spindle afferents in the back muscles may influence motor activity at other spinal levels,[714] contributing to intersegmental reflexes that enable a coordinated muscle response across different spinal levels.

While muscle spindles are believed to be the most important receptors involved in controlling joint position and movement, proprioceptive feedback from other tissues is also likely to contribute. Mechanoreceptors have been identified in a number of spinal tissues, including the intervertebral disc,[1201,1601] apophyseal joint capsule,[262,956] ligaments[1193] and lumbodorsal fascia.[1594] Mechanoreceptors in the disc and joint capsule often have a high mechanical threshold and are therefore activated towards the end of the range of movement when loading becomes more severe.[263,1601] These high-threshold units may contribute to nociception and may also act as limit detectors that protect the spine from excessive movement. However, lower-threshold units which are activated within the normal range of joint movement have been identified in the joint capsule, spinal ligaments and tendons,[1600,1601] and these are thought to act as proprioceptors that may contribute to the reflex control of spinal movement. Direct evidence for such a role has come from studies in anaesthetised patients and animals which have shown that stretching of the supraspinous ligament initiates reflex contractions of the multifidus muscle.[1345] Animal studies have also shown that reflex activity in multifidus and longissimus can be activated by electrical stimulation of afferents in the discs and joint capsules, and this reflex response is augmented if afferents in more than one tissue are stimulated simultaneously.[622,1376]

The above findings suggest that afferent input from mechanoreceptors in a number of spinal tissues may contribute to reflex muscle activation, and it is likely that interaction between these various feedback systems helps to ensure that trunk muscles are activated in such a way as to prevent excessive spinal movements, without generating unnecessarily high compressive forces on the spine.

FACTORS THAT IMPAIR REFLEX CONTROL

There is growing evidence that effects such as soft-tissue creep, muscle fatigue and pain can alter the sensitivity of mechanoreceptor afferents and impair reflex activation of the back muscles.

Creep

Creep involves deformation of a material under constant load, and in soft musculoskeletal tissues is usually due to expulsion of water which causes strain to increase progressively as a function of time even when stress remains constant. (This process is discussed in detail in Chapter 13.) Similarly, if such a tissue is subjected to a constant stretch, fluid expulsion allows the tension within it to fall, a phenomenon known as stress relaxation. In either case, the close correspondence between stress and strain diminishes over time, and this may impair the ability of mechanoreceptors within the tissue to protect it from excessive loads or deformations.

Animal studies have shown that prolonged[1343] or repeated[1344] stretching of the supraspinous ligament causes the normal reflex activation of multifidus to diminish, and then disappear entirely (Fig. 14.4). The fall in reflex activity occurs rapidly but can be reversed by adding a preload to the ligament which immediately restores the reflex response.[1344] However, if the ligament is left to recover naturally, then several hours of recovery time are required for the reflex to be fully restored.[1342] These phenomena can probably be explained in terms of time-dependent changes in the immediate vicinity of mechanoreceptors in ligaments and tendons, so that the receptors are either desensitised from overuse, or else fooled by the manner in which creep stretching removes the normal close correspondence between tissue stress and strain. Whatever the explanation, any loss of stretch reflexes will reduce the ability of the back muscles to protect the lumbar spine by contracting vigorously as the limit of flexion is approached, and it appears that such impairment may persist for several hours.

Muscle spindles can adjust their sensitivity via gamma-motor neurons that innervate the intrafusal fibres, so it is possible that these might accommodate for reduced input from other afferents as a result of soft-tissue creep, so that adequate reflex control would be maintained. However, prolonged or repetitive passive stretching of muscle appears to reduce spindle sensitivity to subsequent stretches.[91,1164] These changes in sensitivity have been attributed to thixotropic effects in the muscle that derive from the formation of stable cross-bridges within the intrafusal fibres. It is proposed that these cross-bridges persist for relatively longer than those that form in the extrafusal fibres during dynamic muscle contraction.[483] As a result, intrafusal fibres that have recently been lengthened become slack when they return to their resting length, and hence less sensitive to a subsequent stretch, whereas fibres that have recently undergone shortening become taut and more sensitive to stretch.[483,1163]

Evidently, prolonged or repeated stretching of spinal soft tissues can alter the firing of muscle spindles and other mechanoreceptor afferents, and this may explain why human volunteers demonstrate impaired spinal position sense[356,1242] and marked delays in reflex activation of the back muscles[1241] following activities that involve sustained lumbar flexion such as sitting in a slumped posture. This delay can be measured as the onset latency in response to a sudden perturbation of the trunk (Fig. 14.5). Following creep, onset latency of the erector spinae muscles can increase by more than 50% (Fig. 14.6). Substantial delays in reflex activation during forward-bending tasks would cause a slower deceleration of the trunk leading to increased levels of lumbar flexion that may increase the risk of tissue injury. These findings therefore have important implications concerning the reflex protection of the spine which appears to be significantly impaired under conditions that lengthen the muscles and induce tensile creep in spinal tissues.

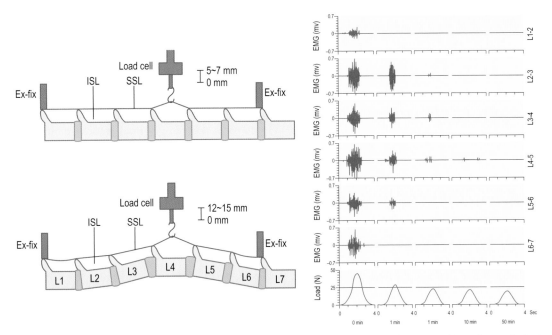

Figure 14.4 (A) Schematic illustration showing how the lumbar spine of an anaethetised cat was subjected to cyclic flexion movements by pulling on the L4–supraspinous ligament. ISL: interspinous ligament, SSL: supraspinous ligament, Ex-fix: external fixator. **(B)** Top six graphs show typical electromyographic (EMG) response from multifidus muscle at L1–2 to L6–7, immediately at the start of the first hour (0 minutes) of cyclic loading, and after 1, 5, 10 and 50 minutes of cyclic loading. The bottom graph shows the peak tensile force pulling on the ligament. Note the gradual decrease in the peak sinusoidal load recorded as time elapses, and the concurrent reduction or disappearance of the EMG response, indicating that the laxity developing in the spine desensitises the mechanoreceptors in the viscoelastic tissues and gradually eliminates the reflexive muscular activity. *(Reproduced from Solomonow et al.[1344] with permission.)*

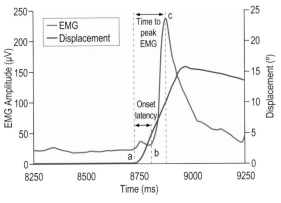

Figure 14.5 A typical trace obtained during the reflex activation test on a healthy volunteer. Displacement is a measure of trunk flexion under gravity in response to the sudden removal of a constraint. The electromyographic (EMG) signal is recorded from the skin surface overlying the erector spinae at L3. Point a indicates the moment of release; b, the onset of erector spinae EMG activity; and c, the peak EMG amplitude of the reflex response. *(Reproduced from Sanchez-Zuriaga et al.[1241] with permission.)*

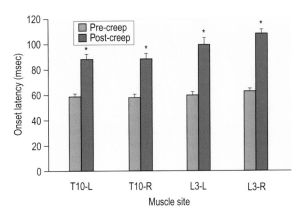

Figure 14.6 Onset latency of the erector spinae muscles during a sudden perturbation of the trunk (see Fig. 14.5) increased significantly after sitting flexed for 1 hour (*$P <$ 0.001), an activity which caused significant creep in spinal tissues. Data shown are the mean values obtained from 15 healthy subjects, recorded from the right (R) and left (L) erector spinae at thoracic (T10) and lumbar (L3) levels. Bars indicate the SEM. *(Data from Sanchez-Zuriaga et al.[1241])*

Muscle fatigue

During dynamic activities, there is also the added potential for fatigue to develop in active muscles, and this may also have adverse effects on sensorimotor function. Fatigue leads to a loss of force in the affected fibres,[139] and provided the muscle is not working maximally, additional motor units would normally be recruited to help maintain contraction force.[139,367,476] As exercise continues, central drive may fall[470] and the muscle can no longer compensate for the loss of contractility in individual fibres, resulting in a loss of force-generating capacity by the muscle.

Metabolic changes within the muscle are generally held responsible for the reduced contractility of muscle fibres. However, they may also affect the sensitivity of muscle afferents leading to altered sensory input and changes in muscle activation that may contribute to central fatigue.[140] Reduced firing of 1a spindle afferents has been reported in human subjects during sustained contractions at moderate load,[865] and this may attenuate reflex activation of the fatigued muscle and affect cortical excitability, thereby influencing higher levels of motor control.[1375] Reduced sensitivity of muscle spindles in fatigued muscles may explain why fatigue is often associated with a loss of coordination and control leading to impaired proprioception,[147,1325,1398] increased postural sway,[322,879,1505] and delays in balance recovery following postural perturbations.[323] However, the effects of fatigue on muscle reflexes are inconsistent, and although several studies found no change in reflex (or onset) latency,[595,1241] the effects on reflex amplitude were more variable, with some studies reporting increases,[553,595,632] decreases[99,477,552] or no change.[1241] Factors such as load and contraction type (static versus dynamic) may explain these conflicting findings since these will determine the degree of ischaemia and the rate at which metabolites accumulate in the muscle. Dynamic contractions will also induce thixotropic effects in muscle spindles, which may act to enhance or reduce spindle sensitivity, as discussed earlier.

Pain

A final factor that may influence reflex control of spinal movements is pain itself, because chronic joint pain and swelling are known to inhibit the recruitment of specific muscles near the joint via a 'short-loop' spinal reflex. This process of reflex inhibition has been described for the knee joint,[1371] but there is also evidence of impaired trunk muscle reflexes in patients with chronic back pain.[1176] Inhibition of specific back muscles may arise from a 'long-loop' reflex involving perceived pain,[604] and there is evidence that pain[616,619] or even the anticipation of pain[1009] can lead to delays in activation of trunk muscles during postural perturbations. Chronic pain can also lead to muscle atrophy[1372] and to fibre-type transformation,[906] both of which are likely to influence the speed and strength of voluntary and reflex muscle contractions. Studies of back muscle cross-sectional area, fibre types and EMG characteristics have attempted to explain selective and generalised back muscle changes in back pain patients in terms of these various interacting mechanisms.[47,604,900,908,1372]

CONSEQUENCES OF IMPAIRED REFLEX CONTROL

The above discussion suggests how creep, muscle fatigue and back pain might alter sensorimotor function, and impair the ability of trunk muscles to protect the underlying spinal tissues from injury. These effects probably explain why repetitive bending and lifting activities lead to increased spinal flexion,[351,359,1428] increased bending stresses on the osteoligamentous spine[359] and increased risk of injury to the spine in general,[923,924] and to intervertebral discs in particular.[732,1287] Time-dependent changes in spinal tissues may also act to increase the risk of acute injury as a result of sudden overload, which normally initiates rapid contraction of the back muscles in order to prevent excessive movement.[899,926,1560] A marked delay in reflex activation of the back muscles caused by creep in the soft tissues of the spine would lead to an impaired ability to respond rapidly to sudden perturbations[1241] and this would reduce muscle protection of the underlying spinal tissues. Some evidence to support this suggestion comes from a longitudinal study in college athletes which found that people with longer trunk muscle response times had an increased risk of sustaining a future back injury.[279]

Chapter | 15 |

Spinal degeneration

INTRODUCTION

Chapter 8 considered the benign and sometimes adaptive changes that occur sooner or later in every ageing spine. These will be contrasted in the present chapter with specific and often painful degenerative conditions that affect some spines, but not others. Degeneration means 'declining to a lower or worse stage of being'[1] and it implies deleterious changes in composition, structure and function. It can often be difficult to distinguish between ageing and degeneration, because ageing is an important risk factor for degeneration, and because degeneration is not always painful, even though it carries an increased risk of pain. However, the attempt is worthwhile for a number of reasons: it focuses attention on which age-related changes are most closely associated with pain, and so are the best targets for therapeutic interventions; it helps epidemiologists identify risk factors for specific diseases[117]; it suggests improved strategies for prevention; and it helps medicolegal experts to distinguish between a disease process and normal constitutional changes.

Apart from age-related sarcopenia (p. 92), and apart from specific diseases which lie outside the scope of this book, there are no degenerative conditions of muscle comparable to those which affect the underlying skeletal tissues. This interesting fact suggests that degeneration of skeletal tissues may be attributable, at least in part, to their poor blood supply, and the relative inability of a small cell population to turn over and repair an extensive extracellular matrix.

INTERVERTEBRAL DISC DEGENERATION

What is disc degeneration?

Disc degeneration can occur at any age, but is much more common in older discs. Many scientists speak of ageing and degeneration as if they were indistinguishable, but this is unhelpful because distinctions can be drawn between them, and a great deal of current research is aimed at making the distinctions clearer still.

Degeneration can involve all of the age-related changes described in Chapter 8, sometimes to an exaggerated extent. Crucially, however, degeneration is also associated with gross structural changes which tend to appear after age 20 years, and which most often affect the annulus and endplate of lower lumbar discs, especially in men.[117,615,979,1482] Typical structural changes, which will be considered in detail below, include circumferential and radial tears in the annulus, inward buckling of the inner annulus, increased radial bulging of the outer annulus, reduced disc height, endplate defects and vertical bulging of the endplates into the adjacent vertebral bodies. We suggest that structural failure should be a defining feature of disc degeneration because, as the following sections will show, it is an easily detected, unambiguous marker of impaired disc function, one which does not occur inevitably with increasing age, and which is more closely related to back pain and sciatica than any other feature of ageing or degenerated discs.

Structural failure is permanent, because the low metabolic rate of adult discs (p. 82) renders them incapable of repairing gross defects. Furthermore, structural failure naturally progresses, by physical and biological mechanisms, and so is a suitable marker for a degenerative process. Physically, damage to one part of a disc increases

load-bearing by adjacent tissue so the damage is likely to spread. This explains crack propagation in engineering materials, and why peripheral rim tears in animal discs progress in towards the nucleus.[1081] Similarly, pathological radial bulging of a disc progresses because compressive forces act to collapse the bulging lamellae. Biological mechanisms of progression depend on the fact that a healthy intervertebral disc equalises pressure within it, whereas a disrupted disc exhibits high concentrations of compressive stress in the annulus, and a decompressed nucleus (Fig. 11.8). Reduced nucleus pressure impairs proteoglycan synthesis,[667] so the aggrecan and water content of a decompressed nucleus would progressively fall. This is the opposite of what is required to restore normal disc function. Similarly, the high stress concentrations generated in the annulus after endplate damage would also be expected to inhibit matrix synthesis, and increase production of matrix metalloproteases (MMPs).[559] In both regions of the disc, therefore, cells would behave inappropriately because structural disruption has uncoupled their local mechanical environment from the overall loading of the disc. Like a collapsed house, a disrupted disc can no longer perform its function, even though its constituent parts remain. Cellular attempts at repair become futile, not because the cells are deficient, but because their local mechanical environment has become abnormal. In this way, structural disruption of the disc progresses by biological mechanisms as well as physical. Low cell density and poor metabolite transport ensure that any healing response is minimal, and likely to be frustrated by repeated mechanical minor injuries.[21] The process of disc degeneration is outlined schematically in Figure 15.1.

Describing disc degeneration in terms of structural failure allows all other features of degenerated discs to be considered as predisposing factors for, or consequences of,

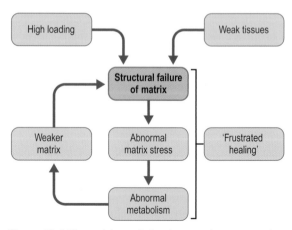

Figure 15.1 The aetiology of disc degeneration: see text for details. *(Adapted from Adams et al.[21])*

the disruption. As discussed below, genetic inheritance, ageing of the matrix, impaired metabolite transport and fatigue damage can all make the disc matrix more vulnerable to injury. Elevated levels of cytokines and MMPs in degenerated discs probably reflect attempted repair, as in other connective tissues, and could be triggered by the abnormal matrix stresses which follow structural disruption (Fig. 11.8). The transport of matrix-degrading molecules would be boosted by the presence of gross fissures, enabling matrix damage to spread, and ingrowth of blood vessels and nerves may be consequences of gross decompression and proteoglycan loss respectively. In healthy discs, a high hydrostatic pressure could collapse hollow blood vessels, keeping them out, and a high proteoglycan content inhibits the growth of nerves and blood vessels.[691,692] Describing disc degeneration in terms of structural failure therefore leads to a simple conceptual framework which incorporates most known features of degenerated discs. It also warns that therapeutic attempts to manipulate disc cell physiology may prove futile unless the cells' mechanical environment is also corrected.

This description of disc degeneration is consistent with the four- or five-point scales conventionally used to grade macroscopic disc degeneration.[17,1020,1127,1416] The first point on these scales refers to young and intact discs, while the final point corresponds to end-stage degeneration, typified by a collapse of disc height (Fig. 10.19). Discograms from such discs reveal increasing internal disruption (Fig. 15.2), and magnetic resonance imaging (MRI) scans reveal decreasing disc height and water content (Fig. 8.15). All of these scales are exercises in pattern recognition, and, although useful, they do not explain or define disc degeneration.

The concept of disc degeneration depicted in Figure 15.1 leads to the following definitions[43]:

- The process of disc degeneration is an aberrant, cell-mediated response to progressive structural failure.
- A degenerated disc is one with structural failure combined with accelerated or advanced signs of ageing. (The second half of this definition distinguishes a degenerated disc from one that has just been injured, and the reference to 'ageing' avoids the practical problem of identifying specific cell-mediated responses to structural failure.)
- Early degenerative changes should refer to accelerated age-related changes in a structurally intact disc.
- Degenerative disc disease should be applied to a degenerated disc which also is painful. (This last definition is consistent with the widespread use of the word 'disease' to denote something which can cause distress or dis-ease.)

Manifestations of structural failure, such as radial fissures, disc prolapse, endplate damage, internal or external collapse of the annulus and disc narrowing, can themselves be defined in pragmatic terms, as is usual in the epidemiological and radiological literature.[412,1346,1489] Cell-mediated responses to structural failure can be regarded as the final common pathway of the disease process.

These definitions of disc degeneration are compatible with previous suggestions: 'mechanical damage which … results in a pattern of morphological and histological changes'[448]; and 'sluggish adaptation to gravity loading

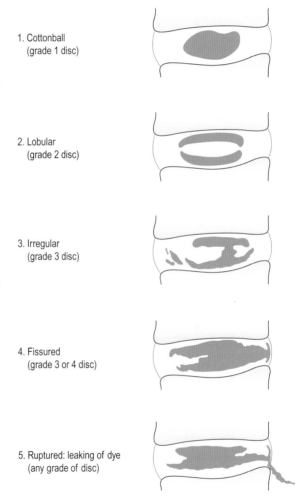

1. Cottonball (grade 1 disc)

2. Lobular (grade 2 disc)

3. Irregular (grade 3 disc)

4. Fissured (grade 3 or 4 disc)

5. Ruptured: leaking of dye (any grade of disc)

Figure 15.2 Diagram showing the stages of disc degeneration, as revealed by discograms.[17] Discograms are radiographs taken after injecting radiopaque material into the nucleus. They reveal internal disorganistion of intervertebral discs better than magnetic resonance imaging scans, but do not indicate tissue water content. 1, Cottonball (grade 1 disc). 2, Lobular (grade 2 disc). 3, Irregular (grade 3 disc). 4, Fissured (grade 3 or 4 disc). 5, Ruptured: leaking of dye (any grade of disc). Grades of disc degeneration 1–4 are shown in Figure 10.19.

followed by obstructed healing'.[850] Epidemiological studies using MRI necessarily equate disc degeneration with associated structural changes.[117] Referring to tendon degeneration, Riley et al. suggest 'an active, cell-mediated process that may result from a failure to regulate specific MMP activities in response to repeated injury or mechanical strain'.[1196] A review of nomenclature made clear distinctions between 'pathological' and 'age-related' changes in discs, and included major structural changes such as radial fissures and disc narrowing in the former category.[412] There is a growing consensus that 'degeneration' involves aberrant cell responses to progressively deteriorating circumstances in their surrounding matrix.

What causes disc degeneration?

Precipitating causes of disc degeneration

The above definitions simplify the issue of causality: excessive mechanical loading causes a disc to degenerate by disrupting its structure and precipitating a cascade of non-reversible cell-mediated responses leading to further disruption. As discussed in Chapter 11, cadaveric experiments and mathematical models show how various combinations of compression, bending and torsion can cause all of the major structural features of disc degeneration, including endplate defects, radial fissures, radial bulging, disc prolapse and internal collapse of the annulus. Damage can be created by injury, or by wear-and-tear 'fatigue' loading. Supporting clinical evidence comes from a large MRI study which reported that a history of back injury is associated with disc degeneration at multiple levels.[274] Similarly, in the cervical spine, prior injury (whiplash) increases the risk of subsequent disc dehydration as visualised by loss of MRI signal intensity.[932] Disc cell apoptosis (programmed cell death) is elevated both in degenerated discs and in discs that have undergone trauma.[1436]

Animal experiments confirm that physical disruption of a disc or endplate always leads to cell-mediated degenerative changes. Animal models can provide a reliable guide to some biological processes within degenerating discs because they preserve the complex mechanical and biochemical environment of disc cells. However, they are less useful for investigating how degenerative changes are initiated in humans, because the interventions (or genetic defects in these animals) may not represent common occurrences in living people. Small-animal models of disc degeneration have particularly severe limitations, because the small (and often young) animal discs have greatly improved metabolite transport, increased cell density and, in many cases, highly active notochordal cells, and so have an improved capacity for repair compared to human discs.[62,777,850] Nevertheless, compressive loading of rodent tail discs can result in cell death, impaired matrix synthesis and disruption of the annulus and vertebral body.[669,877,1524] Forcing rats to walk on their hind limbs can likewise cause

their lumbar discs to degenerate.[827] In larger animals (pigs), surgical disruption of the endplate from the side of the vertebral body causes nucleus decompression, proteoglycan loss and internal disruption of the annulus.[621] Further insights into this model come from an organ culture study which showed that endplate fracture kills some cells in the adjacent disc nucleus, and subsequently causes other cells to synthesise matrix-degrading enzymes and to undergo apoptosis.[577] Uneven complex loading of the annulus can have similar effects.[1527] Also in pigs, incision of the annulus and removal of some nucleus caused immediate nucleus decompression and subsequent internal collapse of the annulus[1125] followed by progressive matrix degeneration.[1077] Cutting into the outer annulus also causes progressive changes in the annulus, nucleus and endplate[968,1001,1081] and shows that degenerative changes (unlike ageing) need not originate in the nucleus. Outer annulus injury has little immediate effect on nucleus pressure[1165] so the degenerative changes in these models may be driven primarily by bleeding and inflammatory changes starting in the periphery. Stabbing the annulus with a needle causes degenerative changes in the discs of large and small animals, and degeneration is more severe if the needle diameter is large enough to compromise disc mechanical function.[396,637] Increased compressive loading without immobilisation affects disc cell metabolism and matrix composition, but does not lead to any architectural degenerative changes.[649]

Disc degeneration in animals can also be initiated by non-mechanical means. Injecting a proteoglycan-degrading enzyme into the goat nucleus pulposus causes a range of biological and biochemical changes over 6 months that mimic human disc degeneration.[626] This suggests that human disc degeneration could be triggered by some genetic impairment in the ability of disc cells to control matrix-degrading enzymes. Cell senescence is probably a consequence of deteriorating circumstances within a degenerated disc, but it could possibly be an initiating factor as well because chemically induced senescence in the discs of sheep results in degeneration-like changes by 3 months.[1630]

Time course of disc degeneration

The time interval for posttraumatic degenerative changes to develop ranges from 1 week for mice[851] to 12–15 months for pigs and sheep.[621,1081] For comparison, a major study of (human) discography showed that, 7–10 years after injection, 35% of the injured discs showed some progression in their degeneration compared to 14% of non-injected discs, and there were more than twice the number of new disc herniations in the injected group.[254] This experiment confirms that injury can cause human disc degeneration. The influence of more natural injuries was investigated on human adolescents who had suffered endplate injury several years previously: a disproportionately high number of affected discs showed degenerative signs at follow-up (mean 3.8 years) at an age when 'natural' degeneration is rare.[739] A later study suggested that vertebral injury does not lead to disc degeneration,[990] but this is probably because: (1) the injuries occurred at upper spinal levels where discs are narrower and have fewer metabolite transport problems; and (2) the follow-up time was so long (40 years) that the influence of the initial injury may have been obscured by a lifetime's 'wear and tear'. Narrowing of degenerated adult human discs progresses at approximately 3% per year[579] so post-traumatic degeneration might be expected to run its course in 1–3 decades. Narrowing of all discs (healthy and degenerated) averages less than 1% per year, and bulging increases by <2% per year.[1490]

Underlying causes of disc degeneration

Although mechanical disruption can precipitate degenerative changes, the most important cause of human disc degeneration could be the various processes which weaken a disc prior to disruption,[547] or which impair its healing response.

As discussed in Chapter 6, genetic inheritance explains 50% of lumbar disc degeneration, probably by weakening disc tissues, but environmental factors such as mechanical loading and nutrition are also important.

Age is a major risk factor for disc degeneration, probably because age-related reductions in proteoglycan and water content (p. 96) reduce the disc's ability to distribute stresses evenly, and increase stress concentration in the annulus. Age-related increases in collagen cross-linking and non-enzymatic glycation make disc tissues stiffer and more vulnerable to impact loading (p. 94).

Inadequate metabolite transport has been proposed as an underlying cause of disc degeneration.[1458] There can be little doubt that low cell density arising from inadequate transport will frustrate any attempts by the disc to heal itself (Fig. 15.1), but the role of inadequate metabolite transport in initiating disc degeneration is not at all clear. Endplate fracture can cause disc degeneration (p. 198), and yet it is associated with increased transport across the endplate, not less.[1181] It is possible that some damaged endplates may subsequently become sclerotic and block metabolite transport across them,[1017] but degenerated human discs are generally associated with thickened rather than denser endplates.[1531] Furthermore, the porosity of human endplates increases with age and disc degeneration, and appears to have little to do with cell density in the nucleus.[1210] When cement injections were used to block endplate transport in dogs, there was little degeneration after 1 year.[650]

It is sometimes implied that cytokines or matrix enzymes can 'cause' disc degeneration, but the increased activity of these agents in degenerated discs probably represents attempted repair rather than an initiating event. The rarity of advanced degenerative changes in thoracic discs[1046] argues strongly against the possibility that disc degeneration is caused by fundamental defects in cell metabolism, because any such defects would affect all discs.

It appears that the combined effects of an unfavourable genetic inheritance, age and inadequate metabolite transport can weaken some discs to such an extent that physical disruption follows some minor incident, or period of repetitive loading. A common example is that of disc herniation following a cough or sneeze. It could be argued that such a weakened disc should be considered degenerated even if it remains structurally sound. However, a disc is unlikely to become painful until it is disrupted, so there is little to be gained by anticipating future events and applying the term 'degeneration' before this actually happens.

Structural features of disc degeneration

Annulus tears or fissures

Three types of tear can be distinguished: (1) circumferential tears or delaminations; (2) peripheral rim tears; and (3) radial fissures (Fig. 15.3). They appear to evolve

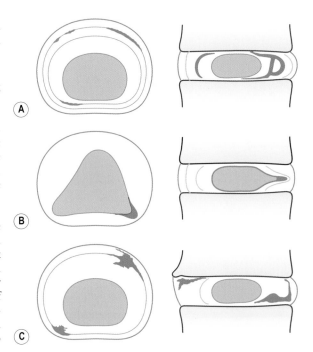

Figure 15.3 Three types of annular tear are common in degenerated intervertebral discs: **(A)** concentric clefts, **(B)** radial fissures and **(C)** peripheral rim lesions. Disrupted tissue is shown in darker shading, and nucleus pulposus is shaded. Left: disc in transverse plane (anterior on top). Right: discs in sagittal plane (anterior on left).

independently of age and of each other,[1483] and all are common by middle age, especially in the lower lumbar spine.[170,615] Circumferential tears may represent the effects of interlaminar shear stresses,[502] possibly arising from compressive stress concentrations in older discs (Fig. 10.18), and they reduce annulus strength in the radial direction in degenerated discs.[456] Peripheral rim tears or rim lesions (Fig. 15.3) consist of focal circumferential avulsions of the peripheral annulus, sometimes with sclerosis and osteophytosis of the adjacent bone. They are twice as common in the anterior annulus compared to the posterior,[1082] and typically affect the upper anterolateral margin of the disc.[608] Mechanical and histological[1082] considerations suggest that they are related to trauma. Radial fissures (Figs 15.3 and 15.4) progress outwards from the nucleus, usually posteriorly or posterolaterally,[615,1082] and this mechanical process can be simulated in cadaveric and animal discs (Ch. 11). Radial fissures are associated with nucleus degeneration[686,1082] and with disc radial bulging,[1622] but it is not clear which comes first. If nucleus pulposus material migrates down a radial fissue, it can sometimes be detected on MRI as a high-intensity zone[80] (Fig. 15.5A). Discography is also good at detecting radial fissures (Fig. 15.5B).

Disc prolapse

When radial fissures allow gross migration of nucleus relative to annulus, to the extent that the disc periphery is affected, then the disc can be said to be prolapsed (or herniated). Prolapsed tissue consists primarily of nucleus pulposus displaced down a radial fissure.[1000] Depending on the extent of nucleus migration, the result can be a protrusion, extrusion or sequestration (Fig. 15.6).[1000,1609]

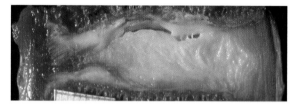

Figure 15.4 Lumbar intervertebral disc sectioned in the mid-sagittal plane (anterior on right). There is a large and complete radial fissure through the posterior annulus, with some penetration of blood in the fissure, apparently from the disc periphery.

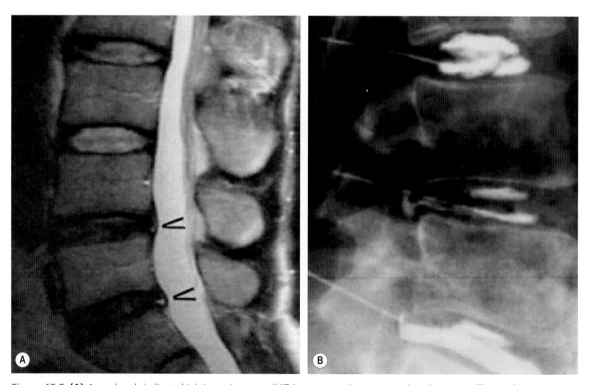

Figure 15.5 (A) Arrowheads indicate high-intensity zones (HIZs) on magnetic resonance imaging scans. These white marks indicate small regions of tissue with a relatively high water content, and correspond to radial fissures as revealed by discograms **(B)**. Provocation discograms on the same patient show that HIZs are also related to painful internal disc disruption. *(Reproduced from Lam et al.[801] with permission of Springer-Verlag, Heidleberg.)*

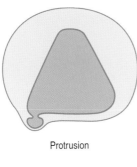

Protrusion

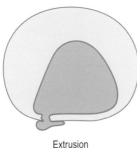

Extrusion

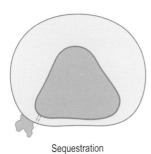

Sequestration

Figure 15.6 Disc prolapses can be categorised as annulus protrusion **(A)**, nucleus extrusion **(B)** and sequestration **(C)**. Disc sections are drawn in the transverse plane, anterior on top. The site of prolapse is usually posterolateral or posterior, but can be lateral or anterior.

In a disc protrusion, the annulus bulges markedly but is not ruptured and so allows no contact between nucleus and the extradiscal space. In an extrusion the annulus is ruptured, but any expelled nucleus is still attached to the rest of the disc and so does not migrate far. In a complete prolapse or sequestration, disc tissue (which may include cartilaginous endplate, especially in older patients[196,566]) is expelled from the disc and is no longer attached to it.

Disc herniation is particularly common at lower lumbar levels, and shows little correlation with age or other signs of spinal degeneration.[1489] In common with other epidemiological evidence this suggests that disc prolapse represents a mechanical injury, or fatigue failure, rather than the end-stage in some age-related degenerative process. Certainly, disc prolapse can be simulated in cadaveric discs

as a result of intense repetitive loading in bending and compression, or by traumatic loading where either bending or compression exceeds physiological limits (Ch. 11). Assymetrical apophyseal joints (facet tropism) show some correlation with disc prolapse, but only in adults, and at L4–5.[818] Herniated discs often show signs of microscopic calcification and neovascularization,[716] although it is not clear if these are causes or consequences of herniation. Inflammatory changes in and around a disc herniation probably contribute to pain (see below) and to ultimate regression of the hernia.[761]

Endplate damage

Vertebral endplates (Fig. 7.22) are the spine's 'weak link' in compression, and accumulating trabecular microdamage[1485] probably explains why the nucleus increasingly bulges into the vertebral bodies in later life,[1445] as shown in Figure 8.9. Endplate damage immediately decompresses the adjacent nucleus and transfers load on to the annulus (Fig. 11.8), causing it to bulge into the nucleus cavity.[22,621] If nucleus pulposus herniates through a damaged endplate, then subsequent calcification can create a Schmorl's node (p. 206).

Internal collapse of annulus

This feature of internal disc disruption[307] involves inwards buckling of the inner annulus, and is more common than prolapse, especially after the age of 40 years (Figs 11.5 and 11.9). Two reports indicate that the anterior annulus is more often affected[542,1403] but a third suggests it is the posterior annulus.[1610] Typically, 20–30% of elderly lumbar discs are affected. It could be caused by nucleus decompression following endplate fracture, as described above. In many elderly discs, the cartilage endplate becomes detached from underlying bone,[1403] presumably because the high internal pressure which presses it against the bone in young discs has been lost.

Disc narrowing, radial bulging and vertebral osteophytes

These three features are closely associated with one another and with the term 'spondylosis' (Fig. 15.7). With increasing age, the nucleus tends to bulge into the vertebral bodies. Nucleus pressure is then reduced,[40,1250] and increased vertical loading of the annulus[40] causes it to bulge radially outwards like a flat tyre,[189] and inwards towards the decompressed nucleus. Moderately degenerated discs have been shown to bulge more in vivo, especially in the posterior annulus when the spine is extended.[1636] Severe degeneration, however, is accompanied by a marked loss of nucleus pressure[1250] and collapse of annulus height (Fig. 10.19D) and bulging may then be reduced.[1636] Annulus height largely determines the

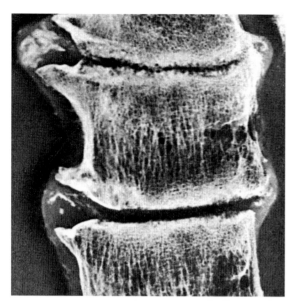

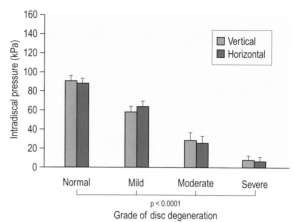

Figure 15.8 Nucleus pressure in living subjects lying prone. Note that the measured pressure falls close to zero in severely degenerated discs. (*Adapted from Sato et al.*[1250] *with permission.*)

Figure 15.7 Radiograph of degenerated lumbar spine (anterior on left). Disc space height has collapsed, and large osteophytes increase the surface area of the vertebral endplates. Note the bony sclerosis adjacent to the endplates, and the preferential loss of horizontal trabeculae. Calcification of the anterior margin of the disc may indicate an early stage in the formation of bridging osteophytes, as shown posteriorly at the upper level.

separation of adjacent neural arches, so narrowed bulging discs are often associated with osteoarthritis (OA) in the apophyseal joints (p. 208) and with osteophytes around the margins of the vertebral bodies (Fig. 15.7).

Other features of degenerated discs

Nerve and blood vessel ingrowth into degenerated discs is described on page 204. Degeneration is associated with several other changes in disc cells and matrix, although it is often difficult to separate ageing from degeneration, or cause from effect. Cell clustering is common in degenerated discs, and the cell proliferation required to cause a cluster increases the proportion of senescent cells that are unable to divide further.[535,811] Senescent cells are more common in the nucleus, and their proportion increases from 0.5% overall in degenerated human discs, to 8.5% in herniated discs, to 25% in cell clusters within herniated discs.[1202] Clustering and senescence seem to counteract each other, because overall cell density does not decrease with progressive ageing and degeneration after skeletal maturity.[830] The proportion of collagen types I and VI increases, and concentric rings rich in type III collagen can appear around some cells.[1204] Elastin content increases from a normal 2% to 9% in the degenerated inner

annulus,[289] possibly to help restore the lamella architecture following abnormally high radial deformations under load. Matrix-degrading enzymes (including the MMPs and aggrecanase) are produced in greater quantity in degenerated discs, both by the indigenous cells[811] and by invading cells, and explain the faster turnover of matrix constituents in degenerated discs.[78,1321,1322] Enzyme levels are particularly high in herniated discs.[1200] Large molecules of fibronectin, which link cartilage cells to their matrix, become more abundant in degenerated discs, and are increasingly fragmented, presumably because of increased enzyme activity.[1062]

Functional changes in degenerated discs

Disc function is affected more by degenerative structural changes than by age-related changes in composition.[40] Normal discs contain a soft deformable nucleus which exhibits a hydrostatic pressure even when old and pigmented. Degenerated and mechanically disrupted discs, however, have either a very small hydrostatic region, or none at all, and exhibit high localised stress concentrations within the annulus (Fig. 10.18). In living people, intrinsic nucleus pressure decreases markedly with grade of disc degeneration (Fig. 15.8). It appears that structural damage destroys the disc's ability to distribute compressive stresses evenly on the adjacent vertebrae, so that different parts of the disrupted tissue resist compression in a more-or-less haphazard way. When nucleus pulposus cells are deformed by non-hydrostatic loading, as they would be in a disrupted disc, then they respond by producing more collagen[933] and this could explain why degenerated discs have such a fibrous nucleus. Other mechanical changes in degenerated discs include an increased neutral zone (region of minimal stiffness) in bending and torsion, combined with a reduced range of bending.[983] The range of axial rotation is increased, possibly because of loss of cartilage in the apophyseal joints.[1089]

Are there two distinct routes to disc degeneration?

There may be two independent routes towards disc degeneration. The first involves radial fissures or herniation, leads to sciatica, is associated with repetitive bending and lifting,[704] mostly affects discs in the lower lumbar spine and develops after age 30 years. The second route involves endplate defects and inward collapse of the annulus, leads to back pain, is associated with compressive injuries such as a fall on the buttocks,[739] mostly affects discs in the upper lumbar and thoracic spine and starts to develop before age 30 years. It is impossible to separate these two routes entirely, especially in the mid-lumbar spine, but the concept of two distinct routes to disc degeneration is supported by the large MRI population study on southern Chinese which shows that associations between Schmorl's nodes (an indicator of endplate fracture: see p. 206) and disc degeneration are much stronger at L1–3 than at L4–S1, and that discs adjacent to Schmorl's nodes are less likely than normal to show evidence of radial fissures or prolapse.[989] Also, this study showed quite distinct age-profiles for Schmorl's nodes and disc degeneration (Fig. 15.9).

This concept is compatible with the biomechanics in Chapters 10 and 11. Lower lumbar discs are intrinsically more vulnerable to bending injuries involving the annulus,

whereas upper lumbar and thoracic discs are vulnerable to endplate fracture in compression. Either type of injury reduces nucleus pressure, and makes the other type of injury less likely in future, as load-bearing is transferred to the neural arch. Endplate injuries have a more direct influence on nucleus pressure, [1165] but only if they occur in middle age rather than in adolescence,[41] so the age of occurrence of disc degeneration from the two routes may be similar. Annulus injuries, on the other hand, may have more effect on discogenic pain because they disturb the outer innervated regions of the disc (see next section). This could explain why complete radial fissures are more closely related to back and sciatic pain than are Schmorl's nodes.

Disc degeneration and pain

Degenerated discs are often painful

There is now compelling evidence from large population studies that the risk of back pain increases in proportion to the severity of disc degeneration[132,273,330](Fig. 15.10). The risk of pain increases further when more than one disc is severely degenerated,[330] presumably because this increases the risk that one of the discs is in a painful stage of degeneration. If disc degeneration is specifically defined by the presence of disc space narrowing, osteophytes and sclerosis, then it is associated with non-specific low-back pain with odds ratios ranging from 1.2 to 3.3.[1439]

The particular features of disc degeneration most closely associated with pain are disc prolapse,[686] disc narrowing[115,330,579,1488] and radial fissures,[994,1488] especially when

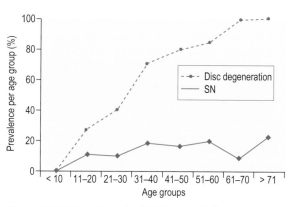

Figure 15.9 Schmorl's nodes (SN) increase in frequency up to the age of about 30 years, but not thereafter, unlike disc degeneration, which continues to increase with age. Data from a large magnetic resonance imaging population study from China. *(Reproduced from Mok et al.[989] with permission.)*

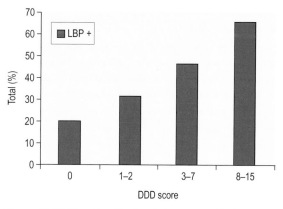

Figure 15.10 The risk of back pain increases with the number of degenerated discs and the severity of degenerative changes. In a large population survey, degenerated disc disease (DDD) was scored 0–3 and then summed over five lumbar discs. Back pain was 'significant pain lasting more than 2 weeks'. Note that 34% of subjects with the highest DDD scores reported no back pain. *(Reproduced from Cheung et al.[273] with permission.)*

they reach the disc exterior and 'leak'.[1494] These changes all involve gross distortions of the outer annulus fibrosus. Other painful features of disc degeneration include osteophytes,[330] internal disc disruption including inwards collapse of the annulus,[1281] endplate fractures and Schmorl's nodes,[557,989] and inflammatory (Modic) changes in adjacent vertebrae.[57] More variably related to pain is disc bulging,[168,557,686,1488] possibly because some radiologists apply the term equally to a slight outward bulge of the annulus, or to a major bulge which could represent a disc herniation. Disc signal intensity on MRI, which correlates strongly with water content but only weakly with proteoglycan content,[915] has little, if any, relationship to pain.[1488]

Pain provocation studies have confirmed that intervertebral discs are often the site of patients' typical back pain[797,1281] and that pain can be reproduced by relatively innocuous mechanical stimulation of the outer posterior annulus and endplate. Painful discs are nearly always structurally disrupted[446,994] and exhibit irregular stress concentrations.[962]

Nerve and blood vessel ingrowth in degenerated discs

Nerve and blood vessel ingrowth is directly (though variably) associated with discogenic pain.[297,446,1120] Nerves rely on blood vessels for nutrition, so these two structures tend to coexist within the disc, although some nerves have been reported in isolation.[446] Only simple capillaries have been described within the disc, without any muscular wall, so any nerves in the disc are likely to be sensory rather than concerned with vasoregulation.

Blood vessels are normally confined to the outer annulus, and to the bony (rather than cartilage) endplate. This is presumably because the central region of a normal disc exhibits a fluid pressure which is well above blood pressure, and so would tend to collapse any ingrowing blood vessels. The fluid-like region of a disc shrinks as it degenerates (Fig. 10.18), and this may explain some slight capillary ingrowth. The distribution of nerves is similar, with terminals of the sinuvertebral nerves (Fig. 4.5) normally penetrating only the outermost 3 mm of annulus.[1094] Reduced proteoglycan concentrations in old and degenerated discs[78] may facilitate some ingrowth, because proteoglycans inhibit the growth of blood vessels[692] and nerves.[691] Nerve ingrowth can also be aided by disc cells synthesising neurotrophic factors such as nerve growth factor that attracts nerve cells,[447,1603] apparently by reducing the inhibitory influence of proteoglycans.[693]

Even in advanced disc degeneration, capillaries do not normally grow right through the annulus to the nucleus.[1034] Some reports of nociceptive nerve ingrowth into the nucleus may refer to vertical growth of just a few millimetres from the endplates,[446] because the central bony endplate has an extensive innervation that probably originates from the mixed sinuvertebral nerve.[95] However, if there is a radial

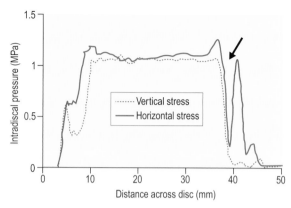

Figure 15.11 Stress profiles through a degenerated intervertebral disc containing a large fissure in the anterior annulus. The region of the fissure (arrow) is marked by a substantial reduction in matrix compressive stress. (*Stress profilometry is explained in* Figure 10.17.)

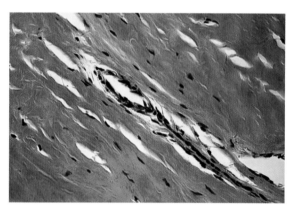

Figure 15.12 Histological section of outer annulus fibrosus in the transverse plane, showing a large blood vessel within a small fissure. Note that the margins of all fissures are stained green (for collagen), indicating that there is focal depletion of proteoglycans which elsewhere cause the tissue to stain red. Small dark oval shapes indicate cell nuclei. Bar indicates 50 μm. (*Adapted from Adams et al.[45] with permission.*)

fissure in the annulus,[297,407,1120,1482] or destruction of the endplate[1034] then further penetration of nerves and blood vessels is possible. Annulus tears represent a protected microenvironment in which matrix compressive stress is reduced (Fig. 15.11) and their inner surfaces are depleted of proteoglycans (Fig. 15.12), leaving a collagenous scaffold that would form an ideal surface for cell migration.[969] This probably explains why granulation tissue has been reported within radial fissures in surgically removed painful discs.[1121] If nociceptive nerves reach the nucleus, they could conceivably be stimulated chemically by the acidic environment which arises from anaerobic respiration.[136] However, they would be unlikely to generate mechanical pain, because central regions of degenerated discs tend to be decompressed, often to a very marked extent (Figs 10.18 and 15.8). Nerves in the middle posterior annulus of a degenerated disc would be in a region that often experiences a particularly high gradient of compressive stress (Fig. 10.18) and this could explain why complete radial fissures are strongly related to back pain.[1494]

Pain sensitisation of nerve roots and intervertebral discs

Pain sensitisation is recognised when a pain response appears disproportionate to the provoking stimulus. An increased response to noxious stimuli is termed hyperalgesia, and to normal stimuli is called allodynia. Evidence for such sensitisation in the spine comes from the pain provocation studies reviewed above, and the mechanisms involved are currently under investigation.

Displaced nucleus pulposus (but not annulus fibrosus[671]) can sensitise adjacent spinal nerve roots. Physical and chemical effects appear to act synergistically to decrease conduction velocity[1076,1400] increase vascular permeability[1070] and induce pain behaviour in laboratory animals.[633,724,1072,1079] Mechanisms can be complicated by the occlusion of blood vessels supplying the nerve root,[636] but they are essentially inflammatory in nature,[546] including an autoimmune response from white blood cells brought into contact with displaced nucleus.[486] Degenerated tissue has a bigger effect on the nerve root than normal tissue,[724] but this is largely unrelated to the acidity (low pH) of the nucleus matrix.[671] Rather, the trigger appears to be the release of certain chemicals from live nucleus cells.[1071]

One such chemical appears to be tumour necrosis factor-alpha (TNF-α). This cytokine is produced by nucleus cells[1073] and is known to mimic the noxious actions of nucleus pulposus better than other cytokines.[79,659] Most importantly, blocking the action of TNF-α also reduces the effects of nucleus pulposus on nerve roots[1075] and diminishes the radicular pain expressed by laboratory animals.[1074,1080,1599] Other chemicals such as nitric oxide (NO) can be induced by TNF-α, and blocking NO also reduces the noxious effects of nucleus pulposus.[192] Some reports suggest that TNF-α cannot be synthesised directly by herniated[713] or degenerated disc tissue,[213] so it is possible that the TNF-α is actually synthesised in the nerve root in response to signals from nucleus cells. TNF-α can influence the discharge thresholds of nerve cells,[269] and preliminary trials of TNF-α blockers in human subjects with sciatica were very promising.[778] However subsequent results were disappointing,[779] possibly because the precise timing of the block is important.[515] Also, caution is warranted when attempting to block systemically an important chemical messenger such as TNF-α.

In a degenerated disc, nucleus pulposus can migrate down a radial fissure and come into contact with nerves in the peripheral annulus. Alternatively, fissures in the outer annulus could allow the ingrowth of nerves towards the nucleus pulposus. Either mechanism could lead to sensitised nerves within the posterior annulus, which is where the highest stress concentrations usually occur in degenerated discs (Fig. 10.18), so either mechanism could explain discogenic back pain. An experiment on rats supports this concept of discogenic pain, although it is difficult to confirm back pain in dumb animals.[1069] Additional support comes from an analysis of surgically removed degenerated human discs, which showed a chronic inflammatory reaction with blood vessel infiltration into the annulus, sometimes reaching the nucleus.[1119] Changes were greater in discs removed from patients diagnosed with discogenic back pain.

The concept of pain sensitisation has been extended to an entire neural pathway, including the spinal cord.[1059] If such central sensitisation could be demonstrated, it would provide a mechanistic basis for chronic pain.

Inflammation and healing in the disc periphery

As discussed above, many of the features of disc degeneration and prolapse resemble an injured tissue that is attempting to repair itself. Increased cellularity, increased levels of cytokines and matrix-degrading enzymes, ingrowth of blood vessels and nerves, increased collagen turnover and decreased proteoglycan synthesis are all indicative of an inflammatory healing response mediated by blood cells.[678,761,1296] Deep within the disc, healing may be frustrated by low cell density, so that a chronic and progressive degenerative condition develops. However, conditions are quite different in the disc periphery, and particularly in the outer posterior annulus. Here, cell density is four times higher than in the nucleus[581] and metabolite transport is boosted by proximity to blood vessels, and by fluid flow (Fig. 7.21). Not surprisingly, effective healing of the outer annulus occurs in animals (Fig. 15.13) with granulation tissue leading to scar formation and, eventually, to some collagen remodelling.[969]

In middle-aged humans, healing processes will be slower, even in the disc periphery, and it is possible that repeated disturbance of the healing tissue could set up an exaggerated inflammatory reaction, as it does in animals that are subjected to repeated injuries.[1452] Pain sensitisation is a purposeful feature of inflammation that promotes healing by prohibiting vigorous loading of the damaged tissue. Perhaps the current fashion of discouraging bed rest as an initial treatment for back pain could actually be making matters worse for those with an injured annulus fibrosus? Traditional approaches to treating large tendon injuries may also be applicable to the outer annulus fibrosus: both tissues are composed predominantly of collagen

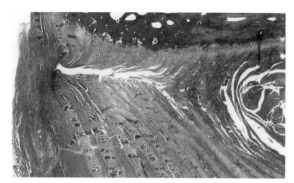

Figure 15.13 Histological section of the annulus of a sheep intervertebral disc in a parasagittal plane. The anterior annulus (left) had been stabbed with a scalpel to a depth of 5 mm. Two months later, the fissure has progressed towards the nucleus pulposus. There is effective healing by scar tissue in the peripheral annulus. *(Reproduced from Osti et al.*[1081] *with permission.)*

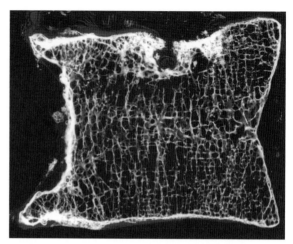

Figure 15.14 Radiograph of a lumbar vertebral body sectioned in the mid-sagittal plane (anterior on left). The upper endplate shows a large Schmorl's node, which represents calcification around some previous vertical herniation of nucleus pulposus. The anterior vertebral body shows large marginal osteophytes.

type I, and both have a poor blood supply and low cell density. According to this view, annulus healing (and discogenic pain) may benefit from an initial period of rest, followed by manual treatments aimed at stimulating annulus cells and boosting metabolite transport.[45]

SCHMORL'S NODES AND MODIC CHANGES

Endplate fracture is often followed by the vertical herniation of nucleus pulposus tissue into the vertebral body (Fig. 11.5). When a calcified shell forms around the displaced tissue, it can be seen on radiographs and it is then referred to as a Schmorl's node (Fig. 15.14). MRI is a more sensitive test of endplate defects because it is able to detect the displaced disc tissue itself, and only 33% of nodes identified by MRI are detected by X-rays.[557] Even smaller endplate irregularities can be detected by cadaveric dissection, and are reported to occur in 76% of spines aged 13–96 years.[609]

Schmorl's nodes are most common near the thoracolumbar junction (Fig. 15.15) and are comparatively rare below L2.[989,1128,1569] Mostly they affect the central part of the endplate,[321] and are more common on the inferior vertebral endplates than on the superior.[321,1128,1569] They increase with age up to approximately 30 years, but do not increase beyond that age, unlike disc degeneration (Fig. 15.9). Age dependence could explain why one or more Schmorl's nodes identified by MRI are reported in 16% of the general population,[989] but in 30% of middle-aged women.[1569]

Risk factors for Schmorl's nodes include being tall, heavy and male,[989] suggesting a mechanical aetiology. However, their close association with inferior vertebral endplates (Fig. 15.9), which normally are mechanically stronger than

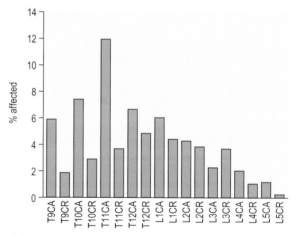

Figure 15.15 Frequency of Schmorl's nodes at different spinal levels, as determined by a large magnetic resonance imaging study on middle-aged women. CA, caudal; CR, cranial surface of the vertebral body on which the Schmorl's node lies. Note that most fractures affect the caudal surface. *(Reproduced from Williams et al.*[1569] *with permission.)*

superior endplates (p. 122), suggests that developmental abnormalities involving the notochord (Fig. 8.2) may play a role in their formation.[989] This could also explain why Schmorl's nodes are influenced strongly by genetic inheritance, with a heritability of 70% being reported for middle-aged women.[1569] (A lower figure would be expected for men involved in heavy manual work.)

Schmorl's nodes are associated with disc degeneration, especially the moderate forms of disc degeneration normally seen near the thoracolumbar junction.[1128] In the lumbar spine, a strong linear correlation has been demonstrated between increasing severity of disc degeneration (averaged over all lumbar levels) and the risk of having a lumbar Schmorl's node.[989] This partially explains why Schmorl's nodes are twice as common in patients with back pain,[557,1569] and why they are linked to both disc degeneration and back pain in young sportsmen.[1390]

Schmorl's nodes could also be painful in their own right, or give rise to pain from the vertebral body.[1118,1639] Endplate defects allow communication between the nucleus pulposus and blood, and could cause a painful inflammatory or autoimmune reaction within the body.[156] Modic et al.[988] identified several distinctive patterns on MRI scans: type 1 changes (decreased signal intensity on T1-weighted spin-echo images and increased signal intensity on T2-weighted images) were seen in a vertebral body in 4% of patients, and type 2 changes (increased signal intensity on T1-weighted images and isointense or slightly increased signal intensity on T2-weighted images) were seen in 16% of patients. In all (type 1 or 2) cases, the adjacent disc was degenerated. Preliminary histology linked the type 1 changes with disruption of the endplates and vascularised fibrous tissue, while type 2 changes were associated with yellow (fat) replacement in the vertebral marrow. Follow-up scans indicated that type 1 (inflammatory) changes convert to type 2 (fatty) changes in 1–3 years, whereas type 2 changes remain stable. Subsequently, several imaging[860] and histological[1064] studies have shown that inflammatory-like changes in the vertebral body, including more nerves,[1064] accompany changes in the adjacent endplate, and are more closely associated with symptoms than the endplate defects themselves.[253,754] A major systematic review reported inflammatory-like endplate changes in 43% of patients with back pain or sciatica, compared to 6% of a non-clinical population.[687] Modic changes in the vertebral body are also associated with disc herniations involving the cartilage endplate[1263]: presumably, stripping some of the cartilage off the bony endplate allows similar communication between nucleus and vertebral body marrow as occurs in endplate fractures. A combination of heavy smoking and a hard physical job leads to a fivefold increased risk of vertebral body inflammation, as indicated by MRI.[814] Discography can be used to identify a painful endplate lesion.[1118]

INSTABILITY

What is spinal instability?

The clinical concept of spinal instability has provoked controversy for over 50 years.[86,760,1004,1148] It is an emotive term which might alarm some patients, but it is also a convenient label for spine changes that bear some relationship to engineering instability (Fig. 11.30). The concept is of little value if applied indiscriminately to most patients with mechanical back pain, but if specific disorders such as trauma, tumours, previous surgery, spondylolysis and scoliosis are first excluded,[660] then the remaining degenerative instability[152] may be a clinically useful concept.[1249] Such instability usually refers to back pain exacerbated by movement, and associated with intersegmental movements that are abnormal or excessive at one or more spinal levels.[382,1249] Abnormal movements can involve angular rotations between vertebrae, or translation movements in which the vertebrae slide past each other at the same orientation, such as in an anterior slip of L5 relative to the sacrum.[660,1135] It has been suggested that horizontal anteroposterior translational movements of more than 3 or 4 mm indicate instability.[154,583]

Laboratory investigations described in Chapter 11 have quantified how each spinal structure resists and limits normal intervertebral movements, and how destruction of restraining structures, and disc degeneration, can create abnormal movements. The biomechanical evidence suggests that segmental instability is best defined in terms of reduced resistance to movement, and that an enlarged neutral zone (see Figure 11.31) is probably more indicative of instability than changes in range of motion.[10,1148,1149,1556] An unusually high range of motion may not necessarily indicate anything wrong, and may simply represent hypermobility.

We therefore propose the following definition: spinal instability is a condition in which a motion segment exhibits an abnormal magnitude or direction of movement when subjected to a normal load. The abnormality may be evident at the end of range, throughout the range of movement, or only somewhere within the range of movement, depending on the cause of instability. Instability at the end of range, or throughout the range, would be expressed as reduced stiffness of the joint. Instability within range would be expressed as an increased neutral zone.

What causes spinal instability?

Theoretically, instability could be caused by injury to any structure which resists or limits spinal movements. Injuries to the supraspinous ligament are relatively easy to detect and the fact that they are common[770] suggests that ligament insufficiency could be a common cause of hypermobility. However, the evidence reviewed above indicates that clinical instability is more often associated with an abnormally low resistance to movement within a normal range of motion, and other explanations must be sought for this.

As described on page 160, intervertebral discs provide most of the spine's intrinsic resistance to small movements, and cadaveric experiments that reproduce early aspects of disc degeneration – water loss and endplate disruption – can simulate segmental instability very well. In living spines, however, complications arise from secondary changes associated with ageing and degeneration, including fibrosis, vertebral osteophytosis and disc resorption.[1477] These reduce spinal mobility, as shown in Table 8.1. This explains why a large MRI study on patients found that translational intervertebral movements increase with degenerative changes in moderately degenerated spines, and yet both translational and rotational movements decrease in the presence of severe degeneration.[773] Finite element modelling[1217] agrees with this evidence, and with the long-standing clinical view of instability as a transitional stage in the degenerative process, lying between some initial dysfunction and subsequent restabilisation or repair.[750,1366] (A more recent finite element model reached different conclusions,[465] but its predictions appear to be dominated by the effects of severe disc narrowing and osteophytosis rather than by ligament laxity.)

Spinal instability and pain

The essentially discogenic origin of spinal instability suggested above provides a ready explanation for associated pain. Disc degeneration,[40] creep-induced loss of water[38] and endplate fracture[22,41] have all been shown to generate high concentrations of compressive stress within the annulus fibrosus, and increase load-bearing by the neural arch.[1142] There is direct evidence linking intradiscal stress concentrations with pain[962] and high load-bearing by the neural arch may also be painful. According to this view, the abnormal movements which characterise spinal instability are not painful in their own right, but serve as markers for underlying degenerative changes which are the true causes of pain. It follows that treatment for segmental instability should be directed towards the degenerative changes rather than the abnormal movements, which may be incidental and harmless.

VERTEBRAL BODY OSTEOPHYTES

An osteophyte (the word means bone plant) is a bony outgrowth that is often found on the anterolateral and posterolateral margins of the vertebral body (Fig. 15.14). The curved shape suggests some association with radial bulging of the disc, and this is supported by MRI studies.[1489] Some authors distinguish between different shapes of vertebral body osteophyte, but there seems little reason to doubt that shape is related to growth, and that osteophytes become more curved as they grow over the bulging surface of the adjacent annulus (Fig. 15.7). They become increasingly common with age, and have been reported in 73% of all lumbar vertebrae in people aged over 50 years.[1173] In extreme cases, osteophytes can form a solid 'bridge' between two vertebrae (Fig. 15.7). They are closely

associated with advanced stages of intervertebral disc degeneration (as indicated by disc space narrowing) and with endplate sclerosis,[1173] although it is not certain which comes first. Large vertebral body osteophytes can have a major clinical impact by trapping nerves and blood vessels, although they are not major risk factors for back pain.

Animal experiments have induced vertebral body osteophytes by cutting into the outer anterior annulus fibrosus. Results suggest that osteophytes arise from proliferating inner annular tissue in which the cells become transformed as their matrix changes gradually from fibrocartilage to hyaline cartilage, then to calcified cartilage, and finally to bone, as in a growth plate.[843] The cells responsible could possibly be derived from the fibrous covering of bone (the periosteum) as it is disturbed by the bulging outer annulus.

Mechanically, osteophytes play a modest role in resisting spinal compression, and a major role in resisting bending. They resist compression by effectively increasing the surface area of the vertebral body (by 10–20%) and they probably resist bending by restricting the lateral bulging of the annulus.[55] In this manner, osteophytes act mainly to stabilise the spine in bending, and because they grow in response to the instability created by a cut into the annulus, their overall effect is to counter the very instability that created them. Hence, vertebral body osteophytes can be considered as adaptive changes rather than degenerative (although the distinction may offer little comfort to a patient with a trapped nerve).

APOPHYSEAL JOINT OSTEOARTHRITIS

OA is the most common degenerative disease to affect synovial joints. There is a huge research literature concerning the disease and its effects on the hip and knee, which are the joints most commonly and seriously affected. The following account attempts to relate the relevant parts of this literature to what is known about OA in the apophyseal joints.

What is osteoarthritis?

OA is characterised by cartilage thinning and fibrillation (surface fissuring), and changes in the subchondral bone which may include marginal osteophytes (bony spurs), sclerosis (thickening) and cysts (cavities). In addition, the syovial tissue that lines the fibrous joint capsule often shows signs of inflammation, so OA is a disorder of the whole joint and not just of its cartilage surface. Within the cartilage, large cell clusters can appear, proteoglycan turnover increases and degradation of the collagen network in the surface zone (Fig. 7.17) allows localised tissue swelling[101] and proteoglycan loss.[1233] In severe OA, the cartilage is lost entirely from some regions of the joint surface and may be replaced by newly regenerated fibrocartilage, which is not suitable as a bearing surface. OA often leads to pain and stiffness, particularly during prolonged load-bearing and after inactivity, but it can also be asymptomatic. In knee OA, the feature that is most closely associated with pain is subchondral bone sclerosis,[1396] which can indicate high focal loading of relatively unprotected bone.

Involvement of the apophyseal joints

Apophyseal joint OA (Fig. 15.16) begins to appear after the age of 25 years and affects at least 40% of cadaveric lumbar spines aged 26–45 years and 90% of spines aged

over 45 years.[824,1406] Joints younger than 30 years can exhibit cartilage fibrillation, generally to a greater extent and prevalence than the knee, hip or ankle joints,[1386] but rarely have severe OA. A condition involving extensive apophyseal joint cartilage loss, but few or no osteophytes, has been likened to chondromalacia patellae, and put forward as a frequent cause of chronic back pain in early middle age.[390] Cartilage damage is predominantly located peripherally on the joint surfaces, superiorly and posteriorly in the concave superior articular surfaces, and inferiorly and posteriorly in the convex inferior articular surfaces.[1386,1420] These regions would be most heavily loaded in lumbar flexion and extension, respectively, and both would be loaded in axial rotation. Indirect evidence suggests that inferior articular processes are affected more

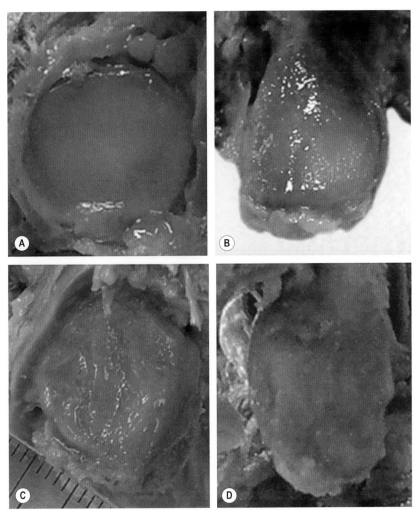

Figure 15.16 Inferior articular processes of human lumbar apophyseal joints, showing progressive degenerative (osteoarthritis) changes from A (normal) to D (severe cartilage loss with osteophytes). *(Reproduced from Tischer et al.[1420] with permission.)*

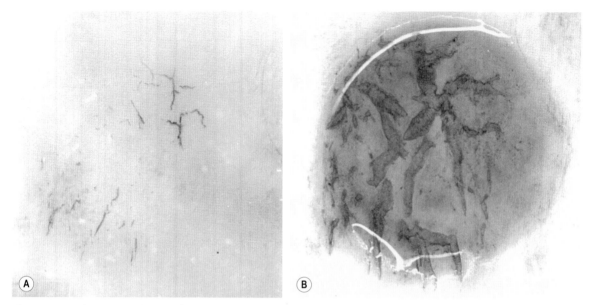

Figure 15.17 Photographs of the surface of bovine articular cartilage. **(A)** Small fissures were created by mechanical overload using a flat circular indenter. Indian ink particles help visualise the fissures. Compare with the 'worm's-eye view' in Figure 7.17. **(B)** Cyclic loading caused these fissures to increase in length and width, although the depth does not increase greatly. *(Reproduced from Kerin et al.[738] with permission.)*

than the superior.[1634] Lower lumbar levels are most frequently affected by OA, with a peak at L4–S1, although L1–2 and L2–3 are more likely to exhibit OA before the age of 45 years.[403,824] Early degenerative changes may explain why adult apophyseal joint cartilage is thinner and softer than knee or hip cartilage, especially around the joint periphery.[1388] Although OA often affects multiple spinal levels, it can also be highly localised, affecting only one level, or one joint in a motion segment. Osteophytes might affect only one of the two articular facets in a given joint.[824] This localisation provides more evidence for the importance of mechanical influences. In the cervical spine, apophyseal joint OA is common at all spinal levels after age 60 years, with cartilage defects being spread over the articular surfaces.[741]

What causes osteoarthritis?

An unfavourable genetic inheritance explains 54–73% of the variance in knee OA in middle-aged women.[1624] As in disc degeneration, the genetic susceptibility probably includes a large number of physical and metabolic influences, such as defective collagen type II[148,1167] and type IX.[744] The simplest explanation for the onset of OA in middle age is that traumatic or repetitive mechanical loading damages the collagen network of articular cartilage,[285,833] creating surface fissures (Fig. 7.17). Subsequent loading can cause increased shearing deformations of the cartilage surface[1586] so that fissures grow in length, width

and number (Fig. 15.17). Collagen damage allows the cartilage to swell up,[239,1426] and a combination of surface damage and swelling facilitates the loss of proteoglycans and water upon which the load-bearing properties of cartilage depend.[353,655] Consequently, stress concentrations appear within the cartilage (Fig. 15.18) and the region of tissue failure progressively increases. Severe mechanical loading can also kill cartilage cells directly, particularly those near the surface.[286,1426] Epidemiological studies reflect the importance of mechanical loading in initiating OA: two of the greatest risk factors include previous joint injury and occupations which involve high loading of particular joints.[421] Also, it is usually the most heavily loaded regions of the joint surface which are worst affected,[197] as indicated above for the apophyseal joints. Rupture of adjacent ligaments is another important cause of OA, both in humans[606] and in animal experiments.[178] This is presumably because the destabilised joint transfers significant load-bearing to regions of the articular surfaces which do not normally experience it. Rupture of the anterior cruciate ligament often precedes painful OA of the knee, but the ligament rupture often goes unrecognised.[606] Relatively low but frequent postural loading of a joint can also cause OA.[1626]

Some scientists believe that OA starts with a stiffening of the subchondral bone,[1177] so that the overlying cartilage is trapped 'between a rock and a hard place'. For this mechanism to work, the bone stiffening must be focal rather then general, so that the region of stiff bone acts

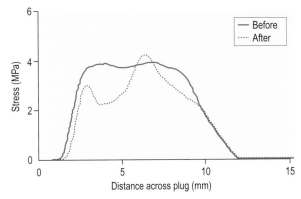

Figure 15.18 Stress concentrations in articular cartilage increase followng water loss. In this plug of human knee cartilage, water loss was effected by creep loading. Compressive stresses were measured within the cartilage, in a direction parallel to the surface, before and after creep. Methods were similar to those described in Figure 10.17. *(After Adams et al.[34])*

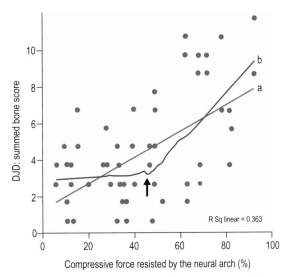

Figure 15.19 High neural arch load-bearing, measured in cadaveric spines, is associated with apophyseal joint osteoarthritis, as indicated by a summed bone score reflecting degenerative joint disease (DJD). The Loess (regression) line (b) suggests that the risk of osteoarthritis increases when the neural arches resist more than 50% of the applied compressive load (arrow). *(Reproduced from Robson-Brown et al.[1209] with permission.)*

like a 'stone in the shoe' to increase stress on the adjacent foot. If bone stiffening is widespread it will have little effect, just as wearing wooden clogs does not hurt the feet. It is reasonable to suppose that degenerative changes in either tissue will adversely affect the other, but evidence from animal models in support of the 'bone-first' hypothesis merely shows that degenerative changes progress more rapidly in bone, which is the more metabolically active tissue (Ch. 7). The subchondral bone plate is actually softer (not stiffer) in OA joints.[825]

Some other influences on OA include age-related non-enzymatic glycation of cartilage (Fig. 8.10) which makes the tissue stiffer[267] and facilitates the onset of OA in animal models of the disease.[335]

Apophyseal joint OA is probably caused by a combination of disc narrowing and lordotic posture leading to abnormally high load-bearing by the apophyseal joints, especially in their inferior regions (Fig. 13.6). Disc degeneration and apophyseal joint OA are closely related,[234,1386] with changes in the disc probably coming first. Cadaveric studies associate high apophyseal joint load-bearing with small hollows of eburnated bone in the laminae, and corresponding osteophytic spurs around the margins of the inferior articular processes.[25,380] In spines aged less than 45 years, facet OA appears unrelated to disc degeneration,[824] and may even precede it,[404] suggesting traumatic origins of early facet OA, possibly involving torsion or shear. Apophyseal joint OA is closely related to vertebral body osteophytes,[824] perhaps reflecting a common origin in spinal instability. No association with articular tropism (asymmetry) was found.[824] In old age, disc degeneration and narrowing cause much of the spinal compressive load to be resisted by the neural arch (Table 8.2), and when this

exceeds 50%, it is associated with apophyseal joint OA (Fig. 15.19). Experiments on sheep confirm that induced disc degeneration and narrowing lead to mild apophyseal joint OA within 2 years.[999] Features of the affected joints included cartilage fibrillation and extensive fibrosis of the joint capsule and synovial folds (Fig. 15.20). Entrapment of such folds between the articular surfaces is a possible cause of back pain in humans,[495] but one that is difficult to demonstrate.

OSTEOPOROSIS AND SENILE KYPHOSIS

Introduction

Normal age-related loss of bone mineral is known as osteopenia (p. 93). If this progresses to the stage where the bone is liable to fracture under the activities of daily living, the condition is known as osteoporosis. (Technically, the bone mineral density (BMD) must fall by more than 2.5 standard deviations below what is normal for a person of that age and gender for the diagnosis to be made.) The spine is particularly vulnerable to osteoporosis because vertebrae contain a high proportion of trabecular bone, which has a high surface area and so can be resorbed by

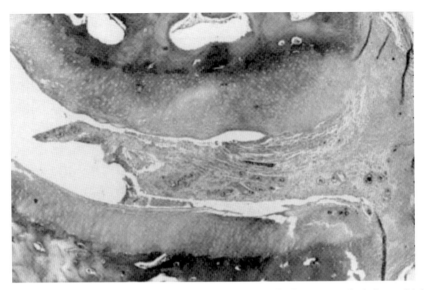

Figure 15.20 Transverse section of a sheep apophyseal joint (posterior on top). The intervertebral disc at this level had been surgically interfered with to cause disc degeneration, and the consequences of this for the apophyseal joint are apparent: there is fissuring and flaking of articular cartilage, and fibrosis affects the joint capsule and the large synovial fold trapped between the articular surfaces. *(From Moore et al.[999] with permission of Lippincott Williams & Wilkins, Philadelphia.)*

the body very quickly. Osteoporotic vertebral fractures become more common as age increases and BMD decreases, and they usually affect the mid-thoracic and upper lumbar levels.[587] They tend to occur either spontaneously or following some minor incident such as opening a window,[1015] and they can sometimes be difficult to detect by conventional means (Fig. 15.21). Consequences can be severe, including pain, deformity, disability, loss of self-esteem and significantly increased mortality.[808]

Three typical fracture patterns can be recognised: anterior wedge fracture, crush fracture and biconcave fractures (Fig. 11.7). Anterior wedge fracture is the most common,[668] and the one most likely to lead to the flexion deformity known as senile kyphosis or 'dowager's hump'[298] (Fig. 15.22).

What causes senile kyphosis?

Elderly people tend to suffer vertebral fractures, not because of gross trauma, but because their vertebrae are already weakened by low BMD and by structural factors such as a thin cortex.[973] Bone weakening is conventionally explained in terms of systemic changes in elderly people, including reduced concentration of circulating sex hormones,[63] reduced physical activity,[972] and an unfavourable genetic inheritance.[582] However, some predisposition to osteoporosis is independent of BMD[261] and systemic factors do not explain why the anterior vertebral body should be affected so frequently and in so characteristic a manner. As described on page 100, disc degeneration can leads to stress-shielding of the anterior vertebral body,

causing it to lose trabecular bone, so that it is vulnerable to fracture when the spine is flexed. This explains the initiation of kyphotic deformity in a previously undamaged spine.

Once formed, an anterior wedge fracture will increase spinal kyphosis and move the centre of gravity of the upper body anteriorly, so that the back muscles must increase their activity in order to prevent spinal flexion (Fig. 9.2). This would increase compressive loading of the deformed spine, increasing the risk of subsequent fractures[261] and accelerating bone 'creep' deformity under constant load (p. 183). Hence kyphotic deformity tends to progress.[182,727]

There is clinical evidence linking senile kyphosis with disc degeneration. Disc narrowing is an unequivocal indicator of disc degeneration, and disc height is inversely proportional to thoracic kyphosis.[909] More explicitly, severe disc narrowing greatly increases the risk of osteoporotic fracture to a neighbouring vertebral body in the same spine.[1347] In this context, it is important to realise that the height of the disc nucleus is an unreliable indicator of degeneration, because nucleus height can be preserved even in a degenerated disc if it causes inwards bulging of a weak adjacent endplate, as in Figure 8.9. Some other clinical evidence argues against a causal link between disc degeneration and vertebral kyphosis, but several confounding factors may explain this.[139] Firstly, some studies[1223] fail to distinguish between anterior wedge fractures and biconcave fractures of the vertebral endplates (Fig. 11.3), even though there are mechanical reasons to

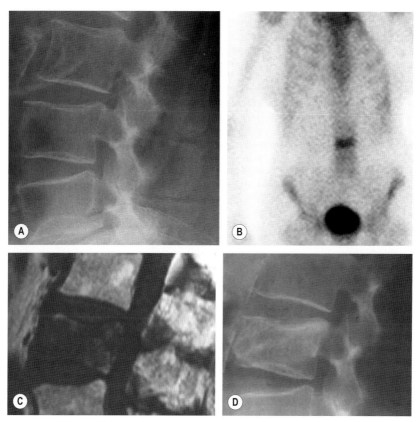

Figure 15.21 Vertebral body fractures in the elderly can be difficult to detect. An 88-year-old woman had a fall: **(A)** radiograph (day 2) shows little; **(B)** bone scintigraphy (3 weeks) shows a 'hot' L3; **(C)** T1-weighted magnetic resonance imaging (3 weeks) shows greatly reduced signal in L3; and **(D)** radiograph (4 months) shows obvious collapse of L3. *(Reproduced from Pham et al.[1130] with permission.)*

suppose that the former are associated with degenerated discs, and the latter with healthy discs. Secondly, some studies assume (quite wrongly) that any disc with a high nucleus is not degenerated, even if its annulus is collapsed. Thirdly, vertebral osteoporosis (and fracture risk) are often assessed on the basis of whole-vertebra BMD measurements taken in the anteroposterior direction, even though these are insensitive to focal bone loss in the anterior vertebral body. Approximately half of the bone mineral in a vertebra lies in the neural arch,[817] so that a potentially dangerous loss of BMD from the anterior vertebral body could be masked by increased BMD in the neural arch following increased load-bearing.

How can senile kyphosis be prevented and treated?

The implications of some of this new research remain to be tested, but it appears that the dramatic loss in BMD and bone quality from the anterior vertebral body in old osteoporotic spines could conceivably be slowed, or even reversed, by exercises which include repetitive flexion movements of the thoracolumbar spine. It may seem paradoxical to recommend flexion exercises to prevent senile kyphosis (and indeed the recommendation should not be made to those who already have anterior wedge fractures because flexion can make them worse[1313]), but it is entirely consistent with the principles of adaptive remodelling (Fig. 7.11). Exercise to build up bone mass would be most effective in earlier life[107] when the tissue is more metabolically active, more responsive to mechanical stimulation and unlikely to 'creep' during sustained flexion (p. 183). Identification of those at risk of senile kyphosis may be improved by performing dual X-ray absorptiometry scans in the sagittal plane[1623,1635] rather than in the frontal plane as at present, in order to detect exaggerated bone loss from the anterior vertebral body. Another approach is to use quantitative computed tomography to assess bone density in specific regions of the vertebrae[1189] such as the anterior vertebral body.

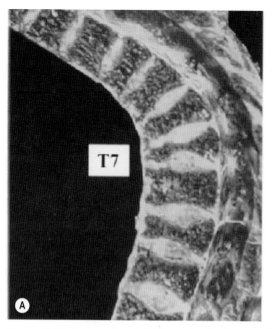
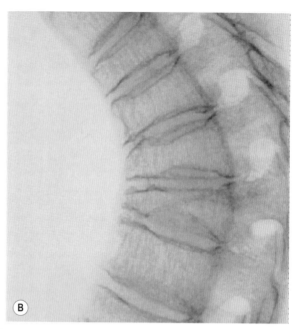

Figure 15.22 Advanced senile kyphosis visualised on a sagittal section of a cadaveric spine **(A)** and on a radiograph **(B)**. Anterior is on the left. Note that several vertebrae have sustained anterior wedge and crush fractures (as defined in Figure 11.7) and that the annulus fibrosus of the adjacent intervertebral discs has collapsed. The nucleus of some discs appears to have normal height, but this is because the central endplate has collapsed into the vertebral body. *(Reproduced from Keller et al.[727] with permission of Lippincott Williams & Wilkins, Philadelphia.)*

Pharmacological treatments for senile kyphosis attempt to slow down the loss of skeletal bone mass that underlies osteoporosis. They target the hormonal control of bone mass,[303] for example by replacing lost oestrogen,[63] so their effects are systemic rather than focal. A more radical solution to senile kyphosis is to inject bone cement into the vertebral body in order to strengthen it (cement augmentation). One procedure, known as vertebroplasty, involves injecting a liquid cement (such as polymethyl methacrylate) into the vertebral body by means of needles inserted down one or both pedicles.[231] A variant of this procedure, kyphoplasty,[1360] seeks to reverse vertebral and spinal deformity by inserting and forcibly inflating a rubber balloon within the vertebral body in order to restore its prefracture dimensions, before cement is injected (Fig. 15.23). These radical treatments have considerable promise, because they are effective at reversing the abnormal load-sharing between vertebral body and neural arch (Fig. 15.24) which contributes to vertebral wedge fractures.

OTHER DISORDERS OF VERTEBRAE

There are several relatively rare diseases of bone which affect ageing vertebrae, including various inflammatory conditions,[435] but they lie outside the scope of this book. However, two conditions should be mentioned briefly: Scheuermann's disease and diffuse idiopathic skeletal hyperostosis (DISH).

Scheuermann's disease is marked by multiple endplate defects and wedged vertebrae in the thoracic and upper lumbar spine, combined with an accentuated thoracic kyphosis and reduced lumbar lordosis. It affects approximately 10% of the adult population,[897] affects both sexes equally and is usually detected before puberty[571] – hence its other common name: adolescent kyphosis. Generally it is not painful.[571,1471] Some changes may be developmental in origin, or involve inflammation of the vertebral growth plates (epiphysitis or osteochondritis). In some cases it may simply represent a childhood incident such as a fall on the buttocks causing vertebral damage at several levels as the impact force travels up the spine. Histological changes similar to those seen in Scheuermann's disease have been reproduced in young rats by intense mechanical loading of their spines.[1192] Also, the fact that Scheuermann's disease in juveniles is often accompanied by degenerative changes in the adjacent discs[589] suggests a common mechanical aetiology, as demonstrated in a study by Kerttula et al.[739] Treatment normally consists of postural advice, possibly bracing and, very rarely, surgery.

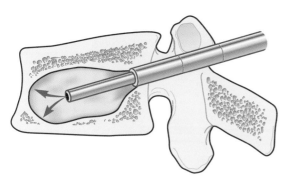

Figure 15.23 In kyphoplasty, a balloon is passed down a cannula inserted through the pedicle, and inflated within the vertebral body to reduce deformity. The balloon is removed, and then cement is injected into the space created within the vertebral body in order to consolidate and stiffen it.

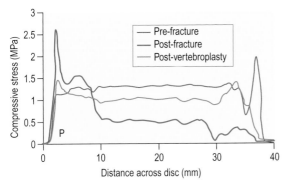

Figure 15.24 Effects of vertebroplasty on load-sharing by the vertebral column. Prefracture, the technique of stress profilometry (Fig. 10.17) shows that compressive loading is spread evenly on to the vertebral body. (Male L1–2, age 74 years.) Vertebral body fracture decompresses the nucleus and anterior annulus, and concentrates loading on to the posterior annulus and vertebral body. Vertebroplasty partially restores normal load-sharing. *(Adapted from Luo et al.[859] with permission.)*

DISH (or Forestier's disease) is characterised by osteophytes on four or more adjacent thoracolumbar vertebrae which are so large and continuous they give the impression of dripping candle wax. Effectively, the anterior longitudinal ligament is ossified. It has been reported in 25% and 15% respectively of men and women aged over 50 years, rising to 35% and 26% of those over 80 years.[1547] Other bony sites can be affected, including the attachment sites (entheses) of large ligaments. Usually it does not result in pain or severe disability, although the spine can feel particularly stiff. The condition is associated with being overweight and with diabetes,[1246] and probably represents a genetic predisposition to exuberant osteophyte growth.

STENOSIS

Spinal stenosis generally refers to a narrowing of the intervertebral foramen through which the spinal nerves must pass. Less often, a central stenosis results from a particularly small vertebral canal (Fig. 15.25). Typical signs are a forward-stooped posture, and reduced ability to move the lumbar spine into extension. Symptoms include aching, a feeling of heaviness, numbness and paresthesia, radiating to the buttock region.[1397] Prevalence of stenosis increases with age, and the condition carries a threefold increased risk of back pain.[706] Symptoms are generally worsened by walking and relieved by sitting, and patients tend to change position frequently in an attempt to get some relief. Some patients experience leg pain akin to sciatica, where the pain has a radicular pattern and is often bilateral and characterised by coming on during walking with concomitant limitation of walking distance. This symptom pattern is known as intermittent (or neurogenic) claudication, and results from the stenosis reducing the available space, thus causing compression of the spinal nerves. Some people experience weakness of leg muscles due to compromise of motor nerves. Patients need to stop walking periodically to recover from the pain; many find best relief from stooping forwards, which opens up the posterior elements, thus reducing neural compromise.

Stenosis is a dynamic condition that changes with posture and movement. A cadaveric study showed that, compared to the neutral posture, the cross-sectional area of the intervertebral foramen increases by 12% in moderate flexion, and decreases by 15% in extension.[666] Nerve root compression in this study was estimated to be 21% in the neutral, 15% in flexed and 33% in extended posture. The aggravation of stenosis by extended postures should be taken into account when giving postural advice to patients: some patients with simple back pain benefit from an exaggerated lordosis[1573] but those suffering from stenosis could be made worse. Nerve root compression can cause morphological as well as functional changes in the afferent (sensory) neurons,[763] even in the absence of pain sensitisation phenomena involving displaced disc material (p. 205). This explains why symptoms sometimes persist after postural change, or even after decompression surgery.

Several tissue changes can contribute to stenosis, including disc bulging and narrowing, disc herniation, spondylolisthesis, osteophytes on the posterior margins of the vertebral body, crush fractures of osteoporotic vertebral bodies[282] and hypertrophy of the ligamentum flavum or apophyseal joint capsule. Gradual compressive creep deformation of intervertebral discs and vertebral bodies (Ch. 13)

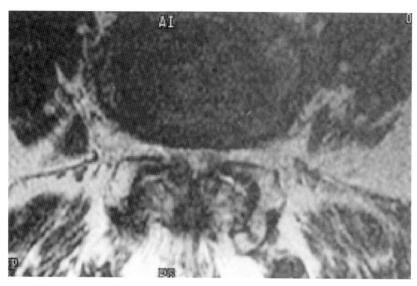

Figure 15.25 Severe spinal stenosis visualised on a magnetic resonance imaging axial T2 scan (anterior on top). The apophyseal joints are just a few millimetres from the posterior wall of the disc, and there is no region of high signal intensity (indicative of cerebrospinal fluid or fat) in the vicinity of the spinal cord or nerve roots. *(Reproduced from Speciale et al.[1349] with permission of Lippincott Williams & Wilkins, Philadelphia.)*

can combine to reduce the height of the intervertebral foramen sufficiently to cause spinal stenosis, according to experiments on elderly cadaveric spines.[1143] This could be considered a dynamic stenosis if all of the creep deformation were reversible, but it is currently not clear just how much of the bone creep is reversible in living people. In the cadaveric experiments, overall spinal creep was greatest when BMD was low[1141] and when intradiscal pressure was low,[1143] suggesting that these may be risk factors for spinal stenosis. However, there was some evidence that total compressive creep deformations were limited by impaction of adjacent neural arches.

Anterior bulging of the ligamentum flavum plays a greater role in narrowing the spinal canal than does posterior bulging of the disc[563] and the extra bulging of the ligament is attributable to the gradual age-related replacement of elastin by collagen,[781] which has less elastic recoil. Individually, these changes occur in many older spines and most can be considered to be part of the normal ageing process. However, if the changes are sufficiently large or combine to cause symptoms, then stenosis should be considered to be a degenerative condition. When hypertrophy of the ligamentum flavum is involved, the ligament generally has a reduced elastin:collagen ratio (which probably makes it less extensible and more likely to buckle when the spine is extended), and can show signs of calcification.[1275] Ligament changes may explain why the nerve roots are compromised in the first place, or they may represent the consequences of reduced movements and a tendency to maintain a moderately flexed posture.

Maintaining a flexed position for long periods probably explains why stenosis is associated with improved endurance characteristics in the paraspinal muscles.[820] Neural structures within the intervertebral foramen can also be affected by the large plexus of the foraminal veins.[636] Pathologic changes within and around the nerve roots include peri- and intraneural fibrosis, oedema of nerve roots and focal demyelination, suggesting that ischaemia arising from venous obstruction may be an important cause of perineural and intraneural fibrosis.

Since lumbar stenosis is a chronic, gradually progressive disorder, many patients are managed conservatively for a longer or shorter period depending on progression and level of symptom severity or disability. Specific non-surgical treatment options are limited. Medication and physical therapy may offer a measure of pain control, whilst epidural steroid injections appear to benefit a minority of patients.[337] For patients who can no longer cope with the pain and activity limitation, surgery becomes an option. The surgical approach will be one of a number of decompression procedures to increase the space available for the neural structures, the precise procedure depending on the individual pathology. The effect on symptoms is usually for the better.[466] It is important to appreciate that decompression surgery is a treatment for leg symptoms rather than back pain, and many patients will experience residual back pain despite reduced leg pain and improved walking distance. Further randomised clinical trials are required, together with more information concerning the natural history of spinal stenosis.[133] In the

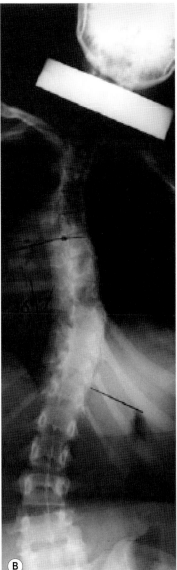
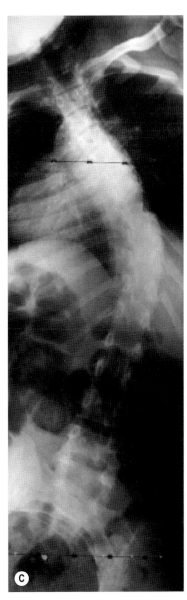

Figure 15.26 Frontal-plane radiographs of a 14-year-old girl with a progressive right thoracic idiopathic scoliosis. **(A)** Normal posture. **(B)** Subject bending to the right. **(C)** Subject bending to the left. It is evident that the scoliosis is structural (permanent) but the spine nevertheless retains some mobility. *(Reproduced from Arlet et al.*[82] *with permission of Springer-Verlag, Heidelberg.)*

meantime, guidelines have been published to improve clinical diagnosis and management.[1536]

SCOLIOSIS

This condition is considered last because it is so poorly understood despite being extensively investigated. One form of scoliosis can be dealt with very briefly: postural scoliosis is simply asymmetrical posture (Ch. 13) and is transient. Real or structural scoliosis involves a fixed tri-planar deformity of the vertebral column. The most characteristic deformity is lateral curvature in the frontal plane (Fig. 15.26), but also generally involves axial twisting and abnormal sagittal-plane curvature, most notably the loss of thoracic kyphosis in idiopathic scoliosis. It is conventional to classify scoliosis as idiopathic (80% of cases) or congenital (involving disturbed vertebral development). Degenerative scoliosis occurs in later life, is sometimes painful and progresses steadily.[930] Degenerative scoliosis may be due to excessive load-bearing by the neural arch following disc collapse (Fig. 8.16), causing coupled twisting movements in other planes, especially if the joints are asymmetrical (Fig. 10.8B).

True idiopathic scoliosis is thought to be a disturbance of postnatal growth (i.e. growth under gravitational loading) and is particularly common in adolescent girls around the growth spurt. In many cases pain is not a significant issue, the patient being unaware of the condition. The main curve is quantified from frontal-plane radiographs by determining the maximum angle between lines drawn parallel to the upper or lower borders of the vertebral bodies at either end of the lateral curve. This angle, the Cobb angle, exceeds 30° in approximately 0.3% of the population. In the great majority of cases, curves remain below 30° and the patient is left with a slight hump to one side of the midline (usually the right) which is best visualised from behind when the patient bends forwards. However, in a proportion of cases the curve will progress to the point when surgery is required. Uncorrected severe curve progression can present serious respiratory compromise and is a surgical necessity. In milder cases the decision to operate is made on a balance of clinical considerations (e.g. Cobb angle, likelihood of achieving a good result, patient preference) and cosmetic grounds. In the latter part of the 20th century, bracing was widely used as a treatment to reduce curve progression, with apparently good results. However, studies have questioned whether bracing does actually reduce the number of patients whose curves will progress and require surgical correction.[505] Physical exercises may help some patients with idiopathic scoliosis, but there is no rigorous evidence that they influence curve progression.[1032]

The origins of the asymmetrical growth remain obscure. Genetic influences are apparent in some families, but not others[550,702] and can involve variants of the oestrogen receptor.[1591] The blood supply to the spine is bilateral (Fig. 4.6), so it is conceivable that some local obstruction could lead to unilateral retarded growth of a vertebra, or rib[1295] or muscle.[1574] Low BMD appears to be a factor in these rapidly growing young people,[826] possibly because it allows increased bone creep, as described on page 183. Other possibilities are that rapid growth generates a defect in the neuromuscular control system,[1476] or that a slowly growing spinal cord initiates a scoliosis by pulling asymmetrically on the vertebrae.[1152]

Once a lateral curvature has developed, muscle tension could act like a bowstring to make matters worse[1367] and the fact that curves are usually concave to the left suggests the involvement of unbalanced muscle forces. Intervertebral discs and vertebral bodies both become wedged,[1364] but changes in scoliotic discs such as increased cell apoptosis,[268] impaired metabolite transport,[135] altered collagen cross-linking[375] and increased collagen II synthesis[76] are probably a consequence of altered stress distributions within the disc[966] rather than an initiating factor, because discs grow much slower than vertebrae. During the growth spurt, lateral wedging progresses more in discs than in the adjacent vertebrae,[1567] although this may represent asymmetrical loading of the deformable discs rather than asymmetrical growth. Changes in the vertebral endplate,[1205] apophyseal joints[1299] and paraspinal muscles[493,907] in scoliosis patients likewise suggest adaptations to altered mechanical loading rather than causal factors. Changes within scoliotic vertebral bodies resemble osteopenia,[271] and may represent adaptations to reduced physical activity in less physically able children.

SACROILIAC JOINT DEGENERATION

Approximately 32% of adults attending a chiropractic clinic for back pain were found to have radiographically demonstrable changes in one or more sacroiliac joints.[1058] One-quarter of these patients were deemed to have inflammatory sacroiliac joint changes; the others were considered degenerative. Inflammatory sacroiliitis was associated with male gender, and buttock pain. Sacroiliac joint changes were poorly correlated with changes in the lumbar spine, suggesting a separate aetiology.

BACK MUSCLES

Although back muscles (and their tendons) are generally acknowledged to be a common cause of transient back pain, it is also recognised that injured muscles heal rapidly, and do not degenerate in the conventional sense. However, an MRI population study showed fat infiltration of the multifidus muscle in 14% of 13-year-olds and 81% of 40-year-olds.[753] Fat infiltration does not appear to alter segmental mobility[773] and so may simply reflect relative muscle disuse in later life. Nevertheless, a strong association between severe fat infiltration and a previous history of low-back pain[753] suggests that back pain may limit physical activity and accelerate disuse atrophy in back muscles.

Chapter |16|

Preventing back pain

INTRODUCTION

This chapter serves to pull together some of the threads in the picture of the biomechanics of back pain by presenting a brief overview of the current knowledge and its interpretation in respect of prevention.

As discussed in Chapter 6, low-back pain (LBP) is a highly prevalent symptom which shows little sign of reduction, despite considerable scientific research across numerous biomedical disciplines. The high rate of disability due to back pain is evidence that we have singularly failed either to prevent or treat the problem satisfactorily.[214] Human beings have experienced back trouble throughout recorded history and before – Oetzi, the so-called Tyrolean ice man who lived 5300 years ago, apparently had degenerative disc disease (http://en.wikipedia.org/wiki/Oetzi). So far as can be ascertained, it is only since the late 19th century that it has become (with few exceptions) a disabling problem consuming substantial healthcare resources; indeed, it is possible that healthcare may have contributed to the problem.[1507] The epidemiological patterns of LBP discussed in Chapter 6 show that the symptom is common across most groups of society, irrespective of age, suggesting that attempts at prevention concentrated in one group or environment are unlikely to have much overall impact. This is, to some extent, evidenced by the huge increase in back-related disability that occurred during the latter half of the 20th century despite a concomitant progressive reduction in the physical stress of work! This rather flies in the face of what most patients tend to believe about back pain, which is that it is caused by lifting and injury.[240] As suggested in Chapter 6, the onset of many episodes of back pain may have some physically stressful element, even if it is trivial and incapable of causing substantial tissue disruption. If that is the case, then one would expect successful preventive interventions to entail reduction of physical stresses on the spine, as suggested in much of the world's health and safety legislation. However, such legislation is based on the premise that occupational physical stresses are the primary cause of most back pain among workers, whereas in many cases the symptoms may simply be associated with work activities, and this needs to be distinguished from the assumption that those activities have initiated significant injury. In other words, the symptoms may be work-relevant for that individual at that time, without the work being in any way noxious. This chapter will look at the evidence and consider the level of support for various preventive interventions in respect of low-back trouble.

EPIDEMIOLOGY REVISITED

It is worth reiterating some of the key epidemiological aspects of low-back trouble relevant to the concept of prevention. The lifetime prevalence of non-specific (common) LBP is estimated at 60–80% in industrialised countries (1-year prevalence 20–60%, adult incidence ~6% per year) (Ch. 6). The prevalence rate during school age approaches that seen in adults, increasing from childhood to adolescence and peaking between ages 35 and 55. Symptoms, pathology and radiological appearances are poorly correlated. Pain cannot be attributed to pathology or neurological encroachment in about 85% of people. A role for a genetic influence on liability to back pain is suggested from recent research.

LBP is an episodic phenomenon often not requiring healthcare, but a minority of people develop chronic pain. The majority of episodes of back pain among workers do not require sick leave, and those that do generally are associated with return to work in a timely fashion; however, around a third are likely to have relapses of work absence,[597] and recurrent and chronic back pain is widely acknowledged to account for a substantial proportion of total workers' absenteeism. About half the days lost from work are accounted for by the 85% of people away from work for short periods (<7 days), whilst the other half is accounted for by the 15% who are off work for >1 month. This is reflected in the social costs of back pain, where some 80% of the healthcare and social costs are for the 10% with chronic pain and disability.[1025] The clinically convenient classification of acute and chronic does not fully reflect the pattern of back pain among the population. The reality of the back pain experience, where back pain and its consequences tend to occur in an episodic manner,[309,331,597,1401,1619] presents interpretive difficulties when considering the matter of prevention. Importantly, back pain should be seen as an issue for all ages, and all sectors of society. Furthermore, it is important to distinguish between the presence of symptoms, care-seeking, work loss and disability. These have different prevalence rates and are influenced by a varying balance of biological, psychological and social factors.

When trying to understand the difficulties surrounding the concept of prevention, it may be helpful to remember that back pain is a common health problem. Common health problems are characterised by their symptoms and the subjectivity of these, and it is not usually possible to demonstrate objectively underlying pathology. The symptoms tend to be recurrent in nature, describing an untidy pattern of episodes having variable frequency, severity and impact, and they tend to coexist with symptoms in other anatomical areas.

When considering just what it is that is to be prevented, it is necessary to define the situation being prevented – the 'case' if you like. For back pain, as for other common

health problems, this becomes very difficult. Most people for most episodes do not seek healthcare and can remain at work. It is almost impossible to differentiate on objective or clinical grounds between those who complain and seek help and those with the same problems who do not. Therefore a 'case' should not be determined simply in terms of the presence of symptoms, but rather by the extent to which the symptoms are sufficiently bothersome to trigger reporting or care-seeking: i.e. at the point where the person is struggling. When a person becomes a case, it is not because he or she has a more severe injury, disease or set of symptoms; rather it is because of the consequences for that person at that time.

Back pain can readily be work-relevant: that is, the symptoms may be felt predominantly at work and may (temporarily) reduce the person's ability to do his or her usual job. This encourages the (often false) belief that work is mainly or wholly responsible. In most cases there is limited objective evidence of injury or disease cogently related to the work exposures: so, in occupational terms it is, again, the consequences that are more important than any (assumed) pathology or injury.

The concept of 'risk' is relevant to how back pain can be most effectively managed or prevented at work. Many factors, both physical and psychological, have been proposed as 'risk factors' (Ch. 6). But, the question is: risk factors for what? For example, psychological factors are frequently mentioned as 'risk factors for back pain'. They clearly do not directly cause musculoskeletal injury (although they may contribute behaviourally to accidents) but they can be related to other outcomes such as reporting patterns or level of disability. Unfortunately, the scientific literature does not always make a distinction between the various outcomes of interest. Throughout much of the existing literature linking work to health outcomes, the term 'risk' is used in a statistical sense that reflects a correlation or non-causal association between work variables and the outcome. There are far fewer studies where the criteria strongly suggestive of true causative relationship are taken into account. The Bradford–Hill criteria for causality are: statistical association; dose–response; temporality; biological plausibility; consistency; experiment; biological coherence; experimental evidence; and analogy.

When an outcome (an injury or disease) is unlikely to occur without some intervening action or exposure to a known and demonstrated hazard (e.g. injury due to a fall from a height; disease due to exposure to asbestos), the exposure can be considered a risk for the occurrence of the outcome. However, as we know, back pain is extremely common irrespective of physical exposure (at work or leisure). Furthermore, back pain does not always occur despite persistent exposure to putative risks. This, combined with the fact that numerous theoretical physical, occupational and psychosocial hazards have turned out to be doubtful causal factors (Ch. 6), renders direct occupational causation for most episodes of back pain difficult to establish. This situation holds true for both physical and psychosocial factors. For this reason, many traditional risk factors reported in the literature might be better termed 'risk indicators' – features noted to be correlated with one or more health outcomes, but without a demonstrable causal link.

The issue of 'risk' for development of LBP is clearly highly relevant to the concept of prevention, but the subject is poorly understood and inconsistently documented. The most powerful risk indicator for a new episode of back pain is a previous history.[598] Beyond that, the most frequently reported risk indicators are heavy physical work, frequent bending, twisting, lifting, pulling and pushing, repetitive work, static postures and vibrations.[74,627] Psychosocial risk indicators include distress, depression, beliefs, job dissatisfaction and mental stress at work.[74,628,840] However, there is limited evidence for these (purported) risk factors and those that are well documented frequently have small effect sizes; logically this will compromise the magnitude of effect from preventive interventions.

PREVENTION IN LOW-BACK PAIN

A multidisciplinary group of European scientists grappled with the prevention problem when developing evidence-based, evidence-linked guidelines on prevention in LBP.[215] These guidelines represent the most recent comprehensive attempt to tackle the issue, and form the basis for this chapter. Despite the problems inherent in systematic reviews (p. 54) there is good justification for concentrating on guidelines which are based on them. Although some management strategies will be omitted from such a guideline because of a lack of scientific evidence, that does not prevent others being discussed here because they are of particular biomechanical interest.

This section will summarise the findings and recommendations of the European Guidelines for Prevention in Low-back Pain.[215] These were produced within the framework of COST Action B13 *Low-back pain: guidelines for its management*, issued by the European Commission, Research Directorate-General, Department of Policy, Co-ordination and Strategy. Under that initiative a multidisciplinary working group was established to develop the guidelines for prevention in LBP; the full guidelines and tables of evidence are available at: www.backpaineurope.org.

Outcomes and interventions

The guidelines working group spent considerable time debating the focus of the guideline, and attempting to produce a working definition of 'prevention'. Taking account of the epidemiology of back pain, they concluded that prevention of the first onset of common LBP is, to all

intents and purposes, likely to be impracticable. It was considered that, overall, non-specific LBP is important not so much for its existence as for its consequences. Therefore, the consequences of common LBP are a primary concern for prevention. They include broad issues such as recurrence (including severity and disability), work loss, care-seeking, health-related quality of life and compensation. Thus, the conceptual focus was prevention of future aspects of LBP, as opposed to manifestations of the current spell. Several aspects of the back pain phenomenon were generally excluded, such as prevention of structural changes and degeneration along with interventions aimed at modification of (purported) risk factors, unless there is concomitant specific influence on back pain outcomes. However, in recognition of widespread interest in back pain among schoolchildren and the possibility of prevention of consequences later in life, consideration of potentially modifiable risk factors for back pain in this population was considered.

There is a vast number of interventions that may 'prevent' (some aspect of) common LBP, and not all possible interventions are included in the guideline because they are idiosyncratic, non-generalisable or untested (though that is not to say they cannot be shown effective at some future date). Clearly, some interventions involve an active element, and some will concern avoidance; some will be physical interventions like supportive belts,[790] whilst others may involve less direct approaches, such as addressing inappropriate beliefs[661] or interfacing with social reorganisation.[1259] Individual interventions may not be universally applicable; rather, they will be variously suited to the general population, workers and school age. Some clinical interventions may have a preventive effect on some outcomes, but therapy is not generally considered prevention; nevertheless, preventive interventions cannot (and should not) exclude people with existing back symptoms. The same basic interventions may apply equally to the different groups, but their nature and location of delivery will differ. It is possible that the evidence will overlap, and may not necessarily come to identical conclusions.

Evidence

The guideline is evidence-based and evidence-linked, relying on systematic searches of the scientific literature up to the end of 2003. In the first instance systematic reviews (and existing guidelines) were sought, supplemented by individual scientific studies where systematic reviews and evidence-based guidelines were not available. The evidence was reviewed and discussed by the entire working group, as were the resultant recommendations; the process is best summarised as systematic searching of the published scientific literature with mixed quantitative/qualitative evaluation of the evidence to produce best-synthesis recommendations.

The strength of the recommendations was based on a four-level rating system:

1. level A: generally consistent findings provided by (a systematic review of) multiple randomised controlled trials (RCTs)
2. level B: generally consistent findings provided by (a systematic review of) multiple weaker scientific studies
3. level C: one RCT/weaker scientific study, or inconsistent findings provided by (a systematic review of) multiple weaker scientific studies
4. level D: no RCTs or no weaker scientific studies.

In the following sections the working group's recommendations are given together with the primary evidence sources. Additional sections of the guideline, representing the discussion of the evidence and formulation of the recommendations, the additional literature considered, and the tables of evidence, can be found in the full guideline at www.backpaineurope.org.

Recommendations

General population

The general population as a focus for prevention in back problems is the largest and most heterogeneous group. It includes different age groups, people with or without back pain, with or without specific spinal disorders, working and non-working people and many other possible subgroups that may or may not be mutually exclusive. Therefore, decisions had to be made about the inclusion criteria for studies in this context. Clearly, people under the age of 18 years were excluded, since this topic is covered in the school-age section. Although the working population is also covered separately, it was decided not to exclude here automatically studies that were undertaken in the working population. One reason is that many studies actually were performed at the worksite, perhaps for ease of conduct and follow-up. This does not necessarily mean that their results are not applicable to a non-working population. In fact, for the purpose of this part of the guideline, interventions at the worksite can be distinguished between those that are specific to the working community (e.g. worksite-based) and those that are more or less generalisable. These potentially valuable studies were included to inform recommendations for the general population, and the significant overlap to the section on workers was accepted.

As indicated in the general introduction, the high prevalence of back pain makes it impractical in most preventive studies to separate people with back pain from asymptomatic people. Therefore, studies dealing with symptomatic people were not excluded.

Physical exercise

Physical exercise is recommended to prevent absence due to back pain and the occurrence or duration of further back pain episodes (level A). The effect size is moderate. There is insufficient evidence to recommend for or against any specific kind of exercise, or the frequency/intensity of training (level B). Water gymnastics may be recommended to reduce (short-term) back pain and extended work loss during and following pregnancy (level C).[688,799,842]

Information/education/training (back schools)

Information and education about back pain, if based on biopsychosocial principles, should be considered for the general population. It improves back beliefs, and can have a positive influence on health and vocational outcomes, though the effect size may be relatively small (level C). Information and education focused principally on a biomedical or biomechanical model cannot be recommended (level C).[207,1468] Back schools based on a biomechanical approach with emphasis on teaching lifting techniques are not recommended (level A). High-intensity back schools, which comprise both an educational/skills programme and exercises, can be recommended for patients with recurrent and persistent pain (level B). The effect sizes of these interventions may be relatively small.[603]

Lumbar supports/back belts

Lumbar supports/back belts are not recommended for prevention in LBP among the general population (level A).[799,842,1461]

Mattresses

There is insufficient robust evidence to recommend for or against any specific mattresses for prevention in back pain (level C), though existing persistent symptoms may reduce with a medium to firm rather than a hard mattress (level C).[785]

Chairs

There is insufficient evidence to recommend for or against any specific chairs for prevention in LBP (level D).

Shoe insoles/correction of leg length discrepancies

The use of shoe insoles or orthoses is not recommended for prevention of back problems (level A). There is insufficient evidence to recommend for or against correction of leg length inequality for prevention in LBP (level D).[418,1424]

Manipulation

No evidence was found to support recommending regular manipulative treatment for the prevention of LBP (level D). There is preliminary evidence that lumbar mobilisation can increase water diffusion in degenerated lumbosacral intervertebral discs,[123] suggesting that slow mobilising exercises such as yoga have the potential to enhance disc nutrition.

Workers

The target population here is workers with or without existing low-back symptoms. Eligible interventions intend to reduce LBP or its consequences among workers in the occupational setting, and can be categorised into: (1) individual focus; (2) physical ergonomics; and (3) organisational ergonomics. Interventions simply to reduce return-to-work time were only included if there was follow-up focusing on recurrence of LBP and/or consequences of LBP. The included interventions are directed predominantly towards workers and their immediate environment. Provision of occupational health services was not considered to be a preventive intervention for the purposes of this guideline, and is the subject of other national guidelines.[1353] However, occupational health has an important role in supporting and enhancing other interventions,[1511] so occupational health interventions concerning return to work were included where the intervention was the provision of modified work for workers sick-listed due to LBP, and the intention was return to regular work.

Four types of factor are commonly found in the literature covering occupational epidemiology and ergonomics: (1) exposure to (purported) risk factors for LBP; (2) perceived exertion, discomfort or fatigue; (3) occurrence and/or recurrence of LBP; and (4) sick leave due to LBP. The evaluation of ergonomic interventions is often based on exposure to risk factors and on perceived exertion, discomfort or fatigue; studies having these outcomes alone were excluded, but studies reporting on the occurrence and/or recurrence of (sick leave due to) LBP were included. Occasionally, the incidence rate of back injuries is used as an outcome measure, but it needs to be acknowledged that use of the concept of injury is imprecise – the reporting of an injury can be driven more by legal and compensation requirements than objectively demonstrable injury. For some recommendations, the wide variety of outcome measures used in studies (e.g. self-reported symptoms, sick leave, occupational back pain, low-back injuries, compensable LBP) necessitated a consensus interpretation.

Physical exercise/physical activity

Physical exercise may be recommended in the prevention of LBP (level A). Furthermore, physical exercise may be recommended in the prevention of recurrence of LBP (level A) and in the prevention of recurrence of sick leave due to LBP (level C).[484,775,799,842,887,1443,1468,1510]

Information/advice/instruction

Traditional information/advice/instruction on biomechanics, lifting techniques and optimal postures is not recommended for prevention of LBP (level A). There is insufficient evidence to recommend for or against psychosocial information delivered at the worksite (level C), but information oriented toward promoting activity and improving coping can promote a positive shift in beliefs (level C). Whilst the evidence is not sufficiently consistent to recommend education in the prevention of recurrence of sick leave due to LBP (level C), incorporating the messages from the accompanying clinical guidelines into workplace information/advice is encouraged.[484,663,775,799,816,842,887,888,1394,1443,1468,1478,1510]

Back belts/lumbar supports

Back belts/lumbar supports are not recommended for prevention of LBP (level A).[790,799,842,887,1443,1468,1510]

Shoe inserts, shoe orthoses, shoe insoles, flooring and mats

Shoe inserts/orthoses are not recommended for prevention in LBP (level A). There is insufficient evidence to recommend for or against shoe insoles, soft shoes, soft flooring or antifatigue floor mats (level D).[806,1010]

Physical ergonomics

There is insufficient consistent evidence to recommend physical ergonomics interventions alone for reduction of the prevalence and severity of LBP (level C). There is insufficient consistent evidence to recommend physical ergonomics interventions alone for the reduction of (reported) back injuries, occupational or compensable LBP (level C). There is some evidence that, to be successful, a physical ergonomics programme would need an organisational dimension and involvement of the workers (level B). There is insufficient evidence to specify precisely the useful content of such interventions (level C) and the size of any effect may be modest.[194,201,405,764,842,919,1088,1331,1553,1608]

Organisational ergonomics

There is insufficient consistent evidence to recommend stand-alone work organisational interventions alone for prevention in LBP (level C), yet such interventions could, in principle, enhance the effectiveness of physical ergonomics programmes.[265,1552]

Multidimensional interventions

Whilst multidimensional interventions at the workplace may be recommended to reduce some aspects of LBP, it is not possible to recommend which dimensions and in what balance (level A). The size of any effect may be modest.[481,1443]

Modified work for return to work after sick leave due to LBP

Temporary modified work (which may include ergonomic workplace adaptations) can be recommended, when needed, in order to facilitate earlier return to work for workers sick-listed due to LBP (level B).[791]

Notwithstanding the evidence on physical and organisational ergonomics specifically to influence outcomes, the working group endorsed the pragmatic view that 'work should be comfortable when we are well, and accommodating when we are ill',[548] and emphasised that ergonomics has a role in formulating modified work to facilitate early return to work.[1511]

School age

While the epidemiology of back pain at young age has been described extensively, studies evaluating the effects of interventions to prevent LBP or the consequences of LBP in schoolchildren are still sparse. As a result, the aim of formulating evidence-based guidelines for prevention in LBP among schoolchildren could not be accomplished. However, the conclusions of the literature search may give guidance for further development and evaluation of preventive interventions during school age. There is limited evidence linking childhood back pain with adult symptoms,[571] but no evidence was found to indicate that modifying childhood back pain would influence its occurrence in adults. The literature review found only studies on school-based interventions that satisfied the criteria for the guideline. Scientific studies that evaluated the efficacy of interventions to modify (purported) risk factors in schoolchildren were conspicuous by their absence. However, it was felt useful to synthesise the available information on modifiable risk factors to inform future research, accepting that risk factor modification without concomitant influence on outcomes cannot be considered prevention.

School-based interventions

There is insufficient evidence to recommend for or against a generalised educational intervention for the prevention of LBP or its consequences in schoolchildren (level C).[97,248,419,974,1374]

Modifiable risk factors

A number of potentially modifiable risk factors/risk indicators was located in the literature. Some have a theoretical causal link with LBP, but others are better described as risk indicators. They fell into four groups: (1) lifestyle factors (overweight/obesity, smoking, alcohol intake, eating habits, working, sports participation, physical inactivity and sedentary activities); (2) physical factors (physical fitness, mobility and flexibility, muscular strength); (3) school-related factors (school bags and school furniture); and (4) psychosocial factors. The association between these purported risk factors/risk indicators and LBP was found to be rather mixed, with no single factor or set of factors predominating. The following statements are thought to reflect the current state of knowledge about back pain prevention during school age. Discussion of the supporting evidence can be found at www.backpaineurope.org:

1. There is no evidence for or against recommending weight control as a preventive action.
2. There is no evidence that antismoking campaigns will have a preventive effect.
3. There is insufficient evidence to recommend for or against modification of eating habits as a preventive measure.
4. There is no evidence for or against recommending modification of alcohol intake as a preventive measure.
5. There is no evidence that performing sports or being physically active has a preventive effect. There is also insufficient evidence to recommend a general limitation of involvement in competitive sports participation as a preventive measure.
6. There is insufficient evidence to recommend for or against modified sitting postures as a preventive action. There is also no evidence that decreasing sedentary activities will have a preventive effect.
7. There is insufficient evidence to recommend for or against modification of mobility and flexibility of muscles and joints as a preventive action.
8. There is insufficient evidence to recommend for or against muscle strengthening as a preventive action.
9. There is no consistent evidence for or against recommending a limit to the weight of schoolbags (or for avoiding their use) or changing the type of schoolbag (or the method of carrying it) as primary preventive measures.
10. There is insufficient evidence to recommend for or against modified school furniture as a preventive measure.
11. There is no evidence that modification of psychological factors may have a preventive effect.

Summary of the concepts of prevention in low-back pain

- The general nature and course of commonly experienced LBP mean that there is limited scope for preventing its incidence (first-time onset). Prevention, in the context of this guideline, is focused primarily on reduction of the impact and consequences of LBP.
- Primary causative mechanisms remain largely undetermined: risk factor modification will not necessarily achieve prevention.
- There is considerable scope, in principle, for prevention of the consequences of LBP, e.g. episodes (recurrence), care-seeking, disability and work loss.
- Different interventions and outcomes will be appropriate for different target populations (general population, workers and children), yet inevitably there is overlap.

Overarching messages from the guidelines

- Overall, there is limited robust evidence for numerous aspects of prevention in LBP.
  - Nevertheless, there is evidence suggesting that prevention of various consequences of LBP is feasible.
  - However, for those interventions where there is acceptable evidence, the effect sizes are rather modest.
  - The most promising approaches seem to involve physical activity/exercise and appropriate (biopsychosocial) education, at least for adults.
  - But no single intervention is likely to be effective in preventing the overall problem of LBP, owing to its multidimensional nature.
- Prevention in LBP is a societal as well as an individual concern.
  - So, optimal progress on prevention in LBP will likely require a cultural shift in the way LBP is viewed, its relationship with activity and work, how it might best be tackled and just what is reasonable to expect from preventive strategies.
  - It is important to get all the players onside, but innovative studies are required to understand better the mechanisms and delivery of prevention in LBP.
  - Anecdotally, individuals may report that various strategies work for them, but in the absence of scientific evidence, that does not mean they can be generally recommended for prevention; it is not known whether some of these strategies have disadvantageous long-term effects.

With special thanks to the members of Working Group 3 of the European Commission's COST Action B13.

UPDATE

The quest for prevention continues, and it is pertinent to look at more recent research to see if it gives any reasons to question the findings of the European guidelines. By and large, it is the same range of risk factors that has been the subject of investigation, and incorporated into systematic reviews.

A review published in 2009,[143] which was based on 20 high-quality controlled trials, found what was described as strong consistent evidence to guide prevention of back pain episodes in working-age adults. In essence, the authors concluded that trials showed exercise interventions to be effective and other interventions not effective. The latter included stress management, shoe inserts, back supports, ergonomic/back education (including reduced

lifting programmes). The issue of training and lifting equipment has been the subject of a Cochrane review.[928,929] This review found no evidence to support the use of advice or training in working techniques with or without lifting equipment for preventing back pain, consequent disability or reduced sick leave, when compared to no intervention or alternative interventions. A similar finding emerged from a review of interventions to prevent back injury in nurses.[326] As pointed out by by Martimo et al., these findings challenge current practice of advising workers on 'correct' lifting techniques.[929] Furthermore, the biomechanical veracity of typical traditional advice can itself be questioned.[526] So whilst training (under ideal circumstances) can temporarily alter the way workers do things, it apparently does not significantly reduce the risk of injury.

The workplace is an obvious location for implementing multidisciplinary prevention programmes. One such was investigated in an RCT among a population of workers in physically demanding jobs in nine large companies across The Netherlands. The prevention programme was based on the principles of the biopsychosocial model, combining individually tailored education and training, immediate treatment of back pain and advice on ergonomic adjustment of the workplace. The results did not show a significant difference between this group and the control group receiving guidelines-based clinical care, and provided no evidence for the adoption of this worksite prevention programme for LBP.[662]

SUMMARY

The epidemiology of back pain (Ch. 6) indicates that primary prevention is an unrealistic goal[214]; there is no single factor (or collection of factors) that, if removed from life, would result in the abolition of back disorders. Numerous studies have reported the apparent success of various interventions in reducing back pain. However, few have been conducted as RCTs, so strong scientific evidence for their effectiveness is often scarce or inconsistent.[215,1509]

The simple notion that reducing physical loading at work would lead to a reduction in back pain has not been realised. Whilst reductions in the physical requirements of work have apparently reduced demonstrable mechanical overload damage to the spine,[187] a corresponding reduction in the prevalence of injuries, symptoms and disability has not followed. Indeed, a large industrial study has shown how a common tool for estimating the loads on the lumbar spine during manual handling (the National Institute of Occupational Safety and Health lifting equation[1534]) does not predict either the prevalence of LBP or the incidence of sickness absence, whether assessed as a composite lifting index or a single task index.[1133] Evidently, much back pain is not caused by work so the impact on the occurrence of back pain from any further ergonomic improvements is likely to be small. That is not to say that ergonomic considerations should not be applied to the design of work: they should (Ch. 17), but not in a vain hope that such action will make any appreciable difference to the development of back pain.

However, people with back pain can find biomechanical demands challenging (or even impossible) until their back pain improves, and in that respect the symptoms may be highly work-relevant. Therefore, workplaces should be provided that are accommodating for symptomatic workers, whilst at the same time being comfortable and pleasant.[548] This approach, whilst not offering anything substantial for primary prevention, has the potential to contribute to reductions in pain, sick leave, compensation and disability.[215,735] Viewed overall, interventions to reduce physical workload have an inconsistent impact on occupational back pain: where there has been an effect it remains unclear if the interventions actually reduced symptoms or injuries, or simply modified reporting patterns and altered what workers do about their back pain.[1509] Stated simply, there is as yet no substantial scientific evidence for the efficacy of ergonomic interventions.[143,842,929] The same holds true for control of physical exposure at the population level; none of the interventions specifically intended to reduce spinal loading has been shown to have discernible preventive capability. Even when an intervention has a beneficial effect in 'small-area' scenarios,[540,1587] it may not be obvious to what extent the results can be generalised.

Scientists are moving away from a narrow view of 'mechanical' back pain towards a broader 'mechanistic' understanding of tissue injury and degeneration, including cellular responses to changes in tissue stress and strain (Fig. 7.11). The focus of research remains on disorders of the intervertebral disc, because the presence of certain features of disc degeneration carries a substantial increased risk of severe back pain (p. 203). Also, it is tempting to associate the unique characteristics of back pain with a unique anatomical structure. However, only time will tell if this endeavour will lead to practical measures to prevent back pain.

One intriguing intervention that was not considered specifically in the European guidelines deserves mention here since it relates to a very specific everyday biomechanical principle potentially related to LBP. An RCT has shown that a simple mechanical intervention can be effective: instructing patients to avoid forward-bending movements of the lumbar spine during the first 3 hours of the day can reduce pain intensity and days in pain.[1340] Presumably this is because it reduces the risk of bending injury to intervertebral discs and ligaments at a time when the discs are swollen with fluid (p. 184). A 3-year follow-up of the experimental intervention subjects showed somewhat equivocal results but suggested that the effects are maintained, especially with continued compliance with the instructions.[1339] It should be borne in mind that the subjects were people who had a long history of LBP (average 17 years), so they had good reason to comply with the intervention instructions; it is unknown if the results can be generalised to people with less intrusive LBP or if it could influence other outcomes, such as the rate of recurrence. Nevertheless, this study can be seen as a stimulus to continue research endeavours into biomechanically based interventions.

The thrust of this chapter has followed the evidence in that it has concentrated on non-specific, common LBP. The literature in respect of specific conditions and diagnoses such as disc herniation, spondylolisthesis and spinal stenosis is much less developed and preventive interventions either have not been proposed or, if they have, remain inadequately tested. Thus, there is scope for further development and testing of biomechanically based interventions directed at specific pathologies. Furthermore, sophisticated interventions involving genetic engineering, perhaps at the cellular level, may hold hope for prevention of certain issues such as spinal degeneration.

Finally, it should perhaps be pointed out that the concern of the European guidelines was prevention of the consequences of LBP such as recurrent episodes, sickness absence and disability. This is quite different from consideration of therapeutic effects, usually measured in terms of reduction of symptoms/disability related to the presenting spell, which is discussed in Chapter 17. Conventional ergonomic and biomechanical interventions have the potential, based on biomechanical concepts, to reduce the incidence of back problems, but that potential has not been demonstrated, and any future impact on the overall incidence rate is unlikely to be large.

POSTSCRIPT: PRACTICAL ADVICE

Some practical advice concerning the prevention and management of back pain has been included at the end of Chapter 17.

Chapter | **17** |

Conservative management of back pain

INTRODUCTION

The focus of this chapter is the conservative treatment and management of so-called non-specific low-back pain (LBP). It should be remembered, though, that most people with an episode of back pain do not seek care. There is some evidence from population-based surveys that females are slightly more likely to seek care, as are those who have had previous episodes. Pain intensity is only slightly associated with care-seeking, whereas patients with high levels of disability are eight times more likely to seek care than patients with lower levels of disability.[426] It seems then that interference with participation is of particular concern to people and a predominant driver of care-seeking, and something that clinicians need to address when considering their treatments – reduction of pain alone is an insufficient outcome.

Because the cause of the pain often cannot be determined,[157] clinicians involved in the treatment of back pain face significant challenges. Although most clinicians give labels that imply a putative pathoanatomy, the evidence that these labels are valid is scant and controversial, and there is a lack of consensus within and between professional groups.[737] That is not to say there is no physical/biomechanical reason for the pain: it is a matter of common sense, as well as common experience, that physical insults can give rise to acute back pain, but such injuries can be considered minor and do not explain all episodes, or persistent pain. Other chapters will show there is substantial scientific evidence for implicating a variety of structures and processes in the generation of LBP, both acute and persistent. Nevertheless, current clinical methods are incapable of reliably identifying these potential causes in the individual patient, leading to considerable uncertainty over the target for therapeutic interventions – pathology, pain or disability? Clinicians are uncomfortable with uncertainty (as indeed are patients!), so it is not surprising that the professions that treat back pain have adopted their own theories about the origin of the symptoms, and have developed their various treatments accordingly.[737,1507] It could be argued that the origins of symptoms are irrelevant if the treatment works, but such an attitude is intellectually unsatisfactory, and makes it difficult to develop and improve the treatment. That said, from a pragmatic perspective the primary focus of research into clinical interventions remains 'effectiveness'. Thus, this chapter juxtaposes the everyday realities of back pain management with the unanswered questions surrounding the source and cause of non-specific symptoms.

What is the best way to determine if a treatment is effective? The currently accepted gold-standard scientific test of efficacy is the randomised controlled trial (RCT).[1023,1234] A treatment that outperforms both a competing treatment and the placebo effect in respect of the chosen outcome measure (reduction of symptoms or disability) and over a chosen time frame can be accepted as preferred practice until a more effective treatment is developed. Because the range of treatment methods is so vast, the present discussion adopts the principles of evidence-based medicine and concentrates on existing systematic reviews and clinical guidelines, with some reference to individual scientific studies where necessary. Inevitably, some management strategies will be omitted because of a lack of scientific evidence for their efficacy in treating LBP, though others are discussed because of their innovative content.

In recognition of the move to evidence-based medicine,[1234] numerous clinical guidelines for the management of back pain have been developed. The developers of guidelines take the RCT as their main source of evidence, and generally rely primarily on systematic reviews that synthesise the published research. The Cochrane Collaboration (www.cochrane.org) is a major source of systematic reviews in the field of back pain therapy through the activities of the Cochrane Back Review Group (www.cochrane.iwh.on.ca), and much useful information comes from that source.

It is appropriate to break down the treatment of back pain into two broad areas: non-surgical (covered in this chapter) and surgical (covered in Chs 18 and 19). The historical and practical reasons for this have been discussed elsewhere.[1507] In principle, surgery should be restricted to those cases where there is an identifiable lesion that (1) is the likely cause of the symptoms and (2) is amenable to surgical correction. That this principle is not always followed in practice is evident from the dramatically different surgery rates across countries and localities.[564] Surgical intervention is generally considered to be appropriate in cases of sciatica due to lumbar disc herniation (Ch. 19), but is regularly performed for back pain in the presence of other lumbar pathologies such as disc degeneration (and associated spinal stenosis), spondylosis, spondylolisthesis and so-called instability. As indicated in Chapter 6, the correlation between symptoms and these pathologies is uncertain, added to which their diagnosis can be difficult.[75] Taking the case of instability (p. 207), the very concept may be spurious[86] and even when diagnosed clinically it cannot be confirmed biomechanically.[218] Similar arguments can be raised about other types of apparently symptomatic lumbar pathology, with the result that it is often treated conservatively, thus blurring the distinction between surgically amenable disorders and other sources of back pain.

In recognition of the move towards evidence-based medicine, many countries have produced clinical guidelines for the treatment of LBP, most often applied to primary care. In common with clinical guidelines for other medical conditions, those for LBP have shown inconsistency in implementation as well as variable influence on outcomes.[129,130,342,510,954,1087] Nevertheless, evidence-based clinical practice will continue to be channelled by guidelines, so this chapter will briefly review the history of clinical guidelines for LBP, and cover in more detail the most recent European guidelines.[1469] These guidelines specifically separate acute and chronic LBP; despite the arguments presented in Chapter 6 that these labels are somewhat inaccurate, there is a pragmatic argument, adopted by the European guidelines management committee, for maintaining the separation when constructing guidelines for clinical management.

Clinical guidelines are, by definition, concerned with treatment regimens (which to some extent are discipline-specific), and seek to advise on what are effective (or cost-effective) interventions for which patients. The outcomes of interest (indicators of effect) are largely clinical in nature (e.g. pain, disability), though vocational and social outcomes (e.g. return to work, beliefs) are not excluded. It is becoming apparent, though, that simple unidimensional outcome measures do not reflect the complex epidemiological patterns of LBP. Those performing RCTs tend to choose numerical outcome measures that are convenient for researchers and scientific methodology, such as the score on a disability questionnaire at a point 12 months after entry to the trial. Whilst such measures are scientifically valid, they may not really capture what is important to patients,[813] and the symptom status at a given point in time may not be appropriate for a fluctuating complaint such as LBP. Assessed against such outcomes, the reality is that most clinical interventions for LBP have a limited effect (see below). There is a case for looking at a broader societal picture, and re-evaluating the process and outcomes of treatment for common health problems,[1511] and a broader-based biopsychosocial approach to back pain management (as opposed to treatment) will be discussed in some detail later in this chapter, including a discussion of the power of beliefs.

When assessing the efficacy of treatment, there are some advantages to specifying a minimal clinically important change in the outcome score, and then reporting the percentage of patients who achieved such a change.[1465] However, this does not invalidate reporting an average improvement score for a group of patients, even if the average improvement is less than the minimal clinically important change, because the average refers to a population rather than an individual.

WORK AS A HEALTH OUTCOME

There is growing interest in the notion that work is an especially important, and often ignored, outcome for people with health problems.[1514] It is well established that work is generally good for our health and wellbeing, and that prolonged periods away from work are detrimental to health.[1513] Furthermore, the longer someone is off work with a health problem, the less likely it is that he or she will return: the chances diminish dramatically beyond about the 3-month point.[1511] There is, then, a strong case for early return to work for those sick-listed for back pain, and a limited window of opportunity to achieve it.[735,1511] Indeed, early return to work is itself therapeutic for common health problems such as back pain.[1514] The concept of work as a health outcome goes beyond simply focusing on early return to work – staying at work is often preferable to sick leave in the first place. Many people with back pain can and do stay at work during recovery, whilst others will need help to do so – that help will involve employers (providing accommodation) and healthcare (eschewing unnecessary sick certification).[735] Sadly, work as a health outcome is rarely a feature of clinical guidelines generally,[578] and is missing from the most recent UK back pain guidelines.[1253] These issues will recur later in the chapter.

A SHORT HISTORY OF BACK PAIN GUIDELINES

Primary care guidelines

A major, highly influential synthesis of the evidence on back pain diagnosis and treatment was undertaken by the Quebec Task Force and published in 1987,[1350] but strictly this did not comprise the development of a clinical guideline. The first true guidelines were produced by the Agency for Healthcare Policy and Research in the USA in 1994. Since then numerous countries have published clinical guidelines for the management of LBP, and those from the Netherlands, Israel, New Zealand, Finland, Australia, the UK, Switzerland, Germany, Denmark and Sweden have been reviewed and compared.[768]

The composition of the guidelines development groups, the way they addressed the subject and the target populations differ somewhat between countries. For example, some countries have focused on acute back pain whilst others have given recommendations for chronic back pain of more than 12 weeks' duration, though generally they did not clearly differentiate between 12 weeks from onset, or 12 weeks from presentation to a healthcare professional. Since the literature available to the guideline developers was international, the various guidelines should give similar recommendations regarding diagnosis and treatment. By and large this is the case,[228,767,768] but differences do occur, and these have been indicated in the following summary of recommendations based on an international comparison.[768]

- All guidelines propose some form of diagnostic triage into: (1) non-specific back pain; (2) sciatica/radicular syndrome; and (3) specific back pain due to a 'red flag' condition such as tumour, infection or fracture. Sciatica was not always categorised separately but was variously included as specific or non-specific back pain.

- There appears to be a consensus that the vast majority of LBP can be managed adequately in primary care, and that X-rays are not a useful investigation in non-specific LBP (although they may reassure patient and clinician alike). Therapeutic recommendations are reasonably consistent for acute LBP, and focused on maintenance or promotion of activity as opposed to passive interventions. Bed rest is discouraged, and advocated only if the pain is severe, and then only for a couple of days.

- There are consistent recommendations that patients should be reassured that they do not have a serious disease, and that the prognosis is generally favourable, though there may be recurrences. The form that the advice should take was not always consistent, but the UK guidelines in particular suggest a format for the messages to be given to patients, and specifically recommended an educational booklet, *The Back Book.*[1218]

- The prescription of medication (perhaps on a time-contingent basis) is essentially for pain control to facilitate return to normal activity. Simple analgesics were recommended by all guidelines as a first choice, with resort to non-steroidal anti-inflammatory drugs (NSAIDs) where analgesics were not sufficient. The use of muscle relaxants and opioids was inconsistently recommended.
- Recommendations for back-specific exercise therapy varied between the guidelines. Some considered they were not useful (Dutch and UK). Low-stress aerobic exercise (USA) and McKenzie exercises (Dutch) were considered to be a therapeutic option. Guidelines that included chronic LBP (CLBP) were consistent in the recommendation that exercise therapy was a useful intervention (Dutch, German and Danish), but the suggested type and intensity were inconsistent.
- Recommendations regarding the use of manipulative therapy showed some variation. In most guidelines, manipulation was considered to be a therapeutic option in the early weeks of an episode, but in some (Dutch, Australian and Israeli) manipulation was not recommended for acute LBP. It was, however, considered useful for CLBP (Dutch and Danish).
- More recently, the UK has issued a clinical guideline for 'early management of persistent non-specific low-back pain', defined as non-specific LBP that has lasted for more than 6 weeks, but for less than 12 months.[1253] The recommendations reflect the uncertainty generated when synthesising the scientific evidence into clinical pathways: no one clinical intervention stands out as superior. This guideline responded by producing an algorithm involving a variety of treatments.
- It was recommended that people be provided with advice and information to promote self-management of their LBP. In addition, one of a number of treatment options should be offered, taking into account patient preference: an exercise programme, a course of manual therapy or a course of acupuncture. Furthermore, if the chosen treatment does not result in satisfactory improvement, the recommendation was made to consider offering another of these options. If people have received at least one less intensive treatment and still have high disability and/or significant psychological distress, referral for a combined physical and psychological treatment programme, comprising around 100 hours over a maximum of 8 weeks, can be considered. Finally, for people who have completed an optimal package of care, including a combined physical and psychological treatment programme, and still have

severe non-specific LBP for which they would consider surgery, referral for an opinion on spinal fusion can be considered. It remains to be seen whether this stepped approach involving patient preferences, which generated some controversy, will be widely implemented or effective.

Occupational health guidelines

To accommodate the different challenges presented by occupational outcomes, primary care guidelines have been supplemented in some countries by guidelines specifically for use within an occupational health context, where work is recognised as an important health outcome. Six national occupational health guidelines were reviewed in an international comparison.[1353]

The countries were Canada, Australia, the USA, New Zealand, the Netherlands and the UK. In general, there is a focus on management of back pain rather than on effective treatments. There is general agreement among the guidelines on numerous issues fundamental to occupational health management of back pain. The assessment recommendations essentially followed the triage advocated by primary care guidelines (see above). In addition, there was general recognition of potential psychosocial obstacles to recovery and workplace obstacles to return to work. The guidelines agreed on advice that LBP is a self-limiting condition and, importantly, that remaining in work or an early (gradual) return to work, if necessary with modified duties, should be encouraged and supported.

The recommendations for the assessment of LBP can be summarised as[257,1353]:

- Carry out diagnostic triage (non-specific LBP, radicular syndrome, specific LBP).
- Exclude 'red flags' and neurological screening.
- Identify psychosocial factors and potential obstacles to recovery.
- Identify workplace factors (physical and psychosocial) that may be related to the LBP problem and return to work.
- Restrict X-rays to suspected cases of specific pathology.

The recommendations regarding information, advice, return-to-work measures and treatment for workers with LBP can be summarised as[257,1353]:

- Reassure the worker and provide adequate information about the self-limiting nature and good prognosis of LBP.
- Advise the worker to continue ordinary activities and working or to return to normal activity and work as soon as possible, even if there is still some pain.
- Most workers with LBP manage to return to more or less normal duties quite rapidly. Consider temporary adaptations of work duties (hours/tasks) only when necessary.

- When a worker fails to return to work within 2–12 weeks (there is considerable variation in the time scale in different guidelines), refer the patient to a gradually increased exercise programme or multidisciplinary rehabilitation (exercises, education, reassurance and pain management following behavioural principles). These rehabilitation programmes should be embedded in an occupational setting.

European guidelines

The European guidelines for the management of LBP were developed within the framework of the COST Action B13 'Low-back pain: guidelines for its management', issued by the European Commission, Research Directorate-General, Department of Policy, Co-ordination and Strategy. Under the direction of a multidisciplinary group representing a dozen European countries, a number of multinational, multidisciplinary working groups were set up to develop the guidelines, which were published at the end of 2004 (available in full at www.backpaineurope.org). Each group comprehensively searched the literature up to 2004, and reviewed and graded the evidence according to standard guidelines development principles, from which evidence-based recommendations were derived.

The two guidelines of interest here are European Guidelines for the Management of Acute Nonspecific Low-back Pain in Primary Care,[1470] and European Guidelines for the Management of Chronic Nonspecific Low-back Pain.[53] Separate European guidelines have been published for the diagnosis and treatment of pelvic girdle pain.[1499] Essentially, these latter guidelines recognise the syndrome as a specific form of LBP that often arises in association with pregnancy, trauma or arthritis. Diagnostic tests are described, and it is suggested that treatment should include individualised exercises. The acute guidelines provided recommendations for diagnosis and treatment of acute non-specific LBP in the primary care setting, which can be summarised as follows[1470]:

Diagnosis of acute non-specific low-back pain

- Case history and brief examination should be carried out.
- If history-taking indicates possible serious spinal pathology or nerve root syndrome, carry out more extensive physical examination, including neurological screening when appropriate.
- Undertake diagnostic triage at the first assessment as the basis for management decisions.
- Be aware of psychosocial factors, and review them in detail if there is no improvement.

- Diagnostic imaging tests (including X-rays, computed tomography (CT) and magnetic resonance imaging (MRI)) are not routinely indicated for non-specific LBP.
- Reassess those patients who are not resolving within a few weeks after the first visit, or those who are following a worsening course.

Treatment of acute non-specific low-back pain

- Give adequate information and reassure the patient.
- Do not prescribe bed rest as a treatment.
- Advise patients to stay active and continue normal daily activities, including work if possible.
- Prescribe medication if necessary for pain relief, preferably to be taken at regular intervals: first choice, paracetamol; second choice, NSAIDs.
- Consider adding a short course of muscle relaxants on its own or added to NSAIDs, if paracetamol or NSAIDs have failed to reduce pain.
- Consider (referral for) spinal manipulation for patients who are failing to return to normal activities.
- Multidisciplinary treatment programmes in occupational settings may be an option for workers with subacute LBP and sick leave for more than 4–8 weeks.

Chronic guidelines: overarching comments

The guidelines for CLBP also provided recommendations for diagnosis and treatment, and in addition discussed some overarching concepts in respect of CLBP. These can be summarised as follows[53]:

- In contrast to acute LBP, very few guidelines exist for the management of CLBP.
- CLBP is not a clinical entity and diagnosis, but rather a symptom in patients with very different stages of impairment, disability and chronicity. Therefore assessment of prognostic factors before treatment is essential.
- Overall, there is limited positive evidence for numerous aspects of diagnostic assessment and therapy in patients with non-specific CLBP.
- In cases of low impairment and disability, simple evidence-based therapies (i.e. exercises, brief interventions and medication) may be sufficient.
- No single intervention is likely to be effective in treating the overall problem of CLBP of longer duration and more substantial disability, owing to its multidimensional nature.
- For most therapeutic procedures, the effect sizes are rather modest.

- The most promising approaches seem to be cognitive-behavioural interventions encouraging activity/exercise.
- It is important to get all the relevant players on side and to provide a consistent approach.

Diagnosis in chronic low-back pain

Patient assessment

Physical examination and case history

The use of diagnostic triage, to exclude specific spinal pathology and nerve root pain, and the assessment of prognostic factors (yellow flags) are recommended. We cannot recommend spinal palpatory tests, soft-tissue tests and segmental range of motion or straight-leg raising tests in the diagnosis of non-specific CLBP.

Imaging

We do not recommend radiographic imaging (plain radiography, CT or MRI), bone scanning, single photon emission CT (SPECT), discography or facet nerve blocks for the diagnosis of non-specific CLBP unless a specific cause is strongly suspected. MRI is the best imaging procedure for use in diagnosing patients with radicular symptoms, or for those in whom discitis or neoplasm is suspected. Plain radiography is recommended for the assessment of structural deformities.

Electromyography

We cannot recommend electromyography for the diagnosis of non-specific CLBP.

Prognostic factors

We recommend the assessment of work-related factors, psychosocial distress, depressive mood, severity of pain and functional impact, prior episodes of LBP, extreme symptom-reporting and patient expectations in the assessment of patients with non-specific CLBP.

Treatment of chronic low-back pain

Conservative treatments

Cognitive-behavioural therapy, supervised exercise therapy, brief educational interventions and multidisciplinary (biopsychosocial) treatment can be recommended for non-specific CLBP. Back schools (for short-term improvement) and short courses of manipulation/mobilisation can also be considered. The use of physical therapies (heat/cold, traction, laser, ultrasound, short-wave, interferential, massage, corsets) cannot be recommended. We do not recommend transcutaneous electrical nerve stimulation.

Pharmacological treatments

The short-term use of NSAIDs and weak opioids can be recommended for pain relief. Noradrenergic or noradrenergic–serotoninergic antidepressants, muscle relaxants and capsicum plasters can be considered for pain relief. We cannot recommend the use of gabapentin.

Invasive treatments

Acupuncture, epidural corticosteroids, intra-articular (facet) steroid injections, local facet nerve blocks, trigger point injections, botulinum toxin, radiofrequency facet denervation, intradiscal radiofrequency lesioning, intradiscal electrothermal therapy, radiofrequency lesioning of the dorsal root ganglion and spinal cord stimulation cannot be recommended for non-specific CLBP. Intradiscal injections and prolotherapy are not recommended. Percutaneous electrical nerve stimulation and neuroreflexotherapy can be considered where available. Surgery for non-specific CLBP cannot be recommended unless 2 years of all other recommended conservative treatments – including multidisciplinary approaches with combined programmes of cognitive intervention and exercises – have failed, or such combined programmes are not available, and only then in carefully selected patients with maximum two-level degenerative disc disease.

What is apparent from the evidence is that many commonly used treatments are of unknown efficacy, whilst others appear to be either ineffective or detrimental, and most of the guidelines have concerns about overmedicalisation and needlessly prolonged treatment for non-specific LBP. Indeed, it has been shown that a single session of evidence-based advice from a physiotherapist is as effective as a median of five sessions of hands-on physiotherapy treatment.[452]

It is also apparent that the effective interventions and treatments for non-specific LBP have small effect sizes on clinical outcomes, and their cost-effectiveness is variable. An interesting example is the UK BEAM trial, which estimated the effect of adding exercise classes and spinal manipulation to 'best care' in general practice for patients consulting with back pain, based on the costs of trial treatments and 12-month healthcare costs (for any reason). A small benefit was found for manipulation, which was of questionable clinical importance but was found to be cost-effective (dependent on purchasing policy).[1450,1451] The societal costs of back pain are accounted for more by sickness absence issues than treatment costs, yet many primary care trials have not been able to include the costs of sickness absence, largely because most patients either do not take sick leave or are not employed. Whilst some treatments may be (somewhat) effective for reducing symptoms, most are quite ineffective at returning people to work once they have been off work for a few weeks.[1511] Since sickness absence accounts for far more of the social cost of back pain than healthcare,[1508] this issue is important, and numerous non-medical agencies are developing an interest in rehabilitation with the hope that it may improve vocational outcomes. The concept owes more to principles of management than specific therapy, not because understanding (biomechanical) causation and treatment aspects of LBP should be abandoned, but because of the need to tackle the societal impact of the back pain phenomenon within the limitations of current knowledge.

REHABILITATION FOR THE MANAGEMENT OF LOW-BACK PAIN

The occupational health guidelines outlined above are naturally concerned with occupational outcomes, in particular return-to-work times, and tend to adopt a multimodal approach to management. This theme can be combined with modern evidence-based principles of rehabilitation to provide a theoretical and conceptual basis for reducing sickness absence and long-term incapacity due to back pain.[1512] LBP and disability may originate from a biological condition, but the development of chronicity and incapacity is subject to powerful psychosocial influences.[735,841,891,1298] There is broad agreement that LBP and disability can only be understood and managed according to a biopsychosocial model (Fig. 6.5) that includes health-related, personal/psychological and social/occupational dimensions and the interactions between them.[1506] 'Bio' refers to the physical or mental health condition; 'psycho' recognises that personal/psychological factors also influence functioning and individuals must take some measure of personal responsibility for their behaviour; and 'social' recognises the importance of the social context, pressures and constraints on behaviour and functioning.

Obstacles to recovery/return to work

Unlike severe medical conditions with permanent impairment, people with non-specific LBP can generally be expected to recover. Epidemiological studies[1025,1523] show that:

- prevalence rates are high among people of working age
- most episodes settle uneventfully with or without formal healthcare (at least enough to return to most normal activities, even if with some persistent or recurrent symptoms)
- most people remain at work, and most who do take time off work return quite quickly (even if still with some symptoms)
- only about 1% go on to long-term incapacity.

These are 'essentially whole people' with a manageable health problem: given the right care, support and encouragement they do have (some) remaining capacity for work. Thus, long-term incapacity is not inevitable. This reverses the question: it is no longer what makes some people take prolonged sick leave, but why do some

people with a problem like non-specific LBP not recover as expected?

As noted earlier, the main driver for care-seeking is the extent of disability/participation associated with back pain, and we know that the longer individuals are disabled/incapacitated, the more difficult it is for them to return to usual participation. We also know that a large proportion of people experiencing back pain will recover and return to participation uneventfully in a short space of time. These facts help to explain the typical recovery curve for back pain, where there is a steep reduction over the first few weeks in the proportion struggling to participate. As time goes by, the curve flattens and the proportion returning to usual participation decreases (Fig. 17.1). The successful management of the back pain phenomenon is all about squashing that curve – early intervention to identify and address obstacles to participation, thus reducing the proportion going on to prolonged disability.

The development of incapacity is a process in which biopsychosocial factors, separately and in combination, aggravate and perpetuate disability.[841,891,1511] Crucially, these factors can also act as obstacles to recovery and return to work.[219,735,914,1298] The logic of rehabilitation then shifts from attempts to overcome, adapt or compensate for impairment to addressing factors that delay or prevent expected recovery. The target for interventions thus shifts to obstacles to the expected recovery or return to work.[1511]

Biological obstacles

Few patients with non-specific LBP have any absolute biological barrier to most jobs in modern society. It is common clinical experience that many were doing the same job with similar symptoms before sickness absence, and/or subsequently return to work despite persisting symptoms.

The main biological obstacles to return to work relate to the physical condition of the back. For many patients this should not be insurmountable, given proper management. Symptoms such as pain and fatigue, in themselves, are often felt to be the main obstacle to work but symptoms correlate poorly with impairment, disability or incapacity for work and do not necessarily imply incapacity.

It is often assumed that the health condition is the obstacle and healthcare the solution, but sometimes healthcare itself may become an obstacle. Inappropriate healthcare for LBP, particularly when combined with unhelpful medical information and advice and inappropriate sick certification, may not only be ineffective but may block more appropriate management and return to work.[1092] Efficacy also requires timely and efficient healthcare delivery, and many reviews have identified health service waiting lists and delays in access to specialist consultations, investigations and therapy as obstacles to return to work.[676]

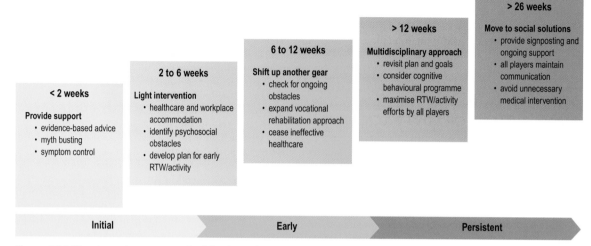

Figure 17.1 The stepped-care approach: doing just what's needed when it's needed. RTW, return to work. *(Adapted with permission from Kendall NAS, Burton AK, Main CJ, et al., on behalf of the Flags Think-Tank. Tackling musculoskeletal problems: a guide for the clinic and workplace – identifying obstacles using the psychosocial flags framework. London: The Stationery Office, 2009, © kendallburton.)*

Personal/psychological obstacles

Personal and psychological factors are central to functioning and disability associated with LBP and they are also important obstacles to recovery. They were originally described as 'yellow flags' for risk of chronicity,[736,890] but it is now clear they act as obstacles to work participation.[735a]

Thoughts

- Catastrophising (focus on worst possible outcome, or interpretation that uncomfortable experiences are unbearable)
- Unhelpful beliefs and expectations about pain, work and healthcare
- Negative expectation of recovery
- Preoccupation with health.

Feelings

- Worry, distress, low mood (may or may not be diagnosable anxiety or depression)
- Fear of movement
- Uncertainty (about what's happened, what's to be done and what the future holds).

Behaviours

- Extreme symptom report
- Passive coping strategies
- Serial ineffective therapy.

There is a further set of perceptions and concerns for workers, which are about the health condition, about work, about the relationship between them, and about 'workability' that are likely to form more specific obstacles for return to work.[735,914,1511] Psychosocial aspects of work are to some extent external characteristics of the job. However, personal perceptions of these working conditions have a more important and direct effect on individual behaviour, whether or not these perceptions are accurate.

Employee

- Fear of reinjury
- Concern about physical job demands
- Low expectation of resuming work
- Low job satisfaction
- Low social support or social dysfunction in workplace
- Perception of stressful job demands.

Workplace

- Lack of job accommodations/modified work
- Lack of employer communication with employees.

Context obstacles

Return to work is not simply a matter of health or healthcare: return to work is a social process that depends on organisational policy, process and practice, which depend

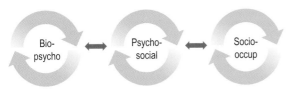

Figure 17.2 Interactions within and between biopsychosocial obstacles to return to work.

in turn upon employers' perceptions and attitudes. These are some of the more important work-related and organisational obstacles to return to work:

- Misunderstandings and disagreements between key players (e.g. employee and employer, or with healthcare)
- Financial and compensation problems
- Process delays (e.g. due to mistakes, waiting lists or claim acceptance)
- Overreactions to sensationalist media reports
- Spouse or family member with negative expectations, fears or beliefs
- Social isolation, social dysfunction
- Unhelpful policies/procedures used by company.

Biopsychosocial interactions

Health-related, personal/psychological and social/ occupational obstacles to return to work all appear to be important, accepting that there is overlap and interaction between the different dimensions (Fig. 17.2), and that their relative importance may vary in different individuals and settings and over time.

Clinical management

The primary goal of healthcare is to relieve symptoms, and it is implicitly assumed this will restore function. Most patients with LBP do recover and return to work quickly, so it may be argued that routine healthcare effectively does rehabilitate. However, for those who do not recover quickly, continued symptomatic treatment alone does not restore function and, in particular, is ineffective for occupational outcomes. It is then necessary to reconsider the goals of clinical management. Relief or at least control of symptoms may require continued healthcare, but management must also maintain or restore function and address occupational outcomes. These goals are closely intertwined, they run concurrently and they are interdependent.

Restoration of function

Almost all successful rehabilitation programmes for LBP (and for other musculoskeletal and cardiorespiratory conditions) include some form of active exercise or graded activity component.[1273,1352] However, increasing activity levels and improving performance may be as much about changing beliefs and behaviour as any physiological change.[841] Personal experience that challenges misconceptions and forces patients to rethink their health problem is a powerful agent for change. The immediate goal is to overcome activity limitations and restore activity levels; the ultimate goal is to improve functioning and social participation.

An occupational focus

Return to work is not only the goal and outcome of successful healthcare: work is generally therapeutic and an essential part of rehabilitation.[432] Too often, health professionals give advice that is unrealistic or frankly harmful, without considering its implications. It is particularly important to avoid fostering inappropriate links between LBP and work (which are often unfounded). All health professionals who treat back pain should not only be interested in, but must also accept some responsibility for, work outcomes.[61] Too many doctors are also unaware of, and fail to consider, the effects of sick certification and extended periods of sickness absence[1255]; it is important to consider the indications and contraindications, its likely impact, and its potential risks and side-effects. It is widely recognised that there is a need for better communication and cooperation between GPs and occupational health professionals,[124,125,1256] but implementing that may require a fundamental shift in the culture of healthcare, in the nature of clinical interventions and in the mind set of clinicians. All health professionals (doctors, nurses, allied health professionals, occupational health personnel) who care for workers with LBP should have an interest in, and accept responsibility for, restoring function and promoting work participation; it goes to the heart of what good clinical management of people of working age is all about.

Stepped care

Although we know that a proportion of patients will fail to recover and return to usual participation in a timely fashion, there are substantial problems when it comes to identifying them at the outset – in essence we currently cannot. There are some interesting initiatives looking at the concept of stratified care – identifying subgroups who may respond to specific early care.[606a] Whilst these approaches are potentially very valuable, they have yet to show that they can be readily and effectively implemented.

Where stratified care is infeasible, the alternative of stepped care can be considered. This is the idea of doing just what's required when it's required, and is applicable when the natural history is favourable for the many and those who will struggle and need more intensive

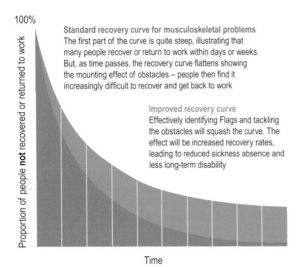

100%

Proportion of people **not** recovered or returned to work

Standard recovery curve for musculoskeletal problems
The first part of the curve is quite steep, illustrating that many people recover or return to work within days or weeks. But, as time passes, the recovery curve flattens showing the mounting effect of obstacles – people then find it increasingly difficult to recover and get back to work

Improved recovery curve
Effectively identifying Flags and tackling the obstacles will squash the curve. The effect will be increased recovery rates, leading to reduced sickness absence and less long-term disability

Time

Figure 17.3 The goal of managing back pain – squashing the back pain recovery curve to reduce prolonged disability. *(Adapted with permission from Kendall NAS, Burton AK, Main CJ, et al., on behalf of the Flags Think-Tank. Tackling musculoskeletal problems: a guide for the clinic and workplace – identifying obstacles using the psychosocial flags framework. London: The Stationery Office, 2009, © kendallburton.)*

intervention cannot be identified at the outset. Stepped care recognises that many people do not need an expensive, complex intervention, and can offer substantial cost–benefits to public healthcare systems. The stepped-care approach fits well for the management of back pain. At the outset, many people will recover rapidly with nothing more than accurate information and advice. Thus fewer people will remain with symptoms/disability at the next stage, say 2–6 weeks, when a light clinical intervention can be considered. Again, that will be sufficient for many. By the 3-month point there is likely to be a small number of people who need a full multidisciplinary approach to rehabilitation, and by 6 months the solutions are social rather than clinical. These steps are illustrated in Figure 17.3.

Occupational management

As noted above, many of the obstacles to return to work lie in and around the workplace, and that is where additional interventions are required to integrate with improved clinical management.

Modified work

The most common occupational intervention, for which there is also most evidence, is to adjust the demands of

work to match (temporarily) reduced capacity.[215,735,791] The principle is simple: 'Work should be comfortable when we are well, and accommodating when we are ill'.[548] The basic idea is to reduce the physical demands of the work, which can be achieved by ergonomic redesign or by reducing exposure times. A key feature seems to be to have a temporal limitation to the modifications, and the phrase 'transitional work arrangments' helps to convey that the process is about facilitation of early return to normal work. However, modified work is not always required: most people with LBP return quickly to normal work without insurmountable difficulty. Clinical advice to return only to modified work may be counterproductive and create obstacles to return if modified work is not available. Implementing transitional work arragements can be problematic; it requires maximum effort from all parties, and demands flexibility.

Examples of helpful workplace accommodations to tackle common obstacles include[735a]

- Alter the work tasks or physical environment to reduce physical demands, e.g. reduce reaching; provide seating; reduce weights; reduce pace of work/frequency; enable help from co-workers; job enlargement (added task variety).
- Alter the work organisation, e.g. flexible start/finish times; reduced work hours/days; additional rest breaks; graded return to work (starting at achievable level, and increasing on a regular quota, or starting with a short week).
- Change the job, e.g. allow someone who cannot drive or use public transport to work at home during the transitional period, or exchange problematic secondary tasks for part of another employee's job description.
- Introduce flexibility, e.g. schedule daily planning sessions with a co-worker at the start of each day to develop achievable goals; allow reasonable time to attend healthcare appointments.

Health at work

Given the nature of LBP, it may be better to address it as a matter of occupational management in the context of health at work. This shifts the perspective from traditional interventions that focus on rehabilitating the individual to a more holistic approach to workers' health. Accepting that LBP will occur, good occupational management is about preventing persistent and disabling consequences.[436,437] This requires employers, unions and insurers to rethink occupational management for LBP. The aim is to improve health at work and alleviate suffering: more specifically, to help workers manage their pain better. The workplace, like healthcare, must then address all of the health, personal and occupational dimensions of health at work, identify obstacles to (return to) work and provide support to overcome them. LBP cannot be left to healthcare workers, and employers must share responsibility for health at work.

Summary

The consequences of LBP among workers raise fundamental questions about clinical and occupational management. More and better healthcare is not the answer. More and better ergonomics is not the answer. It is not a matter just for health professionals or ergonomists: it is equally a matter for employers and workers. Everyone has a part to play, and effective intervention depends on getting all players onside, working together towards a common goal.[436,1298] Getting all the players onside is necessary but not sufficient,[1260] yet implementing these principles, whilst difficult, can improve return-to-work times and reduce absence rates.[216,848] However, it is clear that further progress will require a fundamental cultural shift in how we perceive and manage LBP – in healthcare, in the workplace and in society.

Cultural shifts in the management of low-back pain[1512]

- For most patients with LBP long-term incapacity is not inevitable: given the right care, support and opportunity, most should be able to return to work.
- Strategies (clinical and occupational) should address obstacles to recovery and barriers to (return to) work.
- All health professionals who care for LBP should have an interest in, and accept responsibility for, restoring function and return to work.
- Return to work is not just a matter of healthcare, but a social process that depends on getting all players on side. Clinicians must communicate and cooperate better with occupational health/employers in this process.
- Return to work is not just a matter for healthcare, but a social process that depends on organisational policy, process and practice, which depend in turn upon employers' perceptions and attitudes.
- Workers do not have to wait till they are 100% symptom-free before they return to work. Work is itself therapeutic and an essential part of rehabilitation.
- Maintaining contact with absent workers and the provision of transitional work arrangements are potent return-to-work interventions.
- What is ultimately required is a change in the way the players behave, which will necessitate a change in their perceptions (attitudes and beliefs). To achieve that will variously require

education, training and alterations to social systems.

CULTURAL INTERVENTIONS

It is now clear that psychosocial factors are pivotal to what people do about their back pain experience, and what they do about it has a profound influence on its consequences, irrespective of what might have gone wrong with the back. Beliefs drive behaviour. Beliefs are shaped from childhood onwards, being the product of experience, learning and culture. However, the sources of information that lead to beliefs about back pain (family, health professionals, legal professionals, the media) are not always to be trusted. The sources interact, and an inaccurate set of beliefs generated by one source can readily influence another. People may have a number of fears, such as concerns about damage that may have already occurred, concern about the risk of future damage, concern about the inevitable consequences of the pain, fear that movement will make matters worse and fear of underlying (undetected) serious disease.[1395,1504] Perceptions about the nature of the condition can readily translate into behaviours that may be unhelpful, such as unwarranted care-seeking, demands for investigations, ceasing work and avoiding activity. It has been argued that community actions to correct back pain myths should be useful interventions to prevent the development of long-term disability,[514] but getting the message across is a challenge.

There have been a number of innovative interventions directed at shifting beliefs and behaviours, and they have had some measure of success. A common factor has been that they have tended to demedicalise the back pain experience, and address obstacles to recovery or return to work.

One impressive approach, which targeted the general population and health professionals, was implemented in the state of Victoria, Australia. A major state-wide media campaign including television commercials, outdoor and print advertising, seminars and workplace visits was run for an extended period.[207] In addition, a patient educational booklet (*The Back Book*) was supplied to all clinicians likely to treat back pain, with a recommendation that it should be given to patients. Essentially the campaign promoted, at a population level, the positive messages embodied in *The Back Book*.[1218] The intervention improved beliefs about back pain in the general population, and knowledge and attitudes in GPs, and seemed to influence medical management and reduce disability and workers' compensation costs related to back pain.[207] Interestingly, the population belief shift was found to remain despite the cessation of the campaign. Regrettably, long-term vocational outcomes are not known.[206] A similar public health education campaign has been run in

Scotland using the same messages.[1517] As in Australia, there has been a sustained positive shift in back beliefs at the population level. Furthermore, there has been a change in the advice that doctors give to patients, with a substantial shift away from advising rest to advising an active approach. There are no data available yet on occupational outcomes.[1507]

The uncompromising messages of *The Back Book*, as used in the Australian and Scottish studies, have been found to be effective in changing beliefs and improving clinical outcomes in primary care,[230,301] reducing extended absence in an industrial sample[1394] and improving disability among the elderly.[784] The development of educational material is a complex topic that has been discussed in detail elsewhere,[229] but it should be noted that not all educational material is effective[272]; much seems to depend on the specific content and presentation.

In Ireland, an interesting multimodal intervention has been used in a social security setting. Assessing doctors were trained to use international evidence-based guidelines and consider workplace issues, with the intention of changing their practice in determination of workability.[819] The system was modified such that claimants were invited for an assessment much earlier than previously, and *The Back Book* was made freely available. Interestingly, on receipt of the invitation for assessment, 62% of the claimants came off benefits and returned to work. During the study the assessors declared 64% of those examined fit for work compared with around 20% previously, and there were fewer appeals and fewer successful appeals. Although controlled using only retrospective comparison data, the study does suggest that it is possible, in this setting at least, to change both physician and claimant behaviour at an early stage in the disability process. However, a different sort of social security intervention in Sweden (active sick leave: enablement of return to modified duties with 100% of normal wages) has been less successful.[1259]

Within-company cultural change has also been explored, in which absent workers, from the start of absence, were provided with a workplace supportive network directed at obstacles to return to work. Occupational health nurses were trained to implement a novel intervention protocol which involved very early contact with absent workers, an invitation to attend the occupational health unit for assessment and steps to facilitate return to work. The protocol required them to assess and address psychosocial issues using a cognitive-behavioural approach, to maintain contact with the worker during absence, to liaise with the GP to minimise sick certification and to liaise with the team leader to arrange temporary transitional work arrangements if needed. Treatment beyond attending the GP was specifically excluded. In a controlled trial, the results showed that the protocol, when followed, significantly reduced return-to-work time and also reduced further absence over the ensuing 12 months.[216]

NOVEL NON-SURGICAL THERAPIES FOR BACK DISORDERS

The accelerating pace of research into musculoskeletal disorders is continually throwing up new potential treatments for back pain and the related pathology. Most of these are in the experimental stage only, and have yet to be validated on patients, and they reflect the prevailing research preoccupation with intervertebral discs.[445] Nevertheless they offer hope, and direction for future efforts.

Promoting intervertebral disc healing

Another cultural shift that could help to relieve back pain is to consider painful intervertebral discs as if they were injured and inflamed fibrous connective tissues (which they often are!) and to treat them accordingly. As argued in detail elsewhere,[45] there are many parallels between a disrupted outer annulus fibrosus and injured tendons and ligaments. All of these tissues can give rise to pain as a result of bleeding, inflammation and sensitisation of nerves, and all of them appear to heal by similar mechanisms, albeit at different rates (p. 85). The disc is problematic because of its size, which creates severe metabolite transport difficulties, and because it is difficult to relieve the disc of mechanical loading while the healing takes place. Nevertheless, similar treatment principles should apply. Healing of an injured and painful outer annulus could conceivably by expedited by initial rest, to avoid reinjury, followed by gentle remobilisation to boost collagen synthesis and align the new collagen fibres. Merely stretching a degenerated annulus may protect it from the harmful effects of excessive compressive loading.[852] Animal models support this concept,[536] and many manual therapists already operate on this basis,[742] although the effectiveness of their interventions has not been rigorously assessed. Annulus repair could be aided by technological innovations such as tissue engineering, hydrogels and biological glues,[232,971] and patient selection could possibly be aided by measurements of inflammatory markers in blood.[1604] The cultural shift outlined in the previous section may well benefit patients whose back pain is essentially functional (Ch. 13) or arises from tissue such as muscle that heals very rapidly. But the new paradigm does little to help those with chronic injuries to lumbar discs, ligaments and tendons, and overzealous application of the 'no bed rest' rule could actually do them harm.

New injection therapies for back pain and sciatica

Injection therapies are potentially useful if the tissue origins of pain have been identified. Techniques are avaible to do this (Ch. 5), although they are not

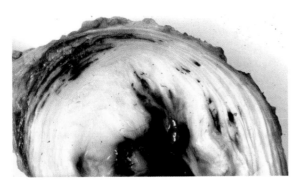

Figure 17.4 Part of a cadaveric intervertebral disc (anterior on the right) showing how an injected blue ionic dye flows freely within the nucleus, and flows more readily between lamellae in the annulus rather than through them. The intact disc was sectioned immediately after injection. The pale blue 'halo' indicates rapid diffusion of dye away from injected locations.

completely reliable, and the method used to identify discogenic back pain (provocation discography[1281]) is now known to carry some risk of accelerating disc degeneration.[254] Recent evidence suggests that injecting the ionic dye methylene blue into a painful disc can be very effective at relieving symptoms for up to 2 years.[1122] Methylene blue disperses rapidly throughout a disc, by fluid flow and diffusion (Fig. 17.4), and it may be able to disable or desensitise any nociceptive nerves it meets. This remarkable study is likely to provoke attempts to reproduce its success, and to develop improved (and patentable!) antinociception agents.

Increasing awareness of an inflammatory involvement in chronic back pain, and treating it with drugs, is likely to be a major growth area, although major obstacles are to identify the right patients and to achieve controlled and sustained drug delivery.[1315] Some help in patient selection is offered by a recent small study which showed that discogenic pain that responds well to surgery can be identified better by blocking the pain in the target disc rather than by provoking it.[1065] Systemic injections of an antibody (infliximab) that blocks the signalling molecule tumour necrosis factor-α (TNF-α) were found to be effective treatment for sciatica in an animal model[1074] and in a pilot study on humans,[718] but not in the subsequent full clinical trial.[779] TNF-α is involved in the sensitisation of nerves and nerve roots, and the timing and delivery of its blocker may be crucial for sucess.[515] A promising development is to inject soluble TNF-α receptors to bind to and inactivate the TNF-α.

Pain arising from osteoarthritis in the apophyseal joints may prove amenable to treatment using recombinant lubricin. This is a synthetic version of the molecule that reduces friction and wear in synovial joints, and it has been shown to reduce cartilage damage and degeneration in the knee joints of rats.[430] Although repeated injections would probably be necessary in human patients, this treatment has the potential to reduce pain and inflammation arising from arthritis. Other injectable compounds include antiapoptotic agents that are able to reduce the progressive cell death that often follows an injury to articular cartilage.[1106]

Sacroiliac joint pain may prove amenable to intraarticular injections of local anaesthetic and/or corticosteroid: a recent uncontrolled trial reported that two-thirds of patients with confirmed sacroiliac joint pain obtained significant pain reduction for more than 6 weeks.[831] A newly developed ultrasound technique may help to ensure accurate needle placement in the sacroiliac joints.[757]

Regenerative medicine

This field is progressing so rapidly that its potential is difficult to assess. It may prove possible to use injected cells to reverse age-related changes in spinal tissues, or to promote healing in them by use of a 'cell bandage'. Intervertebral discs would be a prime, but not only, target. Unfortunately, current techniques are too invasive to justify their use in early-stage disc degeneration, and the implanted cells may die in the hostile environment of a severely degenerated disc. Even if they don't die, additional implanted cells may fail to increase the total production of new proteoglycans if the new cells merely divert nutrients from the existing cell population.[762]

Other

Percutaneous neurotomy using radiofrequency electical current can benefit some patients with chronic back pain arising from an apophyseal joint.[1028] Percutaneous injection of cement into a damaged vertebral body (Fig. 15.23) is able to relieve back pain in some patients, although RCTs show only a marginal clinical benefit.[252] Such cement augmentation reduces movements of a damaged endplate[643] and restores more-or-less normal stress distributions to the adjacent intervertebral disc and neural arch (Fig. 15.24), so it could alleviate pain by a number of mechanisms. It may also provide a means of manipulating the mechanical environment of the adjacent disc so that it can be treated by regenerative medicine (see above). A simple intervention – wearing shock-absorbing insoles – may allieviete back pain somewhat, although it does not prevent future attacks.[1235] Finally, there is good recent evidence that one of the oldest spine treatments of all – yoga – can reduce pain, disability and depression in patients with chronic LBP.[1571]

SUMMARY

So far as therapeutic interventions are concerned, there is strong evidence to support a conservative management strategy based on early activation (or reactivation) in primary care. Specific therapies appear to add only modest benefits when their efficacy is assessed in a statistical sense, although the pain relief is doubtless appreciated by those individuals who do respond to treatment. The potential for psychological interventions to reduce the burden of chronic disability due to back pain has been demonstrated, and there is evidence that exercise therapy is effective in the treatment of chronic LBP. The notion of shifting the culture surrounding back pain in order to tackle social outcomes is attractive, yet current strategies are probably suboptimal.

It is quite striking that no single form of treatment for LBP is able to improve greatly on natural history. This is doubtless due to the extremely heterogeneous nature of LBP, the complex relationships between pathology, pain and pain behaviour, and the practical difficulties of patient selection. Interventions that concentrate on obstacles to recovery rather than on what may have gone wrong are conceptually attractive and deserving of further research. Overall, there is persuasive evidence for demedicalising the management of many patients with LBP, and focusing more on participation outcomes than clinical ones.

Nevertheless, we must not be deterred from trying to develop better treatments for specific patient groups simply because many back pain patients exhibit psychosocial problems. It is instructive to note that psychological distress influences the reporting of knee pain also, and yet distress decreases substantially following knee replacement surgery,[838] presumably because the operation works so well. New treatments for back pain, as well as those currently thought to be unhelpful, may subsequently be shown to be effective once suitable clinical trials are undertaken. The status of specific interventions and therapies for back pain can be found through the Cochrane Back Review Group (www.cochrane.iwh.on.ca), and through the Physiotherapy Evidence Database, PEDro (www.pedro.fhs.usyd.edu.au).

PRACTICAL ADVICE FOR PREVENTING BACK PROBLEMS

The authors of this book strongly endorse the principles of evidence-based medicine, but recognise that systematic reviews (the stuff of evidence-based medicine) can be somewhat nihilistic (p. 55) and can reduce the impact of new ideas. As an aid to the uncertainty likely to be felt by many clinicians over what advice they might give, the authors present some practical steps that could conceivably be of help for individuals. The biomechanical literature reviewed in this book suggests that these simple strategies could help to prevent back pain, although for practical reasons they have not yet been scientifically validated.

- Keep your spine supple. Good mobility reduces peak bending stresses on the spine[357] and appears to reduce the risk of future back pain.[36] This could explain why yoga is beneficial for back pain.[1571]
- Keep your back muscles strong and fatigue-resistant. Fatigued back muscles allow increased bending stresses to act on the spine[359] and may be slower to protect the spine. Fatigue-resistant back muscles protect from future first-time back pain.[900] Having strong muscles does not reduce the risk of future back pain, but training the muscles you already have could be beneficial.
- Avoid spending long periods of time in lordotic or fully flexed postures. Lordotic postures concentrate compressive stresses in the zygapophyseal joints and posterior annulus (Ch. 13). Sustained full flexion can impair the reflexes that enable the back muscles to protect the spine in bending. (p. 192). Lumbar lordosis can be reduced by sitting, or by relaxing the knees when standing.
- Sleep on your side rather than on your back. The fetal position maintains the lumbar spine in moderate flexion, whereas lying supine preserves the lumbar lordosis. Cadaver experiments suggest that flexion aids metabolite transport into the intervertebral discs (p. 180) and equalises stress distributions in the disc and neural arch (Ch. 13). Flexion may also help to keep the spine and back muscles supple.
- Avoid rapid and awkward bending movements, especially in the early morning. Bending injuries to intervertebral discs and ligaments are most easily simulated in vitro when the intervertebral discs are swollen with fluid and when there is a component of lateral bending (Ch. 11). Rapid movements increase internal muscle forces. Avoiding early-morning bending reduces recurrent back pain.[1339,1340]
- Lift slowly, with the spine balanced and slightly bent, muscles relaxed and the weight close to and in front of the body. These factors reduce the peak compressive forces acting on the spine (Ch. 9).
- When starting an arduous job or sporting activity, build up your back strength slowly Muscles can strengthen much faster than the underlying spine, and may cause problems for the discs in particular (p. 85).

PRACTICAL ADVICE FOR COPING WITH BACK PAIN

The following advice (taken from the messages given in *The Back Book*)[1218] is likely to help patients cope with a spell of back pain. Verbal reinforcement of such messages is believed to enhance, though not replace, the effect of giving patients the booklet.

- There is no sign of any serious disease (if applicable).
- The spine is strong. There is no suggestion of any permanent damage (if applicable). Even when it is very painful, hurt does not mean harm.
- Back pain is a symptom that your back is simply not moving and working quite as it should.
- There are a number of treatments that can help to control the pain, but lasting relief depends on your own effort.
- Recovery depends on getting your back moving and working again and restoring normal function and fitness. The sooner you get active, the sooner your back will feel better.
- Positive attitudes are important. Do not let your back take over your life. 'Copers' suffer less at the time, get better quicker and have less trouble in the long run.
- Ask your doctor for a 'fit note' rather than a sick note: use it to show your employer what you can do rather than what you can't.

For patients who have had spinal surgery (discectomy or decompression), the booklet, *Your Back Operation*, has evidence-based information and advice.[1518] For patients with back pain associated with a whiplash injury to the neck, *The Neck Book* or *The Whiplash Book* can be considered. (The Stationery Office, Norwich: www.tsoshop.co.uk)

Chapter |18|

Biomechanics rationale for spinal surgery

instances the biomechanical insults are obvious and real. In others they are potential, conjectural or controversial, and have not been verified empirically, yet remain a theoretical concern.

INTRODUCTION

Surgery is a common form of treatment for low-back pain, but is a momentous undertaking. Unlike other interventions, it involves modifying the structure of the lumbar spine. This requires invading the body and disrupting the surrounding tissues in order to gain access to the target structure. Its effects are irreversible; once anatomy has been altered it cannot be restored. To greater or lesser extents, every surgical procedure carries the risks of failure and of complications. These can be local, such as nerve damage, or systemic, such as infection and blood loss.

In the past, spinal surgery for pain has involved resection or fusion, or a combination of both. Offending structures or lesions, such as osteophytes or disc herniations, could be excised, in an effort to relieve pain. Fusion of individual joints, or of entire motion segments, could be used to eliminate movements that appeared to cause or aggravate pain. Fusion could be used as a supplement to resection if resection threatened the stability of the lumbar spine. A recent innovation is what could be described as reconstructive surgery. This involves replacing offending structures with a prosthesis that preserves the normal function of the lumbar spine. The cardinal example is disc replacement surgery.

Every surgical procedure constitutes an insult to the structure of the lumbar spine. To greater or lesser extents this insult affects the biomechanics of the spine. In some

RESECTION

Resection of any element of the lumbar spine affects its integrity and its operation. The extent to which biomechanics is affected depends on the extent of resection and the functions of the structure or structures affected.

Minimal resections may have little biomechanical effects. Examples include laminotomy, in which only the ligamentum flavum is resected. Since this ligament has only a minor biomechanical role, it can be sacrificed without biomechanical consequence.

To some extent, limited laminectomy can be tolerated. If sufficient bone remains intact, the lamina can continue to serve its function, which is to deliver to the pedicle the controlling forces exerted from the spinous process and from the inferior articular process. However, the pars interarticularis of the lamina is the weakest part of the neural arch. If too much of the lower lamina is removed during laminectomy, it can no longer contribute to bearing forces from the inferior articular process. As a result those forces concentrate on the pars interarticularis, and the risk of pars fracture ensues.

Total laminectomy, or resection of the inferior articular process, may be necessary in order to gain access to the vertebral canal or intervertebral foramen. Without an inferior articular process the segment loses its ability to resist anterior translation on the affected side and axial rotation away from that side. That implies potential instability, and for that reason some surgeons have elected to supplement total laminectomy with segmental arthrodesis – to stabilise the segment prophylactically.

Bilateral laminectomy removes the spinous process. In turn, that removes the site of origin of the multifidus of the affected segment. Without its normal attachment the muscle can no longer contribute its controlling force to the stability of the segment. While this might be tolerable when a single segment is affected, the loss of multifidus becomes more significant if and when multiple segments are resected, as occurs in some treatments of spinal stenosis. Indeed, lumbar spine function is patently impaired unless midline muscle attachments are reconstructed, along with those of the erector spinae aponeurosis and the posterior layer of thoracolumbar fascia (p. 38).

RESECTION

Arthrodesis of the lumbar spine can be accomplished in various ways to various extents. Individual segments or multiple segments can be fused using bone grafts, rods or plates. These can be applied posteriorly, posterolaterally, anteriorly, or in various combinations of each. They can be applied to an otherwise intact spine, or to one in each one or more intervertebral discs have been partially or totally excised.

The biomechanical effect of arthrodesis is elimination of movement at the treated segment or segments. For movement to be eliminated, however, the fusion has to be technically successful. Bone grafts alone may fail to unite consecutive vertebrae. For that reason, surgeons have been motivated to supplement bone grafts with rods or plates, in order to secure fusion and eliminate movement.

The rationale for fusion is insecure. A consistent relationship between the source of pain, the segment treated and the elimination of movement has not been demonstrated. Nor has the benefit of fusion as a treatment for pain been demonstrated empirically.[160] Controlled trials have documented some reduction of pain, but few patients in whom pain is completely relieved.[203,410,450] Moreover, the outcomes attenuate over time.

From a biomechanical perspective, fusion constitutes a substantial impact on the normal operation of the lumbar spine. Although fusion eliminates movement at the treated segment, it does not alter the total loads imposed on the lumbar spine. The same compressive loads continue to be borne by the vertebral column, and the requirements for angular movement must now be met by movements at a reduced number of segments, increasing the bending moments acting on them. The risk arises of untreated segments sustaining greater than normal stresses, and undergoing accelerated degeneration. Avoiding that perceived risk is what prompted the development of reconstructive surgery.

DISC REPLACEMENT

Two factors prompted the development of disc replacement surgery. First was the perception that a degenerated disc was the cause of the patient's symptoms and that, therefore, it should be removed. Second was the recognition that replacing the disc with a bone graft threatened the normal operation of the lumbar spine, particularly with respect to accelerated degeneration of adjacent segments. Consequently, the objectives of reconstructive surgery were to replace the disc with a prosthesis that would mimic the normal function of the disc and preserve the normal function of the lumbar spine.

The extent to which disc replacement surgery has successfully acquitted these objectives is questionable. From a clinical perspective, disc replacement has not been shown to be demonstrably more effective than conventional surgery.[160,985] However, the precepts of biomechanics provide for a more fundamental insight into the design and limitations of disc replacements.

The ideal disc replacement has to be more than a substitute for a bone graft. At the segmental level, the prosthesis has to mimic all the properties of a normal disc, not just its space-filling role.[158] The prosthesis must be able to resist compression; it must allow movements in all three dimensions; but it must also resist those movements. Perhaps most significantly, it must also be compliant in compression.

To date, all varieties of disc prosthesis seem to subserve resistance to compression. They do keep the vertebrae separated. In various ways they also accommodate movements in the sagittal plane. All designs accommodate rotation in the sagittal plane, but they differ in the manner in which, and the extent to which, they accommodate coupled sagittal rotation.

In these respects, the design of prostheses could be summarised as having satisfied the properties of the nucleus of the disc. They subserve resistance to compression and allow sagittal-plane movements. Less attention seems to have been paid to satisfying the properties of the annulus fibrosus. The normal annulus resists translation, bending and axial rotation. Only recently have these properties been deliberately and overtly built into disc prostheses (p. 255). Earlier disc replacements cannot be construed as complete or faithful alternatives to the normal disc because, without those properties, normal function cannot be held to have been preserved or restored.

Perhaps the most significant property of the annulus is its resilience or deformability. The normal disc is able to buffer phasic axial compression by developing tension in response to increased pressure in the annulus. A rigid prosthesis does not have this property. Under axial compression it does not expand radially and thereby dissipate energy into the surrounding annulus. Instead, it transmits load directly and completely from one endplate to the next. In that regard, it concentrates axial loads on the endplates rather than allowing a proportion to be resisted by the neural arch. This correlates with emerging clinical reports that endplate failure is a complication of disc replacement. In effect, the attempt to relieve adjacent segments of increased bending stress has resulted in increased compressive stress being applied to the treated segment.

Yet it is not evident that disc replacement spares adjacent segments. For disc replacement to be deemed as successful in preserving normal function, the axes of rotation of all lumbar segments (Fig. 10.5) should be preserved or restored to normal locations. Designers have attended to the location of axes within segments. They have striven to design prostheses whose axes lie in normal locations under the vertebra that they support. Experiments in cadavers have demonstrated essentially normal movements about normally located axes. However, although prostheses might be accurately designed, they have to be fitted accurately in vivo if they are to have the desired effect on the whole lumbar spine. This has not been demonstrated in outcome studies of disc replacement.

Determining the location of all axes of rotation, during flexion and extension of the lumbar spine, is a practical way of determining the quality of movement of the spine, and the success of disc replacement in restoring or securing normal function. In a successfully reconstructed lumbar spine, the axes at the treated segment and at all other segments would be in normal locations. Conversely, abnormally located axes at one or more segments would indicate that the spine was not operating normally, and that reconstructive surgery had not succeeded in achieving normal function. The abnormal axis would be a sign that abnormal forces were acting on the affected segment.

In this way, the precepts of biomechanics provide criteria that define normal function, and against which satisfaction of the objectives of reconstructive surgery can be assessed. When tested, the successfully reconstructed spine would exhibit normal ranges of movement around normally located axes of movement. Those tests are available for monitoring the professed success of contemporary and future prostheses (Ch. 19).

Chapter 19

Surgery for disc prolapse, spinal stenosis and back pain

INTRODUCTION

Common low-back problems include disc prolapse, spinal stenosis and low-back pain. Disc prolapse commonly presents with pain and numbness radiating to the buttocks and legs. Spinal stenosis may present with an insidious onset of back pain, buttock, thigh and calf pain, usually brought on by standing and walking. It may affect the central canal, lateral recess or neural foramina.

Low-back pain can be subdivided into discogenic pain and facet joint pain. Patients with discogenic pain have pain on bending forward and increased discomfort when sitting. Patients with facet joint arthropathy have pain that is aggravated by extension or standing. A patient with advanced disc degeneration with significant loss of disc height may have a combination of discogenic and facet joint pain.

Young patients with tenderness in the L5–S1 region and pain on extension, particularly if they are involved in sports, may have a condition called spondylolysis which results from repeated stress injury to the pars interarticularis. Spondylolysis can lead to a forward slip of a lumbar vertebra; this is known as spondylolisthesis.

Many patients with low-back problems respond to conservative measures, including simple analgesics, non-steroidal anti-inflammatory medication, increasing activity, and (possibly) physical therapy (Ch. 17). For the minority with high levels of disability, surgical intervention may be indicated. The following sections indicate what surgical interventions might be considered for each of these conditions. The most drastic surgical intervention, spinal fusion, is considered last because it can be indicated for a range of spinal problems.

DISC PROLAPSE

Radicular pain may have a lifetime prevalence of around 5%,[590] but 'surgically important' lumbar disc herniation has a prevalence of approximately 2%.[346] as discussed on p. 56. The onset of annular rupture is conventionally considered to mark the end point of some degenerative process related to genetic susceptibility, although mechanical loading can play a major role (Ch. 11). Major risk factors for disc prolapse include male gender, age (30–50 years), heavy lifting or twisting, stressful occupation, lower income and cigarette smoking (Ch. 6).

It was previously considered that a disc prolapse leads to mechanical deformation of the traversing nerve root producing the symptoms of sciatica. However detailed magnetic resonance imaging (MRI) studies in asymptomatic individuals have shown the presence of disc prolapse without the classic symptoms. It is likely that the symptoms of sciatica (typically caused by an L4–5 or L5–S1 disc prolapse) or femoratica (typically caused by an L3–4 disc prolapse) are indeed initiated by nuclear material coming into physical contact with the nerve root, and not simply due to mechanical deformation. It has been shown that epidural application of nucleus pulposus material induces both structural and functional changes, which relate closely to nerve dysfunction. Leakage of tumour necrosis factor (TNF) from herniated nucleus pulposus can produce a cascade of tissue injury, scar formation and local pain. Such pain sensitisation phenomena are considered on (p. 205).

Disc herniations may be described as a protrusion (contained by the annulus fibrosus), an extrusion (disc material migrating through the annulus fibrosus, but contained by the posterior longitudinal ligament) or sequestered (disc material free in the spinal canal), as shown in Figure 15.6. Ninety-five per cent of lumbar disc herniations occur at L4–5 or L5–S1, with only 5% occurring at L3–4. Disc material may migrate into a central, posterolateral, foraminal or extraforaminal location. A posterolateral disc protrusion will affect the traversing root (e.g. L5–S1 disc protrusion compromises the S1 root). A far-lateral disc protrusion (extraforaminal) on the other hand tends to affect the exiting nerve root (e.g. far-lateral L4–5 disc protrusion compromises the L4 nerve root).

Symptoms typically commence with a period of back pain followed by sciatica. There may be paraesthesia, motor weakness, loss of reflexes and reduction in straight-leg raise. Symptoms resolve spontaneously in up to 70% of cases 3–6 months after onset. The natural history of radicular pain may be aided pharmacologically through epidural steroid and nerve root blocks.[861]

Chemonucleolysis dates back to 1963 when Lyman Smith first injected a purified extract of papaya fruit into the intervertebral disc to treat intervertebral disc prolapse.[1337] There is compelling evidence that chemonucleolysis is a safe and effective treatment for contained herniation of the nucleus pulposus.[503] However, concerns about the risk of anaphylaxis and transverse myelitis have reduced its use and the availability of chymopapain is now extremely limited. As an alternative, manipulation may be considered; it can be as effective as chemonucleolysis for leg pain, and possibly superior for the associated back pain.[225] Others have used an intradiscal catheter with electrothermal energy directed at the disc prolapse to decompress or denervate the disc material. Such procedures can have some mechanical effect,[1140] but clinical results have been disappointing.[333]

More in keeping with the current thoughts on the pathophysiology of sciatica, Karppinen et al.[718] reported the use of anti-TNF-α therapy (p. 205) in 10 patients with severe sciatica secondary to disc herniation. The specific agent used was infliximab and this was administered intravenously. Promising results were achieved, with significant reduction in leg pain sustained at 3 months. The 1-year follow-up confirmed the beneficial effect of a single infusion of 3 mg/kg of infliximab to be sustained in most patients.[778] Furthermore infliximab did not interfere with the spontaneous resorption of disc herniations.

For patients who fail conservative treatment or in whom a progressive neurological deficit is encountered, surgical intervention is indicated. Microdiscectomy is the standard surgical treatment. This may be carried out in the knee–chest position with preoperative fluoroscopic localisation and limited to a partial discectomy (simply removing the offending fragment). Copious irrigation is employed. In this way surgical excision both relieves the pressure on the nerve and reduces the amount of inflammatory cytokines in the vicinity of the nerve. Some authors (Myer et al. personal communication) are now attempting repair of the annulus using microscopic techniques at the time of surgery. The patient is allowed to recover and generally goes home the next day. Extremes of motion are avoided for the first 4–6 weeks whilst the annular lesion seals itself (p. 238). The use of postoperative restrictions is somewhat inconsistent, and their effect on speed and quality of recovery is controversial. A UK survey[348] showed wide variation and inconsistencies in the advice surgeons give about postoperative activity and restrictions, e.g. for sitting, driving or sedentary work. Some surgeons were found still to advocate bed rest for 1–3 days postoperatively, prescribe corsets or restrict sitting for 3–6 months. The evidence favouring activity restrictions is not particularly convincing[952] and the current climate of uncertainty has stimulated development of a booklet to help patients safely reactivate and get on with their lives as soon as possible after discectomy or decompression surgery.[1518] Lifting postoperative restrictions after discectomy allows a shortened time to return to work (mean of 1.2 weeks) without incurring additional complications.[255]

Similar patterns of neurological recovery are reported in all patients treated surgically or conservatively over 10 years,[1540] although patients with moderate or severe sciatica have better outcomes following surgery compared to non-operated patients.[89] Surgery is better than non-operative treatment for disc herniation (at 4 years).[1548]

Cauda equina syndrome

Cauda equina syndrome (CES) secondary to a large disc prolapse is characterised by the onset of severe low-back pain, bilateral or unilateral sciatica, saddle anaesthesia, motor weakness, sensory deficit and urinary incontinence (Fig. 19.1). It may progress to paraplegia and/or permanent incontinence. It is an absolute indication for acute surgical treatment of lumbar disc herniation. A meta-analysis by Ahn et al.[51] showed there was a significant advantage to treating patients within 48 hours versus more than 48 hours after the onset of CES. The authors showed

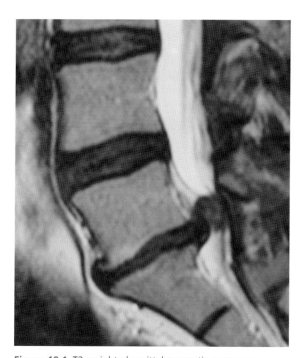

Figure 19.1 T2-weighted sagittal magnetic resonance imaging scan showing a large disc prolapse at L5–S1. The patient had symptoms and signs of cauda equina syndrome and underwent emergency surgery. *(Reproduced from Freeman[444] with permission of Elsevier Ltd, Philadelphia.)*

a significant improvement in sensory and motor deficits as well as urinary and rectal function for those patients undergoing decompression within 48 hours. A review of this paper by Kohles et al.[771] suggested that it understated the value of early surgical intervention, and argued that biologic systems are unlikely to deteriorate in a stepwise fashion, but more in a continuous way. Kohles et al. therefore advocated surgery for this neurological emergency as soon as possible, preferably within 24 hours. Once a diagnosis is confirmed on MRI scan it is advisable to proceed to urgent surgery at the appropriate level.

With an extremely large central disc prolapse, surgical access often can be difficult and it may be necessary to perform a complete laminectomy, identifying the thecal sac and exiting nerve roots before proceeding with the discectomy. Some authors advocate a transdural approach because retraction on the thecal sac and nerve roots may cause further neurological damage. Significant epidural bleeding can be encountered following the removal of disc material as the previously compressed epidural veins now act as a potent source of haemorrhage. A drain is placed in the spinal canal to prevent the formation of potentially compressive haematoma.

LUMBAR SPINAL STENOSIS

Lumbar spinal stenosis is defined as the reduction in the diameter of the spinal canal, lateral nerve canals or neural foramina. This reduction may be due to bony ingrowth, hypertrophy of the ligamentum flavum, disc protrusion, degenerative spondylolisthesis, bone creep (p. 183) or any combination of these elements. Pain in the back and legs caused by compression and ischaemia of nerve roots are the main symptoms. It is one of the most common spinal disorders in people over the age of 65 years.[1351] The natural history of spinal stenosis remains unclear, although there is some evidence that symptoms may progress in up to one third of non-operated patients.[444]

Conservative treatment including non-steroidal anti-inflammatory medication, physiotherapy (including flexion and trunk stabilisation exercises) and general fitness work may improve a patient's symptoms. The use of epidural steroids remains controversial. They may relieve acute pain, but long-term results have been disappointing. Patients who fail conservative treatment and persist with reduced walking distances and moderate or severe intractable leg pain should be considered for surgery. Before proceeding with surgery, radiographic imaging (computed tomography (CT) and/or MRI) should demonstrate clear evidence of neural compression that is congruent with the patient's signs and symptoms. Surgical decompression is limited to the site of neural compromise. This can be achieved by targeted laminotomy procedures, or if the pathology is more extensive, by multiple laminectomy procedures. A unilateral take-down of multifidus followed by spinous process osteotomies at the involved levels will afford an excellent exposure while minimising damage to the paraspinal musculature, the interspinous/supraspinous ligament complex and the facet joints.[1546] Provided the total of one facet joint is retained at each level, spinal instability should not result. Spinal fusion is not required in the vast majority of cases.

Zucherman et al.[1637] introduced an interspinous process decompression system (X-STOP) as an alternative to conservative treatment or decompressive surgery for patients with neurogenic intermittent claudication. The X-STOP device is implanted between the spinous processes and produces localised flexion of the motion segment, leading to an increase in the central canal dimensions. In a randomised controlled trial, the authors compared the X-STOP device to non-operative treatment and showed significantly better outcomes in the surgically treated group at 2 years. Brussee et al. however reported good outcomes in only 31% of patients when the X-STOP was used to treat neurogenic claudication.[205] Similarly, other authors have reported high failure rates when the X-STOP interspinous distraction device was used to treat lumbar spinal stenosis caused by degenerative spondylolisthesis.[1481]

SPONDYLOLYSIS

Spondylolysis is an acquired defect in the pars interarticularis most commonly affecting the L5 vertebra. Mechanical aetiology is considered in Chapter 11. The incidence is approximately 4.5% during the first year of school and is more common in boys than girls.[1237] The incidence of symptomatic pars defects in the young athletic population is much higher and is variously reported between 15% and 47%.[1220,1341] CT imaging suggests a prevalence of 11% in middle-aged adults,[707] which is higher than previous estimates based on plain radiographs, and with a three-times higher prevalence among men.[707] Tissue in the spondylolytic defect is reported to be fibrous, with no innervation,[987] so pain may arise from adjacent structures.

For those who fail conservative care, there are a number of surgical options. Direct repair of the pars defect has been shown to be effective for those with a normal disc, and it preserves intervertebral motion. Many different techniques have been described, including Buck's direct repair[208] (Fig. 19.2), Scott's wiring technique[1045] and Morscher's hook screw.[1007] Successful outcomes have been reported ranging from 63%[684] to 100%.[1423] Predictors of successful surgical outcome include age less than 25 years, spondylolysis of less than 4 mm, absence of disc degeneration, positive response to local anaesthetic infiltration of the pars interarticularis defect, method of surgical repair and motivation of the individual undergoing surgery.[332]

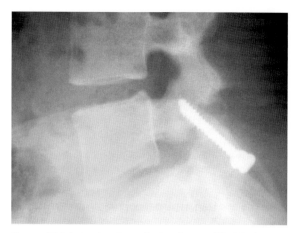

Figure 19.2 Lateral radiograph showing modified Buck's fusion for bilateral spondylolysis of L5. *(Reproduced from Debnath et al.[332] with permission of the British Editorial Society of Bone and Joint Surgery, London.)*

For those patients with established disc degeneration identified on MRI, the disc may be a significant contributor to the patient's pain. In such cases, most surgeons would advocate a spinal fusion to address both the pars defect and the degenerated disc as potential sources of pain.

Biomechanical studies performed on calf lumbar spines have shown that artificially induced bilateral interarticularis defects increase the intervertebral mobility not only at the involved level but also at the upper level adjacent to the spondylolysis.[978] The increased mobility of both the lytic segment and the adjacent level were significantly reduced by the Buck's screw repair. However if a pedicle screw system was applied across the involved segment, the mobility in the adjacent segment was increased. It appears that fixation of the pars defect alone causes less adjacent-level mechanical stress when compared with pedicle screw fixation of the affected motion segment.

Fixation techniques employed for the repair of spondylolytic defects have been compared biomechanically, using calf lumbar spines.[336] Four techniques were compared: (1) Scott's wiring technique (wire loops passed around each transverse process and tightened under the spinous process); (2) modified Scott's technique (wire loops around cortical screws placed in both pedicles and tightened under the spinous process); (3) Buck's technique; and (4) screw-rod-hook fixation. All fixation techniques significantly increased stiffness in the spondylolytic segment. The screw-rod-hook fixation and Buck's technique allowed the least motion across the spondylolytic defect when tested in flexion. The authors suggest that Buck's technique resists forces and movements in all directions, is low-profile and is less expensive than the screw-rod-hook system, but it remains technically demanding.

Screw breakage or nerve root irritation requiring screw removal has occurred following Buck's technique.[208,374] Other experiments have shown that the Buck's screw provides the stiffest and strongest repair followed closely by the Morscher hook screw, with the modified Scott repair being the least stiff.[748] The authors conclude that the Scott wiring of pars defects is a tension band repair that is loaded only in flexion. It is used to repair a defect whose probable cause is repetitive hyperextension of the spine and should be questioned on biomechanical grounds. Nevertheless, it is interesting to note that similar clinical results have been obtained with both Buck's technique and Scott's wiring technique in some reported series.[336]

The advantages of direct repair include a high rate of defect healing, preservation of intervertebral motion by avoidance of fusion across the disc and restoration of anatomy. Buck first reported the direct repair of a pars defect with a 4.5-mm stainless steel AO cortical lag screw in 1970.[208] The defect was packed with cancellous bone graft and the patient was allowed to mobilise immediately following surgery. In a series of 75 patients, satisfactory results were reported in 88%.[209] In 2003, Debnath et al.[332] reported on 22 young athletes who had undergone surgical treatment for lumbar spondylolysis: 19 underwent a Buck's fusion and three underwent a Scott's fusion. Of the 19 who underwent a Buck's fusion followed by a strict rehabilitation programme, 18 (95%) returned to sports activities after a mean of 7 months (range 4–10 months). The outcome in the three patients treated by Scott's fusion was not satisfactory: two patients developed a pseudarthrosis requiring a revision to an instrumented posterolateral fusion, and one showed no improvement in Oswestry Disability Index (ODI) and Short Form-36 (SF-36) scores despite a reverse-gantry CT scan confirming a sound union.

SPONDYLOLISTHESIS

Spondylolisthesis can be described as a shear or gliding displacement of a vertebral body relative to the one below. The most common displacement is a forward or anterior slip of the superior vertebral body. It is reported in 5–6% of caucasian males and 2–3% of caucasian females[1224] and can be classified into five[1582] or six[1583] categories (Table 19.1).

Meyerding in 1932[977] classified spondylolisthesis into grades based on the amount of slippage of the superior vertebral body relative to the vertebra below. Grade I indicates a slip of <25%, grade II 26–50%, grade III 51–75% and grade IV >75%. A complete (grade V) dislocation of L5 on S1 is termed a spondyloptosis. Approximately 60% of cases of spondylolisthesis are classified as grade I, 20–38% as grade II and less than 2% as grade III, IV or V.[1179] Progression of slippage is well documented in the

Table 19.1 Classification of spondylolisthesis[1583]	
Type 1	Congenital or dysplastic spondylolisthesis
Type 2	Isthmic spondylolisthesis
Type 3	Degenerative spondylolisthesis
Type 4	Traumatic spondylolisthesis
Type 5	Pathologic spondylolisthesis
Type 6	Postsurgical spondylolisthesis

skeletally immature. However, once skeletal maturity is reached, further slippage occurs in less than 5%.

Typically patients present with back pain, L5 nerve root pain and/or hamstring spasm. For patients aged over 30 years, it is unusual for spondylolisthesis to produce pain. Usually the pain results from secondary degenerative changes in the discs and facet joints. An MRI scan is essential in any patient with neurological symptoms. Conservative treatment includes exercises focusing on strengthening the back and abdominal muscles and selective foraminal epidural steroid injections for L5 radiculopathy.

For those who fail conservative measures, surgery may be considered. Möller and Hedlund[991] treated 111 patients with isthmic spondylolisthesis. All patients were randomly allocated to an exercise programme ($n = 34$) or to posterolateral fusion with or without transpedicular fixation ($n = 77$). Functional outcome (assessed by the disability rating index) and pain reduction were better in the surgically treated group when compared to the exercise group at both the 1- and 2-year follow-up assessments. Ekman et al.[391] reported a longer-term mean follow-up of 9 years on the same cohort and concluded that surgical treatment of patients with adult isthmic spondylolisthesis resulted in a significant but limited long-term improvement of pain and functional disability. The positive effect of fusion appears to deteriorate with time to a level of pain and functional disability similar to the natural history of symptomatic adult spondylolisthesis. A complicating factor here appears to be increased levels of adjacent-segment disc degeneration following fusion.[392]

For low-grade spondylolisthesis (Meyerding grade I and II), the surgical options include fusion in situ with autologous bone graft, or decompression and fusion in situ for those with objective evidence of radiculopathy, particularly at L5. Pedicle screw fixation has been added to increase fusion rate, although this has not been associated with improved clinical outcome (Fig. 19.3).

For high-grade slips (Meyerding grade III–V), combined anterior and posterior fusion has been suggested, using autogenous bone such as fibula or iliac crest. Slow gradual reduction by means of an external fixator followed by spinal with internal fixation led to 84.5% correction of slip

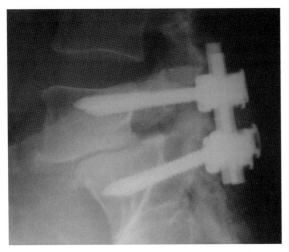

Figure 19.3 Lateral radiograph showing instrumented posterolateral fusion for Meyerding grade II spondylolisthesis at L5–S1. *(Reproduced from Freeman[444] with permission of Elsevier Ltd, Philadelphia.)*

and no neurological complications.[1559] Others have described total resection of L5 and spinal fusion from L4 to S1. The rationale for this surgery is that shortening facilitates the realignment of sagittal balance and reduces the risk of neurological impairment.[463]. However 5/16 patients had permanent neurological motor deficit following this technique. It is clear that attempts to reduce high-grade spondylolithesis should only be made by experienced surgeons in well-equipped centres.

FACET JOINT PAIN

The lumbar facet joints are a potential source of low-back pain and referred leg pain (Ch. 5). The term 'facet syndrome' was first coined by Ghormley in 1933.[490] The prevalence of facet joint involvement in low-back pain varies between 15 and 40%, with back pain caused solely by the facets in only 7%.[674,1283] Disc degeneration is often present with facet joint degeneration, but the relative contribution to low-back pain by either the facet joint or the disc varies, allowing triage of patients into predominantly facet joint pain or predominantly discogenic pain. It is possible to identify, through diagnostic testing, a very select group of patients with facet syndrome that can be treated successfully by radiofrequency facet joint denervation. Some authors use simple injection of local anaesthetic into the facet joint as a diagnostic aid,[411] whereas others emphasise the need to block the medial branch of the posterior primary ramus.[715]

Radiofrequency lumbar facet denervation has been evaluated in a prospective double-blind randomised trial of 31 patients with a history of at least 1 year of chronic low-back pain.[1467] Patients were selected on the basis of a positive response to a diagnostic nerve block and subsequently assigned randomly to one of two treatment groups. Patients in the radiofrequency group ($n = 15$) received an 80°C radiofrequency lesion to the dorsal ramus of the segmental nerve roots of L3–5. Patients in the control group ($n = 16$) underwent the same procedure, but without the use of radiofrequency current. At 3, 6 and 12 months after treatment there were significantly more successfully treated patients in the radiofrequency group than in the sham group.

DISCOGENIC LOW-BACK PAIN

The concept of 'discogenic pain' is not new. Indeed, Inman and Saunders in 1947 refer to pain arising from the disc.[665] In 1948 Lindblom[835] noted that discography could produce low-back pain and somatic referred pain. Crock defined the pathological entity of 'internal disc disruption' in 1970.[306] In this condition the affected disc is rendered painful by changes in its internal structure, while its external appearance remains normal (p. 205).

Provocative lumbar discography can define the internal architecture of the disc[46] and also assess whether discography reproduces typical low-back pain. Clinical outcomes following spinal fusion are improved if the preceding discogram was positive, compared to if it was negative.[292] However, clinical outcomes after circumferential fusion with and without discography were not statistically different.[878] Multiple studies by Carragee et al. have suggested that discography may be an unreliable indicator of the primary cause of illness, especially in the emotionally distressed or pain-sensitised individual,[253] and that the procedure can be harmful to the disc.[254]

There are a number of different treatment options for patients with chronic discogenic low-back pain, including intradiscal electrothermal therapy (IDET), total disc replacement, dynamic stabilisation and spinal fusion. Each of these will now be considered.

Intradiscal electrothermal therapy

The application of heat to thermocoagulate nervous tissue has been used for many years for the treatment of low-back pain. Techniques including percutaneous radiofrequency facet joint denervation have been successful for patients with facet syndrome.[556]

Saal and Saal investigated the treatment of discogenic low-back pain by application of heat. An intradiscal thermal catheter is inserted percutaneously and navigated to the posterior annulus using two-plane fluoroscopic guidance[1231] (Fig. 19.4). The Spinecath intradiscal catheter (NeuroTherm, Wilmington, MA, USA) contains a

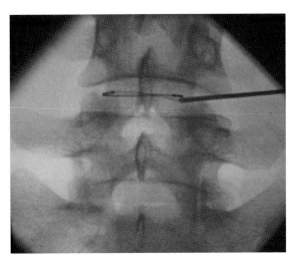

Figure 19.4 Anteroposterior radiograph showing final intradiscal electrothermal therapy catheter position within the L4–5 intervertebral disc. *(Reproduced from Freeman et al.[442] with permission.)*

thermal-resistive heating coil in its terminal 5 cm which can be heated to 90°C. According to Saal and Saal, the standard heating protocol creates annular temperatures of between 60 and 65°C. Following the procedure, patients receive a soft corset for 6 weeks followed initially by stretching exercises and then by trunk stabilisation exercises. IDET improved function and sitting tolerance in 62 patients at 1-year follow-up[1231] and benefits remained at 2 years.[1232] For patients with decreased disc height (>30% loss of disc height) who had treatment at multiple levels, the outcome was less favourable than those with multilevel treatment who had preserved disc height. Karasek and Bogduk[717] reported on 35 patients treated with intradiscal thermal annuloplasty and compared them to a 'convenience control' group of 17 patients who had been denied insurance authorisation for IDET and were subsequently treated with a physical rehabilitation programme. At 3 months only 1 control patient obtained any significant pain relief compared with 23 out of 35 patients in the IDET group. Derby et al.[339] reported a 1-year outcome study on 32 patients undergoing IDET. Overall 62.5% had a favourable outcome, 12.5% non-favourable and 25% no change. Patients with excellent or good catheter positions and those with low-pressure-sensitive discs on preoperative discography had the most favourable outcomes.

The mechanism of action of IDET may involve a combination of thermocoagulation of native nociceptors and ingrown unmyelinated nerve fibres, plus annular collagen shrinkage stabilising annular fissures.[1231,1232] However, Freeman et al.[443] were unable to show denervation of a posterior annular lesion in an animal model. Kleinstueck

et al.[759] showed that IDET increased motion and decreased stiffness in cadaveric lumbar discs. Pollintine et al.[1140] showed that IDET reduced the size of compressive stress concentrations in cadaveric discs and suggested that this could represent an increase in the cohesiveness between regions of disrupted annulus, consistent with a 'welding' effect on the collagen network. However, the exact mechanism whereby IDET exerts its effect is still unknown.

Two randomised controlled trials have compared IDET to a placebo. Pauza et al.[1109] randomised 64 patients – 37 to IDET and 27 to sham treatment – and found that improvements in the IDET group were greater than in the sham group. However, the advantage for IDET patients over sham patients was only 1.3 points on the visual analogue score (VAS) and 7 points on the ODI. There were no significant differences in SF-36 bodily pain or physical function scores between the two groups, and IDET was not a universally successful treatment in this study. Some 50% of patients did not benefit appreciably or at all.

Freeman et al.[442] conducted a prospective randomised double-blind placebo-controlled trial. A total of 57 patients were recruited: 38 were randomised to IDET and 19 to placebo. There were no significant changes in Low-back Outcome Score, Zung Depression Inventory, Modified Somatic Perception Questionnaire or SF-36 scores in either group, and the authors were unable to show any significant benefit of IDET over placebo.

There are important differences between these two studies. The subjects in the Freeman study had higher levels of disability as measured by the ODI and SF-36 physical function scores when compared to the subjects in Pauza's study. Other differences relate to the inclusion criteria, study populations, how the sham procedures were performed, the blinding procedure, and how success and the mean clinically important difference were defined.

It is clear from the literature that highly selected groups of patients are required to show even a marginal benefit from the procedure. IDET appears not to be beneficial for the vast majority of patients with chronic discogenic low-back pain.

Total disc replacement

The attraction of disc replacement is that it removes the putative pain source, entirely and permanently, while retaining (or restoring) normal spinal function. There has been one attempt (in China) to transplant fresh-frozen human cervical discs from cadavers to patients, and this met with moderate success at 5 years.[1225] All other attempts at total disc replacement have used artifical discs of various designs.

The first total disc replacement (Link SB Charité, Waldemar Link, Hamburg, Germany) was implanted in 1984.[839] There has been renewed interest in such devices. The aims of total disc replacement (Ch. 18) include elimination of the discogenic pain source, restoration of disc height and canal volume, retention of the facet joints and restoration of the kinematic and load-sharing properties of the motion segment and for the patient to experience pain relief and return of function. When compared to spinal fusion, total disc replacement may eliminate the unsatisfactory results observed following pseudarthrosis, donor site morbidity, adjacent-level disc degeneration and posterior spinal muscle damage produced by posterior spinal fusions.

There are two main types of total disc replacement:

1. Low-friction total disc replacement, e.g. Charité artificial disc (DePuy Spine, Raynham, MA), ProDisc-L (Synthes Spine, West Chester, PA), FlexiCore intervertebral disc (Stryker Spine, Allendale, NJ)
2. Compliant total disc replacements, e.g. AcroFlex lumbar disc replacement (Depuy Spine, Raynham, MA), CADisc-L (Ranier Technology, Cambridge, UK).

Low-friction total disc replacement

The articulating surfaces for these devices are either metal on polyethylene or metal on metal. The Charité artificial disc comprises two cobalt chromium alloy endplates and an ultra-high molecular weight polyethylene sliding core. The ProDisc-L total disc replacement (Fig. 19.5) comprises two cobalt-chromium molybdenum alloy endplates with central keels and ultra-high-molecular-weight

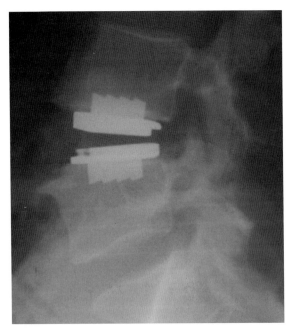

Figure 19.5 Lateral radiograph showing Prodisc-L (Synthes, Switzerland) replacement at L4–5. *(Reproduced from Freeman[444] with permission of Elsevier Ltd, Philadelphia.)*

polyethylene convex inlay, which slides into the inferior endplate and articulates with the superior endplate. The FlexiCore intervertebral disc is a metal-on-metal artificial lumbar total disc replacement composed of a retained ball-and-socket device positioned between two base plates. Three randomised controlled trials and 16 prospective cohort studies have been published relating to total disc replacement.[1464] Blumenthal et al. published the first prospective randomised multicentre study comparing lumbar total disc replacement to lumbar fusion after 2 years.[150] This study involved 304 patients randomised in a 2 : 1 ratio to treatment with the Charité artificial disc or the control group which received an instrumented anterior lumbar interbody fusion. The study demonstrated clinical outcomes following lumbar total disc replacement to be at least equivalent to those observed following anterior lumbar interbody fusion. Guyer et al. reported on the same study with 5-year follow-up: no statistically significant differences in clinical outcomes were identified between groups.[544]

Zigler et al. published a prospective randomised multicentre study of the ProDisc-L total disc replacement compared to circumferential fusion for the treatment of one-level degenerative disc disease, followed up for 2 years.[1631] In this study, the ProDisc-L total disc replacement was found to be safe and efficacious and, in properly chosen patients, the disc replacement group had superior outcomes compared to the circumferential fusion group.

Sasso et al. reported the 2-year preliminary results of a prospective randomised trial of metal-on-metal artificial lumbar total disc replacement.[1248] The authors demonstrated that the FlexiCore lumbar total disc replacement compared favourably to circumferential fusion for the treatment of lumbar degenerative disc disease.

Compliant total disc replacement

The Acroflex elastomeric total disc replacement consists of two titanium endplates bound together by a hexane-based polyolefin rubber core and was designed to replicate the elasticity of the normal human disc. Fraser et al. reviewed the AcroFlex design and clinical results in 28 patients in whom the device was implanted between 1998 and 1999.[439] The mean improvement at 24 months was 23 points using the ODI and 22 points using the low-back outcome score. Complications included one case of autofusion and one case of partial disc expulsion. However, of particular concern was the observation on fine-cut CT of rubber tears in 10/28 (36%) of patients. The majority were mid-substance anteroinferior peripheral tears. Subsequent imaging revealed osteolysis and periannular ossification. Eight of 28 (29%) patients subsequently underwent revision surgery where the implant was removed and an interbody fusion supplemented by pedicle screw fixation and posterolateral grafting was carried out. This study highlighted the potential for wear particle formation with

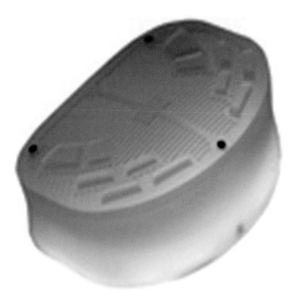

Figure 19.6 A compliant total disc replacement (CADisc-L, Ranier Technology, Cambridge, UK).

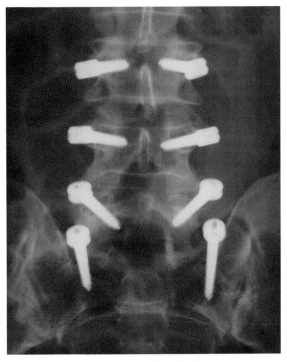

Figure 19.7 Anteroposterior radiograph showing Dynesys (Zimmer, UK) stabilisation of L3–S1. The polyester cords and cylindrical spacers cannot be seen as they are not radiopaque.

resultant osteolysis and secondly the development of peri-annular ossification leading to autofusion. As a result of the disruption of the rubber and the associated osteolysis, the AcroFlex lumbar total disc replacement was withdrawn from the market.[441]

The quest for a viscoelastic device has continued, with attention turning to novel materials such as polycarbonate urethane. The CADisc-L (Ranier Technology, Cambridge, UK) is one such device (Fig. 19.6) with a lower modulus nucleus surrounded by a higher modulus annulus, and even stiffer endplates that allow primary and secondary fixation.[545] Theoretically the graduated interface between the component parts and the lack of moving parts should reduce the risk of long-term fatigue failure. The perceived advantages on device longevity and protection of the adjacent disc will take years to realise, and demand careful long-term follow-up of all patients undergoing this type of procedure. Unpublished clinical results at 1 year were reported to be much better than with previous devices.

Dynamic stabilisation

A number of devices aim to unload the disc and preserve motion while stabilising the motion segment. They may be used alone or in conjunction with rigid stabilisation to 'top off' the proximal segment adjacent to the fusion in order to prevent its accelerated degeneration. Perhaps the best known is the Dynesys or Dynamic Neutralisation System (Zimmer, UK), which consists of titanium alloy pedicle screws, polyester cords and polycarbonate urethane cylindrical spacers[1373] (Fig. 19.7). The cord is passed through the pedicle screw head into the hollow cylindrical spacer and on to the next pedicle screw, thereby preventing excessive compression between the screw heads. The stabilising cord carries tensile forces and the spacers resist compressive forces. The purpose of the system is to establish mobile load transfer and controlled motion of the segment in all planes.

Recent biomechanical studies on cadaveric spines found the Dynesys system to provide greater flexibility in extension and rotation but similar stiffness in flexion and lateral bending when compared to rigid fixation.[1270] Initial clinical results in a multicentre trial by the originators of the device have been encouraging, although screw loosening and adjacent segment disease have been observed. Grob et al.[533] studied 31 patients who had been instrumented with Dynesys. The primary indication for surgery was degenerative disease (disc/stenosis) with associated instability. Thirteen of 31 patients (42%) underwent additional decompression at the time of the original surgery. Within 2 years, six of 31 (19%) had revision surgery. Overall, 67% of patients reported an improvement in their back symptoms, 30% were the same and 3% were worse. Both back and leg pain were moderately high 2 years after instrumentation with Dynesys. Only half of the patients declared the operation had improved their overall quality of life, and fewer than half reported improvements in functional capacity. These results do not support the notion that semirigid fixation results in better patient-oriented outcomes than those typical of spinal fusion. A randomised study is underway, and the results are eagerly awaited.

Spinal fusion

Spinal fusion addresses both disc degeneration and facet joint arthropathy. The aim is to eliminate movement completely from the motion segment in the hope this will provide pain relief and an improvement in functional status. It is the last resort in surgical terms and can have unpredictable results, with satisfactory clinical outcome ranging from 46% to 82% depending on the series.[1418,1554] The most important aspects for the attainment of a solid arthrodesis are meticulous preparation of the graft bed, and accurate placement of an adequate amount of good-quality bone graft material. A wide range of techniques are available to achieve a solid arthrodesis, some of which will now be discussed.

Posterolateral fusion

This may be achieved without the use of instrumentation, using either a midline incision with wide stripping of the erector spinae muscle, or a muscle-splitting approach described by Wiltse et al.[1581] Bone graft is usually harvested from the posterior iliac crest and placed in the posterolateral gutter on the decorticated transverse processes and alar of the sacrum. The patient is placed in a lumbosacral orthosis for 3 months. Pseudarthrosis rates increase with the number of levels fused. Jackson et al.[673] quote a 3.5–10% pseudarthrosis rate for a one-level posterolateral fusion, a 15–20% pseudarthrosis rate for a two-level posterolateral fusion and a 25–33% pseudarthrosis rate for a three-level fusion. The pseudarthrosis rate is higher in individuals who smoke or who take non-steroidal anti-inflammatory medication on a regular basis.

Instrumented posterolateral fusion

The addition of pedicle screw fixation to a posterolateral fusion reduces the risk of pseudarthrosis. Brodsky et al. found that posterolateral fusions without instrumentation led to a 31.5% rate of pseudarthrosis compared to 13% pseudarthrosis with instrumentation.[198]

Posterior lumbar interbody fusion

This technique was popularised by Cloward in 1953.[288] It allows a posterior decompression, restoration of the anterior-column weight-bearing function and a rigid posterior fixation. It has the advantage of removing the disc,

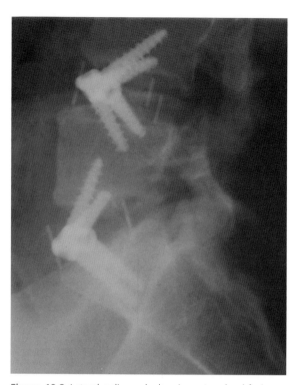

Figure 19.8 Lateral radiograph showing a two-level fusion at L4–5 and L5–S1 for discographically proven discogenic pain. Stand-alone anterior lumbar interbody fusion devices have been used (STALIF, Surgicraft, UK).

which is an important factor bearing in mind that discogenic pain can persist despite a solid posterior fusion.

Anterior lumbar interbody fusion

This is generally carried out via a retroperitoneal approach. Care must be taken in the male as the superior hypogastric plexus may be injured where it lies over the anterior aspect of L5, possibly leading to retrograde ejaculation. The discectomy is carried out and bone graft inserted into the disc space. Several options are available, including cortico-cancellous blocks, milled bone tightly packed in a supporting cage such as titanium mesh, femoral cortical ring allograft and carbon fibre or polyethylethyl ketone implants (Fig. 19.8).

Combined anterior and posterior fusion

Anterior and posterior fusion results in a higher fusion rate,[1055] but this must be balanced against the increased risk of morbidity. In some series of this type of surgery the complication rate can be as high as 30%.[451,955]

Interbody cage devices

Interbody cage devices to assist interbody fusion continue to gain popularity in the surgical management of chronic low-back pain. These devices strive to correct the existing mechanical deformation, provide segmental stability until arthrodesis is obtained, provide the best possible environment for successful arthrodesis and achieve this with limited morbidity.[1545] There are three basic structures: (1) horizontal cylinders; (2) vertical rings; and (3) open-box configurations. Their aim is to restore disc height, lordosis and sagittal balance, while placing the remaining annular fibres under tension. Cages can be made from titanium, carbon fibre composites or allograft such as femoral cortical rings. A major disadvantage of titanium cages is that they prevent adequate radiographic demonstration of fusion. Also the Young's modulus for titanium is approximately 150 GPa, whereas that of cortical bone is approximately 12 GPa. One study comparing femoral ring allograft to a titanium cage in circumferential lumbar spinal fusion[955] showed superior clinical outcome when a femoral ring allograft was used in comparison to a titanium cage. Box cages provide strain and stress-shielding of the incorporated graft and may have a higher incidence of pseudarthrosis. Titanium cages may provide abnormal loading of the endplate. Over time, femoral ring allograft is seen to remodel according to Wolff's law and may allow subtle changes in segmental lordosis over time.

Does spinal fusion reduce discogenic back pain?

Fritzell et al. reported a randomised, controlled multicentre study with 2-year follow-up completed by an independent observer.[450] A total of 294 patients were entered into the study. Patients with spondylolisthesis were excluded from the study. The primary aim was to compare non-surgical treatment (i.e. commonly used physical therapy) to surgical intervention. Seventy-five patients were randomised to physical therapy and 225 patients to surgical intervention. Within the surgical group, 75 patients underwent a non-instrumented posterolateral fusion plus brace, 75 patients underwent an instrumented posterolateral fusion and the remaining 75 underwent a circumferential fusion (instrumented posterolateral fusion plus either anterior lumbar interbody fusion or posterior lumbar interbody fusion) plus brace. The surgical group demonstrated an absolute improvement of 21 points on the VAS, 11.6 points on the ODI and 7.7 points on the Zung depression index. Overall 63% were 'better' or 'much better' and 36% returned to work following surgery. In the non-surgical group the VAS improved only 4.3 points, the ODI improved 2.8 points and the Zung depression index improved by 2.7 points. Twenty-nine per cent of the group were 'much better' or 'better' and 13% returned to work.

The authors conclude that lumbar fusion diminished pain and decreased disability 'more efficiently' than commonly used non-surgical treatment. However, another randomised clinical trial (of lumbar instrumented fusion versus cognitive intervention and exercises) found no significant difference in outcome, although both groups showed significant improvement.[203]

The Medical Research Council spine stabilisation trial recruited 349 participants with chronic low-back pain who were considered candidates for spinal fusion.[410] A total of 176 participants were assigned to surgery and 173 to rehabilitation. Type of surgical intervention was not specified and included posterior stabilisation with the Graf ligament (no longer in use) and all forms of spinal fusion. An intensive rehabilitation programme was based on a 3-week (15-day) model of exercise therapy, spinal stabilisation techniques and education using cognitive-behavioural principles. The mean ODI improved 12.5 points for the surgical group and 8.7 points for the rehabilitation group. The difference only just reached the predefined minimal clinically important difference. The authors concluded that both groups reported reductions in disability during the 2 years of follow-up, possibly unrelated to the interventions. When the potential risk and additional cost of surgery are considered, it is clear that all patients should go through a formal functional restoration programme before committing to surgical intervention.[1199] A number of them may improve sufficiently that surgical intervention can be avoided.

Which type of spinal fusion?

Fritzell et al. compared three surgical techniques of fusion for chronic low-back pain as part of the previously reported randomised controlled trial.[451] A total of 222 patients underwent surgery: 73 received a non-instrumented posterolateral fusion, 74 received a posterolateral fusion combined with an internal fixation device and 75 received a posterolateral fusion with an internal fixation device and interbody fusion, either anterior lumbar interbody fusion or posterior lumbar interbody fusion. All three surgical techniques resulted in a substantial reduction in pain and disability, but there was no significant difference between the groups. The more complex fusions had longer operation times, higher blood transfusion requirements and more days in hospital. Complication rates were 6% for the non-instrumented posterolateral fusion, 16% for the posterolateral fusion combined with internal fixation device and 31% for the posterolateral fusion combined with anterior lumbar interbody fusion or posterior lumbar interbody fusion. Fusion rates were 72%, 87% and 91% respectively. The authors conclude that all fusion techniques used in the study reduced pain and improved function. There was no obvious disadvantage in using the least demanding surgical technique of posterolateral fusion without internal fixation.

SUMMARY

Greater understanding of the pathophysiology underlying the symptoms of sciatica has resulted in a reduction in the number of patients undergoing surgery for this condition. Successful treatment of radicular pain with targeted foraminal epidural steroid injections has resulted in fewer patients requiring lumbar discectomy.[4] Exciting results with anti-TNF agents such as infliximab (p. 239) may mean that sciatica becomes more and more a condition that is treated medically.

Symptoms of CES demand urgent investigation with MRI and represent a neurological emergency. If confirmed on MRI, urgent surgical decompression should be carried out, preferably within 24 hours.

For patients with symptomatic spondylolysis that has not responded to conservative therapy, direct repair of the defect using a modified Buck's fusion appears successful in the majority of cases, provided the intervening disc has not been damaged.

Adult isthmic spondylolisthesis was treated more efficiently by posterolateral fusion than by an exercise programme in at least one randomised controlled trial.[991] However the positive effect of fusion appears to deteriorate with time to a level of pain and functional disability similar to the natural history of symptomatic adult spondylolisthesis.

For newer treatments aimed at discogenic back pain, the evidence is less clear. On the one hand, exciting recent results suggest that discogenic back pain may be treatable by injection therapies aimed at blocking nociception.[1122] On the other hand, there is conflicting evidence on the efficacy of IDET, and it seems unlikely that it will benefit significant numbers of patients. The Charité artificial disc replacement is at least equivalent to lumbar arthrodesis at one level, up to 5 years following surgery. It remains to be seen whether disc replacement is beneficial over two levels and whether the long-term outcome of lumbar disc replacement will be superior to that of spinal fusion. The quest for viscoelastic total disc replacement continues; however biodevice longevity for these devices has yet to be demonstrated. The evidence for dynamic stabilisation of the spine is weak, with no randomised controlled trials currently available.

Spinal fusion for discogenic back pain remains controversial. Whilst there is level 1 evidence showing efficacy of spinal fusion techniques over 'usual physical therapy',[450] there is growing evidence that surgical treatment of patients results in a significant but limited long-term improvement of pain and functional disability. The benefits of spinal fusion appear to deteriorate with time, perhaps reflecting the natural history of symptomatic degenerative disc disease.

There is conflicting evidence regarding the type of spinal fusion. Anterior and posterior fusions appear to have the highest fusion rate but this does not necessarily improve clinical outcome. One must be aware of the increased morbidity associated with this type of invasive surgery.

Although there have been significant advances recently in the technology available to spine surgeons, there is no immediate prospect of a surgical 'quick fix' for all, or even most, patients. News of each novel intervention travels fast, and one of the main challenges for spine surgeons is to ensure that their patients' expectations are realistic, because having one's expectations fulfilled is an important predictor of a good outcome from spinal surgery.[905]

Chapter |20|

Medicolegal considerations

INTRODUCTION

Low-back disorders frequently give rise to litigation concerning medical negligence or occupational causation. Litigation and compensation issues in turn influence the outcomes of low-back disorders. The generic label 'disorder' is used here to encompass both spinal pathology and the pain and disability that may result, but specific terms will be used in certain contexts. The term 'injury' necessarily will apply for claims under workers' compensation systems.

The aim of this chapter is to raise some biomechanical issues and consider the available scientific evidence concerning three common medicolegal questions:

1. Can a given incident or work practice be held responsible for an individual's back disorder?
2. In the absence of such an incident or work practice, would that individual's back be likely to develop the disorder?
3. Would the disorder be likely to place the individual at a disadvantage on the open labour market?

This is a tall order, and there will be no definitive answers, partly because the underlying science is still developing, and partly because there will inevitably be a need for legal interpretation of the facts. The manner in which cases are handled and the courts' function varies from country to country and from context to context but the principle is the same: the Court often requires expert opinion in order to assess the strengths and weaknesses of those facts.

The Court may be faced with reports from a number of experts, and must choose which to accept in coming to a judgement. In the UK, most medicolegal issues are decided under an adversarial system. The process is guided by the Civil Procedure Rules, which are intended to facilitate access to civil justice by giving the Court the power to limit expert evidence to that which it sees as being both pertinent and necessary. What this means in practice is a reduction in the use of experts, often with the appointment of a single joint expert to help the Court decide some lower-value claims. In essence, the Court is now looking for an unbiased opinion that can be substantiated by scientific evidence, rather than an opinion potentially biased in favour of the party paying the expert's fees. It follows that the Court will increasingly favour the evidence from experts who display impartiality and are able to offer a scientific basis for their evidence. In addition, experts are required, where there is a range of opinion, to summarise that range of opinion and give reasons for their own opinion.

This chapter offers a synthesis of the scientific evidence relevant to the questions posed above. It attempts to place the problem of low-back disorders into a scientific perspective that might help experts to comply with their duty to the Court, and may help lawyers to interpret the reports they receive from experts.

There are two fundamental issues in most personal injury claims: causation and liability. A claimant must persuade the Court on both counts to succeed in being awarded damages. The matter of liability for the injury, being context-dependent, is largely outside the scope of this chapter, which concerns only the medical and biological aspects of back disorders without attempting to interpret relevant legislation. However, one intriguing fundamental question relating to liability arises naturally from the evidence in this chapter, and that is: who is liable for genetic predisposition to disease? Is it the patient, the employer or the state? If this wider issue is eventually laid at the door of the state, then medicolegal disputes concerning back injuries could lead to payments by the state to the injured party, because genetic predisposition is arguably the largest underlying cause of back pain and disability (Chs. 6 and 7).

if the circumstances were different? Does the fact that he had been absent from work due to back pain 2 years previously make a difference? What if he regularly worked out at the gym? Would it make a difference if he was aged 55 and had radiographic evidence of lumbar disc degeneration, or magnetic resonance imaging (MRI) evidence of a disc prolapse? Was he likely to develop back pain anyway and, if so, when? Is he at greater risk of future back pain and, if so, when, how frequently and how severe? Is he prevented from returning to a manual job? Would the presence of leg pain make a difference? Suppose that the weights being handled were of the order of 25 kg – would that have an influence? Alternatively, suppose that he had been transferred to the packing job only a few days previously, and his pain came on quite suddenly – are those significant factors? What if he had complained of pain some time before the onset of symptoms – would that be relevant?

These are typical scenarios and questions on which the Court must endeavour to make a fair and reasoned judgement. There are no simple answers, and this chapter does not purport to provide them, for that is rightly the responsibility of the Court.

BACKGROUND ISSUES

A simple mechanistic model of injury suggests that if an exposure is to be implicated in causation, there must be a cogent temporal and biomechanical relationship between exposure and injury. Furthermore, for the injury to be said to have occurred there should be some objective evidence that something has been damaged. This is readily seen in the case of a fractured hip resulting from a fall: there is an exposure to a mechanical force that conceivably could break bone; it occurred at an identifiable point in time prior to the injury; and the resulting damage can be revealed radiographically. Whilst some alleged back disorders can fit such a model, most do not.

For example, take the case of a 35-year-old male book packer who has worked for a printer packing books (in 7-kg packs) for some years. He gradually becomes aware of mild back pain over a period of weeks, which seems to be aggravated at work and gradually deteriorates, culminating in an inability to continue the job because of pain. Evidence presented elsewhere in this book suggests that, in this case, there is a lack of a clear temporal or biomechanical relationship between the exposure and development of symptoms, and there is unlikely to be objectively identifiable mechanical damage. Instead, we have a report of symptoms that are clearly made worse by work, but there is no obvious triggering event and no detectable lesion. The man is convinced that repeatedly taking books from the production line and putting them on a pallet was the cause of his back pain – but is he really injured? What

EPIDEMIOLOGY

Before bringing biomechanics to bear on the matter, it is worth reiterating some of the information from Chapter 6. It is imperative that the issue of causation is viewed against the background of the epidemiology of back pain.

Back pain is a symptom that afflicts most people at some point in their lives, usually in the absence of a relevant, clinically detectable source. For many it is a recurrent complaint, and for a few it results in chronic disability. This pattern does not have a close statistical correlation with exposure to obvious physical stressors (including work); it has been observed in schoolchildren, sedentary workers and non-workers; it is the same in males and females, the physically fit and the unfit; and training in working practices (such as manual handling) has not been shown to influence the pattern substantially. Work loss is certainly related to physical exposures, but it is also related to psychosocial factors. Age-related degenerative changes in the spine, as detected by imaging techniques, are influenced by environmental exposures, but the strength of association is swamped by genetic factors which influence physical and metabolic events within each person's back. Extreme physical demands have been related to reduced intervertebral disc height, which may or may not have been symptomatic.[187] More moderate physical demands (lifting and driving) have been related to symptomatic disc prolapse,[732,1011] but psychosocial factors are also related to pathology and symptoms.[168]

Epidemiology, by the nature of its methods, paints a broad picture – it cannot, nor does it attempt to, explain what actually happens to an individual. Yet its messages cannot be ignored, and it offers an important background to the legal question (in the UK): on the balance of probabilities, was this injury caused by the alleged event/circumstances? It is appropriate to bear in mind the distinction between the presence of symptoms, the reporting of back pain, attributing symptoms to work, reporting an injury, seeking healthcare, loss of time from work and long-term damage (Ch. 6). These matters have different determinants that are important from a medicolegal (as well as clinical) perspective, so they cannot simply be lumped together. It would be irrational to suggest that back injuries do not occur, but what is at issue is whether the particular circumstances of the case are conducive with the alleged injury. Largely leaving aside the difficult matters of diagnostic veracity and consequent disability, the following sections discuss the biomechanical issues pertinent to expert evidence offered to the Court.

UNDERLYING AND PRECIPITATING CAUSES OF BACK DISORDERS

Most back disorders do not have a single cause. Underlying factors (including the influences of genetic inheritance and age) may render certain tissues vulnerable to mechanical loading, so that injury or fatigue failure is then precipitated during a particular activity or incident. Sometimes tissue vulnerability plays the dominant role, so that a back disorder follows normal everyday loading. On other occasions, a back disorder is precipitated by a loading event which is severe enough to injure all but the strongest backs. Generally, however, it is useful to consider both underlying and precipitating causes of the problem.

ALL BACKS ARE MORE OR LESS VULNERABLE TO INJURY

Epidemiological studies suggest that up to 60% of back pain[574,867] and 30–75% of disc degeneration[113,116,117,1240] is associated with genetic inheritance, with the precise heritability depending on factors such as gender, age and the definition of back pain. This statistical jargon just means that two features (back pain and a specific genetic inheritance) are often found together in the same person. An association does not necessarily mean that one feature causes the other.

Although the genetic influence on back disorders is large, it is poorly understood. In rare cases, an unfavourable variety (polymorphism) of a particular gene can be held responsible for a medical problem, such as when a specific mutation of the collagen type II gene leads inexorably to failure of articular cartilage and severe joint disease.[1167] Usually, however, polymorphisms of several or many genes contribute to a greater or lesser extent to a person's predisposition to most common diseases. For example, intervertebral disc degeneration is known to be influenced by variants of the genes for collagen type IX, for proteoglycans and for vitamin D metabolism (p. 61). Another known risk factor for back pain that has some genetic basis is a long stiff back.[36] Other genetic risk factors could possibly include physical characteristics such as small discs, a heavy body or small internal lever arms (which would lead to increased muscle forces, as illustrated in Figure 9.2). Genetically determined risk factors could even involve inadequate proprioception or neuromuscular control, which would increase the risk of accidents, and psychosocial factors, which could increase the risk of them being reported as injuries.

Genetic predisposition to back disorders is important, but rarely decisive. The environment must still play a role, because defective genes are present from the moment of conception, whereas tissue degeneration and failure do not normally occur for a long time after birth (in the case of disc failure, 30–50 years after). Even then it is generally those tissues that are subjected to most mechanical loading that tend to be severely affected, such as the lower lumbar discs. Thoracic discs rarely show advanced degenerative changes,[1046] even though their cells contain the same genes as the lumbar discs. Evidently, environmental influences such as mechanical loading can contribute to tissue failure in addition to genetic predisposition.

Genetic vulnerability is modified by age, which leads to progressive reductions in the strength and stiffness of skeletal tissues.[3,734,1123] Age-related vulnerability to spinal disorders may also include the accumulation of fatigue 'wear-and-tear' damage, and the slow biochemical process of non-enzymatic glycation which leaves cartilaginous tissues more brittle (p. 95). Also, of course, an older person has had more opportunity to become involved in an accident. In the case of intervertebral disc prolapse, tissue vulnerability does not increase relentlessly with age: it appears to peak between 35 and 50 years, and then decreases.[1348] This could be due to the fact that certain disc injuries are less likely to occur when the nucleus pulposus becomes dehydrated, as it generally does in old age.

A closely related cause of tissue vulnerability is fatigue loading, which can propagate microdamage throughout the tissue so that failure occurs at only 30–45% of the normal failure load (Table 11.2). Fatigue damage may partly explain age-related weakening, but the two processes should not be equated. An abrupt increase in the level of physical activity over a period of just a few days or longer could give rise to fatigue damage, even though the age-related changes are negligible in such a time span. A more gradual change to hard physical work could have the opposite effect: it could lead to hypertrophy and strengthening of spinal tissues ('work hardening' or adaptive remodelling: Fig. 7.11) so that the spine becomes less vulnerable to mechanical damage.

A fourth cause of tissue vulnerability is prior injury. Poorly vascularised tissues such as large tendons and intervertebral discs have only a limited capacity to heal (Ch. 7) so that some degree of weakness can remain for years, if not for life. Links between tissue failure and pain are complicated by pain sensitisation effects (p. 205) so it is conceivable that a painful injury could be largely attributable to a previous injury that produced only mild symptoms. This is not very likely, however, if that previous injury involved tissues such as muscle or bone which are capable of rapid and full healing. A previous history of back pain is highly predictive of future pain (p. 57), but it cannot always be assumed that a previous injury predisposes to future injury: it depends very much on the tissue involved, and on the age and health of the individual concerned. And it must be borne in mind that back pain is frequently a recurrent phenomenon unrelated to physical exposures.

Prior injury and fatigue damage are both capable of instigating cell-mediated degenerative changes in affected tissues, leading to inferior biochemical composition and reduced strength (Ch. 15). It is also possible that some primary disease process (other than the ones considered above) could leave a tissue vulnerable to subsequent mechanical damage. However, most of the evidence indicates that cell-mediated degenerative changes usually follow tissue damage rather than precede it, at least in the intervertebral disc (p. 198).

Because there are so many causes of tissue vulnerability, it is inappropriate to label any individual as having either a 'vulnerable' or a 'normal' back. Vulnerability should be assessed on a continuous scale, with a person's position on that scale depending on all of the factors mentioned above. To insist that a back is either vulnerable or normal can lead to circular definitions, such as when a medicolegal report asserts that: 'this disc failed because it was vulnerable (or degenerated)', while at the same time maintaining that 'this disc must have been vulnerable/ degenerated because it failed in response to mechanical loading'. Thinking about the epidemiology, it is perhaps odd that we consider people with back pain to have a bad or weak back when we don't consider people with recurrent headache to have a 'bad head'! In the medicolegal context, it is desirable to attempt to identify the nature and extent of any tissue vulnerability. Medical reports presented to the Court frequently refer to a condition as being 'constitutional', which broadly can be defined as 'something that is inherent in the nature of a person', and is thus not the result of some outside force for which compensation should be awarded. Science is now showing that this seemingly simple concept is far from simple. The concept of vulnerability can impact on issues of liability: for example, should a worker be held responsible for his own

genes, or age, and should his present employer be held responsible for fatigue damage sustained in a previous occupation? These difficult problems will not be considered further here.

MECHANISMS OF INJURY AND FATIGUE FAILURE

Descriptions of injury mechanisms to spinal tissues, and the forces required to cause them, are given in Chapter 11. The site and nature of injury depend on variable factors, including the following:

- the time of day (p. 184)
- the speed of loading (p. 108)
- the curvature (posture) of the lumbar spine at the time of maximal loading (p. 176)
- the age of the subject (p. 96) and the degenerative state of the tissues (see above).

CAN MECHANICAL LOADING CAUSE A NORMAL DISC TO PROLAPSE?

This particular question is often raised in medicolegal cases, even though it has been answered long ago (in the affirmative) by mechanical experiments, albeit on cadaveric and animal tissues (p. 153). The relevance of these experiments to living spines has been justified at length (p. 159), and the mechanism of prolapse has been explained in detail by mathematical models (p. 157). There is, then, a challenge to the previously held view (the stuff of science!); personal dislike, or ignorance, of new evidence should not be confused with scientific debate. The new evidence, from a large and growing number of scientific publications (Ch. 11), indicates that:

- Disc prolapse (or herniation) should never be equated with disc degeneration. Prolapse is a particular feature of some degenerated discs in which there is relative displacement of nucleus pulposus tissue through the retaining annulus fibrosus. Prolapse is more closely related to mechanical loading than most of the other features of a degenerated disc.
- Nor should disc prolapse be equated with disc bulging: all discs bulge to a certain extent, and bulging usually increases with age, but to suggest that every bulging disc is prolapsed would be equivalent to asserting that every middle-aged protruding stomach represents an abdominal hernia. An MRI study reported 'moderate or severe disc prolapse' in 1.6% of middle-aged male discs, as compared to 'disc-bulging' in 15.1%.[1488]

- Most cadaveric lumbar intervertebral discs aged 30–60 years can be made to prolapse in the laboratory if loaded severely in bending and compression (Ch. 11).
- A higher proportion of L4–5 and L5–1 discs aged 40–50 years can be made to prolapse.
- A component of lateral bending and/or torsion facilitates prolapse.
- There is no evidence to suggest that any degenerative condition (other than normal ageing) precedes prolapse in these specimens.
- Either the bending moment or the compressive force must exceed normal limits if prolapse is to occur in the laboratory in a single loading cycle. (Note: all injuries involve, by definition, supraphysiological loading for that person at that time.)
- The magnitude of forces required to cause an individual disc to prolapse cannot reliably be predicted on the basis of gender, age and spinal level.
- Neither bending nor compression need exceed normal limits if cadaveric discs are made to prolapse by repetitive loading.
- Prolapse is easier to obtain in the laboratory when discs are swollen with fluid, as they are at the start of each the day in life.
- Animal experiments show that disc tissues degenerate after mechanical disruption. (It remains possible that disc degeneration precedes mechanical disruption (p. 198) in some humans.)
- Displaced nucleus tissue swells markedly during the 2–3 hours following prolapse in the laboratory, suggesting that symptoms arising from prolapse in life could intensify during this period.

RETROSPECTIVE ANALYSES OF SPINAL LOADING

The broad aim of a biomechanical analysis is to calculate the maximum forces applied to the spine during some incident, and compare them with forces required to injure cadaveric tissues of similar age and gender. Unfortunately, forces and tissue strengths are both difficult to quantify accurately. The present section will explain why it is difficult to quantify peak spinal loading during some fast-moving incident, especially if it is poorly remembered. Spinal loading is discussed at length in Chapter 9, but the following details are particularly relevant to medicolegal cases:

- Most compressive loading of the spine comes from muscle tension (rather than gravity).
- Trunk muscle forces can rise to very high levels during alarming incidents, especially when the spine

is flexed and the muscles are contracting eccentrically. (Trunk muscle forces can crush vertebrae during epileptic fits.[1475])

- Static analyses of peak spinal loading ignore inertial forces associated with accelerations of the spine, which can increase the peak compressive force by up to 60%.[363] Static analyses often ignore antagonistic muscle action, which can account for up to 45% of spinal compression in upright postures.
- Back muscles usually prevent the bending moment on the spine from exceeding physiological limits, but muscle protection is reduced following fatigue, or creep in sustained flexed posture (p. 192).
- The bending moment acting on the spine in the sagittal plane in vivo can be quantified in the laboratory (p. 110), but it is currently impossible to quantify the lateral bending moment, or the axial torque, acting on the spine in vivo.

HOW STRONG IS THE BACK?

The strength of a skeletal structure is the force required to break it. Average values for the strength of the lumbar spine are given in Table 11.1, and the weakening effects of fatigue are shown in Table 11.2. Unfortunately, spinal strength varies so widely between individuals (for reasons explained above) that it is difficult to relate averaged values to any particular individual. In short, it is impossible to say how strong a person's back is: there is just a wide range of likely strengths depending on factors such as age, gender, genetic inheritance and work history. Each case must be assessed on the basis of the available facts, though these may, of course, be limited.

RELATING SPINAL LOADING TO PATHOLOGY AND PAIN

Except in cases involving an obvious traumatic incident, it is rarely possible to state dogmatically that the forces exerted on the spine during a particular incident were sufficient to damage that person's spine, or indeed cause pain. This is partly because of the complications inherent in retrospective analyses of spinal loading in vivo (see above) and partly because of the large interindividual variability in the strength of spinal tissues. Similarly, it is unsafe to insist that a demonstrated spinal pathology is responsible for pain and disability: the relationship is complex and influenced by factors such as pain sensitisation, stress-shielding and the human personality.

Fortunately, medicolegal reports can usually call upon two additional pieces of evidence when attempting to relate mechanical loading to pathology, and pathology to pain, in a particular person. Firstly, there may be evidence from MRI scans to indicate what pathological changes are present. Whilst spinal pathology is a particularly common finding on X-rays and MRI scans, even in painfree people, certain features are more common in those with severe back pain and cannot be considered normal, even though they may not be causing pain in a particular individual. Such features include disc prolapse and a radial fissure in the posterior annulus. Therefore, the medical report does not need to state (for example) whether or not a given loading incident would cause most discs to prolapse; rather, it need only state whether or not the loading could have caused this particular disc to prolapse. Secondly, the report does not need to declare whether or not the pathology is painful (the patient can do that!). The report can give a view on whether the alleged pain and disability are consistent with the demonstrated pathology, but should also acknowledge the general limited correlation between pain and pathology.

If the injured worker is untruthful or exaggerating about the pain, then the report may attribute pain to pathology which is in fact painless. However, it is important that a report from an expert witness should be confined to matters in which the writer is expert, and this should not include judging the truthfulness of a claimant's evidence; that is the responsibility of the Court.

SUMMARY

It is clear that the expert advising the Court on matters of causation faces a significant challenge for which there is no simple solution. We have attempted here to introduce some of the issues the Court may find helpful in reaching a decision – it is for the expert to provide advice and guidance to facilitate that process, by way of presenting a rational opinion based on the available scientific evidence. The major issues that may be pertinent to an expert opinion include the following:

- Back pain is common and likely to recur: sick leave and chronic disability are not inevitable consequences, and occur frequently irrespective of occupational exposures.
- It is not appropriate to deny employment on the basis of a previous history of back pain (though

care should be taken if the job is heavy) and an injured worker need not be symptom-free before returning to work after back pain.[257,1509]
- The relationship between back pain and spinal pathology is complex, and either one can exist without the other. Certain pathological entities such as disc prolapse are associated with an increased risk of symptoms, but in the individual case the symptoms need to be clinically consistent with the pathology for a causative link to be made.
- Symptoms may be experienced predominantly at work and be more severe with specific activities, but that alone does not indicate an injurious mechanism and should not be seen as an indictment of the system of work: there are other important causes contributing to the problem, such as genetics, age or work history.
- Mechanical overload damage to vertebrae and intervertebral discs can occur with especially heavy work, perhaps as a result of 'fatigue failure'. However, that does not necessarily implicate repeated/continual loading as a primary cause.
- In laboratory experiments, most middle-aged lower lumbar intervertebral discs can be made to prolapse by the application of severe or repetitive mechanical loading. Other experiments on human and animal tissues suggest that disc degeneration follows mechanical failure, rather than precedes it.
- Disc prolapse must not be equated with disc degeneration or with disc bulging. Many bulging discs are not degenerated, and most degenerated discs are not prolapsed.
- Most spinal compressive loading comes from back muscles, and forces are likely to rise to high levels during sudden and alarming incidents. These forces are difficult to quantify in retrospective analyses.
- Bending stresses acting on the spine are a potential contributor to injury, particularly to the lower lumbar intervertebral discs. Bending stresses are highest in the early morning and following sustained or repetitive bending.
- Most back injuries should, and generally do, recover (in a clinical sense, if not necessarily in a physiological sense). Persisting disability is best explained by psychosocial influences (Chs 6 and 16).

Chapter |21|

Summary and conclusions

INTRODUCTION

The focus of this book is embodied in its title. It explores the scientific evidence concerning the origins of back pain and attempts to present it in a balanced and rational fashion. Whilst the subject has been approached from a mechanistic perspective, the intention has always been to integrate mechanical, biological and psychological influences into a single comprehensive account of back pain.

The purpose of this final chapter is to provide a brief and (hopefully) clear summary of the most important evidence.

STRUCTURE AND FUNCTION OF THE BACK

What does what?

The S-shaped curves of the spine contribute to shock absorption during locomotion, somewhat in the manner of a bed spring. Muscles of the back and abdomen assist in shock absorption, but their main role is to provide movement, protection against excessive movement and stability in upright postures (p. 114).

Vertebrae make up the rigid component of the vertebral column, giving it shape and strength and anchoring muscles. The vertebral body is largely trabecular bone, and resists compressive loading down the long axis of the spine. The neural arch is a ring of cortical bone which protects the spinal cord, while its processes increase the leverage of muscles and ligaments, which effect and limit movements respectively. Adjacent neural arches articulate by means of the paired zygapophyseal joints, which stabilise the spine and prevent excessive shearing movements or axial rotation between vertebrae (p. 122).

Intervertebral discs are pads of fibrocartilage which allow some intervertebral movment, while distributing forces evenly on the subchondral bone. The normal nucleus pulposus behaves like a pressurised fluid which is restrained by tension in the concentric lamellae of the annulus fibrosus (p. 126).

Motor control

Tension in the trunk muscles is required to stabilise and control the upright spine, and to protect it from excessive movements. If the back muscles become fatigued, or if their tendons become overstretched as a result of sustained spinal flexion, then reflex muscle protection for the underlying spine can be seriously impaired, with full recovery taking up to several hours (p. 192).

SOME BACKS ARE MORE VULNERABLE THAN OTHERS

Only a minority of people relate the onset of their back pain to a major injury, and there is abundant anecdotal evidence that even symptoms relating to a disc prolapse can start with some trivial event such as a sneeze. Conversely, most manual labourers appear to cope well with the rigours of their job. Evidently, some people have, or can develop, weaker or stronger backs than others.

Genetic inheritance predisposes to injury and degeneration

In a statistical sense, genetic inheritance accounts for approximately 50% of back pain, and a similar proportion of various pathologies including disc degeneration, osteoarthritis and osteoporosis (p. 61). However, these conditions do not usually become manifest until middle age, and even then they mostly affect those anatomical sites that are most heavily loaded. The most plausible interpretation is that inherited characteristics make us more vulnerable to environmental influences which then precipitate tissue damage, degeneration and pain. For example, we may inherit genes which produce inferior collagen or proteoglycans in our intervertebral discs, so that mechanical disc failure can then occur at lower load levels than in a person with a more fortunate inheritance.

Genetic predisposition need not involve biochemical composition. It could involve inefficient metabolic pathways; or innate clumsiness (inadequate proprioceptive/neuromuscular control) leading to more accidents; or physical factors such as small discs, a heavy body or short internal lever arms which would lead to higher muscle forces (p. 102).

It is important to realise that genetic predisposition to common musculoskeletal disorders is rarely simple, and rarely decisive. Usually, many genes contribute to a person's predisposition to disease, and the environment must still play an important role.

Ageing contributes to tissue vulnerability

Ageing causes the cells of most skeletal tissues to become less efficient, less responsive to their environment and less able to reproduce. Ageing also causes progressive biochemical changes in the extracellular matrix of spinal tissues which lead to impaired function. For example, loss of proteoglycans from intervertebral discs leads to reduced hydration, and increased stress concentrations within the annulus (Fig. 13.15). The biochemical process of non-enzymatic glycation of collagen (Fig. 8.10) causes an inexorable age-related stiffening in tissues such as cartilage, tendon and annulus fibrosus, which leaves them vulnerable to mechanical impacts.

Loading history

Generally, repeated mechanical loading is good for your back, because all spinal tissues tend to be strengthened by exercise and weakened by inactivity (Ch. 7). However, high levels of repetitive loading can lead to 'fatigue' failure

(Fig. 1.7) if the rate of damage accumulation exceeds the rate at which the tissue can strengthen itself. Fatigue failure is the more likely outcome in poorly vascularised tissues (such as intervertebral discs or large tendons) which have a low density of cells and only a limited capacity for repair. Conversely, adaptive remodelling is the more likely outcome in metabolically active tissues such as muscle and bone, and in young people who have a higher density of viable cells in their tissues. Abrupt increases in the level of physical activity associated with a new job may well cause problems, as discs and ligaments struggle to keep pace with strengthening muscles and bones (p. 85). Old notions concerning the harmful effects of mechanical loading on the spine need to be modified, but not abandoned entirely.

Medicolegal significance

It follows from the above evidence that an individual should not be considered to have a 'vulnerable' or 'normal' back. Rather, all individuals lie on a continuous scale of vulnerability depending on the environment in which they have lived and worked, as well as on their age and genetic inheritance (p. 20). One of the more interesting and important health and medicolegal issues of our times is the problem of genetic predisposition to disease.

BACK INJURIES

Forces acting on the spine

Very high compressive forces can be exerted on the spine during rapid and alarming movements when the back muscles contract vigorously (p. 102). High compression can also result from a fall, when peak forces are proportional to peak deceleration (p. 102). Bending moments on the osteoligamentous spine are highest in the early morning, or following sustained flexion, or during rapid movements, or when the back muscles are fatigued (p. 110).

Epidemiological evidence

Activities that can be associated with (though not necessarily causative of) spinal degeneration and pain include those which involve repetitive or severe spinal loading, especially in bent and twisted postures (p. 62). However, only a minority of patients with back pain associate it with some event or activity involving high loading of the back, and activities that involve regular moderate loading may even benefit the spine. Evidently, the traditional injury model of back pain is inadequate. Only when integrated with the concepts of tissue vulnerability (discussed above) and when the influence of psychosocial factors is acknowledged (below) can a smarter injury model be constructed that is compatible with the epidemiological evidence.

Injury mechanisms

Forces applied to spine specimens in laboratory experiments must reproduce the effects of muscle tension as well as gravitational loading, and experimental loading must match in vivo loading in terms of magnitude, complexity and speed of application. Suitably realistic cadaveric experiments have shown that mechanical loading can cause many spinal injuries similar to those seen in living people. Spinal flexion can injure the posterior intervertebral ligaments, and when combined with high compressive forces can cause an intervertebral disc to prolapse posteriorly (p. 153). Forced axial rotation and backwards bending both cause impaction of the neural arches, and may injure the zyapophyseal joints (p. 149). Compressive overload, acting down the long axis of the spine, tends to injure the vertebral body first, often allowing vertical herniation of disc material into a vertebral body. In elderly people with osteoporosis, patterns of vertebral compression fracture depend on disc degeneration and spinal load-sharing as well as on bone density (p. 100), and vertebral deformity can be accelerated by gradual 'creep' processes (p. 183). Injured discs lose pressure from the nucleus, and allow the annulus to bulge radially outwards or collapse inwards, leading to problems in adjacent tissues (Fig. 11.9). Forward shearing forces can lead to bending of the neural arch, and spondylolysis (p. 162). Vertebral damage can occur during a single loading event, or by the process of accumulating 'fatigue failure', in which the peak forces can be as low as 30–40% of those required for sudden failure (Table 11.2).

Experimentally validated finite element models of injury mechanisms can offer additional insight by predicting the precise location of the highest stresses and strains (Fig. 11.25), and accounting for the influence of variable factors such as age, posture or loading rate.

Healing of back injuries

Well-vascularised tissues respond to injury by healing themselves, whereas poorly vascularised tissues (most notably cartilage) respond inadequately and undergo progressive degeneration (Fig 15.1).

Muscle

Muscle is metabolically very active and can heal fully within days or weeks, with few long-term consequences. Typical eccentric muscle damage due to overexertion causes some pain near the musculotendinous junction (delayed-onset muscle soreness) and stiffness lasting for a few days (p. 72). When healed, the muscle is generally stronger and less likely than before to be injured by a similar insult.

Tendons and ligaments

Adult human tendons and ligaments have a barely adequate blood supply, and low cellularity, so that healing tends to progress steadily over weeks or months. There are too few cells to remodel collagen fibres completely in tendons and ligaments, restoring their crimp structure, so it is unlikely that their mechanical properties are ever fully restored after major injury (though they may be functionally adequate).

Bone

Bone has a plentiful blood supply and tends to heal fully after weeks or months, depending on the age of the individual. However, it is difficult to unload a vertebra during the healing process, so fractured vertebrae often exhibit some residual deformity (e.g. thoracic kyphosis). Incomplete healing within vertebral bodies may explain the inflammatory Modic changes which often accompany endplate defects (p. 206).

Articular cartilage and intervertebral discs

In adult humans, these tissues are avascular and have very low cellularity, so healing after injury is difficult. Furthermore, attempts at healing appear to be frustrated by habitual mechanical loading and reinjuries, resulting in chronic degenerative conditions that may include an inflammatory component (Fig. 15.1). The peripheral annulus is the most metabolically active region of the disc, and is capable of effective healing by scar (Fig. 15.13). However, most disc research is directed towards reversing age-related degenerative changes in the nucleus rather than promoting healing in the peripheral annulus, even though the latter is probably an easier target, and one that is more closely related to pain relief.

AGEING AND DEGENERATION OF THE SPINE

Development and growth

Vertebrae continue to ossify during childhood, with cartilage typically remaining in the pedicles until age 6, and on the tips of the processes until age 18 (Fig. 8.3). Vertebrae grow faster than discs, and the declining ratio of disc:vertebral height contributes to declining spinal mobility during growth. Intervertebral discs lose their metabolically active notochordal cells in childhood, and overall disc cell density decreases throughout growth as metabolite transport difficulties increase (Fig. 8.4). Consequently, the metabolic activity of discs decreases during growth and then remains roughly constant in early adulthood.

Ageing

Bone mineral density peaks around age 30 years, and then declines steadily, with a marked acceleration in women following the menopause. This loss of bone mineral (osteopenia) leads to vertebral deformities (Fig. 11.7) which can occur as a result of both fracture and 'creep' mechanisms. Intervertebral discs do not weaken markedly with age, but the nucleus gradually loses proteoglycans and water, and biochemical changes in disc collagens cause the tissue to become yellow-brown in colour, and noticeably fibrous (Fig. 8.14). Changes in disc composition stiffen the tissues, leading to decreased mobility and increased risk of injury when subjected to impulsive loading. Similar changes affect spinal ligaments and tendons.

Muscles of the back and abdomen become smaller and weaker with age, and the proportion of contractile tissue within them decreases slightly. Age-related loss of muscle mass and strength is known as sarcopenia, and there is increasing evidence that 'sarcopenia drives osteopenia' by providing smaller mechanical stimuli to bone (p. 92). Regular exercise, if sustained, can slow the rate of muscle and bone loss.

Intervertebral disc degeneration

Intervertebral discs frequently show degenerative changes in middle age, especially in the lower lumbar spine (Fig. 10.19). Disc degeneration resembles accelerated ageing, and is influenced strongly by genetic inheritance. However, degeneration is typified by gross failure of disc structure, and degeneration can be initiated by mechanical loading, in both humans and animal models (p. 198). In degenerated discs, the nucleus becomes decompressed, and increased compressive load-bearing disrupts the annulus. Blood vessels and nerves grow into degenerated discs from the peripheral annulus and endplate, following the line of any complete radial fissures (p. 204), but they rarely penetrate more than a few millimetres. Inflammatory-like reactions can be instigated within degenerated discs by blood-borne cells, and also by indigenous cells from the nucleus (p. 205). Inflammation can cause nerves within the disc to become sensitised to mechanical stimulation (p. 205).

Spine 'degenerative cascade'

Disc degeneration often precipitates a 'degenerative cascade' in the spine, as adjacent structures respond adversely to abnormal loading patterns (Ch. 15). The functional aspects of disc degeneration that drive these changes are reduced nucleus volume and pressure, leading to increased radial bulging of the annulus and reduced disc height. The degenerative cascade may possibly be accelerated by a direct outwards spread of inflammatory mediators from a degenerating disc into neighbouring tissues.

Apophyseal joint osteoarthritis

The reduced height of degenerating discs brings the neural arches of adjacent vertebrae closer together so that they become substantially load-bearing (Fig. 8.16). The location of cartilage lesions and bony osteophytes suggests that excessive compressive load-bearing may be a sufficient explanation for osteoarthritis in the apophyseal joints (Fig. 15.16).

Segmental 'instability'

Disc narrowing slackens the outer annulus and intervertebral ligaments, allowing the disc to 'wobble' freely in bending, a condition known as segmental instability (p. 207). Generally, the region of free play (the neutral zone) is increased to a greater extent than the full range of movement, so instability should not be equated with hypermobility. Altered segmental mechanics usually causes the centre of rotation (Fig. 10.5) to migrate posteriorly and inferiorly.

Osteophytosis

Abnormal movements in bending, combined with increased radial bulging of the annulus, give rise to bony outgrowths around the margins of the vertebral body (Fig. 15.14). These osteophytes (the word means bone plants) are probably responding to abnormal stretching of the periosteum which covers the vertebrae. Mechanically, osteophytes restrict movements in bending, effectively reversing segmental instability, so they can be viewed as adaptive rather than degenerative. However, osteophytes can contribute to spinal stenosis.

Spinal stenosis

The space available for spinal nerves becomes restricted by vertebral body osteophytes, by disc narrowing, by radial bulging of the disc and by hypertrophy of the ligamentum flavum. Constriction of nerves, typically in the intervertebral foramen, can give rise to neurogenic pain (see below) and neurogenic claudication involving motor deficit (p. 208).

Osteoporosis and senile kyphosis

Age-related loss of bone (osteoporosis) is a systemic condition associated with reduced levels of sex hormones and physical activity. However, local changes in load-sharing

following disc degeneration can weaken the anterior vertebral body to such an extent (Fig. 8.7) that it results in anterior wedge fractures. Deformity tends to progress under gravity at several vertebral levels until the condition is known as senile kyphosis, or 'dowager's hump' (Fig. 15.22).

BACK PAIN

Pain from disrupted tissues

Although the traditional injury model of back pain is inadequate, it remains true that persisting (chronic) back pain starts as acute back pain, and much acute pain is associated with alterations in spinal tissues. Any innervated structure can become painful if it is physically disrupted, because disruption leads to large deformations in the vicinity of nerve endings. Pain can be amplified if nerves become sensitised by local inflammatory reactions (p. 205).

Muscles

Muscles can be painful when overstretched or 'pulled'. Work in stooped postures could cause pain as a result of eccentric damage to back muscles (Fig. 7.6), particularly near the musculotendinous junctions. Comparisons with other regions of the body suggest that pain from back muscles could be severe, but localised. Probably it would not last more than a few hours or days, because muscle is well vascularised and heals quickly, but repeated insults could lead to a magnified inflammatory response and further pain.

Vertebrae

Vertebral bony endplates and their supporting trabeculae are sometimes damaged in the thoracolumbar spine, so these innervated structures may be a cause of acute back pain. Furthermore, vertebral healing may be frustrated by difficulties in unloading the structure, so that repeated insults and an exaggerated inflammatory response give rise to persisting as well as acute back pain, especially in elderly patients. Inflammatory (Modic) changes are often visualised on magnetic resonance imaging scans of patients with chronic back pain (p. 206).

Zygapophyseal joints

Osteoarthritic changes are extremely common in the apophyseal joints, especially after middle age and following disc narrowing (Fig. 15.16). Osteoarthritis is a major cause of chronic pain in the hip and knee, and evidence from pain provocation/blocking studies suggests that the same is true of apophyseal joints. Cartilage loss can provoke pain from subchondral bone that is subjected to high focal loading. Alternatively, pain could arise from chronic distortions and inflammation of the joint capsule (p. 49).

Sacroiliac joints

Pain provocation and pain-blocking studies confirm that these joints are frequently painful, and that pain is associated with abnormal movements. Tearing and healing of the ligamentous surface (Fig. 2.22) may cause acute pain, with repeated insults causing more inflammatory-led persisting pain (p. 49).

Intervertebral discs

Large population studies have confirmed that disc degeneration is associated with back pain in a dose-related manner (Fig. 15.10). However, many people with severe disc degeneration report no pain, possibly because nerve ingrowth and inflammatory processes are so variable. Repeated minor insults can exaggerate inflammation and pain, and may eventually give rise to central sensitisation effects in the spinal cord and brain (persisting pain), so that pain management becomes the only option. Similar mechanisms could explain pain from ligaments and tendons.

Neurogenic pain

Inflammatory-like mechanisms probably induce sciatica from nerve roots sensitised by blood or herniated nucleus pulposus (p. 205). Physical deformation of a nerve root is more likely to cause radiating paresthesia or motor deficit rather than pain, although direct compression of a nerve root ganglion can be painful. Narrowing of the intervertebral foramen following the spinal degenerative cascade can also contribute to neurogenic claudication, by directly compressing a nerve root or interfering with its blood supply (p. 215).

'Functional' pain

Pain can be elicited from normal tissues if stresses are concentrated within them in an abnormal manner (Ch. 13). This is exemplified by having a stone in your shoe: the stone doesn't cause injury, but hurts because it concentrates an abnormally high portion of body weight on to a very small region of the foot. In a similar manner, certain postures can generate high stress concentrations in regions of the annulus, in the apophyseal joints or in spinal ligaments and muscles. Postural effects can be magnified if held for a long period of time, so that fluid expulsion from soft tissues further reduces their ability to distribute load evenly (Fig. 13.15). 'Functional' back pain does not require any pathological changes in affected

tissues, but if the underlying postural conditions are unrelenting, they may affect tissue metabolism and ultimately tissue morphology, leading to more discomfort and pain.

Psychosocial factors influence pain behaviour

All aspects of pain behaviour are influenced by the intrinsic psychological characteristics of the patient, and by his or her social interactions. Back pain behaviour includes the initial recognition of a discomfort as back pain; the decision to report it as such; to seek and respond to treatment; to become disabled; and to seek financial compensation. Social interactions include those with work colleagues and medical practitioners. Not surprisingly, epidemiological studies of back pain find that psychosocial risk factors feature prominently in predictive models of 'who reports back pain' and 'who progresses to incapacity'. Recognition of the importance of these factors has been termed a 'back pain revolution' and studies of any aspect of back pain behaviour (such as response to pain or its treatment) must consider psychosocial factors if they are to be of much value.

Nevertheless, cause should be distinguished from effect. Psychosocial factors do not predict more than a few per cent of future episodes of first-time back pain, and the back pain they do predict tends to be trivial. The current biopsychosocial model of back pain recognises both the tissue origins of back pain and their psychosocial consequences.

CURRENT AND FUTURE TREATMENT OPTIONS

Manual therapy

Manual therapies may have a non-specific effect on pain, or may have tissue-specific effects. Manual treatment can enhance the healing of damaged muscles by stimulating blood supply and preventing adhesions. They may similarly benefit injured tendons and ligaments by physically stimulating the indigenous cells, increasing metabolite transport to them, and helping to align collagen fibres. However, identifying the specific injured structure in the spine remains problematic (Ch. 5). The potential for manual therapy to treat painful intervertebral discs (or sciatica due to disc herniation) is just beginning to receive formal scientific attention (p. 238). For many years, the achievable goal of speeding up the healing of a painful annulus has been neglected in favour of the rather ambitious aim of reversing age-related degenerative changes in the nucleus.

Surgery

Despite some scepticism, spinal surgery remains an effective treatment for several spinal disorders, including spondylolisthesis, spinal stenosis and disc prolapse (Ch. 19). It is not so good for non-specific or discogenic back pain, probably because multifactorial origins reduce the chances of success. There is limited evidence that the latest designs of disc prosthesis, which contain no moving parts (Fig. 19.6), can be effective.

Drugs

Increasing awareness of an inflammatory involvement in chronic back pain should lead to several approaches to pain relief. Blocking cell signalling by tumour necrosis factor-α appeared to give effective pain relief in animals, and was mirrored in an early pilot study on humans, yet results from the follow-up randomised controlled trial were disappointing (p. 239). Accurate selection of patients, and treating them at the right time, is probably crucial. Recent unique evidence suggests that injecting the ionic dye methylene blue into painful discs can relieve symptoms for up to 2 years. Methylene blue can disperse rapidly throughout a disc, by fluid flow and diffusion (Fig. 17.4), and may be able to desensitise (or incapacitate) any nociceptive nerves it meets.

Regenerative medicine

It may become possible to use implanted cells and tissues to reverse age-related changes in the spine, or to promote healing by use of a 'cell bandage'. However, current techniques are too invasive to justify their use in early-stage disc degeneration, and implanted cells may die in the hostile environment of severely degenerated discs (p. 239).

Cognitive-behavioural therapy (CBT)

If back pain fails to respond to several weeks of simple therapeutic intervention, patients should be helped to cope with their residual pain in order to minimise impact on their behaviour and quality of life. Consideration of multidisciplinary approaches, including CBT, should be offered. Importantly, though, it is now clear that it is not simply the psychological status of the patient that is important; rather the beliefs and behaviours of all the players in this complex biopsychosocial phenomenon are important determinants of what happens to people with back pain (Ch. 17). Interactions between peripheral pain and functions of the central nervous system are only now being explored, so the full potential of CBT may increase.

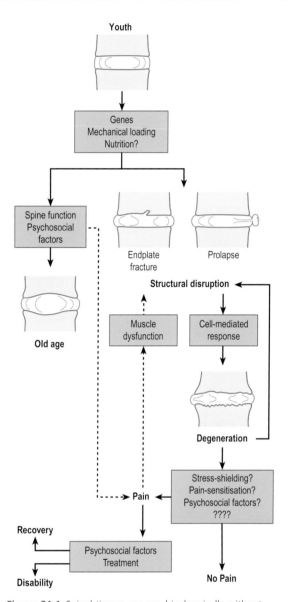

Figure 21.1 Spinal tissues can age biochemically without becoming degenerated or painful (left). However, genetic predisposition, combined with mechanical loading which is excessive for that spine, can disrupt spinal tissues (in this example, an intervertebral disc). Degeneration follows as the tissue's cells respond to their altered mechanical environment in an inappropriate way. This can lead to further tissue weakness and disruption. Degeneration can lead to pain, but this depends on variable factors such as stress-shielding and chemical sensitisation of damaged tissues. The patient's responses to pain and treatment are greatly influenced by psychosocial factors, and pain-induced alterations in muscle function may possibly contribute to reinjury.

Exercise

Chronic back pain involves complex interactions between mind and body, with altered muscle function perhaps playing an intermediary role. Rehabilitation programmes which involve active exercise are able to reduce the severity of pain in many chronic sufferers, and help others back to normal activity and work (p. 235). These programmes work directly on the body by increasing factors such as mobility, muscle strength, muscle endurance and cardiovascular fitness. In addition, they will have psychological benefits through fostering self-belief, reducing fear and increasing motivation.

Other

Injecting bone cement into a damaged vertebral body (Fig. 15.23) is able to relieve back pain in some patients, although randomised controlled trials have shown only a marginal benefit. Cement augmentation of a vertebra can restore more-or-less-normal stress distributions to the adjacent intervertebral disc (Fig. 15.24) and neural arch, and could alleviate pain by a number of mechanisms. The technique evidently needs to be optimised in respect of cement type, volume and placement, whilst patient selection doubtless will prove important.

CONCLUDING REMARKS

A typical natural history of spinal ageing, degeneration and pain is summarised in Figure 21.1. For many patients, a blend of physical and psychological strengthening may be sufficient to bring each episode of back pain to a natural conclusion. For others, the organic problems that often underlie chronic back pain will require more specific interventions, from manual therapy to surgery. There is no reason to believe that back pain is fundamentally different from other joint pain, or that it cannot be treated successfully, but the practical problems inherent in treating such a deep and complicated structure as the vertebral column will take some time to overcome. Nevertheless, successful treatments for back pain are finally beginning to emerge, and parallel improvements in imaging technology and diagnostic procedures are helping to match the patient to the treatment.

Hopefully, these advances will stimulate continued attempts to identify rigorous explanations for those patterns of back pain currently referred to as 'non-specific',[1638] leading in turn to better targeting of treatments and improved and more predictable outcomes. That said, the principles of tackling psychosocial obstacles to recovery and participation apply whatever the cause or treatment. There is good evidence that the psychosocial characteristics of many patients with chronic back pain are not the underlying cause of the problem; rather they are a response to vague diagnosis, ineffective treatment and a 'compensation culture'. Persistent back pain starts as acute pain, and if that pain can be dealt with early, then there will be less need to abandon patients to overzealous clinicians and lawyers. The authors of this book hope that their efforts will encourage others to adopt an integrative approach to back pain, and to believe that spinal degeneration and pain can be explained rigorously and treated successfully.

References

1. Oxford English Dictionary (online), published by Oxford University Press, 2012. Website http://www.oed.com/

2. Abelin K, Vialle R, Lenoir T, et al. The sagittal balance of the spine in children and adolescents with osteogenesis imperfecta. Eur Spine J 2008;17:1697–704.

3. Acaroglu ER, Iatridis JC, Setton LA, et al. Degeneration and aging affect the tensile behavior of human lumbar annulus fibrosus. Spine 1995;20:2690–701.

4. Adams CI, Freeman BJC, Clark AJ, et al. Targeted foraminal epidural steroid injection for radicular pain: A Kaplan–Meier survival analysis. Orthopaedic Proceedings. J Bone Joint Surg 2005;87-B:243.

5. Adams M. 'Masonry arch' model of the spine [letter] [see comments]. Spine 1989;14:1272.

6. Adams M. Re: Spine stability: the six blind men and the elephant. Clin Biomech 2007;22:486; author reply 7–8.

7. Adams MA. The mechanical properties of lumbar intervertebral joints with special reference to the causes of low-back pain. PhD thesis. London, U.K.: Polytechnic of Central London; 1980.

8. Adams MA. Letter to the Editor. Proc Instn Mech Egrs 1995:135.

9. Adams MA. Mechanical testing of the spine. An appraisal of methodology, results, and conclusions. Spine 1995;20:2151–6.

10. Adams MA. Biomechanics of the intervertebral disc, vertebra and ligaments. In: Szpalski M, Gunzburg R, Pope MH, editors. Lumbar segmental instability. Philadelphia, U.S.A.: Lippincott Williams & Wilkins; 1999.

11. Adams MA. The mechanical environment of chondrocytes in articular cartilage. Biorheology 2006;43:537–45.

12. Adams MA. Point of view. Spine (Phila Pa) 2006;31:E525–6; discussion E7.

13. Adams MA, Dolan P. A technique for quantifying the bending moment acting on the lumbar spine in vivo. J Biomech 1991;24:117–26.

14. Adams MA, Dolan P. Time-dependent changes in the lumbar spine's resistance to bending. Clin Biomech 1996;11:194–200.

15. Adams MA, Dolan P. Could sudden increases in physical activity cause degeneration of intervertebral discs? Lancet 1997;350:734–5.

16. Adams MA, Dolan P. Spine biomechanics. J Biomech 2005;38:1972–83.

17. Adams MA, Dolan P, Hutton WC. The stages of disc degeneration as revealed by discograms. J Bone Joint Surg [Br] 1986;68:36–41.

18. Adams MA, Dolan P, Hutton WC. Diurnal variations in the stresses on the lumbar spine. Spine 1987;12:130–7.

19. Adams MA, Dolan P, Hutton WC. The lumbar spine in backward bending. Spine 1988;13:1019–26.

20. Adams MA, Dolan P, Marx C, et al. An electronic inclinometer technique for measuring lumbar curvature. Clin Biomech 1986;1:130–4.

21. Adams MA, Dolan P, McNally DS. The internal mechanical functioning of intervertebral discs and articular cartilage, and its relevance to matrix biology. Matrix Biol 2009;28:384–9.

22. Adams MA, Freeman BJ, Morrison HP, et al. Mechanical initiation of intervertebral disc degeneration. Spine 2000;25:1625–36.

23. Adams MA, Green TP. Tensile properties of the annulus fibrosus. Part I The contribution of fibre–matrix interactions to tensile stiffness and strength. Eur Spine J 1993;2:203–8.

24. Adams MA, Green TP, Dolan P. The strength in anterior bending of lumbar intervertebral discs. Spine 1994;19:2197–203.

25. Adams MA, Hutton WC. The effect of posture on the role of the apophysial joints in resisting intervertebral compressive forces. J Bone Joint Surg [Br] 1980;62:358–62.

26. Adams MA, Hutton WC. The relevance of torsion to the mechanical derangement of the lumbar spine. Spine 1981;6:241–8.

27. Adams MA, Hutton WC. Prolapsed intervertebral disc. A hyperflexion injury 1981 Volvo Award in Basic Science. Spine 1982;7:184–91.

28. Adams MA, Hutton WC. The effect of posture on the fluid content of lumbar intervertebral discs. Spine 1983;8:665–71.

29. Adams MA, Hutton WC. The mechanical function of the lumbar apophyseal joints. Spine 1983;8:327–30.

30. Adams MA, Hutton WC. Gradual disc prolapse. Spine 1985;10:524–31.

31. Adams MA, Hutton WC. The effect of posture on diffusion into lumbar intervertebral discs. J Anat 1986;147:121–34.

32. Adams MA, Hutton WC. Has the lumbar spine a margin of safety in forward bending? Clin Biomech 1986;1:3–6.

33. Adams MA, Hutton WC, Stott JR. The resistance to flexion of the lumbar intervertebral joint. Spine 1980;5:245–53.

34. Adams MA, Kerin AJ, Bhatia LS, et al. Experimental determination of stress distributions in articular cartilage before and after sustained loading. Clin Biomech 1999;14:88–96.

35. Adams MA, Kerin AJ, Wisnom MR. Sustained loading increases the compressive strength of articular cartilage. Connect Tissue Res 1998;39:245–56.

36. Adams MA, Mannion AF, Dolan P. Personal risk factors for first-time low-back pain. Spine 1999;24:2497–505.

37. Adams MA, May S, Freeman BJ, et al. Effects of backward bending on lumbar intervertebral discs. Relevance to physical therapy treatments for low-back pain. Spine 2000;25:431–7; discussion 8.

38. Adams MA, McMillan DW, Green TP, et al. Sustained loading generates stress concentrations in lumbar intervertebral discs. Spine 1996;21:434–8.

39. Adams MA, McNally DS, Chinn H, et al. Posture and the compressive strength of the lumbar spine. Clin Biomech 1994;9:5–14.

40. Adams MA, McNally DS, Dolan P. 'Stress' distributions inside intervertebral discs. The effects of age and degeneration. J Bone Joint Surg Br 1996; 78:965–72.

41. Adams MA, McNally DS, Wagstaff J, et al. Abnormal stress concentrations in lumbar intervertebral discs following damage to the vertebral body: a cause of disc failure. Eur Spine J 1993;1:214–21.

42. Adams MA, Pollintine P, Tobias JH, et al. Intervertebral disc degeneration can predispose to anterior vertebral fractures in the thoracolumbar spine. J Bone Miner Res 2006;21: 1409–16.

43. Adams MA, Roughley PJ. What is Intervertebral Disc Degeneration, and What Causes It? Spine 2006;31:2151–61.

44. Adams MA, Silver IA. Early enhanced exercise: damaging or beneficial to joints? Equine Vet J 2009;41:515–6.

45. Adams MA, Stefanakis M, Dolan P. Healing of a painful intervertebral disc should not be confused with reversing disc degeneration: implications for physical therapies for discogenic back pain. Clin Biomech 2010;25:961–71.

46. Agorastides ID, Lam KS, Freeman BJ, et al. The Adams classification for cadaveric discograms: inter- and intra-observer error in the clinical setting. Eur Spine J 2002;11:76–9.

47. Ahern DK, Follick MJ, Council JR, et al. Comparison of lumbar paravertebral EMG patterns in chronic low-back pain patients and non-patient controls. Pain 1988;34:153–60.

48. Ahern DK, Hannon DJ, Goreczny AJ, et al. Correlation of chronic low-back pain behavior and muscle function examination of the flexion–relaxation response. Spine 1990; 15:92–5.

49. Ahlgren BD, Vasavada A, Brower RS, et al. Annular incision technique on the strength and multidirectional flexibility of the healing intervertebral disc. Spine 1994;19:948–54.

50. Ahmed AM, Duncan NA, Burke DL. The effect of facet geometry on the axial torque-rotation response of lumbar motion segments. Spine 1990;15: 391–401.

51. Ahn UM, Ahn NU, Buchowski JM, et al. Cauda equina syndrome secondary to lumbar disc herniation: a meta-analysis of surgical outcomes. Spine 2000;25:1515–22.

52. Aigner T, Gresk-otter KR, Fairbank JC, et al. Variation with age in the pattern of type X collagen expression in normal and scoliotic human intervertebral discs. Calcif Tissue Int 1998;63:263–8.

53. Airaksinen O, Brox JL, Cedraschi C, et al. European guidelines for the management of chronic nonspecific low-back pain. EC Cost Action B13. Available online at: www.backpaineurope.org. 2004.

54. Akerblom B. Standing and sitting posture. With special reference to the construction of chairs. Stockholm: Nordiska Bokhandeln; 1948.

55. Al-Rawahi M, Luo J, Pollintine P, et al. Mechanical function of vertebral body osteophytes, as revealed by experiments on cadaveric spines. Spine (Phila Pa) 2011;36:770–7.

56. Aladin DM, Cheung KM, Chan D, et al. Expression of the Trp2 allele of COL9A2 is associated with alterations in the mechanical properties of human intervertebral discs. Spine 2007;32:2820–6.

57. Albert HB, Manniche C. Modic changes following lumbar disc herniation. Eur Spine J 2007;16:977–82.

58. Alexander LA, Hancock E, Agouris I, et al. The response of the nucleus pulposus of the lumbar intervertebral discs to functionally loaded positions. Spine 2007;32:1508–12.

59. Alexander RM. Elastic mechanisms in animal movement. Cambridge: Cambridge University Press; 1988.

60. Alexander RM. Elasticity in human and animal backs. In: Vleeming A, Mooney V, Dorman T, et al, editors. Movement, Stability and Low-back Pain. Edinburgh: Churchill Livingstone; 1997.

61. Alexanderson K, Norlund A. Sickness absence – causes, consequences and physicians' sickness certification practice. A systematic literature review by the Swedish Council on Technology Assessment in Healthcare (SBU).

Scand J Public Health Suppl 2004;32:1–263.

62. Alini M, Eisenstein SM, Ito K, et al. Are animal models useful for studying human disc disorders/degeneration? Eur Spine J 2008;17:2–19.

63. Aloia JF, Cohn SH, Vaswani A, et al. Risk factors for postmenopausal osteoporosis. Am J Med 1985;78:95–100.

64. Althoff I, Brinckmann P, Frobin W, et al. An improved method of stature measurement for quantitative determination of spinal loading. Application to sitting postures and whole body vibration. Spine 1992;17:682–93.

65. Andersen TB, Simonsen EB. Sudden loading during a dynamic lifting task: a simulation study. J Biomech Eng 2005;127:108–13.

66. Anderson AL, McIff TE, Asher MA, et al. The effect of posterior thoracic spine anatomical structures on motion segment flexion stiffness. Spine 2009;34:441–6.

67. Anderson CK, Chaffin DB, Herrin GD, et al. A biomechanical model of the lumbosacral joint during lifting activities. J Biomech 1985;18:571–84.

68. Anderson DG, Li X, Tannoury T, et al. A fibronectin fragment stimulates intervertebral disc degeneration in vivo. Spine 2003;28:2338–45.

69. Andersson BJ, Ortengren R, Nachemson AL, et al. The sitting posture: an electromyographic and discometric study. Orthop Clin North Am 1975;6:105–20.

70. Andersson G, Bogduk N, et al. Muscle: clinical perspectives. In: Frymoyer JW, Gordon SL, editors. New perspectives on low-back pain. Park Ridge, Illinois: American Academy of Orthopaedic Surgeons; 1989. p. 293–334.

71. Andersson GB. Epidemiology of low-back pain. Acta Orthop Scand Suppl 1998;281:28–31.

72. Andersson GB, Murphy RW, Ortengren R, et al. The influence of backrest inclination and lumbar support on lumbar lordosis. Spine 1979;4:52–8.

73. Andersson GB, Schultz AB. Effects of fluid injection on mechanical properties of intervertebral discs. J Biomech 1979;12:453–8.

74. Andersson GBJ. The epidemiology of spinal disorders. In: Frymoyer JW, editor. The adult spine: principles and practice. Philadelphia: Lippincott-Raven; 1997. p. 93–141.

75. Andersson GBJ, Deyo R. Sensitivity, specificity and predictive value. In: Frymoyer JW, editor. The adult spine: principles and practice. 2nd ed. Philadelphia: Lippincott-Raven, 1997. p. 308–10.

76. Antoniou J, Arlet V, Goswami T, et al. Elevated synthetic activity in the convex side of scoliotic intervertebral discs and endplates compared with normal tissues. Spine 2001;26:E198–206.

77. Antoniou J, Goudsouzian NM, Heathfield TF, et al. The human lumbar endplate. Evidence of changes in biosynthesis and denaturation of the extracellular matrix with growth, maturation, aging, and degeneration. Spine 1996;21:1153–61.

78. Antoniou J, Steffen T, Nelson F, et al. The human lumbar intervertebral disc: evidence for changes in the biosynthesis and denaturation of the extracellular matrix with growth, maturation, ageing, and degeneration. J Clin Invest 1996;98:996–1003.

79. Aoki Y, Rydevik B, Kikuchi S, et al. Local application of disc-related cytokines on spinal nerve roots. Spine 2002;27:1614–7.

80. Aprill C, Bogduk N. High-intensity zone: a diagnostic sign of painful lumbar disc on magnetic resonance imaging. Br J Radiol 1992;65:361–9.

81. Argoubi M, Shirazi-Adl A. Poroelastic creep response analysis of a lumbar motion segment in compression. J Biomech 1996;29:1331–9.

82. Arlet V, Papin P, Marchesi D, et al. Adolescent idiopathic thoracic scoliosis: apical correction with specialized pedicle hooks. Eur Spine J 1999;8:266–71.

83. Armstrong RB, Ogilvie RW, Schwane JA. Eccentric exercise-induced injury to rat skeletal muscle. J Appl Physiol 1983;54:80–93.

84. Arokoski JP, Jurvelin JS, Vaatainen U, et al. Normal and pathological adaptations of articular cartilage to joint loading. Scand J Med Sci Sports 2000;10:186–98.

85. Arun R, Freeman BJ, Scammell BE, et al. 2009 ISSLS Prize Winner: What influence does sustained mechanical load have on diffusion in the human intervertebral disc? An in vivo study using serial postcontrast magnetic resonance imaging. Spine (Phila Pa) 2009;34:2324–37.

86. Ashton-Miller JA, Schultz AB. Spine instability and segmental hypermobility biomechanics: a call for the definition and standard use of terms. Semin Spine Surg 1991;3:136–48.

87. Aspden RM. The spine as an arch. A new mathematical model [see comments]. Spine 1989;14:266–74.

88. Atkinson PJ. Variation in trabecular structure of vertebrae with age. Calcif Tissue Res 1967;1:24–32.

89. Atlas SJ, Keller RB, Chang Y, et al. Surgical and nonsurgical management of sciatica secondary to a lumbar disc herniation: five-year outcomes from the Maine Lumbar Spine Study. Spine 2001;26:1179–87.

90. Autio RA, Karppinen J, Niinimaki J, et al. Determinants of spontaneous resorption of intervertebral disc herniations. Spine 2006;31:1247–52.

91. Avela J, Kyrolainen H, Komi PV. Altered reflex sensitivity after repeated and prolonged passive muscle stretching. J Appl Physiol 1999;86:1283–91.

92. Aylott CEW, Nicholls P, Kilburn-Topping F, et al. The effect of changing spinous process morphology and patterns of neoarticulation on spinal deformity and association with back pain. Liverpool, U.K.; Britspine; 2010.

93. Bailey AJ. Molecular mechanisms of ageing in connective tissues. Mech Ageing Dev 2001;122:735–55.

94. Bailey AJ, Sims TJ, Ebbesen EN, et al. Age-related changes in the biochemical properties of human cancellous bone collagen: relationship to bone strength. Calcif Tissue Int 1999;65:203–10.

95. Bailey JF, Liebenberg E, Degmetich S, et al. Innervation patterns of PGP 9.5-positive nerve fibers within the human lumbar vertebra. J Anat 2011;218:263–70.

96. Balagopal P, Rooyackers OE, Adey DB, et al. Effects of aging on in vivo synthesis of skeletal muscle myosin heavy-chain and sarcoplasmic protein in humans. Am J Physiol 1997;273:E790–800.

97. Balague F, Nordin M, Dutoit G, et al. Primary prevention, education, and low-back pain among school children. Bull Hosp Jt Dis 1996;55:130–4.

98. Baldwin ML, Johnson WG, Butler RJ. The error of using returns-to-work to measure the outcomes of healthcare. Am J Ind Med 1996;29:632–41.

99. Balestra C, Duchateau J, Hainaut K. Effects of fatigue on the stretch reflex in a human muscle. Electroencephalogr Clin Neurophysiol 1992;85:46–52.

100. Bank RA, Bayliss MT, Lafeber FP, et al. Ageing and zonal variation in post-translational modification of collagen in normal human articular cartilage. The age-related increase in non-enzymatic glycation affects biomechanical properties of cartilage. Biochem J 1998;330:345–51.

101. Bank RA, Soudry M, Maroudas A, et al. The increased swelling and instantaneous deformation of osteoarthritic cartilage is highly correlated with collagen degradation. Arthritis Rheum 2000;43:2202–10.

102. Barker PJ, Briggs CA, Bogeski G. Tensile transmission across the lumbar fasciae in unembalmed cadavers: effects of tension to various muscular attachments. Spine 2004;29:129–38.

103. Barnsley L, Lord SM, Wallis BJ, et al. The prevalence of chronic cervical zygapophyseal joint pain after whiplash. Spine 1995;20:20–5; discussion 6.

104. Bartelink DL. The role of abdominal pressure in relieving the pressure on the lumbar intervertebral discs. J Bone Joint Surg [Br] 1957;39:718–25.

105. Bartys S, Burton K, Main C. A prospective study of psychosocial risk factors and absence due to musculoskeletal disorders – implications for occupational screening. Occup Med (Lond) 2005;55:375–9.

106. Bass EC, Duncan NA, Hariharan JS, et al. Frozen storage affects the compressive creep behavior of the porcine intervertebral disc. Spine 1997;22:2867–76.

107. Bass S, Pearce G, Bradney M, et al. Exercise before puberty may confer residual benefits in bone density in adulthood: studies in active prepubertal and retired female gymnasts. J Bone Miner Res 1998;13:500–7.

108. Bassey EJ. Exercise in primary prevention of osteoporosis in women. Ann Rheum Dis 1995;54:861–2.

109. Bassey EJ, Ramsdale SJ. Increase in femoral bone density in young women following high-impact exercise. Osteoporos Int 1994;4:72–5.

110. Bassey EJ, Rothwell MC, Littlewood JJ, et al. Pre- and postmenopausal women have different bone mineral density responses to the same high-impact exercise. J Bone Miner Res 1998;13:1805–13.

111. Battie MC, Bigos SJ, Fisher LD, et al. Anthropometric and clinical measures as predictors of back pain complaints in industry: a prospective study. J Spinal Disord 1990;3:195–204.

112. Battie MC, Levalahti E, Videman T, et al. Heritability of Lumbar Flexibility and the Role of Disc Degeneration and Body Weight. J Appl Physiol 2007;104:379–85.

113. Battie MC, Videman T, Gibbons LE, et al. 1995 Volvo Award in clinical sciences. Determinants of lumbar disc degeneration. A study relating lifetime exposures and magnetic resonance imaging findings in identical twins. Spine 1995;20:2601–12.

114. Battie MC, Videman T, Gill K, et al. 1991 Volvo Award in clinical sciences. Smoking and lumbar intervertebral disc degeneration: an MRI study of identical twins. Spine 1991;16:1015–21.

115. Battie MC, Videman T, Levalahti E, et al. Heritability of low-back pain and the role of disc degeneration. Pain 2007;131:272–80.

116. Battie MC, Videman T, Levalahti E, et al. Genetic and environmental effects on disc degeneration by phenotype and spinal level: a multivariate twin study. Spine 2008;33:2801–8.

117. Battie MC, Videman T, Parent E. Lumbar disc degeneration: epidemiology and genetic influences. Spine 2004;29:2679–90.

118. Bayliss MT, Urban JP, Johnstone B, et al. In vitro method for measuring synthesis rates in the intervertebral disc. J Orthop Res 1986;4:10–7.

119. Bazrgari B, Shirazi-Adl A, Arjmand N. Analysis of squat and stoop dynamic liftings: muscle forces and internal spinal loads. Eur Spine J 2007;16:687–99.

120. Bazrgari B, Shirazi-Adl A, Kasra M. Seated whole body vibrations with high-magnitude accelerations – relative roles of inertia and muscle forces. J Biomech 2008;41:2639–46.

121. Bazrgari B, Shirazi-Adl A, Lariviere C. Trunk response analysis under sudden forward perturbations using a kinematics-driven model. J Biomech 2009;42:1193–200.

122. Bearn JG. The significance of the activity of the abdominal muscles in weight lifting. Acta Anat 1961;45:83–9.

123. Beattie PF, Donley JW, Arnot CF, et al. The change in the diffusion of water in normal and degenerative lumbar intervertebral discs following joint mobilization compared to prone lying. J Orthop Sports Phys Ther 2009;39:4–11.

124. Beaumont D. Rehabilitation and retention in the workplace – the interaction between general practitioners and occupational health professionals: a consensus statement. Occup Med (Lond) 2003;53:254–5.

125. Beaumont DG. The interaction between general practitioners and occupational health professionals in relation to rehabilitation for work: a Delphi study. Occup Med (Lond) 2003;53:249–53.

126. Becker CK, Savelberg HH, Barneveld A. In vitro mechanical properties of the accessory ligament of the deep digital flexor tendon in horses in relation to age. Equine Vet J 1994;26:454–9.

127. Beighton P, Solomon L, Soskolne CL. Articular mobility in an African population. Ann Rheum Dis 1973;32:413–8.

128. Bejia I, Abid N, Ben Salem K, et al. Low-back pain in a cohort of 622 Tunisian schoolchildren and adolescents: an epidemiological study. Eur Spine J 2005;14:331–6.

129. Bekkering GE, Hendriks HJ, van Tulder MW, et al. Prognostic factors for low-back pain in patients referred for physiotherapy: comparing outcomes and varying modeling techniques. Spine 2005;30: 1881–6.

130. Bekkering GE, van Tulder MW, Hendriks EJ, et al. Implementation of clinical guidelines on physical therapy for patients with low-back pain: randomized trial comparing patient outcomes after a standard and active implementation strategy. Phys Ther 2005;85:544–55.

131. Belcastro AN, Shewchuk LD, Raj DA. Exercise-induced muscle injury: a calpain hypothesis. Mol Cell Biochem 1998;179:135–45.

132. Bendix T, Kjaer P, Korsholm L. Burned-out discs stop hurting: fact or fiction? Spine 2008;33:E962–7.

133. Benoist M. The natural history of lumbar degenerative spinal stenosis. Joint Bone Spine 2002;69:450–7.

134. Bernick S, Walker JM, Paule WJ. Age changes to the annulus fibrosus in human intervertebral discs. Spine 1991;16:520–4.

135. Bibby SR, Fairbank JC, Urban MR, et al. Cell viability in scoliotic discs in relation to disc deformity and nutrient levels. Spine 2002;27:2220–8; discussion 7–8.

136. Bibby SR, Jones DA, Ripley RM, et al. Metabolism of the intervertebral disc: effects of low levels of oxygen, glucose, and pH on rates of energy metabolism of bovine nucleus pulposus cells. Spine 2005;30:487–96.

137. Bible JE, Simpson AK, Emerson JW, et al. Quantifying the effects of degeneration and other patient factors on lumbar segmental range of motion using multivariate analysis. Spine 2008;33:1793–9.

138. Biering-Sorensen F. Physical measurements as risk indicators for low-back trouble over a one-year period. Spine 1984;9:106–19.

139. Bigland-Ritchie B, Cafarelli E, Vollestad NK. Fatigue of submaximal static contractions. Acta Physiol Scand Suppl 1986;556:137–48.

140. Bigland-Ritchie BR, Dawson NJ, Johansson RS, et al. Reflex origin for the slowing of motoneurone firing rates in fatigue of human voluntary contractions. J Physiol 1986;379:451–9.

141. Bigland B, Lippold OC. The relationship between force, velocity and integrated electrical activity in human muscles. J Physiol 1954;123:214–20.

142. Bigos SJ, Battie MC, Fisher LD, et al. A prospective evaluation of preemployment screening methods for acute industrial back pain. Spine 1992;17:922–6.

143. Bigos SJ, Holland J, Holland C, et al. High-quality controlled trials on preventing episodes of back problems: systematic literature review in working-age adults. Spine J 2009;9: 147–68.

144. Birch HL, Wilson AM, Goodship AE. The effect of exercise-induced localised hyperthermia on tendon cell survival. J Exp Biol 1997;200:1703–8.

145. Bishop JB, Szpalski M, Ananthraman SK, et al. Classification of low-back pain from dynamic motion characteristics using an artificial neural network. Spine 1997;22:2991–8.

146. Bishop PB, Pearce RH. The proteoglycans of the cartilaginous end-plate of the human intervertebral disc change after maturity. J Orthop Res 1993;11:324–31.

147. Bjorklund M, Crenshaw AG, Djupsjobacka M, et al. Position sense acuity is diminished following repetitive low-intensity work to fatigue in a simulated occupational setting. Eur J Appl Physiol 2000;81:361–7.

148. Bleasel JF, Poole AR, Heinegard D, et al. Changes in serum cartilage marker levels indicate altered cartilage metabolism in families with the osteoarthritis-related type II collagen gene COL2A1 mutation. Arthritis Rheum 1999;42:39–45.

149. Blouin JS, Inglis JT, Siegmund GP. Auditory startle alters the response of human subjects exposed to a single whiplash-like perturbation. Spine 2006;31:146–54.

150. Blumenthal S, McAfee PC, Guyer RD, et al. A prospective, randomized, multicenter Food and Drug Administration investigational device exemptions study of lumbar total disc replacement with the CHARITE artificial disc versus lumbar fusion: part I: evaluation of clinical outcomes. Spine 2005;30: 1565–75; discussion E387–91.

151. Boden SD, Davis DO, Dina TS, et al. Abnormal magnetic-resonance scans of the lumbar spine in asymptomatic subjects. A prospective investigation. J Bone Joint Surg [Am] 1990;72:403–8.

152. Boden SD, Frymoyer JW. Segmental instability: overview and classification. In: Frymoyer JW, editor. The adult spine: principles and practice. Philadelphia: Lippincott-Raven; 1997.

153. Boden SD, Riew KD, Yamaguchi K, et al. Orientation of the lumbar facet joints: association with degenerative disc disease. J Bone Joint Surg Am 1996;78:403–11.

154. Boden SD, Wiesel SW. Lumbosacral segmental motion in normal individuals. Have we been measuring instability properly? Spine 1990;15:571–6.

155. Bogduk N. The lumbar disc and low-back pain. Neurosurg Clin North Am 1991;2:791–806.

156. Bogduk N. Clinical anatomy of the lumbar spine. 3rd ed. Edinburgh, U.K.: Churchill Livingstone; 1997.

157. Bogduk N. What's in a name? The labelling of back pain. Med J Aust 2000;173:400–1.

158. Bogduk N. Functional anatomy of the disc and lumbar spine. In: Buttner-Janz K, Hochschuller SH, McAfee PC, editors. The Artificial Disc. Berlin: Springer; 2003. p. 19–32.

159. Bogduk N. Evidence-informed management of chronic low-back pain with facet injections and radiofrequency neurotomy. Spine J 2008;8:56–64.

160. Bogduk N, Andersson G. Is spinal surgery effective for back pain? F1000 Med Rep 2009;1.

161. Bogduk N, Johnson G, Spalding D. The morphology and biomechanics of latissimus dorsi. Clin Biomech 1998;13:377–85.

162. Bogduk N, Lord SM. Commentary on: Donelson, R., Aprill, C., Medcalf, R. Grant, W. (1997). A prospective study of centralization of lumbar and referred pain. Pain Med J Club J 1997;3:246–8.

163. Bogduk N, Macintosh JE. The applied anatomy of the thoracolumbar fascia. Spine 1984;9:164–70.

164. Bogduk N, Macintosh JE, Pearcy MJ. A universal model of the lumbar back muscles in the upright position. Spine 1992;17:897–913.

165. Bogduk N, Mercer S. Biomechanics of the cervical spine. I: Normal kinematics. Clin Biomech 2000;15:633–48.

166. Bogduk N, Pearcy M, Hadfield G. Anatomy and biomechanics of psoas major. Clin Biomech 1992;7:109–19.

167. Bongers PM, de Winter CR, Kompier MA, et al. Psychosocial factors at work and musculoskeletal disease. Scand J Work Environ Health 1993;19:297–312.

168. Boos N, Rieder R, Schade V, et al. 1995 Volvo Award in clinical sciences. The diagnostic accuracy of magnetic resonance imaging, work perception, and psychosocial factors in identifying symptomatic disc herniations. Spine 1995;20:2613–25.

169. Boos N, Semmer N, Elfering A, et al. Natural history of individuals with asymptomatic disc abnormalities in magnetic resonance imaging: predictors of low-back pain-related medical consultation and work incapacity. Spine 2000;25:1484–92.

170. Boos N, Weissbach S, Rohrbach H, et al. Classification of age-related changes in lumbar intervertebral discs: 2002 Volvo Award in basic science. Spine 2002;27:2631–44.

171. Boszczyk BM, Boszczyk AA, Boos W, et al. An immunohistochemical study of the tissue bridging adult spondylolytic defects – the presence and significance of fibrocartilaginous entheses. Eur Spine J 2006;15:965–71.

172. Botsford DJ, Esses SI, Ogilvie-Harris DJ. In vivo diurnal variation in intervertebral disc volume and morphology. Spine 1994;19:935–40.

173. Boulay C, Tardieu C, Hecquet J, et al. Sagittal alignment of spine and pelvis regulated by pelvic incidence: standard values and prediction of lordosis. Eur Spine J 2006;15:415–22.

174. Bovenzi M, Hulshof CT. An updated review of epidemiologic studies on the relationship between exposure to whole-body vibration and low-back pain (1986–1997). Int Arch Occup Environ Health 1999;72:351–65.

175. Bradbury N, Wilson LF, Mulholland RC. Adolescent disc protrusions. A long-term follow-up of surgery compared to chymopapain. Spine 1996;21: 372–7.

176. Bradford DS, Oegema Jr TR, Cooper KM, et al. Chymopapain, chemonucleolysis, and nucleus pulposus regeneration. A biochemical and biomechanical study. Spine 1984;9:135–47.

177. Braithwaite I, White J, Saifuddin A, et al. Vertebral end-plate (Modic) changes on lumbar spine MRI: correlation with pain reproduction at lumbar discography. Eur Spine J 1998;7:363–8.

178. Brandt KD, Braunstein EM, Visco DM, et al. Anterior (cranial) cruciate ligament transection in the dog: a bona fide model of osteoarthritis, not merely of cartilage injury and repair. J Rheumatol 1991;18:436–46.

179. Brattberg G. Do pain problems in young school children persist into early adulthood? A 13-year follow-up. Eur J Pain 2004; 8:187–99.

180. Bressler HB, Keyes WJ, Rochon PA, et al. The prevalence of low-back pain in the elderly. A systematic review of the literature. Spine 1999;24:1813–9.

181. Brickley-Parsons D, Glimcher MJ. Is the chemistry of collagen in intervertebral discs an expression of Wolff's law? A study of the human lumbar spine. Spine 1984;9:148–63.

182. Briggs AM, Greig AM, Wark JD. The vertebral fracture cascade in osteoporosis: a review of aetiopathogenesis. Osteoporos Int 2007;18:575–84.

183. Brinckmann P. Injury of the annulus fibrosus and disc protrusions. An in vitro investigation on human lumbar discs. Spine 1986;11:149–53.

184. Brinckmann P, Biggemann M, Hilweg D. Fatigue fracture of human lumbar vertebrae. Clin Biomech 1988;3(Suppl. 1).

185. Brinckmann P, Biggemann M, Hilweg D. Prediction of the compressive strength of human lumbar vertebrae. Clin Biomech 1989;4:(Suppl. 2).

186. Brinckmann P, Biggemann M, Hilweg D. Prediction of the

compressive strength of human lumbar vertebrae. Spine 1989;14: 606–10.

187. Brinckmann P, Frobin W, Biggemann M, et al. Quantification of overload injuries to the thoracolumbar spine in persons exposed to heavy physical exertions or vibration at the workplace: Part 2 – Occurrence and magnitude of overload injury in exposed cohorts. Clin Biomech 1998;13:s(2)1–s(2)36.

188. Brinckmann P, Frobin W, Hierholzer E, et al. Deformation of the vertebral end-plate under axial loading of the spine. Spine 1983;8:851–6.

189. Brinckmann P, Grootenboer H. Change of disc height, radial disc bulge, and intradiscal pressure from discectomy. An in vitro investigation on human lumbar discs. Spine 1991; 16:641–6.

190. Brinckmann P, Horst M. The influence of vertebral body fracture, intradiscal injection, and partial discectomy on the radial bulge and height of human lumbar discs. Spine 1985; 10:138–45.

191. Brinckmann P, Porter RW. A laboratory model of lumbar disc protrusion. Fissure and fragment [see comments]. Spine 1994; 19:228–35.

192. Brisby H, Byrod G, Olmarker K, et al. Nitric oxide as a mediator of nucleus pulposus-induced effects on spinal nerve roots. J Orthop Res 2000;18:815–20.

193. Brisby H, Wei AQ, Molloy T, et al. The effect of running exercise on intervertebral disc extracellular matrix production in a rat model. Spine (Phila Pa) 2010;35: 1429–36.

194. Brisson C, Montreuil S, Punnett L. Effects of an ergonomic training program on workers with video display units. Scand J Work Environ Health 1999;25: 255–63.

195. Broberg KB. Slow deformation of intervertebral discs. J Biomech 1993;26:501–12.

196. Brock M, Patt S, Mayer HM. The form and structure of the

extruded disc. Spine 1992;17:1457–61.

197. Brocklehurst R, Bayliss MT, Maroudas A, et al. The composition of normal and osteoarthritic articular cartilage from human knee joints. With special reference to unicompartmental replacement and osteotomy of the knee. J Bone Joint Surg [Am] 1984;66:95–106.

198. Brodsky AE, Kovalsky ES, Khalil MA. Correlation of radiologic assessment of lumbar spine fusions with surgical exploration. Spine 1991;16:S261–5.

199. Broom ND, Silyn-Roberts H. The three-dimensional 'knit' of collagen fibrils in articular cartilage. Connect Tissue Res 1989;23:261–77.

200. Broom ND, Silyn-Roberts H. Collagen-collagen versus collagen-proteoglycan interactions in the determination of cartilage strength. Arthritis Rheum 1990;33:1512–7.

201. Brophy MO, Achimore L, Moore-Dawson J. Reducing incidence of low-back injuries reduces cost. American Journal of Occupational and Environmental Health and Safety 2001;62: 508–11.

202. Brown MF, Hukkanen MV, McCarthy ID, et al. Sensory and sympathetic innervation of the vertebral endplate in patients with degenerative disc disease. J Bone Joint Surg Br 1997;79:147–53.

203. Brox JI, Sorensen R, Friis A, et al. Randomized clinical trial of lumbar instrumented fusion and cognitive intervention and exercises in patients with chronic low-back pain and disc degeneration. Spine 2003;28:1913–21.

204. Bruehlmann SB, Matyas JR, Duncan NA. ISSLS prize winner: Collagen fibril sliding governs cell mechanics in the annulus fibrosus: an in situ confocal microscopy study of bovine discs. Spine 2004;29:2612–20.

205. Brussee P, Hauth J, Donk RD, et al. Self-rated evaluation of outcome of the implantation of

interspinous process distraction (X-Stop) for neurogenic claudication. Eur Spine J 2008;17:200–3.

206. Buchbinder R, Jolley D. Population based intervention to change back pain beliefs: three year follow up population survey. BMJ 2004;328:321.

207. Buchbinder R, Jolley D, Wyatt M. Population based intervention to change back pain beliefs and disability: three part evaluation. BMJ 2001;322:1516–20.

208. Buck JE. Direct repair of the defect in spondylolisthesis. Preliminary report. J Bone Joint Surg Br 1970;52:432–7.

209. Buck JE. Further thoughts on direct repair of the defect in spondylolisthesis. J Bone Joint Surg Br 1979;61:123.

210. Buckley JM, Kuo CC, Cheng LC, et al. Relative strength of thoracic vertebrae in axial compression versus flexion. Spine J 2009;9: 478–85.

211. Buckwalter JA. Aging and degeneration of the human intervertebral disc. Spine 1995;20:1307–14.

212. Burdorf A, Sorock G. Positive and negative evidence of risk factors for back disorders. Scand J Work Environ Health 1997;23:243–56.

213. Burke JG, Watson RW, Conhyea D, et al. Human nucleus pulposis can respond to a pro-inflammatory stimulus. Spine 2003;28:2685–93.

214. Burton AK. Back injury and work loss. Biomechanical and psychosocial influences. Spine 1997;22:2575–80.

215. Burton AK, Balague F, Eriksen HR et al. European Guidelines for Prevention in Low-back Pain. EC Cost Action B13. Available online at: www.backpaineurope.org. 2004.

216. Burton AK, Bartys S, Wright IA, et al. Obstacles to recovery from musculoskeletal disorders in industry. (Research Report 323). London: HSE books; 2005.

217. Burton AK, Clarke RD, McClune TD, et al. The natural history of low-back pain in adolescents. Spine 1996;21:2323–8.

218. Burton AK, Leivseth G. Manipulative therapy. In: Szpalski

M, Gunzburg R, Pope MH, editors. Lumbar Segmental Instability. Philadelphia: Lippincott Williams and Wilkins; 1998. p. 153–8.

219. Burton AK, Main CJ. Obstacles to recovery from work-related musculoskeletal disorders. In: Karwowski W, editor. International Encyclopedia of Ergonomics and Human Factors. London: Taylor and Francis; 2000. p. 1542–4.

220. Burton AK, Main CJ. Relevance of biomechanics in occupational musculoskeletal disorders. In: Mayer TG, Gatchel RJ, Polatin PB, editors. Occupational musculoskeletal disorders: function, outcomes and evidence. Philadelphia: Lippincott-Raven; 2000. p. 157–66.

221. Burton AK, McClune TD, Clarke RD, et al. Long-term follow-up of patients with low-back pain attending for manipulative care: outcomes and predictors. Man Ther 2004;9:30–5.

222. Burton AK, Symonds TL, Zinzen E, et al. Is ergonomic intervention alone sufficient to limit musculoskeletal problems in nurses? Occup Med (Lond) 1997;47:25–32.

223. Burton AK, Tillotson KM. Reference values for 'normal' regional lumbar sagittal mobility. Clin Biomech 1988;3:106–13.

224. Burton AK, Tillotson KM, Boocock MG. Estimation of spinal loads in overhead work. Ergonomics 1994;37:1311–21.

225. Burton AK, Tillotson KM, Cleary J. Single-blind randomised controlled trial of chemonucleolysis and manipulation in the treatment of symptomatic lumbar disc herniation. Eur Spine J 2000;9:202–7.

226. Burton AK, Tillotson KM, Symonds TL, et al. Occupational risk factors for the first-onset and subsequent course of low-back trouble. A study of serving police officers. Spine 1996;21:2612–20.

227. Burton AK, Tillotson KM, Troup JD. Variation in lumbar sagittal mobility with low-back trouble. Spine 1989;14:584–90.

228. Burton AK, Waddell G. Clinical guidelines in the management of low-back pain. Bailliere's Clin Rheumatol 1998;12:17–35.

229. Burton AK, Waddell G. Educational and informational approaches. In: Linton SJ, editor. New avenues for the prevention of chronic musculoskeletal pain and disability. Amsterdam: Elsevier Science; 2002. p. 245–58.

230. Burton AK, Waddell G, Tillotson KM, et al. Information and advice to patients with back pain can have a positive effect. A randomized controlled trial of a novel educational booklet in primary care. Spine 1999;24: 2484–91.

231. Burton AW, Rhines LD, Mendel E. Vertebroplasty and kyphoplasty: a comprehensive review. Neurosurg Focus 2005;18:e1.

232. Buser Z, Kuelling F, Liu J, et al. Biological and biomechanical effects of fibrin injection into porcine intervertebral discs. Spine (Phila Pa) 2011.

233. Busscher I, van Dieen JH, Kingma I, et al. Biomechanical characteristics of different regions of the human spine: an in vitro study on multilevel spinal segments. Spine (Phila Pa) 2009;34:2858–64.

234. Butler D, Trafimow JH, Andersson GB, et al. Discs degenerate before facets. Spine 1990;15:111–3.

235. Byrod G, Rydevik B, Nordborg C, et al. Early effects of nucleus pulposus application on spinal nerve root morphology and function. Eur Spine J 1998;7:445–9.

236. Cady LD, Bischoff DP, O'Connell ER, et al. Strength and fitness and subsequent back injuries in firefighters. J Occup Med 1979;21:269–72.

237. Caligaris M, Ateshian GA. Effects of sustained interstitial fluid pressurization under migrating contact area, and boundary lubrication by synovial fluid, on cartilage friction. Osteoarthritis Cartilage 2008;16:1220–7.

238. Callaghan JP, McGill SM. Frozen storage increases the ultimate compressive load of porcine vertebrae. J Orthop Res 1995;13: 809–12.

239. Calvo E, Palacios I, Delgado E, et al. High-resolution MRI detects cartilage swelling at the early stages of experimental osteoarthritis. Osteoarthritis Cartilage 2001;9:463–72.

240. Campbell C, Muncer SJ. The causes of low-back pain: a network analysis. Soc Sci Med 2005;60:409–19.

241. Canepari M, Rossi R, Pellegrino MA, et al. Effects of resistance training on myosin function studied by the in vitro motility assay in young and older men. J Appl Physiol 2005;98:2390–5.

242. Cannon JG. Intrinsic and extrinsic factors in muscle aging. Ann N Y Acad Sci 1998;854:72–7.

243. Cannon JG, Meydani SN, Fielding RA, et al. Acute phase response in exercise. II. Associations between vitamin E, cytokines, and muscle proteolysis. Am J Physiol 1991;260:R1235–40.

244. Cannon JG, St Pierre BA. Cytokines in exertion-induced skeletal muscle injury. Mol Cell Biochem 1998;179:159–67.

245. Cao DY, Khalsa PS, Pickar JG. Dynamic responsiveness of lumbar paraspinal muscle spindles during vertebral movement in the cat. Exp Brain Res 2009;197:369–77.

246. Cao DY, Pickar JG, Ge W, et al. Position sensitivity of feline paraspinal muscle spindles to vertebral movement in the lumbar spine. J Neurophysiol 2009;101:1722–9.

247. Cardon G, Balague F. Low-back pain prevention's effects in schoolchildren. What is the evidence? Eur Spine J 2004;13:663–79.

248. Cardon GM, De Clercq DL, De Bourdeaudhuij IM. Back education efficacy in elementary schoolchildren: a 1-year follow-up study. Spine 2002;27:299–305.

249. Carey TS, Garrett JM, Jackman A, et al. Recurrence and care-seeking after acute back pain: results of a

long- term follow-up study. North Carolina Back Pain Project. Med Care 1999;37:157–64.

250. Carosella AM, Lackner JM, Feuerstein M. Factors associated with early discharge from a multidisciplinary work rehabilitation program for chronic low-back pain. Pain 1994;57:69–76.

251. Carragee E, Alamin T, Cheng I, et al. Does minor trauma cause serious low-back illness? Spine 2006;31:2942–9.

252. Carragee EJ. The vertebroplasty affair: the mysterious case of the disappearing effect size. Spine J 2010;10:191–2.

253. Carragee EJ, Alamin TF, Miller JL, et al. Discographic, MRI and psychosocial determinants of low-back pain disability and remission: a prospective study in subjects with benign persistent back pain. Spine J 2005;5:24–35.

254. Carragee EJ, Don AS, Hurwitz EL, et al. 2009 ISSLS Prize Winner: Does discography cause accelerated progression of degeneration changes in the lumbar disc: a ten-year matched cohort study. Spine (Phila Pa) 2009;34:2338–45.

255. Carragee EJ, Han MY, Yang B, et al. Activity restrictions after posterior lumbar discectomy. A prospective study of outcomes in 152 cases with no postoperative restrictions. Spine 1999; 24:2346–51.

256. Carragee EJ, Paragioudakis SJ, Khurana S. 2000 Volvo Award winner in clinical studies: Lumbar high-intensity zone and discography in subjects without low-back problems. Spine (Phila Pa) 2000;25:2987–92.

257. Carter JT, Birrell LN. Occupational health guidelines for the management of low-back pain at work – principal recommendations. London: Faculty of Occupational Medicine; 2000.

258. Cassidy JD, Yong-Hing K, Kirkaldy-Willis WH, et al. A study of the effects of bipedism and upright posture on the lumbosacral spine and paravertebral muscles of the Wistar rat. Spine 1988; 13:301–8.

259. Cassidy JJ, Hiltner A, Baer E. Hierarchical structure of the intervertebral disc. Connect Tissue Res 1989;23:75–88.

260. Cassisi JE, Robinson ME, O'Conner P, et al. Trunk strength and lumbar paraspinal muscle activity during isometric exercise in chronic low-back pain patients and controls. Spine 1993; 18:245–51.

261. Cauley JA, Hochberg MC, Lui LY, et al. Long-term risk of incident vertebral fractures. Jama 2007;298:2761–7.

262. Cavanaugh JM, Ozaktay AC, Yamashita HT, et al. Lumbar facet pain: biomechanics, neuroanatomy and neurophysiology. J Biomech 1996;29:1117–29.

263. Cavanaugh JM, Ozaktay AC, Yamashita T, et al. Mechanisms of low-back pain: a neurophysiologic and neuroanatomic study. Clin Orthop 1997;335:166–80.

264. Chaffin D. Computerised biomechanical models – development and use in studying gross body actions. J Biomech 1969;2:429–41.

265. Charney W. The lift team method for reducing back injuries. A 10 hospital study. Journal of the American Association of Occupational Health Nurses 1997;45:300–4.

266. Cheadle A, Franklin G, Wolfhagen C, et al. Factors influencing the duration of work-related disability: a population-based study of Washington State workers' compensation. Am J Public Health 1994;84:190–6.

267. Chen AC, Temple MM, Ng DM, et al. Induction of advanced glycation end products and alterations of the tensile properties of articular cartilage. Arthritis Rheum 2002;46:3212–7.

268. Chen B, Fellenberg J, Wang H, et al. Occurrence and regional distribution of apoptosis in scoliotic discs. Spine 2005;30:519–24.

269. Chen C, Cavanaugh JM, Song Z, et al. Effects of nucleus pulposus on nerve root neural activity, mechanosensitivity, axonal morphology, and sodium channel expression. Spine 2004;29:17–25.

270. Chen SM, Liu MF, Cook J, et al. Sedentary lifestyle as a risk factor for low-back pain: a systematic review. Int Arch Occup Environ Health 2009; 82:797–806.

271. Cheng JC, Tang SP, Guo X, et al. Osteopenia in adolescent idiopathic scoliosis: a histomorphometric study. Spine 2001;26:E19–23.

272. Cherkin DC, Deyo RA, Battie M, et al. A comparison of physical therapy, chiropractic manipulation, and provision of an educational booklet for the treatment of patients with low-back pain. N Engl J Med 1998;339:1021–9.

273. Cheung KM, Karppinen J, Chan D, et al. Prevalence and pattern of lumbar magnetic resonance imaging changes in a population study of one thousand forty-three individuals. Spine 2009; 34:934–40.

274. Cheung KM, Samartzis D, Karppinen J, et al. Intervertebral disc degeneration: New insights based on 'skipped' level disc pathology. Arthritis Rheum 2010;62:2392–400.

275. Cholewicki J, Crisco 3rd JJ, Oxland TR, et al. Effects of posture and structure on three-dimensional coupled rotations in the lumbar spine. A biomechanical analysis. Spine 1996;21:2421–8.

276. Cholewicki J, McGill SM. Lumbar posterior ligament involvement during extremely heavy lifts estimated from fluoroscopic measurements. J Biomech 1992;25:17–28.

277. Cholewicki J, McGill SM, Norman RW. Comparison of muscle forces and joint load from an optimization and EMG assisted lumbar spine model: towards development of a hybrid approach. J Biomech 1995;28:321–31.

278. Cholewicki J, Reeves NP. All abdominal muscles must be considered when evaluating the intra-abdominal pressure contribution to trunk extensor moment and spinal loading. J Biomech 2004;37:953–4.

279. Cholewicki J, Silfies SP, Shah RA, et al. Delayed trunk muscle reflex responses increase the risk of low-back injuries. Spine 2005;30:2614–20.

280. Chow DH, Luk KD, Leong JC, et al. Torsional stability of the lumbosacral junction. Significance of the iliolumbar ligament. Spine 1989;14:611–5.

281. Chu JY, Skrzypiec D, Pollintine P, et al. Can compressive stress be measured experimentally within the annulus fibrosus of degenerated intervertebral discs? Proc Inst Mech Eng [H] 2008;222:161–70.

282. Chung SK, Lee SH, Kim DY, et al. Treatment of lower lumbar radiculopathy caused by osteoporotic compression fracture: the role of vertebroplasty. J Spinal Disord Tech 2002;15:461–8.

283. Clarke JM. The organisation of collagen in cryofractured rabbit articular cartilage: a scanning electron microscopic study. J Orthop Res 1985;3:17–29.

284. Clarkson PM, Kroll W, McBride TC. Maximal isometric strength and fiber type composition in power and endurance athletes. Eur J Appl Physiol Occup Physiol 1980;44:35–42.

285. Clements K, Hollander A, Sharif M, et al. Cyclic Loading Can Denature Type II Collagen in Articular Cartilage. Connect Tissue Res 2004;45:174–80.

286. Clements KM, Bee ZC, Crossingham GV, et al. How severe must repetitive loading be to kill chondrocytes in articular cartilage? Osteoarthritis Cartilage 2001;9:499–507.

287. Clouet J, Grimandi G, Pot-Vaucel M, et al. Identification of phenotypic discriminating markers for intervertebral disc cells and articular chondrocytes. Rheumatology (Oxf) 2009;48:1447–50.

288. Cloward RR. The treatment of ruptured lumbar intervertebral disc by interbody fusion. Indications, operative technique, aftercare. J Neurosurg 1953;10:154–68.

289. Cloyd JM, Elliott DM. Elastin content correlates with human disc degeneration in the annulus fibrosus and nucleus pulposus. Spine 2007;32:1826–31.

290. Coggan D, Rose G, Barker DJP. Epidemiology for the uninitiated. London: BMJ Publishing Group; 1997.

291. Cohen RE, Hooley CJ, McCrum NG. Viscoelastic creep of collagenous tissue. J Biomech 1976;9:175–84.

292. Colhoun E, McCall IW, Williams L, et al. Provocation discography as a guide to planning operations on the spine. J Bone Joint Surg Br 1988;70:267–71.

293. Collee G, Dijkmans BA, Vandenbroucke JP, Cats A. Iliac crest pain syndrome in low-back pain: frequency and features. J Rheumatol 1991;18:1064–7.

294. Colombini D, Occhipinti E, Grieco A, et al. Estimation of lumbar disc areas by means of anthropometric parameters [published erratum appears in Spine 1989 May;14(5):533]. Spine 1989;14:51–5.

295. Conley KE, Esselman PC, Jubrias SA, et al. Ageing, muscle properties and maximal O(2) uptake rate in humans. J Physiol 2000;526:211–7.

296. Conley KE, Jubrias SA, Esselman PC. Oxidative capacity and ageing in human muscle. J Physiol 2000;526:203–10.

297. Coppes MH, Marani E, Thomeer RT, et al. Innervation of 'painful' lumbar discs. Spine 1997;22:2342–9; discussion 9–50.

298. Cortet B, Houvenagel E, Puisieux F, et al. Spinal curvatures and quality of life in women with vertebral fractures secondary to osteoporosis. Spine 1999;24:1921–5.

299. Cossette JW, Farfan HF, Robertson GH, et al. The instantaneous center of rotation of the third lumbar intervertebral joint. J Biomech 1971;4:149–53.

300. Costi JJ, Stokes IA, Gardner-Morse M, et al. Direct measurement of intervertebral disc maximum shear strain in six degrees of freedom: motions that place disc tissue at risk of injury. J Biomech 2007;40:2457–66.

301. Coudeyre E, Rannou F, Coriat F, et al. Impact of The Back Book on acute low-back pain outcome. Presented to the International Society for the Study of the Lumbar Spine, New York, 2005.

302. Cox VM, Williams PE, Wright H, et al. Growth induced by incremental static stretch in adult rabbit latissimus dorsi muscle. Exp Physiol 2000;85:193–202.

303. Crans GG, Silverman SL, Genant HK, et al. Association of severe vertebral fractures with reduced quality of life: reduction in the incidence of severe vertebral fractures by teriparatide. Arthritis Rheum 2004;50:4028–34.

304. Cresswell AG. Responses of intra-abdominal pressure and abdominal muscle activity during dynamic trunk loading in man. Eur J Appl Physiol Occup Physiol 1993;66:315–20.

305. Cribb GL, Jaffray DC, Cassar-Pullicino VN. Observations on the natural history of massive lumbar disc herniation. J Bone Joint Surg Br 2007;89:782–4.

306. Crock HV. A reappraisal of intervertebral disc lesions. Med J Aust 1970;1:983–9.

307. Crock HV. Internal disc disruption. A challenge to disc prolapse fifty years on. Spine 1986;11:650–3.

308. Croft P, Papageorgiou AC, McNally R. Low-back pain. In: Stevens A, Rafferty J, editors. Healthcare Needs Assessment. 2nd series. Oxford: Radcliffe Medical Press; 1997. p. 129–82.

309. Croft PR, Macfarlane GJ, Papageorgiou AC, et al. Outcome of low-back pain in general practice: a prospective study. BMJ 1998;316:1356–9.

310. Croft PR, Papageorgiou AC, Ferry S, et al. Psychologic distress and low-back pain. Evidence from a prospective study in the general population. Spine 1995;20:2731–7.

311. Currey JD. Anelasticity in Bone and Echinoderm Skeletons. J Exp Biol 1965;43:279–92.

312. Cvijanovic O, Bobinac D, Zoricic S, et al. Age- and region-dependent changes in human lumbar vertebral bone: a histomorphometric study. Spine 2004;29:2370–5.

313. Cyron BM, Hutton WC. The fatigue strength of the lumbar neural arch in spondylolysis. J Bone Joint Surg [Br] 1978;60-B:234–8.

314. Cyron BM, Hutton WC. Variations in the amount and distribution of cortical bone across the partes interarticulares of L5. A predisposing factor in spondylolysis? Spine 1979;4:163–7.

315. Cyron BM, Hutton WC. Articular tropism and stability of the lumbar spine. Spine 1980;5:168–72.

316. Cyron BM, Hutton WC. The behaviour of the lumbar intervertebral disc under repetitive forces. Int Orthop 1981;5:203–7.

317. Cyron BM, Hutton WC. The tensile strength of the capsular ligaments of the apophyseal joints. J Anat 1981;132:145–50.

318. Cyron BM, Hutton WC, Troup JD. Spondylolytic fractures. J Bone Joint Surg [Br] 1976;58-B:462–6.

319. Daggfeldt K, Thorstensson A. The mechanics of back-extensor torque production about the lumbar spine. J Biomech 2003;36:815–25.

320. Damien E, Price JS, Lanyon LE. Mechanical strain stimulates osteoblast proliferation through the estrogen receptor in males as well as females. J Bone Miner Res 2000;15:2169–77.

321. Dar G, Masharawi Y, Peleg S, et al. Schmorl's nodes distribution in the human spine and its possible etiology. Eur Spine J 2010;19:670–5.

322. Davidson BS, Madigan ML, Nussbaum MA. Effects of lumbar extensor fatigue and fatigue rate on postural sway. Eur J Appl Physiol 2004;93:183–9.

323. Davidson BS, Madigan ML, Nussbaum MA, et al. Effects of localized muscle fatigue on recovery from a postural perturbation without stepping. Gait Posture 2009;29:552–7.

324. Davis KG, Heaney CA. The relationship between psychosocial work characteristics and low-back pain: underlying methodological issues. Clin Biomech 2000;15:389–406.

325. Davis PR, Troup JDG, Burnard JH. Movements of the thoracic and lumbar spine when lifting: a chrono-cyclophotographic study. J Anat 1965;99:13–26.

326. Dawson AP, McLennan SN, Schiller SD, et al. Interventions to prevent back pain and back injury in nurses: a systematic review. Occup Environ Med 2007;64:642–50.

327. Day R, Puustjarvi K, Adams MA. Can physical exercise strengthen intervertebral discs? Presented to the Society for Back Pain Research; 1999; Cardiff, U.K.; 1999.

328. de Looze MP, Visser B, Houting I, et al. Weight and frequency effect on spinal loading in a bricklaying task. J Biomech 1996;29:1425–33.

329. De Pukey P. The physiological oscillation of the length of the body. Acta Orthop Scand 1935;6:338.

330. de Schepper EI, Damen J, van Meurs JB, et al. The association between lumbar disc degeneration and low-back pain: the influence of age, gender, and individual radiographic features. Spine (Phila Pa) 2010;35:531–6.

331. de Vet HC, Heymans MW, Dunn KM, et al. Episodes of low-back pain: a proposal for uniform definitions to be used in research. Spine 2002;27:2409–16.

332. Debnath UK, Freeman BJ, Gregory P, et al. Clinical outcome and return to sport after the surgical treatment of spondylolysis in young athletes. J Bone Joint Surg Br 2003;85:244–9.

333. Deen HG, Fenton G. Electro-thermal disc decompression. Preliminary experience. Presented at the IITS meeting, May 19–24 2004; Munich, Germany; 2004.

334. DeGroot J, Verzijl N, Bank RA, et al. Age-related decrease in proteoglycan synthesis of human articular chondrocytes: the role of nonenzymatic glycation. Arthritis Rheum 1999;42:1003–9.

335. DeGroot J, Verzijl N, Wenting-Van Wijk MJ, et al. Accumulation of advanced glycation end products as a molecular mechanism for aging as a risk factor in osteoarthritis. Arthritis Rheum 2004;50:1207–15.

336. Deguchi M, Rapoff AJ, Zdeblick TA. Biomechanical comparison of spondylolysis fixation techniques. Spine 1999;24:328–33.

337. Delport EG, Cucuzzella AR, Marley JK, et al. Treatment of lumbar spinal stenosis with epidural steroid injections: a retrospective outcome study. Arch Phys Med Rehabil 2004;85:479–84.

338. Denis F. The three column spine and its significance in the classification of acute thoracolumbar spinal injuries. Spine 1983;8:817–31.

339. Derby R, Eek B, Chen Y. Intradiscal electrothermal annuloplasty (IDET); A novel approach for treating chronic discogenic back pain. Neuromodulation 2000;3:82–8.

340. Devereux JJ, Buckle PW, Vlachonikolis IG. Interactions between physical and psychosocial risk factors at work increase the risk of back disorders: an epidemiological approach. Occup Environ Med 1999;56:343–53.

341. Devor ST, Faulkner JA. Regeneration of new fibers in muscles of old rats reduces contraction- induced injury. J Appl Physiol 1999;87:750–6.

342. Dey P, Simpson CW, Collins SI, et al. Implementation of RCGP guidelines for acute low-back pain: a cluster randomised controlled trial. Br J Gen Pract 2004;54:33–7.

343. Deyo RA. Practice variations, treatment fads, rising disability. Do we need a new clinical research paradigm? Spine 1993;18:2153–62.

344. Deyo RA, Diehl AK. Cancer as a cause of back pain: frequency,

clinical presentation, and diagnostic strategies. J Gen Intern Med 1988;3:230–8.

345. Deyo RA, Rainville J, Kent DL. What can the history and physical examination tell us about low-back pain? JAMA 1992;268:760–5.

346. Deyo RA, Tsui-Wu YJ. Descriptive epidemiology of low-back pain and its related medical care in the United States. Spine 1987;12:264–8.

347. Dhillon N, Bass EC, Lotz JC. Effect of frozen storage on the creep behavior of human intervertebral discs. Spine 2001;26:883–8.

348. Dicken BJ, McGregor AH, Jamrozik KD. Trends in the management of post-operative back pain. J Bone Joint Surg 2005;87-B(Suppl. 1):38.

349. Dickey JP, Kerr DJ. Effect of specimen length: are the mechanics of individual motion segments comparable in functional spinal units and multisegment specimens? Med Eng Phys 2003;25: 221–7.

350. Dieen van JH, Creemers M, Draisma I, et al. Repetitive lifting and spinal shrinkage, effects of age and lifting technique. Clin Biomech 1994;9:367–74.

351. Dieen van JH, van der Burg P, Raaijmakers TAJ, et al. Effects of repetitive lifting on kinematics: inadequate anticipatory control or adaptive changes? J Motor Behav 1998;30:20–32.

352. Dietz V. Human neuronal control of automatic functional movements: interaction between central programs and afferent input. Physiol Rev 1992;72: 33–69.

353. DiMicco MA, Patwari P, Siparsky PN, et al. Mechanisms and kinetics of glycosaminoglycan release following in vitro cartilage injury. Arthritis Rheum 2004;50: 840–8.

354. Dionne CE. Low-back pain. In: Crombie IK, editor. Epidemiology of pain. Seattle: IASP Press; 1999. p. 283–97.

355. Doherty TJ, Vandervoort AA, Brown WF. Effects of ageing on the motor unit: a brief review. Can J Appl Physiol 1993;18:331–58.

356. Dolan KJ, Green A. Lumbar spine reposition sense: the effect of a 'slouched' posture. Man Ther 2006;11:202–7.

357. Dolan P, Adams MA. Influence of lumbar and hip mobility on the bending stresses acting on the lumbar spine. Clin Biomech 1993;8:185–92.

358. Dolan P, Adams MA. The relationship between EMG activity and extensor moment generation in the erector spinae muscles during bending and lifting activities. J Biomech 1993;26:513–22.

359. Dolan P, Adams MA. Repetitive lifting tasks fatigue the back muscles and increase the bending moment acting on the lumbar spine. J Biomech 1998;31:713–21.

360. Dolan P, Adams MA. Recent advances in lumbar spinal mechanics and their significance for modelling. Clin Biomech 2001;16:S8–S16.

361. Dolan P, Adams MA, Hutton WC. The short-term effects of chymopapain on intervertebral discs. J Bone Joint Surg [Br] 1987;69:422–8.

362. Dolan P, Adams MA, Hutton WC. Commonly adopted postures and their effect on the lumbar spine. Spine 1988;13:197–201.

363. Dolan P, Earley M, Adams MA. Bending and compressive stresses acting on the lumbar spine during lifting activities. J Biomech 1994;27:1237–48.

364. Dolan P, Kingma I, De Looze MP, et al. An EMG technique for measuring spinal loading during asymmetric lifting. Clin Biomech 2001;16:S17–24.

365. Dolan P, Kingma I, van Dieen J, et al. Dynamic forces acting on the lumbar spine during manual handling. Can they be estimated using electromyographic techniques alone? Spine 1999;24:698–703.

366. Dolan P, Mannion AF, Adams MA. Passive tissues help the back muscles to generate extensor moments during lifting. J Biomech 1994;27:1077–85.

367. Dolan P, Mannion AF, Adams MA. Fatigue of the erector spinae muscles. A quantitative assessment using 'frequency banding' of the surface electromyography signal. Spine 1995;20:149–59.

368. Dolan P, Mannion AF, Adams MA. 'Schober test' measurements do not correlate well with angular movements of the lumbar spine. In: International Society for the Study of the Lumbar Spine; 1995; Helsinki, Finland; 1995.

369. Dolan P, Shandall S, Hodges K, et al. 'Creep' in spinal tissues impairs spinal proprioception and delays activation of the back muscles. In: Orthopaedic Research Society; Washington, USA; 2005.

370. Donelson R, Aprill C, Medcalf R, et al. A prospective study of centralization of lumbar and referred pain. A predictor of symptomatic discs and annular competence. Spine 1997;22:1115–22.

371. Dore D, Quinn S, Ding C, et al. Subchondral bone and cartilage damage: a prospective study in older adults. Arthritis Rheum 2010;62:1967–73.

372. Dressler MR, Butler DL, Wenstrup R, et al. A potential mechanism for age-related declines in patellar tendon biomechanics. J Orthop Res 2002;20:1315–22.

373. Dreyfuss P, Michaelsen M, Pauza K, et al. The value of medical history and physical examination in diagnosing sacroiliac joint pain [see comments]. Spine 1996;21:2594–602.

374. Dreyzin V, Esses SI. A comparative analysis of spondylolysis repair. Spine 1994;19:1909–14; discussion 15.

375. Duance VC, Crean JK, Sims TJ, et al. Changes in collagen cross-linking in degenerative disc disease and scoliosis. Spine 1998;23:2545–51.

376. Dumas GA, Beaudoin L, Drouin G. In situ mechanical behavior of posterior spinal ligaments in the lumbar region. An in vitro study. J Biomech 1987;20:301–10.

377. Dumas GA, Reid JG, Wolfe LA, et al. Exercise, posture, and back pain during pregnancy. Clin Biomech 1995;10:104–9.

378. Duncan NA. Cell deformation and micromechanical environment in the intervertebral disc. J Bone Joint Surg Am 2006;88(Suppl. 2):47–51.

379. Duncan NA, Ahmed AM. The role of axial rotation in the etiology of unilateral disc prolapse. An experimental and finite-element analysis. Spine 1991;16:1089–98.

380. Dunlop RB, Adams MA, Hutton WC. Disc space narrowing and the lumbar facet joints. J Bone Joint Surg [Br] 1984;66:706–10.

381. Dunn KM, Croft PR. Epidemiology and natural history of low-back pain. Eura Medicophys 2004;40:9–13.

382. Dupuis PR, Yong-Hing K, Cassidy JD, et al. Radiologic diagnosis of degenerative lumbar spinal instability. Spine 1985;10:262–76.

383. Dvorak J, Panjabi MM, Chang DG, et al. Functional radiographic diagnosis of the lumbar spine. Flexion- extension and lateral bending. Spine 1991;16:562–71.

384. Dvorak J, Vajda EG, Grob D, et al. Normal motion of the lumbar spine as related to age and gender. Eur Spine J 1995;4:18–23.

385. Ebara S, Iatridis JC, Setton LA, et al. Tensile properties of nondegenerate human lumbar annulus fibrosus. Spine 1996;21:452–61.

386. Egund N, Olsson TH, Schmid H, et al. Movements in the sacroiliac joints demonstrated with roentgen stereophotogrammetry. Acta Radiol [Diagn] 1978;19:833–46.

387. Eie N. Load capacity of the low-back. J Oslo City Hosp 1966;16:73–98.

388. Eie N. Recent measurements of the intra-abdominal pressure. In: Kenedi RM, editor. Perspectives in Biomedical Engineering. London: MacMillan Press; 1973. p. 121.

389. Eisenstein S. Spondylolysis. A skeletal investigation of two population groups. J Bone Joint Surg [Br] 1978;60-B:488–94.

390. Eisenstein SM, Parry CR. The lumbar facet arthrosis syndrome. Clinical presentation and articular surface changes. J Bone Joint Surg Br 1987;69:3–7.

391. Ekman P, Moller H, Hedlund R. The long-term effect of posterolateral fusion in adult isthmic spondylolisthesis: a randomized controlled study. Spine J 2005;5:36–44.

392. Ekman P, Moller H, Shalabi A, et al. A prospective randomised study on the long-term effect of lumbar fusion on adjacent disc degeneration. Eur Spine J 2009;18:1175–86.

393. El-Metwally A, Mikkelsson M, Stahl M, et al. Genetic and environmental influences on non-specific low-back pain in children: a twin study. Eur Spine J 2008;17:502–8.

394. El Mahdi MA, Latif FYA, Janko M. The spinal nerve root innervation, and a new concept of the clinicopathological interrelations in back pain and sciatica. Neurochirurgia 1981;24:137–41.

395. Elders LA, Heinrich J, Burdorf A. Risk factors for sickness absence because of low-back pain among scaffolders: a 3-year follow-up study. Spine 2003;28:1340–6.

396. Elliott DM, Yerramalli CS, Beckstein JC, et al. The effect of relative needle diameter in puncture and sham injection animal models of degeneration. Spine 2008;33:588–96.

397. Ennion S, Sant'ana Pereira J, Sargeant AJ, et al. Characterization of human skeletal muscle fibres according to the myosin heavy chains they express. J Muscle Res Cell Motil 1995;16:35–43.

398. Ensink FB, Saur PM, Frese K, et al. Lumbar range of motion: influence of time of day and individual factors on measurements. Spine 1996;21:1339–43.

399. Eriksen W, Bruusgaard D, Knardahl S. Work factors as predictors of intense or disabling low-back pain; a prospective study of nurses' aides. Occup Environ Med 2004;61:398–404.

400. Errington RJ, Puustjarvi K, White IR, et al. Characterisation of cytoplasm-filled processes in cells of the intervertebral disc. J Anat 1998;192:369–78.

401. Esola MA, McClure PW, Fitzgerald GK, et al. Analysis of lumbar spine and hip motion during forward bending in subjects with and without a history of low-back pain. Spine 1996;21:71–8.

402. Eswaran SK, Gupta A, Adams MF, et al. Cortical and trabecular load sharing in the human vertebral body. J Bone Miner Res 2006;21:307–14.

403. Eubanks JD, Lee MJ, Cassinelli E, et al. Does Lumbar Facet Arthrosis Precede Disc Degeneration?: A Postmortem Study. Clin Orthop Relat Res 2007;464:184–9.

404. Eubanks JD, Lee MJ, Cassinelli E, et al. Prevalence of lumbar facet arthrosis and its relationship to age, sex, and race: an anatomic study of cadaveric specimens. Spine 2007;32:2058–62.

405. Evanoff BA, Bohr PC, Wolf LD. Effects of a participatory ergonomics team among hospital orderlies. Am J Ind Med 1999;35:358–65.

406. Eyre DR, Muir H. Quantitative analysis of types I and II collagens in human intervertebral discs at various ages. Biochim Biophys Acta 1977;492:29–42.

407. Fagan AB, Sarvestani G, Moore RJ, et al. Innervation of annulus tears: an experimental animal study. Spine (Phila Pa) 2010;35:1200–5.

408. Fahrni WH. Conservative treatment of lumbar disc degeneration: our primary responsibility. Orthop Clin North Am 1975;6:93–103.

409. Fahrni WH, Trueman GE. Comparative radiological study of the spines of a primitive population with North Americans and North Europeans. J Bone Joint Surg [Br] 1965;47:552–5.

410. Fairbank J, Frost H, Wilson-MacDonald J, et al. Randomised

controlled trial to compare surgical stabilisation of the lumbar spine with an intensive rehabilitation programme for patients with chronic low-back pain: the MRC spine stabilisation trial. BMJ 2005;330:1233.

411. Fairbank JC, Park WM, McCall IW, et al. Apophyseal injection of local anesthetic as a diagnostic aid in primary low-back pain syndromes. Spine 1981;6:598–605.

412. Fardon DF. Nomenclature and classification of lumbar disc pathology. Spine 2001;26:461–2.

413. Farfan HF, Cossette JW, Robertson GH, et al. The effects of torsion on the lumbar intervertebral joints: the role of torsion in the production of disc degeneration. J Bone Joint Surg [Am] 1970;52:468–97.

414. Farfan HF, Huberdeau RM, Dubow HI. Lumbar intervertebral disc degeneration: the influence of geometrical features on the pattern of disc degeneration – a post mortem study. J Bone Joint Surg [Am] 1972;54:492–510.

415. Farfan HF, Sullivan JD. The relation of facet orientation to intervertebral disc failure. Can J Surg 1967;10:179–85.

416. Fathallah FA, Marras WS, Parnianpour M. An assessment of complex spinal loads during dynamic lifting tasks. Spine 1998;23:706–16.

417. Fathallah FA, Marras WS, Parnianpour M. The role of complex, simultaneous trunk motions in the risk of occupation-related low-back disorders. Spine 1998;23:1035–42.

418. Fauno P, Kalund S, Andreasen I, et al. Soreness in lower extremities and back is reduced by use of shock absorbing heel inserts. Int J Sports Med 1993;14:288–90.

419. Feingold AJ, Jacobs K. The effect of education on backpack wearing and posture in a middle school population. Work 2002;18:287–94.

420. Feinstein B, Langton JNK, Jameson RM, et al. Experiments on pain referred from deep somatic tissues. J Bone Joint Surg 1954;35 A:981–7.

421. Felson DT, Hannan MT, Naimark A, et al. Occupational physical demands, knee bending, and knee osteoarthritis: results from the Framingham Study. J Rheumatol 1991;18:1587–92.

422. Ferguson SA, Marras WS. A literature review of low-back disorder surveillance measures and risk factors. Clin Biomech 1997;12:211–26.

423. Ferguson SA, Marras WS, Waters TR. Quantification of back motion during asymmetric lifting. Ergonomics 1992;35:845–59.

424. Ferguson SJ, Ito K, Nolte LP. Fluid flow and convective transport of solutes within the intervertebral disc. J Biomech 2004;37:213–21.

425. Ferrando AA, Sheffield-Moore M, Yeckel CW, et al. Testosterone administration to older men improves muscle function: molecular and physiological mechanisms. Am J Physiol Endocrinol Metab 2002;282:E601–7.

426. Ferreira V, Brito C, Portela M, et al. DOTS in primary care units in the city of Rio de Janeiro, Southeastern Brazil. Rev Saude Publica 2011;45:40–8.

427. Fiatarone MA, O'Neill EF, Ryan ND, et al. Exercise training and nutritional supplementation for physical frailty in very elderly people. N Engl J Med 1994;330:1769–75.

428. Finigan J, Greenfield DM, Blumsohn A, et al. Risk factors for vertebral and nonvertebral fracture over 10 years: a population-based study in women. J Bone Miner Res 2008;23:75–85.

429. Fishbain DA, Cutler RB, Rosomoff HL, et al. Impact of chronic pain patients' job perception variables on actual return to work. Clin J Pain 1997;13:197–206.

430. Flannery CR, Zollner R, Corcoran C, et al. Prevention of cartilage degeneration in a rat model of osteoarthritis by intraarticular treatment with recombinant lubricin. Arthritis Rheum 2009;60:840–7.

431. Floyd WF, Silver PHS. The function of the erectores spinae muscles in certain movements and postures in man. J Physiol 1955;129:184–203.

432. Fordyce WE. Back pain in the workplace: management of disability in non-specific conditions. Seattle: IASP Press; 1995.

433. Foreman TK, Troup JDG. Diurnal variations in spinal loading and the effects on stature: a preliminary study of nursing activities. Clin Biomech 1987;2:48–54.

434. Fortin JD, Dwyer AP, West S, et al. Sacroiliac joint: pain referral maps upon applying a new injection/arthrography technique. Part I: Asymptomatic volunteers. Spine 1994;19:1475–82.

435. Fournie B. Pathology and clinico-pathologic correlations in spondyloarthropathies. Joint Bone Spine 2004;71:525–9.

436. Frank J, Sinclair S, Hogg-Johnson S, et al. Preventing disability from work-related low-back pain. New evidence gives new hope – if we can just get all the players onside. Cmaj 1998;158:1625–31.

437. Frank JW, Brooker AS, DeMaio SE, et al. Disability resulting from occupational low-back pain. Part II: What do we know about secondary prevention? A review of the scientific evidence on prevention after disability begins. Spine 1996;21:2918–29.

438. Frank JW, Kerr MS, Brooker AS, et al. Disability resulting from occupational low-back pain. Part I: What do we know about primary prevention? A review of the scientific evidence on prevention before disability begins. Spine 1996;21:2908–17.

439. Fraser RD, Ross ER, Lowery GL, et al. AcroFlex design and results. Spine J 2004;4:245S–51S.

440. Fredrickson BE, Edwards WT, Rauschning W, et al. Vertebral burst fractures: an experimental, morphologic, and radiographic study. Spine 1992;17:1012–21.

441. Freeman BJ, Davenport J. Total disc replacement in the lumbar

spine: a systematic review of the literature. Eur Spine J 2006;15(Suppl. 3):S439–47.

442. Freeman BJ, Fraser RD, Cain CM, et al. A randomized, double-blind, controlled trial: intradiscal electrothermal therapy versus placebo for the treatment of chronic discogenic low-back pain. Spine 2005;30:2369–77; discussion 78.

443. Freeman BJ, Walters RM, Moore RJ, et al. Does intradiscal electrothermal therapy denervate and repair experimentally induced posterolateral annular tears in an animal model? Spine 2003;28:2602–8.

444. Freeman BJC. The Spine and Spinal Cord. In: Burnand KG, editor. The New Aird's Companion in Surgical Studies. 3rd ed. China: Elsevier-Churchill Livingstone; 2005. p. 1014–29.

445. Freemont AJ. The cellular pathobiology of the degenerate intervertebral disc and discogenic back pain. Rheumatology (Oxf) 2009;48:5–10.

446. Freemont AJ, Peacock TE, Goupille P, et al. Nerve ingrowth into diseased intervertebral disc in chronic back pain. Lancet 1997;350:178–81.

447. Freemont AJ, Watkins A, Le Maitre C, et al. Nerve growth factor expression and innervation of the painful intervertebral disc. J Pathol 2002;197:286–92.

448. Freemont AJ, Watkins A, Le Maitre C, et al. Current understanding of cellular and molecular events in intervertebral disc degeneration: implications for therapy. J Pathol 2002;196:374–9.

449. Friden J, Sjostrom M, Ekblom B. Myofibrillar damage following intense eccentric exercise in man. Int J Sports Med 1983;4:170–6.

450. Fritzell P, Hagg O, Wessberg P, et al. 2001 Volvo Award Winner in Clinical Studies: Lumbar fusion versus nonsurgical treatment for chronic low-back pain: a multicenter randomized controlled trial from the Swedish Lumbar Spine Study Group. Spine 2001;26:2521–32; discussion 32–4.

451. Fritzell P, Hagg O, Wessberg P, et al. Chronic low-back pain and fusion: a comparison of three surgical techniques: a prospective multicenter randomized study from the Swedish lumbar spine study group. Spine 2002; 27:1131–41.

452. Frost H, Lamb SE, Doll HA, et al. Randomised controlled trial of physiotherapy compared with advice for low-back pain. BMJ 2004;329:708.

453. Frost HM. Bone 'mass' and the 'mechanostat': a proposal. Anat Rec 1987;219:1–9.

454. Fuchs RK, Allen MR, Ruppel ME, et al. In situ examination of the time-course for secondary mineralization of Haversian bone using synchrotron Fourier transform infrared microspectroscopy. Matrix Biol 2008;27:34–41.

455. Fujii R, Sakaura H, Mukai Y, et al. Kinematics of the lumbar spine in trunk rotation: in vivo three-dimensional analysis using magnetic resonance imaging. Eur Spine J 2007;16:1867–74.

456. Fujita Y, Duncan NA, Lotz JC. Radial tensile properties of the lumbar annulus fibrosus are site and degeneration dependent. J Orthop Res 1997;15:814–9.

457. Fujiwara A, Lim TH, An HS, et al. The effect of disc degeneration and facet joint osteoarthritis on the segmental flexibility of the lumbar spine. Spine 2000;25:3036–44.

458. Fujiwara A, Tamai K, An HS, et al. The interspinous ligament of the lumbar spine. Magnetic resonance images and their clinical significance. Spine 2000;25:358–63.

459. Fukui S, Ohseto K, Shiotani M, et al. Distribution of referred pain from the lumbar zygapophyseal joints and dorsal rami. Clin J Pain 1997;13:303–7.

460. Fukushima M, Kaneoka K, Ono K, et al. Neck injury mechanisms during direct face impact. Spine 2006;31:903–8.

461. Furlan AD, Clarke J, Esmail R, et al. Critical Review of Reviews on the Treatment of Chronic Low-back Pain. Spine 2001;26:E155–E62.

462. Gagnon D, Gagnon M. The influence of dynamic factors on triaxial net muscular moments at the L5/S1 joint during asymmetrical lifting and lowering. J Biomech 1992;25:891–901.

463. Gaines RW, Nichols WK. Treatment of spondyloptosis by two stage L5 vertebrectomy and reduction of L4 on to S1. Spine 1985;10:680–6.

464. Galante JO. Tensile properties of the human lumbar annulus fibrosus. Acta Orthop Scand 1967;(Suppl):1–91.

465. Galbusera F, Schmidt H, Neidlinger-Wilke C, et al. The mechanical response of the lumbar spine to different combinations of disc degenerative changes investigated using randomized poroelastic finite element models. Eur Spine J 2011;20:563–71.

466. Galiano K, Obwegeser AA, Gabl MV, et al. Long-term outcome of laminectomy for spinal stenosis in octogenarians. Spine 2005;30:332–5.

467. Gallagher D, Ruts E, Visser M, et al. Weight stability masks sarcopenia in elderly men and women. Am J Physiol Endocrinol Metab 2000;279:E366–75.

468. Gallagher D, Visser M, De Meersman RE, et al. Appendicular skeletal muscle mass: effects of age, gender, and ethnicity. J Appl Physiol 1997;83:229–39.

469. Gallagher S. Letter to the Editor. Spine 2002;27:1378–9.

470. Gandevia SC, Allen GM, Butler JE, et al. Supraspinal factors in human muscle fatigue: evidence for suboptimal output from the motor cortex. J Physiol 1996;490:529–36.

471. Gao Y, Kostrominova TY, Faulkner JA, et al. Age-related changes in the mechanical properties of the epimysium in skeletal muscles of rats. J Biomech 2008;41:465–9.

472. Gardner-Morse MG, Stokes IA. The effects of abdominal muscle coactivation on lumbar spine

stability. Spine 1998;23:86–91; discussion -2.

473. Gardner-Morse MG, Stokes IA. Physiological axial compressive preloads increase motion segment stiffness, linearity and hysteresis in all six degrees of freedom for small displacements about the neutral posture. J Orthop Res 2003;21:547–52.

474. Garg A, Moore JS. Epidemiology of low-back pain in industry. Occup Med 1992;7:593–608.

475. Garg A, Moore JS. Prevention strategies and the low-back in industry. Occup Med 1992;7:629–40.

476. Garland SJ, Enoka RM, Serrano LP, et al. Behavior of motor units in human biceps brachii during a submaximal fatiguing contraction. J Appl Physiol 1994;76:2411–9.

477. Garland SJ, McComas AJ. Reflex inhibition of human soleus muscle during fatigue. J Physiol 1990;429:17–27.

478. Garras DN, Carothers JT, Olson SA. Single-leg-stance (flamingo) radiographs to assess pelvic instability: how much motion is normal? J Bone Joint Surg Am 2008;90:2114–8.

479. Garrett Jr WE, Seaber AV, Boswick J, et al. Recovery of skeletal muscle after laceration and repair. J Hand Surg [Am] 1984;9:683–92.

480. Gatton ML, Pearcy MJ. Kinematics and movement sequencing during flexion of the lumbar spine. Clin Biomech 1999;14:376–83.

481. Gatty CM, Turner M, Buitendorp DJ, et al. The effectiveness of back pain and injury prevention programs in the workplace. Work 2003;20:257–66.

482. Ge W, Long CR, Pickar JG. Vertebral position alters paraspinal muscle spindle responsiveness in the feline spine: effect of positioning duration. J Physiol 2005;569(Pt 2):655–65.

483. Ge W, Pickar JG. Time course for the development of muscle history in lumbar paraspinal muscle spindles arising from changes in vertebral position. Spine J 2008;8:320–8.

484. Gebhardt WA. Effectiveness of training to prevent job-related back pain: a meta-analysis. Br J Clin Psychol 1994;33: 571–4.

485. Gedalia U, Solomonow M, Zhou BH, et al. Biomechanics of increased exposure to lumbar injury caused by cyclic loading. Part 2. Recovery of reflexive muscular stability with rest. Spine 1999;24:2461–7.

486. Geiss A, Larsson K, Junevik K, et al. Autologous nucleus pulposus primes T cells to develop into interleukin-4-producing effector cells: an experimental study on the autoimmune properties of nucleus pulposus. J Orthop Res 2009;27:97–103.

487. Gelb DE, Lenke LG, Bridwell KH, et al. An analysis of sagittal spinal alignment in 100 asymptomatic middle and older aged volunteers. Spine 1995;20:1351–8.

488. Gercek E, Hartmann F, Kuhn S, et al. Dynamic angular three-dimensional measurement of multisegmental thoracolumbar motion in vivo. Spine 2008;33:2326–33.

489. Gertzbein SD, Seligman J, Holtby R, et al. Centrode patterns and segmental instability in degenerative disc disease. Spine 1985;10:257–61.

490. Ghormley K. Low-back pain with special reference to the articular facets, with presentation of an operative procedure. JAMA 1933;101:1773–7.

491. Gibala MJ, MacDougall JD, Tarnopolsky MA, et al. Changes in human skeletal muscle ultrastructure and force production after acute resistance exercise. J Appl Physiol 1995;78:702–8.

492. Gibson JN, Halliday D, Morrison WL, et al. Decrease in human quadriceps muscle protein turnover consequent upon leg immobilization. Clin Sci (Colch) 1987;72:503–9.

493. Gibson JN, McMaster MJ, Scrimgeour CM, et al. Rates of muscle protein synthesis in paraspinal muscles: lateral disparity in children with idiopathic scoliosis. Clin Sci (Colch) 1988;75:79–83.

494. Gibson JN, Smith K, Rennie MJ. Prevention of disuse muscle atrophy by means of electrical stimulation: maintenance of protein synthesis. Lancet 1988;2:767–70.

495. Giles LG, Taylor JR, Cockson A. Human zygapophyseal joint synovial folds. Acta Anat (Basel) 1986;126:110–4.

496. Gilgil E, Kacar C, Butun B, et al. Prevalence of low-back pain in a developing urban setting. Spine 2005;30:1093–8.

497. Gill K, Videman T, Shimizu T, et al. The effect of repeated extensions on the discographic dye patterns in cadaveric lumbar motion segments. Clin Biomech 1987;2:205–10.

498. Gill KP, Bennett SJ, Savelsbergh GJ, et al. Regional changes in spine posture at lift onset with changes in lift distance and lift style. Spine 2007;32:1599–604.

499. Gillespie KA, Dickey JP. Biomechanical role of lumbar spine ligaments in flexion and extension: determination using a parallel linkage robot and a porcine model. Spine 2004;29:1208–16.

500. Giori NJ, Beaupre GS, Carter DR. Cellular shape and pressure may mediate mechanical control of tissue composition in tendons. J Orthop Res 1993;11:581–91.

501. Goel VK, Kong W, Han JS, et al. A combined finite element and optimization investigation of lumbar spine mechanics with and without muscles. Spine 1993;18:1531–41.

502. Goel VK, Monroe BT, Gilbertson LG, et al. Interlaminar shear stresses and laminae separation in a disc. Finite element analysis of the L3–L4 motion segment subjected to axial compressive loads. Spine 1995;20:689–98.

503. Gogan WJ, Fraser RD. Chymopapain. A 10-year, double-blind study. Spine 1992;17:388–94.

504. Goh S, Tan C, Price RI, et al. Influence of age and gender on thoracic vertebral body shape and disc degeneration: an MR

investigation of 169 cases. J Anat 2000;197:647–57.

505. Goldberg CJ, Moore DP, Fogarty EE, et al. Adolescent idiopathic scoliosis: the effect of brace treatment on the incidence of surgery. Spine 2001;26:42–7.

506. Goldspink G. Cellular and molecular aspects of adaptation in skeletal muscle. In: Komi PV, editor. The Encyclopaedia of Sports Medicine III: Strength and Power in Sport. Oxford: Blackwell Science; 1992. p. 211–29.

507. Goldspink G, Ward PS. Changes in rodent muscle fibre types during post-natal growth, undernutrition and exercise. J Physiol 1979;296:453–69.

508. Goldspink G, Waterson SE. The effect of growth and inanition on the total amount of nitroblue tetrazolium deposited in individual muscle fibres of fast and slow rat skeletal muscle. Acta Histochem 1971;40:16–22.

509. Goldspink G, Williams PE. The nature of the increased passive resistance in muscle following immobilization of the mouse soleus muscle [proceedings]. J Physiol 1979;289:55P.

510. Gonzalez-Urzelai V, Palacio-Elua L, Lopez-de-Munain J. Routine primary care management of acute low-back pain: adherence to clinical guidelines. Eur Spine J 2003;12:589–94.

511. Goodship AE, Birch HL, Wilson AM. The pathobiology and repair of tendon and ligament injury. Vet Clin North Am Equine Pract 1994;10:323–49.

512. Goodship AE, Lanyon LE, McFie H. Functional adaptation of bone to increased stress. An experimental study. J Bone Joint Surg [Am] 1979;61:539–46.

513. Gordon SJ, Yang KH, Mayer PJ, et al. Mechanism of disc rupture. A preliminary report. Spine 1991;16:450–6.

514. Goubert L, Crombez G, De Bourdeaudhuij I. Low-back pain, disability and back pain myths in a community sample: prevalence and interrelationships. Eur J Pain 2004;8:385–94.

515. Goupille P, Mulleman D, Paintaud G, et al. Can sciatica induced by disc herniation be treated with tumor necrosis factor alpha blockade? Arthritis Rheum 2007;56:3887–95.

516. Gracovetsky S, Farfan H. The optimum spine. Spine 1986;11:543–73.

517. Gracovetsky S, Farfan H, Helleur C. The abdominal mechanism. Spine 1985;10:317–24.

518. Gracovetsky S, Farfan HF, Lamy C. A mathematical model of the lumbar spine using an optimized system to control muscles and ligaments. Orthop Clin North Am 1977;8:135–53.

519. Granata KP, Marras WS. An EMG-assisted model of loads on the lumbar spine during asymmetric trunk extensions. J Biomech 1993;26:1429–38.

520. Granata KP, Marras WS. The influence of trunk muscle coactivity on dynamic spinal loads. Spine 1995;20:913–9.

521. Granata KP, Marras WS. Cost-benefit of muscle cocontraction in protecting against spinal instability. Spine 2000;25:1398–404.

522. Granata KP, Marras WS, Davis KG. Biomechanical assessment of lifting dynamics, muscle activity and spinal loads while using three different styles of lifting belt. Clin Biomech 1997;12:107–15.

523. Granata KP, Marras WS, Davis KG. Variation in spinal load and trunk dynamics during repeated lifting exertions. Clin Biomech 1999;14:367–75.

524. Granhed H, Jonson R, Hansson T. The loads on the lumbar spine during extreme weight lifting. Spine 1987;12:146–9.

525. Granhed H, Jonson R, Hansson T. Mineral content and strength of lumbar vertebrae. A cadaver study. Acta Orthop Scand 1989;60:105–9.

526. Graveling RA, Melrose AS, Hanson MA. The principles of good manual handing: achieving a consensus (HSE RR 97). London: HSE Books; 2003.

527. Green HJ, Thomson JA, Daub WD, et al. Fiber composition, fiber size and enzyme activities in vastus lateralis of elite athletes involved in high intensity exercise. Eur J Appl Physiol Occup Physiol 1979;41:109–17.

528. Green TP, Adams MA, Dolan P. Tensile properties of the annulus fibrosus. Part II Ultimate tensile strength and fatigue life. Eur Spine J 1993;2:209–14.

529. Green TP, Allvey JC, Adams MA. Spondylolysis. Bending of the inferior articular processes of lumbar vertebrae during simulated spinal movements. Spine 1994;19:2683–91.

530. Greenough CG, Fraser RD. The effects of compensation on recovery from low-back injury. Spine 1989;14:947–55.

531. Gregersen GG, Lucas DB. An in vivo study of the axial rotation of the human thoracolumbar spine. J Bone Joint Surg [Am] 1967;49:247–62.

532. Grimby G, Saltin B. The ageing muscle. Clin Physiol 1983;3:209–18.

533. Grob D, Benini A, Junge A, et al. Clinical experience with the Dynesys semirigid fixation system for the lumbar spine: surgical and patient-oriented outcome in 50 cases after an average of 2 years. Spine 2005;30:324–31.

534. Grotle M, Brox JI, Veierod MB, et al. Clinical course and prognostic factors in acute low-back pain: patients consulting primary care for the first time. Spine 2005;30:976–82.

535. Gruber HE, Ingram JA, Norton HJ, et al. Senescence in cells of the aging and degenerating intervertebral disc: immunolocalization of senescence-associated beta-galactosidase in human and sand rat discs. Spine 2007;32:321–7.

536. Guehring T, Omlor GW, Lorenz H, et al. Disc distraction shows evidence of regenerative potential in degenerated intervertebral discs as evaluated by protein expression, magnetic resonance imaging, and messenger ribonucleic acid expression analysis. Spine 2006;31:1658–65.

537. Guehring T, Wilde G, Sumner M, et al. Notochordal intervertebral disc cells: sensitivity to nutrient

deprivation. Arthritis Rheum 2009;60:1026–34.

538. Guilak F. Compression-induced changes in the shape and volume of the chondrocyte nucleus. J Biomech 1995;28:1529–41.

539. Guilak F, Ting-Beall HP, Baer AE, et al. Viscoelastic properties of intervertebral disc cells. Identification of two biomechanically distinct cell populations. Spine 1999;24:2475–83.

540. Gundewall B, Liljeqvist M, Hansson T. Primary prevention of back symptoms and absence from work. A prospective randomized study among hospital employees. Spine 1993;18:587–94.

541. Gunzburg R, Hutton W, Fraser R. Axial rotation of the lumbar spine and the effect of flexion. An in vitro and in vivo biomechanical study. Spine 1991;16:22–8.

542. Gunzburg R, Parkinson R, Moore R, et al. A cadaveric study comparing discography, magnetic resonance imaging, histology, and mechanical behavior of the human lumbar disc. Spine 1992;17:417–26.

543. Gupta A. Analyses of myo-electrical silence of erectors spinae. J Biomech 2001;34:491–6.

544. Guyer RD, McAfee PC, Banco RJ, et al. Prospective, randomized, multicenter Food and Drug Administration investigational device exemption study of lumbar total disc replacement with the CHARITE artificial disc versus lumbar fusion: five-year follow-up. Spine J 2009;9:374–86.

545. Gwynne JH, Cameron RE. Using small angle X-ray scattering to investigate the variation in composition across a graduated region within an intervertebral disc prosthesis. J Mater Sci Mater Med 2010;21:787–95.

546. Habtemariam A, Virri J, Gronblad M, et al. Inflammatory cells in full-thickness annulus injury in pigs. An experimental disc herniation animal model. Spine 1998;23:524–9.

547. Hadjipavlou AG, Tzermiadianos MN, Bogduk N, et al. The pathophysiology of disc degeneration: a critical review. J Bone Joint Surg Br 2008;90:1261–70.

548. Hadler NM. Back pain in the workplace. What you lift or how you lift matters far less than whether you lift or when. Spine 1997;22:935–40.

549. Hadler NM. Backache: predicament at home, nemesis at work. In: Hadler NM, editor. Occupational musculoskeletal disorders. 2nd ed. Philadelphia: Lippincott Williams & Wilkins; 1999. p. 7–17.

550. Hadley Miller N. Spine update: genetics of familial idiopathic scoliosis. Spine 2000;25:2416–8.

551. Haefeli M, Kalberer F, Saegesser D, et al. The course of macroscopic degeneration in the human lumbar intervertebral disc. Spine 2006;31:1522–31.

552. Hagbarth KE, Bongiovanni LG, Nordin M. Reduced servo-control of fatigued human finger extensor and flexor muscles. J Physiol 1995;485:865–72.

553. Hakkinen K, Komi PV. Electromyographic and mechanical characteristics of human skeletal muscle during fatigue under voluntary and reflex conditions. Electroencephalogr Clin Neurophysiol 1983;55: 436–44.

554. Haldorsen EM, Indahl A, Ursin H. Patients with low-back pain not returning to work. A 12-month follow-up study. Spine 1998;23:1202–7; discussion 8.

555. Hall AC, Urban JP, Gehl KA. The effects of hydrostatic pressure on matrix synthesis in articular cartilage. J Orthop Res 1991; 9:1–10.

556. Hall DJ. Facet joint denervation; a minimally invasive treatment for low-back pain in selected patients. In: Herkowitz HN, editor. The Lumbar Spine. 3rd ed. Philadelphia: Lippincott, Williams and Wilkins; 2004. p. 307–11.

557. Hamanishi C, Kawabata T, Yosii T, et al. Schmorl's nodes on magnetic resonance imaging. Their incidence and clinical relevance. Spine 1994;19:450–3.

558. Hampton D, Laros G, McCarron R, et al. Healing potential of the annulus fibrosus. Spine 1989;14:398–401.

559. Handa T, Ishihara H, Ohshima H, et al. Effects of hydrostatic pressure on matrix synthesis and matrix metalloproteinase production in the human lumbar intervertebral disc. Spine 1997;22:1085–91.

560. Hansen U, Zioupos P, Simpson R, et al. The effect of strain rate on the mechanical properties of human cortical bone. J Biomech Eng 2008;130:011011.

561. Hansson T, Roos B. The amount of bone mineral and Schmorl's nodes in lumbar vertebrae. Spine 1983;8:266–71.

562. Hansson T, Roos B, Nachemson A. The bone mineral content and ultimate compressive strength of lumbar vertebrae. Spine 1980;5:46–55.

563. Hansson T, Suzuki N, Hebelka H, et al. The narrowing of the lumbar spinal canal during loaded MRI: the effects of the disc and ligamentum flavum. Eur Spine J 2009;18:679–86.

564. Hansson TH, Hansson EK. The effects of common medical interventions on pain, back function, and work resumption in patients with chronic low-back pain: A prospective 2-year cohort study in six countries. Spine 2000;25:3055–64.

565. Hansson TH, Keller TS, Spengler DM. Mechanical behavior of the human lumbar spine. II. Fatigue strength during dynamic compressive loading [published erratum appears in J Orthop Res 1988;6:465]. J Orthop Res 1987;5:479–87.

566. Harada Y, Nakahara S. A pathologic study of lumbar disc herniation in the elderly. Spine 1989;14:1020–4.

567. Hardcastle P, Annear P, Foster DH, et al. Spinal abnormalities in young fast bowlers. J Bone Joint Surg [Br] 1992;74:421–5.

568. Harding IJ, Charosky S, Vialle R, et al. Lumbar disc degeneration below a long arthrodesis (performed for scoliosis in

adults) to L4 or L5. Eur Spine J 2008;17:250–4.

569. Harkness EF, Macfarlane GJ, Nahit ES, et al. Risk factors for new-onset low-back pain amongst cohorts of newly employed workers. Rheumatology (Oxf) 2003;42:959–68.

570. Harkness EF, Macfarlane GJ, Silman AJ, et al. Is musculoskeletal pain more common now than 40 years ago?: Two population-based cross-sectional studies. Rheumatology (Oxf) 2005;44: 890–5.

571. Harreby M, Neergaard K, Hesselsoe G, et al. Are radiologic changes in the thoracic and lumbar spine of adolescents risk factors for low-back pain in adults? A 25-year prospective cohort study of 640 school children. Spine 1995; 20:2298–302.

572. Hartigan C, Miller L, Liewehr SC. Rehabilitation of acute and subacute low-back and neck pain in the work- injured patient. Orthop Clin North Am 1996;27:841–60.

573. Hartvigsen J, Christensen K, Frederiksen H. Back and Neck Pain Exhibit Many Common Features in Old Age: A Population-Based Study of 4,486 Danish Twins 70–102 Years of Age. Spine 2004;29:576–80.

574. Hartvigsen J, Christensen K, Frederiksen H, et al. Genetic and environmental contributions to back pain in old age: a study of 2108 Danish twins aged 70 and older. Spine 2004;29:897–901; discussion 2.

574a. Hartvigsen J, Christensen K. Pain in the back and neck are with us until the end: a nationwide interview-based survey of Danish 100-year-olds. Spine 2008;33:909–13.

575. Hartvigsen J, Leboeuf-Yde C, Lings S, et al. Is sitting-while-at-work associated with low-back pain? A systematic, critical literature review. Scand J Public Health 2000;28:230–9.

576. Hasberry S, Pearcy MJ. Temperature dependence of the tensile properties of interspinous ligaments of sheep. J Biomed Eng 1986;8:62–6.

577. Haschtmann D, Stoyanov JV, Gedet P, et al. Vertebral endplate trauma induces disc cell apoptosis and promotes organ degeneration in vitro. Eur Spine J 2008;17:289–99.

578. Hashtroudi A, Paterson H. Occupational health advice in NICE guidelines. Occup Med 2009;59:353–6.

579. Hassett G, Hart DJ, Manek NJ, et al. Risk factors for progression of lumbar spine disc degeneration: the Chingford Study. Arthritis Rheum 2003;48:3112–7.

580. Hasten DL, Pak-Loduca J, Obert KA, et al. Resistance exercise acutely increases MHC and mixed muscle protein synthesis rates in 78–84 and 23–32 yr olds. Am J Physiol Endocrinol Metab 2000;278:E620–6.

581. Hastreiter D, Ozuna RM, Spector M. Regional variations in certain cellular characteristics in human lumbar intervertebral discs, including the presence of alpha-smooth muscle actin. J Orthop Res 2001;19:597–604.

582. Havill LM, Mahaney MC, L Binkley T, et al. Effects of genes, sex, age, and activity on BMC, bone size, and areal and volumetric BMD. J Bone Miner Res 2007;22:737–46.

583. Hayes MA, Howard TC, Gruel CR, et al. Roentgenographic evaluation of lumbar spine flexion–extension in asymptomatic individuals. Spine 1989;14:327–31.

584. Hazard RG, Haugh LD, Reid S, et al. Early physician notification of patient disability risk and clinical guidelines after low-back injury: a randomized, controlled trial. Spine 1997;22: 2951–8.

585. Healey EL, Burden AM, McEwan IM, et al. The impact of increasing paraspinal muscle activity on stature recovery in asymptomatic people. Arch Phys Med Rehabil 2008;89:749–53.

586. Healey EL, Fowler NE, Burden AM, et al. Raised paraspinal muscle activity reduces rate of stature recovery after loaded exercise in individuals with chronic low-back pain. Arch Phys Med Rehabil 2005; 86:710–5.

587. Hedlund LR, Gallagher JC, Meeger C, et al. Change in vertebral shape in spinal osteoporosis. Calcif Tissue Int 1989;44:168–72.

588. Hedtmann A, Steffen R, Methfessel J, et al. Measurement of human lumbar spine ligaments during loaded and unloaded motion. Spine 1989;14:175–85.

589. Heithoff KB, Gundry CR, Burton CV, et al. Juvenile discogenic disease. Spine 1994;19:335–40.

590. Heliovaara M. Body height, obesity, and risk of herniated lumbar intervertebral disc. Spine 1987;12:469–72.

591. Hemingway H, Shipley MJ, Stansfeld S, et al. Sickness absence from back pain, psychosocial work characteristics and employment grade among office workers. Scand J Work Environ Health 1997;23: 121–9.

592. Heneghan P, Riches PE. Determination of the strain-dependent hydraulic permeability of the compressed bovine nucleus pulposus. J Biomech 2008;41:903–6.

593. Heneweer H, Vanhees L, Picavet HSJ. Physical activity and low-back pain: a u-shaped relation? Pain 2009;143:21–5.

594. Herring SW, Grimm AF, Grimm BR. Regulation of sarcomere number in skeletal muscle: a comparison of hypotheses. Muscle Nerve 1984;7:161–73.

595. Herrmann CM, Madigan ML, Davidson BS, et al. Effect of lumbar extensor fatigue on paraspinal muscle reflexes. J Electromyogr Kinesiol 2006;16:637–41.

596. Hestbaek L, Iachine IA, Leboeuf-Yde C, et al. Heredity of low-back pain in a young population: a classical twin study. Twin Res 2004;7:16–26.

597. Hestbaek L, Leboeuf-Yde C, Engberg M, et al. The course of low-back pain in a general population. Results from a 5-year

prospective study. J Manipulative Physiol Ther 2003;26:213–9.

598. Hestbaek L, Leboeuf-Yde C, Manniche C. Low-back pain: what is the long-term course? A review of studies of general patient populations. Eur Spine J 2003;12:149–65.

599. Heuer F, Schmidt H, Claes L, et al. A new laser scanning technique for imaging intervertebral disc displacement and its application to modeling nucleotomy. Clin Biomech 2008;23:260–9.

600. Heuer F, Schmidt H, Wilke HJ. The relation between intervertebral disc bulging and annular fiber associated strains for simple and complex loading. J Biomech 2008;41:1086–94.

601. Heuer F, Schmitt H, Schmidt H, et al. Creep associated changes in intervertebral disc bulging obtained with a laser scanning device. Clin Biomech 2007;22:737–44.

602. Heylings DJ. Supraspinous and interspinous ligaments of the human lumbar spine. J Anat 1978;125:127–31.

603. Heymans MW, van Tulder MW, Esmail R, et al. Back schools for non-specific low-back pain. Cochrane Database Syst Rev 2004:CD000261.

604. Hides JA, Stokes MJ, Saide M, et al. Evidence of lumbar multifidus muscle wasting ipsilateral to symptoms in patients with acute/subacute low-back pain. Spine 1994;19:165–72.

605. Hill AB. The environment and disease: association or causation? Proc R Soc Med 1965;58:295–300.

606. Hill CL, Seo GS, Gale D, et al. Cruciate ligament integrity in osteoarthritis of the knee. Arthritis Rheum 2005;52:794–9.

606a. Hill J, Dunn KM, Lewis M, et al. A primary care back pain screening tool: identifying patient subgroups for initial treatment. Arthritis Care & Research 2008;59:632–41.

607. Hills BA. Boundary lubrication in vivo. Proc Inst Mech Eng [H] 2000;214:83–94.

608. Hilton RC, Ball J. Vertebral rim lesions in the dorsolumbar spine. Ann Rheum Dis 1984; 43:302–7.

609. Hilton RC, Ball J, Benn RT. Vertebral end-plate lesions (Schmorl's nodes) in the dorsolumbar spine. Ann Rheum Dis 1976;35:127–32.

610. Hilton RC, Ball J, Benn RT. In vitro mobility of the lumbar spine. Ann Rheum Dis 1979;38:378–83.

611. Hindle RJ, Pearcy MJ, Cross A. Mechanical function of the human lumbar interspinous and supraspinous ligaments. J Biomed Eng 1990;12:340–4.

612. Hindle RJ, Pearcy MJ, Cross AT, et al. Three-dimensional kinematics of the human back. Clin Biomech 1990;5:218–28.

613. Hirsch C, Inglemark B, Miller M. The anatomical basis for low-back pain. Acta Orthop Scand 1963;33:1–17.

614. Hirsch C, Nachemson A. Clinical observations on the spine in ejected pilots. Acta Orthop Scand 1961;31:135–45.

615. Hirsch C, Schajowicz F. Studies on structural changes in the lumbar annulus fibrosus. Acta Orthop Scand 1953;22:184–231.

616. Hodges P. Changes in motor planning of feedforward postural responses of the trunk muscles in low-back pain. Exp Brain Res 2001;141:261–6.

617. Hodges P, Kaigle Holm A, Holm S, et al. Intervertebral stiffness of the spine is increased by evoked contraction of transversus abdominis and the diaphragm: in vivo porcine studies. Spine 2003;28:2594–601.

618. Hodges PW, Cresswell AG, Daggfeldt K, et al. In vivo measurement of the effect of intra-abdominal pressure on the human spine. J Biomech 2001;34:347–53.

619. Hodges PW, Moseley GL, Gabrielsson A, et al. Experimental muscle pain changes feedforward postural responses of the trunk muscles. Exp Brain Res 2003;151:262–71.

620. Holdsworth FW. Fractures, dislocations and

fracture-dislocations of the spine. J Bone Joint Surg [Br] 1963;45:6–20.

621. Holm S, Holm AK, Ekstrom L, et al. Experimental disc degeneration due to endplate injury. J Spinal Disord Tech 2004;17:64–71.

622. Holm S, Indahl A, Solomonow M. Sensorimotor control of the spine. J Electromyogr Kinesiol 2002;12:219–34.

623. Holm S, Nachemson A. Nutritional changes in the canine intervertebral disc after spinal fusion. Clin Orthop 1982: 243–58.

624. Holmes AD, Hukins DW, Freemont AJ. End-plate displacement during compression of lumbar vertebra-disc- vertebra segments and the mechanism of failure. Spine 1993; 18:128–35.

625. Honeyman PT, Jacobs EA. Effects of culture on back pain in Australian aboriginals. Spine 1996;21:841–3.

626. Hoogendoorn R, Doulabi BZ, Huang CL, et al. Molecular changes in the degenerated goat intervertebral disc. Spine 2008;33:1714–21.

627. Hoogendoorn WE, Bongers PM, de Vet HC, et al. Flexion and rotation of the trunk and lifting at work are risk factors for low-back pain: results of a prospective cohort study. Spine 2000;25:3087–92.

628. Hoogendoorn WE, van Poppel MN, Bongers PM, et al. Systematic review of psychosocial factors at work and private life as risk factors for back pain. Spine 2000;25:2114–25.

629. Hoppeler H, Lindstedt SL. Malleability of skeletal muscle in overcoming limitations: structural elements. J Exp Biol 1985;115:355–64.

630. Horner HA, Urban JP. 2001 Volvo Award Winner in Basic Science Studies: Effect of nutrient supply on the viability of cells from the nucleus pulposus of the intervertebral disc. Spine 2001;26:2543–9.

631. Horowits R. The physiological role of titin in striated muscle.

Rev Physiol Biochem Pharmacol 1999;138:57–96.

632. Hortobagyi T, Lambert NJ, Kroll WP. Voluntary and reflex responses to fatigue with stretch-shortening exercise. Can J Sport Sci 1991;16:142–50.

633. Hou SX, Tang JG, Chen HS, et al. Chronic inflammation and compression of the dorsal root contribute to sciatica induced by the intervertebral disc herniation in rats. Pain 2003;105:255–64.

634. Hou Y, Luo Z. A study on the structural properties of the lumbar endplate: histological structure, the effect of bone density, and spinal level. Spine (Phila Pa) 2009;34:E427–33.

635. Hoy D, Toole MJ, Morgan D, et al. Low-back pain in rural Tibet. Lancet 2003;361:225–6.

636. Hoyland JA, Freemont AJ, Jayson MI. Intervertebral foramen venous obstruction. A cause of periradicular fibrosis? Spine 1989;14:558–68.

637. Hsieh AH, Hwang D, Ryan DA, et al. Degenerative annular changes induced by puncture are associated with insufficiency of disc biomechanical function. Spine 2009;34:998–1005.

638. Hukins DW, Aspden RM, Yarker YE. Fibre reinforcement and mechanical stability in articular cartilage. Eng Med 1984;13:153–6.

639. Hukins DW, Kirby MC, Sikoryn TA, et al. Comparison of structure, mechanical properties, and functions of lumbar spinal ligaments. Spine 1990;15:787–95.

640. Hukins DWL. Disc structure and function. In: Ghosh P, editor. The Biology of the Intervertebral Disc. Boca Raton, Florida: CRC Press; 1988. p. 24–7.

641. Hukins DWL, Aspden RM. Composition and properties of connective tissue. TIBS 1985;10:260–4.

642. Hulme PA, Boyd SK, Ferguson SJ. Regional variation in vertebral bone morphology and its contribution to vertebral fracture strength. Bone 2007;41:946–57.

643. Hulme PA, Boyd SK, Heini PF, et al. Differences in endplate deformation of the adjacent and augmented vertebra following cement augmentation. Eur Spine J 2009;18:614–23.

644. Hunter CJ, Matyas JR, Duncan NA. The functional significance of cell clusters in the notochordal nucleus pulposus: survival and signaling in the canine intervertebral disc. Spine 2004;29:1099–104.

645. Hunter SK, Thompson MW, Adams RD. Relationships among age-associated strength changes and physical activity level, limb dominance, and muscle group in women. J Gerontol A Biol Sci Med Sci 2000;55:B264–73.

645a. Hüppe A, Müller K, Raspe H. Is the occurrence of back pain in Germany decreasing? Two regional postal surveys a decade apart. Eur J Public Health 2007;17:318–22.

646. Huser CA, Davies ME. Validation of an in vitro single-impact load model of the initiation of osteoarthritis-like changes in articular cartilage. J Orthop Res 2006;24:725–32.

647. Hutton WC, Adams MA. Can the lumbar spine be crushed in heavy lifting? Spine 1982;7:586–90.

648. Hutton WC, Cyron BM, Stott JR. The compressive strength of lumbar vertebrae. J Anat 1979;129:753–8.

649. Hutton WC, Ganey TM, Elmer WA, et al. Does long-term compressive loading on the intervertebral disc cause degeneration? Spine 2000;25:2993–3004.

650. Hutton WC, Murakami H, Li J, et al. The effect of blocking a nutritional pathway to the intervertebral disc in the dog model. J Spinal Disord Tech 2004;17:53–63.

651. Hutton WC, Stott JRR, Cyron BM. Is spondylolysis a fatigue fracture? Spine 1977;2:202–9.

652. Hutton WC, Toribatake Y, Elmer WA, et al. The effect of compressive force applied to the intervertebral disc in vivo. A study of proteoglycans and collagen. Spine 1998;23:2524–37.

653. Huxley AF. Muscle structure and theories of contraction. Prog Biophys 1957;7:255–318.

654. Huxley HE. The mechanism of muscular contraction. Sci Am 1965;213:18–27.

655. Hwang J, Bae WC, Shieu W, et al. Increased hydraulic conductance of human articular cartilage and subchondral bone plate with progression of osteoarthritis. Arthritis Rheum 2008;58:3831–42.

656. Iatridis JC, MacLean JJ, O'Brien M, et al. Measurements of proteoglycan and water content distribution in human lumbar intervertebral discs. Spine 2007;32:1493–7.

657. Iatridis JC, Mente PL, Stokes IA, et al. Compression-induced changes in intervertebral disc properties in a rat tail model. Spine 1999; 24:996–1002.

658. Iatridis JC, Weidenbaum M, Setton LA, et al. Is the nucleus pulposus a solid or a fluid? Mechanical behaviors of the nucleus pulposus of the human intervertebral disc. Spine 1996;21:1174–84.

659. Igarashi T, Kikuchi S, Shubayev V, et al. 2000 Volvo Award winner in basic science studies: Exogenous tumor necrosis factor-alpha mimics nucleus pulposus-induced neuropathology. Molecular, histologic, and behavioral comparisons in rats. Spine 2000;25:2975–80.

660. Iguchi T, Kanemura A, Kasahara K, et al. Age distribution of three radiologic factors for lumbar instability: probable aging process of the instability with disc degeneration. Spine 2003;28:2628–33.

661. Ihlebaek C, Eriksen HR. Are the 'myths' of low-back pain alive in the general Norwegian population? Scand J Public Health 2003;31:395–8.

662. Ijzelenberg H, Meerding WJ, Burdorf A. Effectiveness of a back pain prevention program: A cluster randomized controlled trial in an occupational setting. Spine 2007;32:711–9.

663. Indahl A, Haldorsen EH, Holm S, et al. Five-year follow-up study of a controlled clinical trial using light mobilization and an informative approach to low-back pain. Spine 1998;23: 2625–30.

664. Infante-Rivarde C, Lortie M. Relapse and short sickness absence for back pain in the six months after returning to work. Occup Environ Med 1997;54:328–34.

665. Inman VT, Saunders GBM. Anatomico-physiological aspects of injuries to the intervertebral disc. J Bone Joint Surg 1947;29B:461–8.

666. Inufusa A, An HS, Lim TH, et al. Anatomic changes of the spinal canal and intervertebral foramen associated with flexion–extension movement. Spine 1996;21 :2412–20.

667. Ishihara H, McNally DS, Urban JP, et al. Effects of hydrostatic pressure on matrix synthesis in different regions of the intervertebral disk. J Appl Physiol 1996;80: 839–46.

668. Ismail AA, Cooper C, Felsenberg D, et al. Number and type of vertebral deformities: epidemiological characteristics and relation to back pain and height loss. European Vertebral Osteoporosis Study Group. Osteoporos Int 1999;9:206–13.

669. Issever AS, Walsh A, Lu Y, et al. Micro-computed tomography evaluation of trabecular bone structure on loaded mice tail vertebrae. Spine 2003;28:123–8.

670. Ito M, Incorvaia KM, Yu SF, et al. Predictive signs of discogenic lumbar pain on magnetic resonance imaging with discography correlation. Spine 1998;23:1252–8; discussion 9–60.

671. Iwabuchi M, Rydevik B, Kikuchi S, et al. Effects of annulus fibrosus and experimentally degenerated nucleus pulposus on nerve root conduction velocity: relevance of previous experimental investigations using normal nucleus pulposus. Spine 2001;26:1651–5.

672. Jackson DW, Wiltse LL, Cirincoine RJ. Spondylolysis in the female gymnast. Clin Orthop 1976:68–73.

673. Jackson RK, Boston DA, Edge AJ. Lateral mass fusion. A prospective study of a consecutive series with long-term follow-up. Spine 1985;10:828–32.

674. Jackson RP, Jacobs RR, Montesano PX. 1988 Volvo award in clinical sciences. Facet joint injection in low- back pain. A prospective statistical study. Spine 1988;13:966–71.

675. Jackson RP, McManus AC. Radiographic analysis of sagittal plane alignment and balance in standing volunteers and patients with low-back pain matched for age, sex, and size. A prospective controlled clinical study. Spine 1994;19:1611–8.

676. James P, Cunningham I, Dibben P. Absence management and the issues of job retention and return to work. Hum Res Manage J 2002;12:82–94.

677. Janevic J, Ashton-Miller JA, Schultz AB. Large compressive preloads decrease lumbar motion segment flexibility. J Orthop Res 1991;9:228–36.

678. Jansen NW, Roosendaal G, Bijlsma JW, et al. Degenerated and healthy cartilage are equally vulnerable to blood-induced damage. Ann Rheum Dis 2008;67:1468–73.

679. Janssen I, Heymsfield SB, Wang ZM, et al. Skeletal muscle mass and distribution in 468 men and women aged 18–88 yr. J Appl Physiol 2000;89:81–8.

680. Jarvik JG, Deyo RA. Imaging of lumbar intervertebral disk degeneration and aging, excluding disk herniations. Radiol Clin North Am 2000;38:1255–66, vi.

681. Jarvik JG, Hollingworth W, Heagerty PJ, et al. Three-year incidence of low-back pain in an initially asymptomatic cohort: clinical and imaging risk factors. Spine 2005;30:1541–8; discussion 9.

682. Jarvinen TA, Jarvinen TL, Kannus P, et al. Collagen fibres of the spontaneously ruptured human tendons display decreased thickness and crimp angle. J Orthop Res 2004;22:1303–9.

683. Jay GD, Torres JR, Rhee DK, et al. Association between friction and wear in diarthrodial joints lacking lubricin. Arthritis Rheum 2007;56:3662–9.

684. Jeanneret B. Direct repair of spondylolysis. Acta Orthop Scand 1933;151:111–5.

685. Jeffery AK, Blunn GW, Archer CW, et al. Three-dimensional collagen architecture in bovine articular cartilage. J Bone Joint Surg [Br] 1991;73:795–801.

686. Jensen MC, Brant-Zawadzki MN, Obuchowski N, et al. Magnetic resonance imaging of the lumbar spine in people without back pain. N Engl J Med 1994;331: 69–73.

687. Jensen TS, Karppinen J, Sorensen JS, et al. Vertebral endplate signal changes (Modic change): a systematic literature review of prevalence and association with non-specific low-back pain. Eur Spine J 2008;17:1407–22.

688. Jewell D, Young G. Interventions for nausea and vomiting in early pregnancy. Cochrane Database Syst Rev 2003: CD000145.

689. Jiang G, Luo J, Pollintine P, et al. Vertebral fractures in the elderly may not always be 'osteoporotic'. Bone 2010;47:111–6.

690. Jiang H, Raso JV, Moreau MJ, et al. Quantitative morphology of the lateral ligaments of the spine. Assessment of their importance in maintaining lateral stability. Spine 1994;19:2676–82.

691. Johnson WE, Caterson B, Eisenstein SM, et al. Human intervertebral disc aggrecan inhibits nerve growth in vitro. Arthritis Rheum 2002;46 :2658–64.

692. Johnson WE, Caterson B, Eisenstein SM, et al. Human intervertebral disc aggrecan inhibits endothelial cell adhesion and cell migration in vitro. Spine 2005;30:1139–47.

693. Johnson WE, Sivan S, Wright KT, et al. Human intervertebral disc cells promote nerve growth over substrata of human intervertebral

disc aggrecan. Spine 2006;31:1187–93.

694. Johnstone B, Urban JP, Roberts S, et al. The fluid content of the human intervertebral disc. Comparison between fluid content and swelling pressure profiles of discs removed at surgery and those taken postmortem. Spine 1992;17:412–6.

695. Jonck LM, Van Niekerk JM. A roentgenological study of the motion of the lumbar spine of the Bantu. S A J Lab Clin Med 1961;7:67–71.

696. Jones DA, Newham DJ, Round JM, et al. Experimental human muscle damage: morphological changes in relation to other indices of damage. J Physiol 1986;375:435–48.

697. Jones GT, Macfarlane GJ. Epidemiology of low-back pain in children and adolescents. Arch Dis Child 2005;90:312–6.

698. Jones HH, Priest JD, Hayes WC, et al. Humeral hypertrophy in response to exercise. J Bone Joint Surg [Am] 1977;59:204–8.

699. Jones JR, Hodgson JT, Clegg TA, et al. Self-reported work-related illness in 1995. Results from a household survey. Norwich: Her Majesty's Stationery Office; 1998.

700. Jones MA, Stratton G, Reilly T, et al. A school-based survey of recurrent non-specific low-back pain prevalence and consequences in children. Health Educ Res 2004;19:284–9.

701. Junger S, Gantenbein-Ritter B, Lezuo P, et al. Effect of limited nutrition on in situ intervertebral disc cells under simulated-physiological loading. Spine 2009;34:1264–71.

702. Justice CM, Miller NH, Marosy B, et al. Familial idiopathic scoliosis: evidence of an X-linked susceptibility locus. Spine 2003;28:589–94.

703. Kaapa E, Han X, Holm S, et al. Collagen synthesis and types I, III, IV, and VI collagens in an animal model of disc degeneration. Spine 1995;20:59–66; discussion -7.

704. Kaila-Kangas L, Leino-Arjas P, Karppinen J, et al. History of

physical work exposures and clinically diagnosed sciatica among working and nonworking Finns aged 30 to 64. Spine 2009;34:964–9.

705. Kaila-Kangas L, Leino-Arjas P, Riihimaki H, et al. Smoking and overweight as predictors of hospitalization for back disorders. Spine 2003;28:1860–8.

706. Kalichman L, Cole R, Kim DH, et al. Spinal stenosis prevalence and association with symptoms: the Framingham Study. Spine J 2009;9:545–50.

707. Kalichman L, Guermazi A, Li L, et al. Facet orientation and tropism: associations with spondylolysis. J Spinal Disord Tech 2010;23:101–5.

708. Kanayama M, Abumi K, Kaneda K, et al. Phase lag of the intersegmental motion in flexion–extension of the lumbar and lumbosacral spine. An in vivo study. Spine 1996;21:1416–22.

709. Kanayama M, Tadano S, Kaneda K, et al. A cineradiographic study on the lumbar disc deformation during flexion and extension of the trunk. Clin Biomech 1995;10:193–9.

710. Kaneoka K, Ono K, Inami S, et al. Motion analysis of cervical vertebrae during whiplash loading. Spine 1999;24:763–9; discussion 70.

711. Kanerva A, Kommonen B, Gronblad M, et al. Inflammatory cells in experimental intervertebral disc injury. Spine 1997;22:2711–5.

712. Kang CH, Kim YH, Lee SH, et al. Can magnetic resonance imaging accurately predict concordant pain provocation during provocative disc injection? Skeletal Radiol 2009;38:877–85.

713. Kang JD, Georgescu HI, McIntyre-Larkin L, et al. Herniated lumbar intervertebral discs spontaneously produce matrix metalloproteinases, nitric oxide, interleukin-6, and prostaglandin E_2. Spine 1996;21:271–7.

714. Kang YM, Choi WS, Pickar JG. Electrophysiologic evidence for

an intersegmental reflex pathway between lumbar paraspinal tissues. Spine 2002;27:E56–63.

715. Kaplan M, Dreyfuss P, Halbrook B, et al. The ability of lumbar medial branch blocks to anesthetize the zygapophyseal joint. A physiologic challenge. Spine 1998;23:1847–52.

716. Karamouzian S, Eskandary H, Faramarzee M, et al. Frequency of lumbar intervertebral disc calcification and angiogenesis, and their correlation with clinical, surgical, and magnetic resonance imaging findings. Spine (Phila Pa) 2010;35:881–6.

717. Karasek M, Bogduk N. Twelve-month follow-up of a controlled trial of intradiscal thermal anuloplasty for back pain due to internal disc disruption. Spine 2000;25:2601–7.

718. Karppinen J, Korhonen T, Malmivaara A, et al. Tumor Necrosis Factor-alpha Monoclonal Antibody, Infliximab, Used to Manage Severe Sciatica. Spine 2003;28:750–3.

719. Kasashima Y, Smith RK, Birch HL, et al. Exercise-induced tendon hypertrophy: cross-sectional area changes during growth are influenced by exercise. Equine Vet J Suppl 2002:264–8.

720. Kastelic J, Galeski A, Baer E. The multicomposite structure of tendon. Connect Tissue Res 1978;6:11–23.

721. Katake K. Studies on the strength of human skeletal muscles. J Kyoto Pref Med Univ 1961;69:463–83.

722. Kawaguchi Y, Kanamori M, Ishihara H, et al. The association of lumbar disc disease with vitamin-D receptor gene polymorphism. J Bone Joint Surg Am 2002;84-A:2022–8.

723. Kawaguchi Y, Osada R, Kanamori M, et al. Association between an aggrecan gene polymorphism and lumbar disc degeneration. Spine 1999;24:2456–60.

724. Kawakami M, Hashizume H, Nishi H, et al. Comparison of neuropathic pain induced by the application of normal and mechanically compressed nucleus

pulposus to lumbar nerve roots in the rat. J Orthop Res 2003;21:535–9.

725. Kayama S, Konno S, Olmarker K, et al. Incision of the annulus fibrosus induces nerve root morphologic, vascular, and functional changes. An experimental study. Spine 1996;21:2539–43.

726. Keller TS, Hansson TH, Holm SH, et al. In vivo creep behaviour of the normal and degenerated porcine intervertebral disc: a preliminary report. J Spinal Disord 1989;1:267–78.

727. Keller TS, Harrison DE, Colloca CJ, et al. Prediction of osteoporotic spinal deformity. Spine 2003;28:455–62.

728. Keller TS, Holm SH, Hansson TH, et al. 1990 Volvo Award in experimental studies. The dependence of intervertebral disc mechanical properties on physiologic conditions. Spine 1990;15:751–61.

729. Kellgren JH. Observations on referred pain arising from muscle. Clin Sci 1938;3:175–90.

730. Kellgren JH. On the distribution of pain arising from deep somatic structures with charts of segmental pain areas. Clin Sci 1939;4:35–46.

731. Kelsey JL, Githens PB, O'Conner T, et al. Acute prolapsed lumbar intervertebral disc. An epidemiologic study with special reference to driving automobiles and cigarette smoking. Spine 1984;9:608–13.

732. Kelsey JL, Githens PB, White AAd et al. An epidemiologic study of lifting and twisting on the job and risk for acute prolapsed lumbar intervertebral disc. J Orthop Res 1984;2:61–6.

733. Kelsey JL, Hardy RJ. Driving of motor vehicles as a risk factor for acute herniated lumbar intervertebral disc. Am J Epidemiol 1975;102:63–73.

734. Kempson GE. Age-related changes in the tensile properties of human articular cartilage: a comparative study between the femoral head of the hip joint and the talus of the ankle joint. Biochim Biophys Acta 1991;1075:223–30.

735. Kendall NAS, Burton AK, Main CJ, et al. Tackling musculokeletal problems: a guide for clinic and workplace – identifying obstacles using the psychosoical flags framework. London: TSO; 2009.

735a. Kendall NAS, Burton AK, Main CJ, Watson PJ, on behalf of the Flags Think-Tank. Tackling musculoskeletal problems: a guide for the clinic and workplace – identifying obstacles using the psychosocial flags framework. London: The Stationery Office; 2009.

736. Kendall NAS, Linton SJ, Main CJ. Guide to assessing psychosocial yellow flags in acute low-back pain: Risk factors for long-term disability and work loss. Wellington, NZ: Accident Rehabilitation & Compensation Insurance Corporation of New Zealand and the National Health Committee; 1997.

737. Kent P, Keating JL. Classification in nonspecific low-back pain: what methods do primary care clinicians currently use? Spine 2005;30:1433–40.

738. Kerin AJ, Coleman A, Wisnom MR, et al. Propagation of surface fissures in articular cartilage in response to cyclic loading in vitro. Clin Biomech 2003;18:960–8.

739. Kerttula LI, Serlo WS, Tervonen OA, et al. Post-traumatic findings of the spine after earlier vertebral fracture in young patients: clinical and MRI study. Spine 2000;25:1104–8.

740. Kettler A, Rohlmann F, Ring C, et al. Do early stages of lumbar intervertebral disc degeneration really cause instability? Evaluation of an in vitro database. Eur Spine J 2011;20:578–84.

741. Kettler A, Werner K, Wilke HJ. Morphological changes of cervical facet joints in elderly individuals. Eur Spine J 2007;16:987–92.

742. Key S. Sarah Key's Back Sufferers' Bible. Australia: Allen & Unwin; 2007.

743. Kim KW, Lim TH, Kim JG, et al. The origin of chondrocytes in the nucleus pulposus and histologic findings associated with the transition of a notochordal nucleus pulposus to a fibrocartilaginous nucleus pulposus in intact rabbit intervertebral discs. Spine 2003;28:982–90.

744. Kimura T, Nakata K, Tsumaki N, et al. Progressive degeneration of articular cartilage and intervertebral discs. An experimental study in transgenic mice bearing a type IX collagen mutation. Int Orthop 1996;20:177–81.

745. Kingma I, Baten CT, Dolan P, et al. Lumbar loading during lifting: a comparative study of three measurement techniques. J Electromyogr Kinesiol 2001;11:337–45.

746. Kingma I, de Looze MP, Toussaint HM, et al. Validation of a full body 3-D dynamic linked segment model. Hum Move Science 1996;15:833–60.

747. Kingma I, van Dieen JH, de Looze M, et al. Asymmetric low-back loading in asymmetric lifting movements is not prevented by pelvic twist [see comments]. J Biomech 1998;31:527–34.

748. Kip PC, Esses SI, Doherty BI, et al. Biomechanical testing of pars defect repairs. Spine 1994;19:2692–7.

749. Kippers V, Parker AW. Posture related to myoelectric silence of erectores spinae during trunk flexion. Spine 1984;9:740–5.

750. Kirkaldy-Willis WH, Farfan HF. Instability of the lumbar spine. Clin Orthop 1982:110–23.

751. Kissling RO, Jacob HAC. The mobility of sacroiliac joints in healthy subjects. In: Vleeming A et al, editor. Movement, Stability and Low-back Pain. Edinburgh: Churchill Livingstone; 1997.

752. Kjaer P. Low-back pain in relation to lumbar spine abnormalities as identified by MRI. (PhD thesis). Odense: University of Southern Denmark; 2004.

753. Kjaer P, Bendix T, Sorensen JS, et al. Are MRI-defined fat infiltrations in the multifidus muscles associated with low-back pain? BMC med 2007;5:2.

754. Kjaer P, Korsholm L, Bendix T, et al. Modic changes and their

associations with clinical findings. Eur Spine J 2006;15: 1312–9.

755. Kjaer P, Leboeuf-Yde C, Sorensen JS, et al. An epidemiologic study of MRI and low-back pain in 13-year-old children. Spine 2005;30:798–806.

756. Klaber Moffett JA, Hughes GI, Griffiths P. A longitudinal study of low-back pain in student nurses. Int J Nursing Studies 1993;30:197–212.

757. Klauser A, De Zordo T, Feuchtner G, et al. Feasibility of ultrasound-guided sacroiliac joint injection considering sonoanatomic landmarks at two different levels in cadavers and patients. Arthritis Rheum 2008;59:1618–24.

758. Klein JA, Hukins DW. Collagen fibre orientation in the annulus fibrosus of intervertebral disc during bending and torsion measured by x-ray diffraction. Biochim Biophys Acta 1982;719:98–101.

759. Kleinstueck FS, Diederich CJ, Nau WH, et al. Acute biomechanical and histological effects of intradiscal electrothermal therapy on human lumbar discs. Spine 2001;26:2198–207.

760. Knutson F. The instability associated with disc degeneration in the lumbar spine. Acta Radiol 1944;25:593–609.

761. Kobayashi S, Meir A, Kokubo Y, et al. Ultrastructural analysis on lumbar disc herniation using surgical specimens: role of neovascularization and macrophages in hernias. Spine 2009;34:655–62.

762. Kobayashi S, Meir A, Urban J. Effect of cell density on the rate of glycosaminoglycan accumulation by disc and cartilage cells in vitro. J Orthop Res 2008;26:493–503.

763. Kobayashi S, Yoshizawa H, Yamada S. Pathology of lumbar nerve root compression. Part 2: morphological and immunohistochemical changes of dorsal root ganglion. J Orthop Res 2004;22:180–8.

764. Koda S, Nakagiri S, Yasuda N, et al. A follow-up study of preventive effects on low-back pain at worksites by providing a participatory occupational safety and health program. Ind Health 1997;35:243–8.

765. Koeller W, Funke F, Hartmann F. Biomechanical behavior of human intervertebral discs subjected to long lasting axial loading. Biorheology 1984; 21:675–86.

766. Koeller W, Muehlhaus S, Meier W, et al. Biomechanical properties of human intervertebral discs subjected to axial dynamic compression – influence of age and degeneration. J Biomech 1986;19:807–16.

767. Koes BW, van Tulder M, Lin CWC, et al. An updated overview of clinical guidelines for the management of non-specific low-back pain in primary care. Eur Spine J 2010; 19:2075–94.

768. Koes BW, van Tulder MW, Ostelo R, et al. Clinical guidelines for the management of low-back pain in primary care: an international comparison. Spine 2001;Submitted.

769. Koh TJ, Herzog W. Excursion is important in regulating sarcomere number in the growing rabbit tibialis anterior. J Physiol 1998;508:267–80.

770. Kohler R. Contrast examination of lumbar interspinous ligaments. Acta Orthop Scand 1962; (Suppl. 55).

771. Kohles SS, Kohles DA, Karp AP, et al. Time-dependent surgical outcomes following cauda equina syndrome diagnosis: comments on a meta-analysis. Spine 2004;29:1281–7.

772. Komori H, Shinomiya K, Nakai O, et al. The natural history of herniated nucleus pulposus with radiculopathy. Spine 1996;21:225–9.

773. Kong MH, Morishita Y, He W, et al. Lumbar segmental mobility according to the grade of the disc, the facet joint, the muscle, and the ligament pathology by using kinetic magnetic resonance imaging. Spine (Phila Pa) 2009;34:2537–44.

774. Kongsted A, Sorensen JS, Andersen H, et al. Are early MRI findings correlated with long-lasting symptoms following whiplash injury? A prospective trial with 1-year follow-up. Eur Spine J 2008;17:996–1005.

775. Kool J, de Bie R, Oesch P, et al. Exercise reduces sick leave in patients with non-acute non-specific low-back pain: a meta-analysis. J Rehabil Med 2004;36:49–62.

776. Kopsidas G, Kovalenko SA, Heffernan DR, et al. Tissue mitochondrial DNA changes. A stochastic system. Ann N Y Acad Sci 2000;908:226–43.

777. Korecki CL, Kuo CK, Tuan RS, et al. Intervertebral disc cell response to dynamic compression is age and frequency dependent. J Orthop Res 2009;27:800–6.

778. Korhonen T, Karppinen J, Malmivaara A, et al. Efficacy of infliximab for disc herniation-induced sciatica: one-year follow-up. Spine 2004;29: 2115–9.

779. Korhonen T, Karppinen J, Paimela L, et al. The treatment of disc herniation-induced sciatica with infliximab: one-year follow-up results of FIRST II, a randomized controlled trial. Spine 2006;31:2759–66.

780. Korkala O, Gronblad M, Liesi P, et al. Immunohistochemical demonstration of nociceptors in the ligamentous structures of the lumbar spine. Spine 1985;10: 156–7.

781. Kosaka H, Sairyo K, Biyani A, et al. Pathomechanism of loss of elasticity and hypertrophy of lumbar ligamentum flavum in elderly patients with lumbar spinal canal stenosis. Spine 2007;32:2805–11.

782. Kotani Y, Cunningham BW, Cappuccino A, et al. The effects of spinal fixation and destabilization on the biomechanical and histologic properties of spinal ligaments. An in vivo study. Spine 1998;23:672–82; discussion 82–3.

783. Kouwenhoven JW, Smit TH, van der Veen AJ, et al. Effects of dorsal versus ventral shear loads on the rotational stability of the thoracic spine: a biomechanical

porcine and human cadaveric study. Spine 2007;32:2545–50.

784. Kovacs F, Abraira V, Santos S, et al. A comparison of two short education programs for improving low-back pain-related disability in the elderly: A cluster randomized controlled trial. Spine 2007;32:1053–9.

785. Kovacs FM, Gestoso M, Gil del Real MT, et al. Risk factors for non-specific low-back pain in schoolchildren and their parents: a population based study. Pain 2003;103:259–68.

786. Kraemer J, Kolditz D, Gowin R. Water and electrolyte content of human intervertebral discs under variable load. Spine 1985;10:69–71.

787. Kraemer WJ, Patton JF, Gordon SE, et al. Compatibility of high-intensity strength and endurance training on hormonal and skeletal muscle adaptations. J Appl Physiol 1995;78:976–89.

788. Krag MH, Cohen MC, Haugh LD, et al. Body height change during upright and recumbent posture. Spine 1990;15:202–7.

789. Krajcarski SR, Potvin JR, Chiang J. The in vivo dynamic response of the spine to perturbations causing rapid flexion: effects of pre-load and step input magnitude. Clin Biomech 1999;14:54–62.

790. Kraus JF, Schaffer KB, Rice T, et al. A field trial of back belts to reduce the incidence of acute low-back injuries in New York City home attendants. Int J Occup Environ Health 2002;8:97–104.

791. Krause N, Ragland DR, Fisher JM, et al. Psychosocial job factors, physical workload, and incidence of work- related spinal injury: a 5-year prospective study of urban transit operators. Spine 1998;23:2507–16.

792. Krause N, Rugulies R, Ragland DR, et al. Physical workload, ergonomic problems, and incidence of low-back injury: a 7.5-year prospective study of San Francisco transit operators. Am J Ind Med 2004;46:570–85.

793. Krismer M, Haid C, Rabl W. The contribution of annulus fibers to

torque resistance. Spine 1996; 21:2551–7.

794. Kujala UM, Oksanen A, Taimela S, et al. Training does not increase maximal lumbar extension in healthy adolescents. Clin Biomech 1997;12:181–4.

795. Kumar S. The physiological cost of three different methods of lifting in sagittal and lateral planes. Ergonomics 1984; 27:425–33.

796. Kuo YL, Tully EA, Galea MP. Video analysis of sagittal spinal posture in healthy young and older adults. J Manipul Physiol Ther 2009;32:210–5.

797. Kuslich SD, Ulstrom CL, Michael CJ. The tissue origin of low-back pain and sciatica: a report of pain response to tissue stimulation during operations on the lumbar spine using local anesthesia. Orthop Clin North Am 1991; 22:181–7.

798. Kutzner I, Heinlein B, Graichen F, et al. Loading of the knee joint during activities of daily living measured in vivo in five subjects. J Biomech 2010;43: 2164–73.

799. Lahad A, Malter AD, Berg AO, et al. The effectiveness of four interventions for the prevention of low-back pain. Jama 1994; 272:1286–91.

800. Laible JP, Pflaster DS, Krag MH, et al. A poroelastic-swelling finite element model with application to the intervertebral disc. Spine 1993;18:659–70.

801. Lam KS, Carlin D, Mulholland RC. Lumbar disc high-intensity zone: the value and significance of provocative discography in the determination of the discogenic pain source. Eur Spine J 2000;9: 36–41.

802. Lancourt J, Kettelhut M. Predicting return to work for lower back pain patients receiving worker's compensation. Spine 1992;17:629–40.

803. Lane RJM. Handbook of muscle disease. New York: Marcel Dekker; 1996.

804. Lansade C, Laporte S, Thoreux P, et al. Three-dimensional analysis of the cervical spine kinematics: effect of age and gender in

healthy subjects. Spine (Phila Pa) 2009;34:2900–6.

805. Lanyon LE, Rubin CT. Static vs dynamic loads as an influence on bone remodelling. J Biomech 1984;17:897–905.

806. Larsen K, Weidich F, Leboeuf-Yde C. Can custom-made biomechanic shoe orthoses prevent problems in the back and lower extremities? A randomized, controlled intervention trial of 146 military conscripts. J Manipul Physiol Ther 2002;25:326–31.

807. Larsson L. Physical training effects on muscle morphology in sedentary males at different ages. Med Sci Sports Exerc 1982;14: 203–6.

808. Lau E, Ong K, Kurtz S, et al. Mortality following the diagnosis of a vertebral compression fracture in the Medicare population. J Bone Joint Surg Am 2008;90:1479–86.

809. Lavender SA, Shakeel K, Andersson GB, et al. Effects of a lifting belt on spine moments and muscle recruitments after unexpected sudden loading. Spine 2000;25: 1569–78.

810. Lavender SA, Tsuang YH, Hafezi A, et al. Coactivation of the trunk muscles during asymmetric loading of the torso. Hum Factors 1992;34:239–47.

811. Le Maitre CL, Freemont AJ, Hoyland JA. Accelerated cellular senescence in degenerate intervertebral discs: a possible role in the pathogenesis of intervertebral disc degeneration. Arthritis Res Ther 2007;9:R45.

812. Leboeuf-Yde C. Smoking and low-back pain. A systematic literature review of 41 journal articles reporting 47 epidemiologic studies. Spine 1999;24:1463–70.

813. Leboeuf-Yde C, Gronstvedt A, Borge JA, et al. The Nordic back pain subpopulation program: a 1-year prospective multicenter study of outcomes of persistent low-back pain in chiropractic patients. J Manipul Physiol Ther 2005;28:90–6.

814. Leboeuf-Yde C, Kjaer P, Bendix T, et al. Self-reported hard physical work combined with heavy smoking or overweight may result in so-called Modic changes. BMC musculoskeletal disorders 2008;9:5.

815. Leboeuf-Yde C, Wedderkopp N, Andersen LB, et al. Back pain reporting in children and adolescents: the impact of parents' educational level. J Manipul Physiol Ther 2002;25:216–20.

816. Leclaire R, Esdaile JM, Suissa S, et al. Back school in a first episode of compensated acute low-back pain: a clinical trial to assess efficacy and prevent relapse. Arch Phys Med Rehabil 1996;77:673–9.

817. Lee DC, Campbell PP, Gilsanz V, et al. Contribution of the vertebral posterior elements in anterior-posterior DXA spine scans in young subjects. J Bone Miner Res 2009;24:1398–403.

818. Lee DY, Ahn Y, Lee SH. The influence of facet tropism on herniation of the lumbar disc in adolescents and adults. J Bone Joint Surg Br 2006;88:520–3.

819. Leech C. Preventing chronic disability from low-back pain – Renaissance Project. Dublin: The Stationery Office (Government Publications Office); 2004.

820. Leinonen V, Maatta S, Taimela S, et al. Paraspinal muscle denervation, paradoxically good lumbar endurance, and an abnormal flexion–extension cycle in lumbar spinal stenosis. Spine 2003;28:324–31.

821. Leivseth G, Drerup B. Spinal shrinkage during work in a sitting posture compared to work in a standing posture. Clin Biomech 1997;12:409–18.

822. Leong JC, Luk KD, Chow DH, et al. The biomechanical functions of the iliolumbar ligament in maintaining stability of the lumbosacral junction. Spine 1987;12:669–74.

823. Leppilahti J, Puranen J, Orava S. Incidence of Achilles tendon rupture. Acta Orthop Scand 1996;67:277–9.

824. Lewin T. Osteoarthritis in lumbar synovial joints. A morphologic study. Acta Orthop Scand 1964;(Suppl. 73).

825. Li B, Aspden RM. Mechanical and material properties of the subchondral bone plate from the femoral head of patients with osteoarthritis or osteoporosis. Ann Rheum Dis 1997;56:247–54.

826. Li XF, Li H, Liu ZD, et al. Low bone mineral status in adolescent idiopathic scoliosis. Eur Spine J 2008;17(11):1431–40.

827. Liang QQ, Zhou Q, Zhang M, et al. Prolonged upright posture induces degenerative changes in intervertebral discs in rat lumbar spine. Spine 2008;33:2052–8.

828. Lieber RL, Friden J. Selective damage of fast glycolytic muscle fibres with eccentric contraction of the rabbit tibialis anterior. Acta Physiol Scand 1988;133:587–8.

829. Lieber RL, Friden J. Mechanisms of muscle injury after eccentric contraction. J Sci Med Sport 1999;2:253–65.

830. Liebscher T, Haefeli M, Wuertz K, et al. Age-related variation in cell density of human lumbar intervertebral disc. Spine 2011;36:153–9.

831. Liliang PC, Lu K, Weng HC, et al. The therapeutic efficacy of sacroiliac joint blocks with triamcinolone acetonide in the treatment of sacroiliac joint dysfunction without spondyloarthropathy. Spine 2009;34:896–900.

832. Lim CH, Jee WH, Son BC, et al. Discogenic lumbar pain: association with MR imaging and CT discography. Eur J Radiol 2005;54:431–7.

833. Lin PM, Chen CT, Torzilli PA. Increased stromelysin-1 (MMP-3), proteoglycan degradation (3B3- and 7D4) and collagen damage in cyclically load-injured articular cartilage. Osteoarthritis Cartilage 2004;12:485–96.

834. Lin TW, Cardenas L, Soslowsky LJ. Biomechanics of tendon injury and repair. J Biomech 2004;37:865–77.

835. Lindblom K. Diagnostic puncture of intervertebral disks in sciatica. Acta Orthop Scand 1948;17:231–9.

836. Lindblom K. Experimental ruptures of intervertebral discs in rats' tails. J Bone Joint Surg [Am] 1952;34:123–8.

837. Lindblom K. Intervertebral disc degeneration considered as a pressure atrophy. J Bone Joint Surg [Am] 1957;39:933–45.

838. Lingard EA, Riddle DL. Impact of psychological distress on pain and function following knee arthroplasty. J Bone Joint Surg Am 2007;89:1161–9.

839. Link HD. History, design and biomechanics of the LINK SB Charite artificial disc. Eur Spine J 2002;11(Suppl. 2):S98-S105.

840. Linton SJ. A review of psychological risk factors in back and neck pain. Spine 2000;25:1148–56.

841. Linton SJ. New avenues for the prevention of chronic musculoskeletal pain and disability. Amsterdam: Elsevier Science; 2002.

842. Linton SJ, van Tulder MW. Preventive interventions for back and neck pain problems: what is the evidence? Spine 2001;26:778–87.

843. Lipson SJ, Muir H. Vertebral osteophyte formation in experimental disc degeneration. Morphologic and proteoglycan changes over time. Arthritis Rheum 1980;23:319–24.

844. Little CB, Flannery CR, Hughes CE, et al. Aggrecanase versus matrix metalloproteinases in the catabolism of the interglobular domain of aggrecan in vitro. Biochem J 1999;344(Pt 1):61–8.

845. Liu YK, Goel VK, Dejong A, et al. Torsional fatigue of the lumbar intervertebral joints. Spine 1985;10:894–900.

846. Liu YK, Njus G, Buckwalter J, et al. Fatigue response of lumbar intervertebral joints under axial cyclic loading. Spine 1983;8:857–65.

847. Liyang D, Yinkan X, Wenming Z, et al. The effect of flexion–extension motion of the lumbar spine on the capacity of the

spinal canal. An experimental study. Spine 1989;14:523–5.

848. Loisel P, Lemaire J, Poitras S, et al. Cost-benefit and cost-effectiveness analysis of a disability prevention model for back pain management: a six year follow up study. Occup Environ Med 2002;59:807–15.

849. Lord MJ, Small JM, Dinsay JM, et al. Lumbar lordosis. Effects of sitting and standing. Spine 1997; 22:2571–4.

850. Lotz JC. Animal models of intervertebral disc degeneration: lessons learned. Spine 2004;29:2742–50.

851. Lotz JC, Colliou OK, Chin JR, et al. Compression-induced degeneration of the intervertebral disc: an in vivo mouse model and finite-element study. Spine 1998;23:2493–506.

852. Lotz JC, Hadi T, Bratton C, et al. Annulus fibrosus tension inhibits degenerative structural changes in lamellar collagen. Eur Spine J 2008;17:1149–59.

853. Lu Y, Markel MD, Swain C, et al. Development of partial thickness articular cartilage injury in an ovine model. J Orthop Res 2006; 24:1974–82.

854. Lu YM, Hutton WC, Gharpuray VM. Can variations in intervertebral disc height affect the mechanical function of the disc? Spine 1996;21:2208–16; discussion 17.

855. Lu YM, Hutton WC, Gharpuray VM. Do bending, twisting, and diurnal fluid changes in the disc affect the propensity to prolapse? A viscoelastic finite element model. Spine 1996;21:2570–9.

856. Lucas N, Macaskill P, Irwig L, et al. Reliability of physical examination for diagnosis of myofascial trigger points: a systematic review of the literature. Clin J Pain 2009;25:80–9.

857. Lundin O, Ekstrom L, Hellstrom M, et al. Injuries in the adolescent porcine spine exposed to mechanical compression. Spine 1998;23:2574–9.

858. Luo J, Pollintine P, Dolan P, et al. Atraumatic vertebral deformity arising from an accelerated 'creep' mechanism. European Spine Journal 2012 (accepted for publication).

859. Luo J, Skrzypiec DM, Pollintine P, et al. Mechanical efficacy of vertebroplasty: Influence of cement type, BMD, fracture severity, and disc degeneration. Bone 2007;40:1110–9.

860. Luoma K, Vehmas T, Gronblad M, et al. MRI follow-up of subchondral signal abnormalities in a selected group of chronic low-back pain patients. Eur Spine J 2008;17:1300–8.

861. Lutz GE, Vad VB, Wisneski RJ. Fluoroscopic transforaminal lumbar epidural steroids: an outcome study. Arch Phys Med Rehabil 1998;79:1362–6.

862. Ma H, Leskinen T, Alen M, et al. Long-term leisure time physical activity and properties of bone: a twin study. J Bone Miner Res 2009;24:1427–33.

863. Mac-Thiong JM, Berthonnaud E, Dimar 2nd JR, et al. Sagittal alignment of the spine and pelvis during growth. Spine 2004;29: 1642–7.

864. Mac-Thiong JM, Labelle H, Berthonnaud E, et al. Sagittal spinopelvic balance in normal children and adolescents. Eur Spine J 2007;16:227–34.

865. Macefield G, Hagbarth KE, Gorman R, et al. Decline in spindle support to alpha-motoneurones during sustained voluntary contractions. J Physiol 1991;440:497–512.

866. Macfarlane GJ, Thomas E, Papageorgiou AC, et al. Employment and physical work activities as predictors of future low-back pain. Spine 1997;22: 1143–9.

867. MacGregor AJ, Andrew T, Sambrook PN, et al. Structural, psychological, and genetic influences on low-back and neck pain: a study of adult female twins. Arthritis Rheum 2004; 51:160–7.

868. Macintosh J, Bogduk N. The biomechanics of the lumbar multifidus. Clin Biomech 1986;1:205–13.

869. Macintosh J, Valencia F, Bogduk N, et al. The morphology of the human lumbar multifidus. Clin Biomech 1986;1:196–204.

870. MacIntosh JE, Bogduk N. The biomechanics of the lumbar multifidus. Clin Biomech 1986;1:205–13.

871. Macintosh JE, Bogduk N. 1987 Volvo award in basic science. The morphology of the lumbar erector spinae. Spine 1987;12:658–68.

872. Macintosh JE, Bogduk N. The attachments of the lumbar erector spinae. Spine 1991;16: 783–92.

873. MacIntosh JE, Bogduk N, Gracovetsky S. The biomechanics of the thoracolumbar fascia.. Clin Biomech 1987;2:78–83.

874. Macintosh JE, Bogduk N, Pearcy MJ. The effects of flexion on the geometry and actions of the lumbar erector spinae. Spine 1993;18:884–93.

875. Macintosh JE, Pearcy MJ, Bogduk N. The axial torque of the lumbar back muscles: torsion strength of the back muscles. Aust N Z J Surg 1993;63:205–12.

876. Mackay C, Burton K, Boocock M, et al. Musculoskeletal disorders in supermarket cashiers. Norwich: Her Majesty's Stationery Office; 1998.

877. MacLean JJ, Lee CR, Grad S, et al. Effects of immobilization and dynamic compression on intervertebral disc cell gene expression in vivo. Spine 2003;28:973–81.

878. Madan S, Gundanna M, Harley JM, et al. Does provocative discography screening of discogenic back pain improve surgical outcome? J Spinal Disord Tech 2002;15:245–51.

879. Madigan ML, Davidson BS, Nussbaum MA. Postural sway and joint kinematics during quiet standing are affected by lumbar extensor fatigue. Hum Mov Sci 2006;25:788–99.

880. Maeda S, Kokubun S. Changes with age in proteoglycan synthesis in cells cultured in vitro from the inner and outer rabbit annulus fibrosus. Responses to interleukin-1 and interleukin-1 receptor antagonist protein. Spine 2000;25:166–9.

881. Maganaris CN, Narici MV, Reeves ND. In vivo human tendon mechanical properties: effect of resistance training in old age. J Musculoskelet Neuronal Interact 2004;4:204–8.

882. Magnusson ML, Aleksiev A, Wilder DG, et al. Unexpected load and asymmetric posture as etiologic factors in low-back pain. Eur Spine J 1996;5:23–35.

883. Magnusson ML, Aleksiev AR, Spratt KF, et al. Hyperextension and spine height changes. Spine 1996;21:2670–5.

884. Magnusson ML, Bishop JB, Hasselquist L, et al. Range of motion and motion patterns in patients with low-back pain before and after rehabilitation. Spine 1998;23:2631–9.

885. Magnusson ML, Pope MH, Hasselquist L, et al. Cervical electromyographic activity during low-speed rear impact. Eur Spine J 1999;8:118–25.

886. Magora A. Investigation of the relation between low-back pain and occupation. IV. Physical requirements: bending, rotation, reaching and sudden maximal effort. Scand J Rehabil Med 1973;5:186–90.

887. Maher CG. A systematic review of workplace interventions to prevent low-back pain. Aust J Physiother 2000;46:259–69.

888. Maier-Riehle B, Harter M. The effects of back schools – a meta-analysis. Int J Rehabil Res 2001;24:199–206.

889. Maigne JY, Aivaliklis A, Pfefer F. Results of sacroiliac joint double block and value of sacroiliac pain provocation tests in 54 patients with low-back pain. Spine 1996;21:1889–92.

890. Main CJ, Burton AK. Economic and occupational influences on pain and disability. In: Main CJ, Spanswick CC, editors. Pain management An interdisciplinary approach. Edinburgh: Churchill Livingstone; 2000.

891. Main CJ, Spanswick CC. Pain management. An interdisciplinary approach. Edinburgh: Churchill Livingstone; 2000.

892. Malham GM, Ackland HM, Varma DK, et al. Traumatic cervical discoligamentous injuries: correlation of magnetic resonance imaging and operative findings. Spine (Phila Pa) 2009;34:2754–9.

893. Malinsky J. The ontogenetic development of nerve terminations in the intervertebral discs of man. Acta Anat 1959;38:96–113.

894. Malko JA, Hutton WC, Fajman WA. An in vivo magnetic resonance imaging study of changes in the volume (and fluid content) of the lumbar intervertebral discs during a simulated diurnal load cycle. Spine 1999;24:1015–22.

895. Malone AM, Anderson CT, Tummala P, et al. Primary cilia mediate mechanosensing in bone cells by a calcium-independent mechanism. Proc Natl Acad Sci U S A 2007;104:13325–30.

896. Manek NJ, MacGregor AJ. Epidemiology of back disorders: prevalence, risk factors, and prognosis. Curr Opin Rheumatol 2005;17:134–40.

897. Mann T, Oviatt SK, Wilson D, et al. Vertebral deformity in men. J Bone Miner Res 1992;7:1259–65.

898. Mannion AF, Adams MA, Dolan P. People who load their spines heavily during standard lifting tasks are more likely to develop low-back pain. Presented to the International Society for the Study of the Lumbar Spine; 1997; Singapore; 1997.

899. Mannion AF, Adams MA, Dolan P. Sudden and unexpected loading generates high forces on the lumbar spine. Spine 2000;25:842–52.

900. Mannion AF, Connolly B, Wood K, et al. The use of surface EMG power spectral analysis in the evaluation of back muscle function. J Rehabil Res Dev 1997;34:427–39.

901. Mannion AF, Dolan P. The effects of muscle length and force output on the EMG power spectrum of the erector spinae. J Electromyogr Kinesiol 1996;6:159–68.

902. Mannion AF, Dolan P. Relationship between myoelectric and mechanical manifestations of fatigue in the quadriceps femoris muscle group. Eur J Appl Physiol 1996;74:411–9.

903. Mannion AF, Dolan P, Adams MA. Psychological questionnaires: do 'abnormal' scores precede or follow first-time low-back pain? Spine 1996;21:2603–11.

904. Mannion AF, Dumas GA, Cooper RG, et al. Muscle fibre size and type distribution in thoracic and lumbar regions of erector spinae in healthy subjects without low-back pain: normal values and sex differences. J Anat 1997;190:505–13.

905. Mannion AF, Junge A, Elfering A, et al. Great expectations: really the novel predictor of outcome after spinal surgery? Spine (Phila Pa) 2009;34:1590–9.

906. Mannion AF, Kaser L, Weber E, et al. Influence of age and duration of symptoms on fibre type distribution and size of the back muscles in chronic low-back pain patients. Eur Spine J 2000;9:273–81.

907. Mannion AF, Meier M, Grob D, et al. Paraspinal muscle fibre type alterations associated with scoliosis: an old problem revisited with new evidence. Eur Spine J 1998;7:289–93.

908. Mannion AF, Weber BR, Dvorak J, et al. Fibre type characteristics of the lumbar paraspinal muscles in normal healthy subjects and in patients with low-back pain. J Orthop Res 1997;15:881–7.

909. Manns RA, Haddaway MJ, McCall IW, et al. The relative contribution of disc and vertebral morphometry to the angle of kyphosis in asymptomatic subjects. Clin Radiol 1996;51:258–62.

910. Manolio TA, Collins FS, Cox NJ, et al. Finding the missing heritability of complex diseases. Nature 2009;461:747–53.

911. Mansell JP, Bailey AJ. Increased metabolism of bone collagen in post-menopausal female osteoporotic femoral heads. Int J Biochem Cell Biol 2003;35:522–9.

912. Marchand F, Ahmed AM. Mechanical properties and failure mechanisms: constituent components of the annulus

fibrosus. Proceedings of the 10th Annual Conference of the Canadian Biomaterials Society, Montreal, Canada, June 1989; p. 74–7.

913. Marchand F, Ahmed AM. Investigation of the laminate structure of lumbar disc annulus fibrosus. Spine 1990;15:402–10.

914. Marhold C, Linton SJ, Melin L. Identification of obstacles for chronic pain patients to return to work: evaluation of a questionnaire. J Occup Rehabil 2002;12:65–75.

915. Marinelli NL, Haughton VM, Munoz A, et al. T2 relaxation times of intervertebral disc tissue correlated with water content and proteoglycan content. Spine 2009;34:520–4.

916. Markolf KL, Morris JM. The structural components of the intervertebral disc. A study of their contributions to the ability of the disc to withstand compressive forces. J Bone Joint Surg Am 1974;56:675–87.

917. Maroudas A, Rigler D, Schneiderman R. Young and aged cartilage differ in their response to dynamic compression as far as the rate of glycosaminoglycan synthesis is concerned. Presented to the Orthopaedic Research Society; 1999; Anaheim, California; 1999.

918. Maroudas A, Stockwell RA, Nachemson A, et al. Factors involved in the nutrition of the human lumbar intervertebral disc: cellularity and diffusion of glucose in vitro. J Anat 1975;120:113–30.

919. Marras WS, Allread WG, Burr DL, et al. Prospective validation of a low-back disorder risk model and assessment of ergonomic interventions associated with manual materials handling tasks. Ergonomics 2000;43: 1866–86.

920. Marras WS, Davis KG, Heaney CA, et al. The influence of psychosocial stress, gender, and personality on mechanical loading of the lumbar spine. Spine 2000;25:3045–54.

921. Marras WS, Granata KP. A biomechanical assessment and model of axial twisting in the thoracolumbar spine. Spine 1995;20:1440–51.

922. Marras WS, Jorgensen MJ, Granata KP, et al. Female and male trunk geometry: size and prediction of the spine loading trunk muscles derived from MRI. Clin Biomech 2001;16: 38–46.

923. Marras WS, Lavender SA, Ferguson SA, et al. Quantitative dynamic measures of physical exposure predict low-back functional impairment. Spine (Phila Pa) 2010;35:914–23.

924. Marras WS, Lavender SA, Leurgans SE, et al. The role of dynamic three-dimensional trunk motion in occupationally- related low-back disorders. The effects of workplace factors, trunk position, and trunk motion characteristics on risk of injury. Spine 1993; 18:617–28.

925. Marras WS, Mirka GA. Intra- abdominal pressure during trunk extension motions. Clin Biomech 1996;11:267–74.

926. Marras WS, Rangarajulu SL, Lavender SA. Trunk loading and expectation. Ergonomics 1987; 30:551–62.

927. Marras WS, Sommerich CM. A three-dimensional motion model of loads on the lumbar spine: I. Model structure. Hum Factors 1991;33:123–37.

928. Martimo KP, Verbeek J, Karppinen J, et al. Manual material handling advice and assistive devices for preventing and treating back pain in workers (Cochrane Review). In: Cochrane Database of Systematic Reviews, Issue 3. Chichester: John Wiley & Sons; 2007.

929. Martimo KP, Verbeek J, Karppinen J, et al. Effect of training and lifting equipment for preventing back pain in lifting and handling: systematic review. BMJ 2008;336:429–31.

930. Marty-Poumarat C, Scattin L, Marpeau M, et al. Natural history of progressive adult scoliosis. Spine 2007;32:1227–34; discussion 35.

931. Masharawi Y, Dar G, Peleg S, et al. A morphological adaptation of the thoracic and lumbar vertebrae to lumbar hyperlordosis in young and adult females. Eur Spine J 2010;19:768–73.

932. Matsumoto M, Okada E, Ichihara D, et al. Prospective Ten-Year Follow-up Study Comparing Patients With Whiplash- Associated Disorders and Asymptomatic Subjects Using Magnetic Resonance Imaging. Spine (Phila Pa) 2010; 35(18):1684–90.

933. Matsumoto T, Kawakami M, Kuribayashi K, et al. Cyclic mechanical stretch stress increases the growth rate and collagen synthesis of nucleus pulposus cells in vitro. Spine 1999;24:315–9.

934. Maul I, Laubli T, Klipstein A, et al. Course of low-back pain among nurses: a longitudinal study across eight years. Occup Environ Med 2003;60:497–503.

935. Mayer T, Tabor J, Bovasso E, et al. Physical progress and residual impairment quantification after functional restoration. Part I: Lumbar mobility. Spine 1994;19:389–94.

936. McBroom RJ, Hayes WC, Edwards WT, et al. Prediction of vertebral body compressive fracture using quantitative computed tomography. J Bone Joint Surg [Am] 1985;67:1206–14.

937. McCall IW, Park WM, O'Brien JP. Induced pain referral from posterior lumbar elements in normal subjects. Spine 1979;4:441–6.

938. McComas AJ. 1998 ISEK Congress Keynote Lecture: Motor units: how many, how large, what kind? International Society of Electrophysiology and Kinesiology. J Electromyogr Kinesiol 1998;8:391–402.

939. McGill S, Juker D, Kropf P. Appropriately placed surface EMG electrodes reflect deep muscle activity (psoas, quadratus lumborum, abdominal wall) in the lumbar spine. J Biomech 1996;29:1503–7.

940. McGill S, Seguin J, Bennett G. Passive stiffness of the lumbar torso in flexion, extension, lateral bending, and axial rotation.

Effect of belt wearing and breath holding. Spine 1994;19:696–704.

941. McGill SM. Electromyographic activity of the abdominal and low-back musculature during the generation of isometric and dynamic axial trunk torque: implications for lumbar mechanics. J Orthop Res 1991; 9:91–103.

942. McGill SM. The influence of lordosis on axial trunk torque and trunk muscle myoelectric activity. Spine 1992;17:1187–93.

943. McGill SM. A myoelectrically based dynamic three-dimensional model to predict loads on lumbar spine tissues during lateral bending. J Biomech 1992;25:395–414.

944. McGill SM, Brown S. Creep response of the lumbar spine to prolonged full flexion. Clin Biomech 1992;7:43–6.

945. McGill SM, Kippers V. Transfer of loads between lumbar tissues during the flexion-relaxation phenomenon. Spine 1994;19:2190–6.

946. McGill SM, Norman RW. Dynamically and statically determined low-back moments during lifting. J Biomech 1985;18:877–85.

947. McGill SM, Norman RW. Partitioning of the L4-L5 dynamic moment into disc, ligamentous, and muscular components during lifting [see comments]. Spine 1986; 11:666–78.

948. McGill SM, Norman RW. Effects of an anatomically detailed erector spinae model on L4/L5 disc compression and shear. J Biomech 1987; 20:591–600.

949. McGill SM, Norman RW, Sharratt MT. The effect of an abdominal belt on trunk muscle activity and intra- abdominal pressure during squat lifts. Ergonomics 1990;33:147–60.

950. McGill SM, Yingling VR, Peach JP. Three-dimensional kinematics and trunk muscle myoelectric activity in the elderly spine – a database compared to young people. Clin Biomech 1999;14: 389–95.

951. McGorry RW, Hsiang SM, Fathallah FA, et al. Timing of activation of the erector spinae and hamstrings during a trunk flexion and extension task. Spine 2001;26:418–25.

952. McGregor AH, Burton AK, Sell P, et al. The development of an educational booklet for patients following spinal surgery. Presented to the International Society for the Study of the Lumbar Spine; New York; 2005.

953. McGregor AH, McCarthy ID, Dore CJ, et al. Quantitative assessment of the motion of the lumbar spine in the low-back pain population and the effect of different spinal pathologies of this motion. Eur Spine J 1997; 6:308–15.

954. McGuirk B, King W, Govind J, et al. Safety, efficacy, and cost effectiveness of evidence-based guidelines for the management of acute low-back pain in primary care. Spine 2001;26: 2615–22.

955. McKenna PJ, Freeman BJ, Mulholland RC, et al. A prospective, randomised controlled trial of femoral ring allograft versus a titanium cage in circumferential lumbar spinal fusion with minimum 2-year clinical results. Eur Spine J 2005;14:727–37.

956. McLain RF, Pickar JG. Mechanoreceptor endings in human thoracic and lumbar facet joints. Spine 1998;23:168–73.

957. McMillan DW, Garbutt G, Adams MA. Effect of sustained loading on the water content of intervertebral discs: implications for disc metabolism. Ann Rheum Dis 1996;55:880–7.

958. McMillan DW, McNally DS, Garbutt G, et al. Stress distributions inside intervertebral discs: the validity of experimental 'stress profilometry'. Proc Inst Mech Eng [H] 1996;210:81–7.

959. McNally DS, Adams MA. Internal intervertebral disc mechanics as revealed by stress profilometry. Spine 1992;17:66–73.

960. McNally DS, Adams MA, Goodship AE. Development and validation of a new transducer for intradiscal pressure measurement. J Biomed Eng 1992;14:495–8.

961. McNally DS, Adams MA, Goodship AE. Can intervertebral disc prolapse be predicted by disc mechanics? Spine 1993;18:1525–30.

962. McNally DS, Shackleford IM, Goodship AE, et al. In vivo stress measurement can predict pain on discography. Spine 1996;21:2580–7.

963. McNeil PL, Khakee R. Disruptions of muscle fiber plasma membranes. Role in exercise-induced damage. Am J Pathol 1992;140:1097–109.

964. McNeill T, Warwick D, Andersson G, et al. Trunk strengths in attempted flexion, extension, and lateral bending in healthy subjects and patients with low-back disorders. Spine 1980;5: 529–38.

965. Meakin JR, Smith FW, Gilbert FJ, et al. The effect of axial load on the sagittal plane curvature of the upright human spine in vivo. J Biomech 2008;41:2850–4.

966. Meir A, McNally DS, Fairbank JC, et al. The internal pressure and stress environment of the scoliotic intervertebral disc – a review. Proc Inst Mech Eng [H] 2008;222:209–19.

967. Mellin GP. Comparison between tape measurements of forward and lateral flexion of the spine. Clin Biomech 1989;4:121–3.

968. Melrose J, Ghosh P, Taylor TK, et al. A longitudinal study of the matrix changes induced in the intervertebral disc by surgical damage to the annulus fibrosus. J Orthop Res 1992; 10:665–76.

969. Melrose J, Roberts S, Smith S, et al. Increased nerve and blood vessel ingrowth associated with proteoglycan depletion in an ovine annular lesion model of experimental disc degeneration. Spine 2002;27:1278–85.

970. Melrose J, Smith SM, Appleyard RC, et al. Aggrecan, versican and type VI collagen are components of annular translamellar crossbridges in the intervertebral disc. Eur Spine J 2008;17:314–24.

303

References

971. Melrose J, Smith SM, Little CB, et al. Recent advances in annular pathobiology provide insights into rim-lesion mediated intervertebral disc degeneration and potential new approaches to annular repair strategies. Eur Spine J 2008;17:1131–48.

972. Melton 3rd LJ, Riggs BL, Achenbach SJ, et al. Does reduced skeletal loading account for age-related bone loss? J Bone Miner Res 2006;21:1847–55.

973. Melton 3rd LJ, Riggs BL, Keaveny TM, et al. Structural determinants of vertebral fracture risk. J Bone Miner Res 2007;22:1885–92.

974. Mendez FJ, Gomez-Conesa A. Postural hygiene program to prevent low-back pain. Spine 2001;26:1280–6.

975. Mercer S, Bogduk N. The ligaments and annulus fibrosus of human adult cervical intervertebral discs. Spine 1999;24:619–26; discussion 27–8.

976. Merskey H, Bogduk N. Classification of chronic pain: descriptions of chronic pain syndromes and definitions of pain terms. 2nd ed. Seattle: IASP Press; 1994.

977. Meyerding HW. Spondylolisthesis. Surg gynaecol obstet 1932;54:371–7.

978. Mihara H, Onari K, Cheng BC, et al. The biomechanical effects of spondylolysis and its treatment. Spine 2003;28:235–8.

979. Miller JA, Schmatz C, Schultz AB. Lumbar disc degeneration: correlation with age, sex, and spine level in 600 autopsy specimens. Spine 1988;13:173–8.

980. Miller JA, Schultz AB, Andersson GB. Load-displacement behavior of sacroiliac joints. J Orthop Res 1987;5:92–101.

981. Miller JA, Schultz AB, Warwick DN, et al. Mechanical properties of lumbar spine motion segments under large loads. J Biomech 1986;19:79–84.

982. Miller SA, Mayer T, Cox R, et al. Reliability problems associated with the modified Schober technique for true lumbar flexion measurement. Spine 1992;17:345–8.

983. Mimura M, Panjabi MM, Oxland TR, et al. Disc degeneration affects the multidirectional flexibility of the lumbar spine. Spine 1994;19:1371–80.

984. Minajeva A, Neagoe C, Kulke M, et al. Titin-based contribution to shortening velocity of rabbit skeletal myofibrils. J Physiol 2002;540:177–88.

985. Mirza SK, Deyo RA. Systematic review of randomized trials comparing lumbar fusion surgery to nonoperative care for treatment of chronic back pain. Spine 2007;32:816–23.

986. Miyamoto K, Iinuma N, Maeda M, et al. Effects of abdominal belts on intra-abdominal pressure, intra-muscular pressure in the erector spinae muscles and myoelectrical activities of trunk muscles. Clin Biomech 1999;14:79–87.

987. Miyauchi A, Baba I, Sumida T, et al. Relationship between the histological findings of spondylolytic tissue, instability of the loose lamina, and low-back pain. Spine 2008;33:687–93.

988. Modic MT, Steinberg PM, Ross JS, et al. Degenerative disk disease: assessment of changes in vertebral body marrow with MR imaging. Radiology 1988;166:193–9.

989. Mok FP, Samartzis D, Karppinen J, et al. ISSLS prize winner: Prevalence, determinants, and association of Schmorl nodes of the lumbar spine with disc degeneration: a population-based study of 2449 individuals. Spine (Phila Pa) 2010;35:1944–52.

990. Moller A, Maly P, Besjakov J, et al. A vertebral fracture in childhood is not a risk factor for disc degeneration but for Schmorl's nodes: a mean 40-year observational study. Spine 2007;32:2487–92.

991. Möller H, Hedlund R. Surgery versus conservative management in adult isthmic spondylolisthesis – a prospective randomized study: part 1. Spine 2000;25:1711–5.

992. Monemi M, Eriksson PO, Kadi F, et al. Opposite changes in myosin heavy chain composition of human masseter and biceps brachii muscles during aging. J Muscle Res Cell Motil 1999;20:351–61.

993. Monemi M, Kadi F, Liu JX, et al. Adverse changes in fibre type and myosin heavy chain compositions of human jaw muscle vs. limb muscle during ageing. Acta Physiol Scand 1999;167:339–45.

994. Moneta GB, Videman T, Kaivanto K, et al. Reported pain during lumbar discography as a function of annular ruptures and disc degeneration. A re-analysis of 833 discograms. Spine 1994;19:1968–74.

995. Moon DK, Woo SL, Takakura Y, et al. The effects of refreezing on the viscoelastic and tensile properties of ligaments. J Biomech 2006;39:1153–7.

996. Mooney V, Robertson J. The facet syndrome. Clin Orthop 1976;115:149–56.

997. Moore DR, Phillips SM, Babraj JA, et al. Myofibrillar and collagen protein synthesis in human skeletal muscle in young men after maximal shortening and lengthening contractions. Am J Physiol Endocrinol Metab 2005;288:E1153–9.

998. Moore RJ. The vertebral end-plate: what do we know? Eur Spine J 2000;9:92–6.

999. Moore RJ, Crotti TN, Osti OL, et al. Osteoarthrosis of the facet joints resulting from annular rim lesions in sheep lumbar discs. Spine 1999;24:519–25.

1000. Moore RJ, Vernon-Roberts B, Fraser RD, et al. The origin and fate of herniated lumbar intervertebral disc tissue. Spine 1996;21:2149–55.

1001. Moore RJ, Vernon-Roberts B, Osti OL, et al. Remodeling of vertebral bone after outer annular injury in sheep. Spine 1996;21:936–40.

1002. Morales AJ, Haubrich RH, Hwang JY, et al. The effect of six months treatment with a 100 mg daily dose of dehydroepiandrosterone (DHEA) on circulating sex steroids, body composition and muscle strength in age-advanced men and women. Clin Endocrinol (Oxf) 1998;49:421–32.

1003. Moreton RD. Spondylolysis. Jama 1966;195:671–4.

1004. Morgan FP, King T. Primary instability of lumbar vertebrae as a common cause of low-back pain. J Bone Joint Surg Br 1957;39-B:6–22.

1005. Morley JE. Anorexia, sarcopenia, and aging. Nutrition 2001;17:660–3.

1006. Morley JE, Baumgartner RN, Roubenoff R, et al. Sarcopenia. J Lab Clin Med 2001;137:231–43.

1007. Morscher E, Gerber B, Fasel J. Surgical treatment of spondylolisthesis by bone grafting and direct stabilization of spondylolysis by means of a hook screw. Arch Orthop Trauma Surg 1984;103:175–8.

1008. Mosekilde L. Normal vertebral body size and compressive strength: relations to age and to vertebral and iliac trabecular bone compressive strength. Bone 1986;7:207–12.

1009. Moseley GL, Nicholas MK, Hodges PW. Does anticipation of back pain predispose to back trouble? Brain 2004;127: 2339–47.

1010. Mundermann A, Stefanyshyn DJ, Nigg BM. Relationship between footwear comfort of shoe inserts and anthropometric and sensory factors. Med Sci Sports Exerc 2001;33:1939–45.

1011. Mundt DJ, Kelsey JL, Golden AL, et al. An epidemiologic study of non-occupational lifting as a risk factor for herniated lumbar intervertebral disc. The Northeast Collaborative Group on Low-back Pain. Spine 1993;18: 595–602.

1012. Muraki S, Oka H, Akune T, et al. Prevalence of radiographic lumbar spondylosis and its association with low-back pain in elderly subjects of population-based cohorts: the ROAD study. Ann Rheum Dis 2009;68:1401–6.

1013. Murray RC, Zhu CF, Goodship AE, et al. Exercise affects the mechanical properties and histological appearance of equine articular cartilage. J Orthop Res 1999;17:725–31.

1014. Mustard CA, Kalcevich C, Frank JW, et al. Childhood and early adult predictors of risk of incident back pain: Ontario Child Health Study 2001 follow-up. Am J Epidemiol 2005; 162:779–86.

1015. Myers ER, Wilson SE. Biomechanics of osteoporosis and vertebral fracture. Spine 1997;22:25S–31S.

1016. Myklebust JB, Pintar F, Yoganandan N, et al. Tensile strength of spinal ligaments. Spine 1988;13:526–31.

1017. Nachemson A, Lewin T, Maroudas A, et al. In vitro diffusion of dye through the end-plates and the annulus fibrosus of human lumbar inter-vertebral discs. Acta Orthop Scand 1970;41: 589–607.

1018. Nachemson A, Morris JM. In vivo measurements of intradiscal pressure. J Bone Joint Surg [Am] 1964;46:1077–92.

1019. Nachemson A, Vingard E. Influences of individual factors and smoking on neck and low-back pain. In: Nachemson AL, Jonsson E, editors. Neck and back pain: the scientific evidence of causes, diagnosis and treatment. Philadelphia: Lippincott Williams & Wilkins; 2000. p. 79–96.

1020. Nachemson AL. Lumbar intradiscal pressure. Acta Orthop Scand 1960;(Suppl. 43).

1021. Nachemson AL. The influence of spinal movements on the lumbar intradiscal pressure and on the tensile stresses in the annulus fibrosus. Acta Orthop Scand 1963;33:183–207.

1022. Nachemson AL. Disc pressure measurements. Spine 1981;6: 93–7.

1023. Nachemson AL. Introduction to treatment of neck and back pain. In: Nachemson AL, Jonsson E, editors. Neck and back pain: the scientific evidence of causes, diagnosis and treatment. Philadelphia: Lippincott Williams and Wilkins; 2000. p. 237–40.

1024. Nachemson AL, Evans JH. Some mechanical properties of the third human lumbar interlaminar ligament (ligamentum flavum). J Biomech 1968;1:211–20.

1025. Nachemson AL, Jonsson E. Neck and back pain: the scientific evidence of causes, diagnosis and treatment. Philadelphia: Lippincott Williams & Wilkins; 2000.

1026. Nahit ES, Macfarlane GJ, Pritchard CM, et al. Short term influence of mechanical factors on regional musculoskeletal pain: a study of new workers from 12 occupational groups. Occup Environ Med 2001;58:374–81.

1027. Nakamura N, Hart DA, Boorman RS, et al. Decorin antisense gene therapy improves functional healing of early rabbit ligament scar with enhanced collagen fibrillogenesis in vivo. J Orthop Res 2000;18:517–23.

1028. Nath S, Nath CA, Pettersson K. Percutaneous lumbar zygapophyseal (Facet) joint neurotomy using radiofrequency current, in the management of chronic low-back pain: a randomized double-blind trial. Spine 2008;33:1291–7; discussion 8.

1029. Nazarian A, Hermannsson BJ, Muller J, et al. Effects of tissue preservation on murine bone mechanical properties. J Biomech 2009;42:82–6.

1030. Neagoe C, Opitz CA, Makarenko I, et al. Gigantic variety: expression patterns of titin isoforms in striated muscles and consequences for myofibrillar passive stiffness. J Muscle Res Cell Motil 2003;24:175–89.

1031. Neame RL, Muir K, Doherty S, et al. Genetic risk of knee osteoarthritis: a sibling study. Ann Rheum Dis 2004;63:1022–7.

1032. Negrini S, Antonini G, Carabalona R, et al. Physical exercises as a treatment for adolescent idiopathic scoliosis. A systematic review. Pediatr Rehabil 2003;6:227–35.

1033. Nelson JM, Walmsley RP, Stevenson JM. Relative lumbar and pelvic motion during loaded spinal flexion/extension. Spine 1995;20:199–204.

1034. Nerlich AG, Schaaf R, Walchli B, et al. Temporo-spatial distribution of blood vessels in human lumbar intervertebral discs. Eur Spine J 2007;16: 547–55.

1035. Nerlich AG, Schleicher ED, Boos N. 1997 Volvo Award winner in basic science studies. Immunohistologic markers for age-related changes of human lumbar intervertebral discs. Spine 1997;22:2781–95.

1036. Neumann P, Keller T, Ekstrom L, et al. Structural properties of the anterior longitudinal ligament. Correlation with lumbar bone mineral content. Spine 1993;18:637–45.

1037. Neumann P, Keller TS, Ekstrom L, et al. Effect of strain rate and bone mineral on the structural properties of the human anterior longitudinal ligament. Spine 1994;19:205–11.

1038. Neumann P, Nordwall A, Osvalder AL. Traumatic instability of the lumbar spine. A dynamic in vitro study of flexion-distraction injury. Spine 1995;20:1111–21.

1039. Neumann P, Osvalder AL, Nordwall A, et al. The mechanism of initial flexion-distraction injury in the lumbar spine. Spine 1992;17:1083–90.

1040. Newham DJ, Jones DA, Clarkson PM. Repeated high-force eccentric exercise: effects on muscle pain and damage. J Appl Physiol 1987;63:1381–6.

1041. Newham DJ, Jones DA, Edwards RH. Large delayed plasma creatine kinase changes after stepping exercise. Muscle Nerve 1983;6:380–5.

1042. Newham DJ, McPhail G, Mills KR, et al. Ultrastructural changes after concentric and eccentric contractions of human muscle. J Neurol Sci 1983;61:109–22.

1043. Newton M, Thow M, Somerville D, et al. Trunk strength testing with iso-machines. Part 2: Experimental evaluation of the Cybex II Back Testing System in normal subjects and patients with chronic low-back pain. Spine 1993;18:812–24.

1044. Newton M, Waddell G. Trunk strength testing with iso-machines. Part 1: Review of a decade of scientific evidence [see comments]. Spine 1993;18:801–11.

1045. Nicol RO, Scott JH. Lytic spondylolysis. Repair by wiring. Spine 1986;11:1027–30.

1046. Niemelainen R, Battie MC, Gill K, et al. The prevalence and characteristics of thoracic magnetic resonance imaging findings in men. Spine 2008;33:2552–9.

1047. Nightingale RW, Carol Chancey V, Ottaviano D, et al. Flexion and extension structural properties and strengths for male cervical spine segments. J Biomech 2007;40:535–42.

1048. NIOSH. Low-back musculoskeletal disorders: evidence for work-relatedness. Musculoskeletal disorders and workplace factors. Cincinatti, U.S.A.: National Institute of Occupational Safety and Health; 1997.

1049. Nitz AJ, Peck D. Comparison of muscle spindle concentrations in large and small human epaxial muscles acting in parallel combinations. Am Surg 1986;52: 273–7.

1050. Njoo KH, van der Does E, Stam HJ. Interobserver agreement on iliac crest pain syndrome in general practice. J Rheumatol 1995;22:1532–5.

1051. Nordin M, et al. Early predictors of delayed return to work in patients with low-back pain. J Musculoskeletal Pain 1997;5:5–27.

1052. Noren R, Trafimow J, Andersson GB, et al. The role of facet joint tropism and facet angle in disc degeneration. Spine 1991;16:530–2.

1053. Norman R, Wells R, Neumann P, et al. A comparison of peak vs cumulative physical work exposure risk factors for the reporting of low-back pain in the automotive industry. Clin Biomech 1998;13:561–73.

1054. Nyman T, Mulder M, Iliadou A, et al. Physical workload, low-back pain and neck-shoulder pain: a Swedish twin study. Occup Environ Med 2009;66:395–401.

1055. O'Brien JP, Dawson MH, Heard CW, et al. Simultaneous combined anterior and posterior fusion. A surgical solution for failed spinal surgery with a brief review of the first 150 patients. Clin Orthop Relat Res 1986: 191–5.

1056. O'Connell GD, Johannessen W, Vresilovic EJ, et al. Human internal disc strains in axial compression measured noninvasively using magnetic resonance imaging. Spine 2007;32:2860–8.

1057. O'Hara BP, Urban JP, Maroudas A. Influence of cyclic loading on the nutrition of articular cartilage. Ann Rheum Dis 1990;49:536–9.

1058. O'Shea FD, Boyle E, Salonen DC, et al. Inflammatory and degenerative sacroiliac joint disease in a primary back pain cohort. Arthritis Care Res (Hoboken) 2010;62:447–54.

1059. Obata K, Tsujino H, Yamanaka H, et al. Expression of neurotrophic factors in the dorsal root ganglion in a rat model of lumbar disc herniation. Pain 2002;99:121–32.

1060. Ochia RS, Inoue N, Takatori R, et al. In vivo measurements of lumbar segmental motion during axial rotation in asymptomatic and chronic low-back pain male subjects. Spine 2007;32:1394–9.

1061. Oda K, Shibayama Y, Abe M, et al. Morphogenesis of vertebral deformities in involutional osteoporosis. Age-related, three-dimensional trabecular structure. Spine 1998;23:1050–5, discussion 6.

1062. Oegema Jr TR, Johnson SL, Aguiar DJ, et al. Fibronectin and its fragments increase with degeneration in the human intervertebral disc. Spine 2000;25:2742–7.

1063. Ogon M, Bender BR, Hooper DM, et al. A dynamic approach to spinal instability. Part II: Hesitation and giving-way during interspinal motion. Spine 1997;22:2859–66.

1064. Ohtori S, Inoue G, Ito T, et al. Tumor necrosis factor-immunoreactive cells and PGP 9.5-immunoreactive nerve fibers in vertebral endplates of patients with discogenic low-back Pain and Modic Type 1 or Type 2 changes on MRI. Spine 2006; 31:1026–31.

1065. Ohtori S, Kinoshita T, Yamashita M, et al. Results of surgery for discogenic low-back pain: a randomized study using discography versus discoblock for diagnosis. Spine (Phila Pa) 2009;34:1345–8.

1066. Okawa A, Shinomiya K, Komori H, et al. Dynamic motion study of the whole lumbar spine by videofluoroscopy. Spine 1998;23:1743–9.

1067. Oleinick A, Gluck JV, Guire K. Factors affecting first return to work following a compensable occupational back injury. Am J Ind Med 1996;30:540–55.

1068. Oliver MJ, Twomey LT. Extension creep in the lumbar spine. Clin Biomech 1995;10:363–8.

1069. Olmarker K. Puncture of a lumbar intervertebral disc induces changes in spontaneous pain behavior: an experimental study in rats. Spine 2008;33: 850–5.

1070. Olmarker K, Blomquist J, Stromberg J, et al. Inflammatogenic properties of nucleus pulposus. Spine 1995;20:665–9.

1071. Olmarker K, Brisby H, Yabuki S, et al. The effects of normal, frozen, and hyaluronidase-digested nucleus pulposus on nerve root structure and function. Spine 1997;22:471–5; discussion 6.

1072. Olmarker K, Iwabuchi M, Larsson K, et al. Walking analysis of rats subjected to experimental disc herniation. Eur Spine J 1998;7:394–9.

1073. Olmarker K, Larsson K. Tumor necrosis factor alpha and nucleus-pulposus-induced nerve root injury. Spine 1998;23: 2538–44.

1074. Olmarker K, Nutu M, Storkson R. Changes in spontaneous behavior in rats exposed to experimental disc herniation are blocked by selective TNF-alpha inhibition. Spine 2003;28:1635–41; discussion 42.

1075. Olmarker K, Rydevik B. Selective inhibition of tumor necrosis factor-alpha prevents nucleus pulposus-induced thrombus formation, intraneural edema, and reduction of nerve conduction velocity: possible implications for future pharmacologic treatment strategies of sciatica. Spine 2001;26:863–9.

1076. Olmarker K, Rydevik B, Nordborg C. Autologous nucleus pulposus induces neurophysiologic and histologic changes in porcine cauda equina nerve roots [see comments]. Spine 1993;18:1425–32.

1077. Omlor GW, Nerlich AG, Wilke HJ, et al. A new porcine in vivo animal model of disc degeneration: response of annulus fibrosus cells, chondrocyte-like nucleus pulposus cells, and notochordal nucleus pulposus cells to partial nucleotomy. Spine (Phila Pa) 2009;34:2730–9.

1078. Omokhodion FO, Sanya AO. Risk factors for low-back pain among office workers in Ibadan, Southwest Nigeria. Occup Med (Lond) 2003;53:287–9.

1079. Onda A, Murata Y, Rydevik B, et al. Nerve growth factor content in dorsal root ganglion as related to changes in pain behavior in a rat model of experimental lumbar disc herniation. Spine 2005;30:188–93.

1080. Onda A, Yabuki S, Kikuchi S. Effects of neutralizing antibodies to tumor necrosis factor-alpha on nucleus pulposus-induced abnormal nociresponses in rat dorsal horn neurons. Spine 2003;28:967–72.

1081. Osti OL, Vernon-Roberts B, Fraser RD. 1990 Volvo Award in experimental studies. Annulus tears and intervertebral disc degeneration. An experimental study using an animal model. Spine 1990;15:762–7.

1082. Osti OL, Vernon-Roberts B, Moore R, et al. Annular tears and disc degeneration in the lumbar spine. A postmortem study of 135 discs. J Bone Joint Surg Br 1992;74:678–82.

1083. Osvalder AL, Neumann P, Lovsund P, et al. Ultimate strength of the lumbar spine in flexion – an in vitro study. J Biomech 1990;23:453–60.

1084. Osvalder AL, Neumann P, Lovsund P, et al. A method for studying the biomechanical load response of the (in vitro) lumbar spine under dynamic flexion-shear loads. J Biomech 1993; 26:1227–36.

1085. Otsuki S, Brinson DC, Creighton L, et al. The effect of glycosaminoglycan loss on chondrocyte viability: a study on porcine cartilage explants. Arthritis Rheum 2008;58: 1076–85.

1086. Otterness IG, Eskra JD, Bliven ML, et al. Exercise protects against articular cartilage degeneration in the hamster. Arthritis Rheum 1998;41:2068–76.

1087. Overmeer T, Linton SJ, Holmquist L, et al. Do evidence-based guidelines have an impact in primary care? A cross-sectional study of Swedish physicians and physiotherapists. Spine 2005;30: 146–51.

1088. Owen BD, Keene K, Olson S. An ergonomic approach to reducing back/shoulder stress in hospital nursing personnel: a five year follow up. Int J Nurs Stud 2002;39:295–302.

1089. Oxland TR, Lund T, Jost B, et al. The relative importance of vertebral bone density and disc degeneration in spinal flexibility and interbody implant performance. An in vitro study. Spine 1996;21:2558–69.

1090. Oxland TR, Panjabi MM. The onset and progression of spinal injury: a demonstration of neutral zone sensitivity. J Biomech 1992;25:1165–72.

1091. Paassilta P, Lohiniva J, Goring HH, et al. Identification of a novel common genetic risk factor for lumbar disk disease. JAMA 2001;285:1843–9.

1092. Page LA, Wessely S. Medically unexplained symptoms: exacerbating factors in the doctor-patient encounter. J R Soc Med 2003;96:223–7.

1093. Palmer KT, Walsh K, Bendall H, et al. Back pain in Britain: comparison of two prevalence surveys at an interval of 10 years. BMJ 2000;320:1577–8.

1094. Palmgren T, Gronblad M, Virri J, et al. An immunohistochemical study of nerve structures in the annulus fibrosus of human normal lumbar intervertebral discs. Spine 1999;24:2075–9.

1095. Panjabi M, Brown M, Lindahl S, et al. Intrinsic disc pressure as a measure of integrity of the lumbar spine [see comments]. Spine 1988;13:913–7.

1096. Panjabi M, Yamamoto I, Oxland T, et al. How does posture affect coupling in the lumbar spine? Spine 1989;14:1002–11.

1097. Panjabi MM. The stabilizing system of the spine. Part II. Neutral zone and instability hypothesis. J Spinal Disord 1992;5:390–6; discussion 7.

1098. Panjabi MM, Andersson GB, Jorneus L, et al. In vivo measurements of spinal column vibrations. J Bone Joint Surg [Am] 1986;68:695–702.

1099. Panjabi MM, Cholewicki J, Nibu K, et al. Mechanism of whiplash injury. Clin Biomech 1998;13: 239–49.

1100. Panjabi MM, Goel VK, Takata K. Physiologic strains in the lumbar spinal ligaments. An in vitro biomechanical study 1981 Volvo Award in Biomechanics. Spine 1982;7:192–203.

1101. Panjabi MM, Ivancic PC, Maak TG, et al. Multiplanar cervical spine injury due to head-turned rear impact. Spine 2006;31:420–9.

1102. Panjabi MM, Krag M, Summers D, et al. Biomechanical time-tolerance of fresh cadaveric human spine specimens. J Orthop Res 1985;3:292–300.

1103. Panjabi MM, Oxland TR, Lin RM, et al. Thoracolumbar burst fracture. A biomechanical investigation of its multidirectional flexibility. Spine 1994;19:578–85.

1104. Papageorgiou AC, Croft PR, Thomas E, et al. Influence of previous pain experience on the episode incidence of low-back pain: results from the South Manchester Back Pain Study. Pain 1996;66:181–5.

1105. Papageorgiou AC, Macfarlane GJ, Thomas E, et al. Psychosocial factors in the workplace – do they predict new episodes of low-back pain? Evidence from the South Manchester Back

Pain Study. Spine 1997;22: 1137–42.

1106. Pascual Garrido C, Hakimiyan AA, Rappoport L, et al. Anti-apoptotic treatments prevent cartilage degradation after acute trauma to human ankle cartilage. Osteoarthritis Cartilage 2009;17: 1244–51.

1107. Patt S, Brock M, Mayer HM, et al. Nucleus pulposus regeneration after chemonucleolysis with chymopapain? Spine 1993;18:227–31.

1108. Patwardhan AG, Havey RM, Meade KP, et al. A follower load increases the load-carrying capacity of the lumbar spine in compression. Spine 1999;24: 1003–9.

1109. Pauza KJ, Howell S, Dreyfuss P, et al. A randomized, placebo-controlled trial of intradiscal electrothermal therapy for the treatment of discogenic low-back pain. Spine J 2004;4: 27–35.

1110. Pearcy M, Portek I, Shepherd J. Three-dimensional x-ray analysis of normal movement in the lumbar spine. Spine 1984;9: 294–7.

1111. Pearcy M, Portek I, Shepherd J. The effect of low-back pain on lumbar spinal movements measured by three-dimensional X-ray analysis. Spine 1985;10:150–3.

1112. Pearcy MJ. Twisting mobility of the human back in flexed postures. Spine 1993;18:114–9.

1113. Pearcy MJ, Bogduk N. Instantaneous axes of rotation of the lumbar intervertebral joints. Spine 1988;13:1033–41.

1114. Pearcy MJ, Gill JM, Whittle MW, et al. Dynamic back movement measured using a three-dimensional television system. J Biomech 1987;20:943–9.

1115. Pearcy MJ, Hindle RJ. New method for the non-invasive three-dimensional measurement of human back movement. Clin Biomech 1989;4:73–9.

1116. Pearcy MJ, Tibrewal SB. Axial rotation and lateral bending in the normal lumbar spine measured by three-dimensional radiography. Spine 1984;9:582–7.

1117. Pearcy MJ, Tibrewal SB. Lumbar intervertebral disc and ligament deformations measured in vivo. Clin Orthop 1984:281–6.

1118. Peng B, Chen J, Kuang Z, et al. Diagnosis and surgical treatment of back pain originating from endplate. Eur Spine J 2009;18:1035–40.

1119. Peng B, Chen J, Kuang Z, et al. Expression and role of connective tissue growth factor in painful disc fibrosis and degeneration. Spine (Phila Pa) 2009;34:E178–82.

1120. Peng B, Hao J, Hou S, et al. Possible pathogenesis of painful intervertebral disc degeneration. Spine 2006;31:560–6.

1121. Peng B, Hou S, Wu W, et al. The pathogenesis and clinical significance of a high-intensity zone (HIZ) of lumbar intervertebral disc on MR imaging in the patient with discogenic low-back pain. Eur Spine J 2006;15:583–7.

1122. Peng B, Pang X, Wu Y, et al. A randomized placebo-controlled trial of intradiscal methylene blue injection for the treatment of chronic discogenic low-back pain. Pain 2010;149:124–9.

1123. Perey O. Fracture of the vertebral endplate. A biomechanical investigation. Acta Orthop Scand 1957.

1124. Pezowicz CA, Robertson PA, Broom ND. Intralamellar relationships within the collagenous architecture of the annulus fibrosus imaged in its fully hydrated state. J Anat 2005;207:299–312.

1125. Pfeiffer M, Griss P, Franke P, et al. Degeneration model of the porcine lumbar motion segment: effects of various intradiscal procedures. Eur Spine J 1994;3: 8–16.

1126. Pfirrmann CW, Metzdorf A, Elfering A, et al. Effect of aging and degeneration on disc volume and shape: A quantitative study in asymptomatic volunteers. J Orthop Res 2006;24:1086–94.

1127. Pfirrmann CW, Metzdorf A, Zanetti M, et al. Magnetic resonance classification of lumbar intervertebral disc degeneration. Spine 2001;26:1873–8.

1128. Pfirrmann CW, Resnick D. Schmorl nodes of the thoracic and lumbar spine: radiographic-pathologic study of prevalence, characterization, and correlation with degenerative changes of 1,650 spinal levels in 100 cadavers. Radiology 2001;219: 368–74.

1129. Pflaster DS, Krag MH, Johnson CC, et al. Effect of test environment on intervertebral disc hydration. Spine 1997;22:133–9.

1130. Pham T, Azulay-Parrado J, Champsaur P, et al. 'Occult' osteoporotic vertebral fractures: vertebral body fractures without radiologic collapse. Spine 2005; 30:2430–5.

1131. Phillips S, Mercer S, Bogduk N. Anatomy and biomechanics of quadratus lumborum. Proc Inst Mech Eng 2008; 222:151–9.

1132. Pincus T, Burton AK, Vogel S, et al. A systematic review of psychological factors as predictors of chronicity/disability in prospective cohorts of low-back pain. Spine 2002;27:E109–20.

1133. Pinder ADJ, Frost GA. The 1991 NIOSH lifting equation does not predict low-back pain. In: Proceedings of the XXIst Annual International Occupational Ergonomics and Safety Conference Dallas, Texas, USA, 11–2 June 2009. International Society of Occupational Ergonomics and Safety; 2009.

1134. Pintar FA, Yoganandan N, Myers T, et al. Biomechanical properties of human lumbar spine ligaments. J Biomech 1992;25: 1351–6.

1135. Pitkanen M, Manninen H. Sidebending versus flexion–extension radiographs in lumbar spinal instability. Clin Radiol 1994;49:109–14.

1136. Plamondon A, Gagnon M, Gravel D. Moments at the L(5)/S(1) joint during asymmetrical lifting: effects of different load trajectories and initial load positions. Clin Biomech 1995;10:128–36.

1137. Pocock SJ, Collier TJ, Dandreo KJ, et al. Issues in the reporting of epidemiological studies: a survey of recent practice. BMJ 2004;329: 883.

1138. Pokharna HK, Phillips FM. Collagen crosslinks in human lumbar intervertebral disc aging. Spine 1998;23:1645–8.

1139. Pollintine P, Dolan P, Tobias JH, et al. Intervertebral disc degeneration can lead to 'stress-shielding' of the anterior vertebral body: a cause of osteoporotic vertebral fracture? Spine 2004;29:774–82.

1140. Pollintine P, Findlay G, Adams MA. Intradiscal electrothermal therapy can alter compressive stress distributions inside degenerated intervertebral discs. Spine 2005;30:E134–9.

1141. Pollintine P, Luo J, Offa-Jones B, et al. Bone creep can cause progressive vertebral deformity. Bone 2009;45:466–72.

1142. Pollintine P, Przybyla AS, Dolan P, et al. Neural arch load-bearing in old and degenerated spines. J Biomech 2004;37:197–204.

1143. Pollintine P, van Tunen MS, Luo J, et al. Time-dependent compressive deformation of the ageing spine: relevance to spinal stenosis. Spine (Phila Pa) 2010;35:386–94.

1144. Pollock RD, Woledge RC, Mills KR, et al. Muscle activity and acceleration during whole body vibration: Effect of frequency and amplitude. Clin Biomech 2010;25:840–6.

1145. Pope MH, Broman H, Hansson T. Impact response of the standing subject – a feasibility study. Clin Biomech 1989;4:195–200.

1146. Pope MH, Kaigle AM, Magnusson M, et al. Intervertebral motion during vibration. Proc Inst Mech Eng [H] 1991;205:39–44.

1147. Pope MH, Magnusson M, Wilder DG. Kappa Delta Award. Low-back pain and whole body vibration. Clin Orthop 1998: 241–8.

1148. Pope MH, Ogon M, Okawa A. Biomechanical measurements. In: Szpalski M, Gunzburg R, Pope MH, editors. Lumbar segmental instability. Philadelphia, U.S.A.: Lippincott Williams & Wilkins; 1999.

1149. Pope MH, Panjabi M. Biomechanical definitions of spinal instability. Spine 1985;10:255–6.

1150. Portek I, Pearcy MJ, Reader GP, et al. Correlation between radiographic and clinical measurement of lumbar spine movement. Br J Rheumatol 1983;22:197–205.

1151. Porter JL, Wilkinson A. Lumbar-hip flexion motion. A comparative study between asymptomatic and chronic low-back pain in 18- to 36-year-old men. Spine 1997;22:1508–13; discussion 13–4.

1152. Porter RW. The pathogenesis of idiopathic scoliosis: uncoupled neuro-osseous growth? Eur Spine J 2001;10:473–81; discussion 82–9.

1153. Porter RW, Adams MA, Hutton WC. Physical activity and the strength of the lumbar spine. Spine 1989;14:201–3.

1154. Porter RW, Trailescu IF. Diurnal changes in straight leg raising [see comments]. Spine 1990;15:103–6.

1155. Potvin JR, McGill SM, Norman RW. Trunk muscle and lumbar ligament contributions to dynamic lifts with varying degrees of trunk flexion [see comments]. Spine 1991;16: 1099–107.

1156. Potvin JR, Norman RW. Quantification of erector spinae muscle fatigue during prolonged, dynamic lifting tasks. Eur J Appl Physiol Occup Physiol 1993;67: 554–62.

1157. Potvin JR, Norman RW, McGill SM. Reduction in anterior shear forces on the L4/L5 disc by the lumbar musculature. Clin Biomech 1991;6:88–96.

1158. Potvin JR, Norman RW, McGill SM. Mechanically corrected EMG for the continuous estimation of erector spinae muscle loading during repetitive lifting. Eur J Appl Physiol Occup Physiol 1996;74:119–32.

1159. Prado LG, Makarenko I, Andresen C, et al. Isoform diversity of giant proteins in relation to passive and active contractile properties of rabbit skeletal muscles. J Gen Physiol 2005;126:461–80.

1160. Preuschoft H, Hayama S, Gunther MM. Curvature of the lumbar spine as a consequence of mechanical necessities in Japanese macaques trained for bipedalism. Folia Primatol 1988;50:42–58.

1161. Prista A, Balague F, Nordin M, et al. Low-back pain in Mozambican adolescents. Eur Spine J 2004;13:341–5.

1162. Proske U, Morgan DL. Muscle damage from eccentric exercise: mechanism, mechanical signs, adaptation and clinical applications. J Physiol 2001;537:333–45.

1163. Proske U, Morgan DL, Gregory JE. Muscle history dependence of responses to stretch of primary and secondary endings of cat soleus muscle spindles. J Physiol 1992;445:81–95.

1164. Proske U, Stuart GJ. The initial burst of impulses in responses of toad muscle spindles during stretch. J Physiol 1985;368:1–17.

1165. Przybyla A, Pollintine P, Bedzinski R, et al. Outer annulus tears have less effect than endplate fracture on stress distributions inside intervertebral discs: Relevance to disc degeneration. Clin Biomech 2006;21:1013–9.

1166. Przybyla AS, Skrzypiec D, Pollintine P, et al. Strength of the cervical spine in compression and bending. Spine 2007;32: 1612–20.

1167. Pun YL, Moskowitz RW, Lie S, et al. Clinical correlations of osteoarthritis associated with a single-base mutation (arginine519 to cysteine) in type II procollagen gene. A newly defined pathogenesis. Arthritis Rheum 1994;37:264–9.

1168. Purslow PP. Strain-induced reorientation of an intramuscular connective tissue network: implications for passive muscle elasticity. J Biomech 1989;22:21–31.

1169. Putto E, Tallroth K. Extension-flexion radiographs for motion studies of the lumbar spine. A comparison of two methods. Spine 1990;15:107–10.

1170. Puustjarvi K. Exercise-induced alterations in the metabolism of intervertebral disc matrix, vertebral mineral density and spinal muscle fibre types. [PhD]. Kuopio, Finland: University of Kuopio; 1994.

1171. Puustjarvi K, Lammi M, Kiviranta I, et al. Proteoglycan synthesis in canine intervertebral discs after long- distance running training. J Orthop Res 1993;11:738–46.

1172. Puustjarvi K, Tammi M, Reinikainen M, et al. Running training alters fiber type composition in spinal muscles. Eur Spine J 1994;3:17–21.

1173. Pye SR, Reid DM, Lunt M, et al. Lumbar disc degeneration: association between osteophytes, end-plate sclerosis and disc space narrowing. Ann Rheum Dis 2007;66:330–3.

1174. Quinn KP, Bauman JA, Crosby ND, et al. Anomalous fiber realignment during tensile loading of the rat facet capsular ligament identifies mechanically induced damage and physiological dysfunction. J Biomech 2010;43:1870–5.

1175. Rabischong P, Louis R, Vignaud J, et al. The intervertebral disc. Anat Clin 1978;1:55–64.

1176. Radebold A, Cholewicki J, Polzhofer GK, et al. Impaired postural control of the lumbar spine is associated with delayed muscle response times in patients with chronic idiopathic low-back pain. Spine 2001;26:724–30.

1177. Radin EL, Rose RM. Role of subchondral bone in the initiation and progression of cartilage damage. Clin Orthop 1986:34–40.

1178. Radin EL, Yang KH, Riegger C, et al. Relationship between lower limb dynamics and knee joint pain [published erratum appears in J Orthop Res 1991 Sep;9(5):776]. J Orthop Res 1991;9:398–405.

1179. Rainville J. Non-degenerative spondylolisthesis: epidemiology and natural history, classification, history and physical examination, and non-operative treatment of adults. In: Herkowitz HN, editor. The Lumbar Spine. 3rd ed. Philadelphia: Lippincott, Williams and Wilkins; 2004. p. 556–64.

1180. Rajapakse CS, Thomsen JS, Espinoza Ortiz JS, et al. An expression relating breaking stress and density of trabecular bone. J Biomech 2004;37:1241–9.

1181. Rajasekaran S, Babu JN, Arun R, et al. ISSLS prize winner: A study of diffusion in human lumbar discs: a serial magnetic resonance imaging study documenting the influence of the endplate on diffusion in normal and degenerate discs. Spine 2004; 29:2654–67.

1182. Ranatunga KW. Sarcomeric visco-elasticity of chemically skinned skeletal muscle fibres of the rabbit at rest. J Muscle Res Cell Motil 2001;22:399–414.

1183. Ranu HS. Multipoint determination of pressure-volume curves in human intervertebral discs. Ann Rheum Dis 1993;52:142–6.

1184. Rao RD, Singrakhia MD. Painful osteoporotic vertebral fracture. Pathogenesis, evaluation, and roles of vertebroplasty and kyphoplasty in its management. J Bone Joint Surg Am 2003;85-A:2010–22.

1185. Raspe H, Hueppe A, Neuhauser H. Back pain, a communicable disease? Int J Epidemiol 2008;37:69–74.

1186. Raspe H, Matthis C, Croft P, et al. Variation in back pain between countries: the example of Britain and Germany. Spine 2004;29:1017–21; discussion 21.

1187. Rauschning W, Jonsson H. Injuries of the cervical spine in automobile accidents: pathoanatomic and clinical aspects. In: Gunzburg R, Szpalski M, editors. Whiplash Injuries. Philadelphia, U.S.A.: Lippincott-Raven; 1998.

1188. Reeves NP, Narendra KS, Cholewicki J. Spine stability: the six blind men and the elephant. Clin Biomech 2007;22:266–74.

1189. Rehman Q, Lang T, Modin G, et al. Quantitative computed tomography of the lumbar spine, not dual x-ray absorptiometry, is an independent predictor of prevalent vertebral fractures in postmenopausal women with osteopenia receiving long-term glucocorticoid and hormone-replacement therapy. Arthritis Rheum 2002;46:1292–7.

1190. Reigo T. The nature of back pain in a general population: a longitudinal study. PhD thesis. Linkoping: Linkoping University; 2001.

1191. Reihsner R, Menzel EJ. Two-dimensional stress-relaxation behavior of human skin as influenced by non-enzymatic glycation and the inhibitory agent aminoguanidine. J Biomech 1998;31:985–93.

1192. Revel M, Andre-Deshays C, Roudier R, et al. Effects of repetitive strains on vertebral endplates in young rats. Clin Orthop 1992:303–9.

1193. Rhalmi S, Yahia LH, Newman N, et al. Immunohistochemical study of nerves in lumbar spine ligaments. Spine 1993;18:264–7.

1194. Ricketson R, Simmons JW, Hauser BO. The prolapsed intervertebral disc. The high-intensity zone with discography correlation. Spine (Phila Pa) 1996;21:2758–62.

1195. Riihimaki H, Wickstrom G, Hanninen K, et al. Predictors of sciatic pain among concrete reinforcement workers and house painters – a five-year follow-up. Scand J Work Environ Health 1989;15:415–23.

1196. Riley GP, Curry V, DeGroot J, et al. Matrix metalloproteinase activities and their relationship with collagen remodelling in tendon pathology. Matrix Biol 2002;21:185–95.

1197. Rimnac CM, Petko AA, Santner TJ, et al. The effect of temperature, stress and microstructure on the creep of compact bovine bone. J Biomech 1993;26:219–28.

1198. Rissanen PM. The surgical anatomy and pathology of the supraspinous and interspinous ligaments of the lumbar spine with special reference to ligament

ruptures. Acta Orthop Scand 1960;(Suppl. 46).

1199. Rivero-Arias O, Campbell H, Gray A, et al. Surgical stabilisation of the spine compared with a programme of intensive rehabilitation for the management of patients with chronic low-back pain: cost utility analysis based on a randomised controlled trial. BMJ 2005;330:1239.

1200. Roberts S, Caterson B, Menage J, et al. Matrix metalloproteinases and aggrecanase: their role in disorders of the human intervertebral disc. Spine 2000;25:3005–13.

1201. Roberts S, Eisenstein SM, Menage J, et al. Mechanoreceptors in intervertebral discs. Morphology, distribution, and neuropeptides [see comments]. Spine 1995;20:2645–51.

1202. Roberts S, Evans EH, Kletsas D, et al. Senescence in human intervertebral discs. Eur Spine J 2006;15(Suppl. 15):312–6.

1203. Roberts S, McCall IW, Menage J, et al. Does the thickness of the vertebral subchondral bone reflect the composition of the intervertebral disc? Eur Spine J 1997;6:385–9.

1204. Roberts S, Menage J, Duance V, et al. 1991 Volvo Award in basic sciences. Collagen types around the cells of the intervertebral disc and cartilage endplate: an immunolocalization study. Spine 1991;16:1030–8.

1205. Roberts S, Menage J, Eisenstein SM. The cartilage end-plate and intervertebral disc in scoliosis: calcification and other sequelae. J Orthop Res 1993;11:747–57.

1206. Roberts S, Menage J, Urban JP. Biochemical and structural properties of the cartilage end-plate and its relation to the intervertebral disc. Spine 1989;14: 166–74.

1207. Roberts S, Urban JP, Evans H, et al. Transport properties of the human cartilage endplate in relation to its composition and calcification. Spine 1996;21:415–20.

1208. Robin S, Skalli W, Lavaste F. Influence of geometrical factors

on the behavior of lumbar spine segments: a finite element analysis. Eur Spine J 1994;3: 84–90.

1209. Robson-Brown K, Pollintine P, Adams MA. Biomechanical implications of degenerative joint disease in the apophyseal joints of human thoracic and lumbar vertebrae. Am J Phys Anthropol 2008;136:318–26.

1210. Rodriguez AG, Slichter CK, Acosta FL, et al. Human disc nucleus properties and vertebral endplate permeability. Spine (Phila Pa) 2011;36:512–20.

1211. Roffey DM, Wai EK, Bishop P, et al. Causal assessment of awkward occupational postures and low-back pain: results of a systematic review. Spine J 2010; 10:89–99.

1212. Roffey DM, Wai EK, Bishop P, et al. Causal assessment of occupational pushing or pulling and low-back pain: results of a systematic review. Spine J 2010; 10:544–53.

1213. Roffey DM, Wai EK, Bishop P, et al. Causal assessment of occupational sitting and low-back pain: results of a systematic review. Spine J 2010;10:252–61.

1214. Roffey DM, Wai EK, Bishop P, et al. Causal assessment of occupational standing or walking and low-back pain: results of a systematic review. Spine J 2010; 10:262–72.

1215. Roffey DM, Wai EK, Bishop P, et al. Causal assessment of workplace manual handling or assisting patients and low-back pain: results of a systematic review. Spine J 2010; 10:639–51.

1216. Rogers BA, Murphy CL, Cannon SR, et al. Topographical variation in glycosaminoglycan content in human articular cartilage. J Bone Joint Surg Br 2006;88:1670–4.

1217. Rohlmann A, Zander T, Schmidt H, et al. Analysis of the influence of disc degeneration on the mechanical behaviour of a lumbar motion segment using the finite element method. J Biomech 2006;39:2484–90.

1218. Roland M, Waddell G, Klaber-Moffett J, et al. The back book.

References

Norwich: The Stationery Office; 1996.

1219. Roos MR, Rice CL, Vandervoort AA. Age-related changes in motor unit function. Muscle Nerve 1997;20:679–90.

1220. Rossini F, Dragoni S. Lumbar spondylolysis: occurrence in competitive athletes. Updated achievements in a series of 390 cases. J Sports Med Phys Fitness 1990;30:450–2.

1221. Roubenoff R, Harris TB, Abad LW, et al. Monocyte cytokine production in an elderly population: effect of age and inflammation. J Gerontol A Biol Sci Med Sci 1998;53: M20–6.

1222. Roughley PJ. Biology of intervertebral disc aging and degeneration: involvement of the extracellular matrix. Spine 2004; 29:2691–9.

1223. Roux C, Fechtenbaum J, Briot K, et al. Inverse relationship between vertebral fractures and spine osteoarthritis in postmenopausal women with osteoporosis. Ann Rheum Dis 2008;67:224–8.

1224. Rowe GG, Roche MB. The etiology of separate neural arch. J Bone Joint Surg 1953; 35A: 102–10.

1225. Ruan D, He Q, Ding Y, et al. Intervertebral disc transplantation in the treatment of degenerative spine disease: a preliminary study. Lancet 2007;369:993–9.

1226. Rubin CT, Lanyon LE. Regulation of bone formation by applied dynamic loads. J Bone Joint Surg [Am] 1984;66:397–402.

1227. Rubin CT, Lanyon LE. Regulation of bone mass by mechanical strain magnitude. Calcif Tissue Int 1985;37:411–7.

1228. Ruff S. Brief acceleration: less than one second. In: German aviation medicine, World War II: Washington DC, U.S.A.; Government Printing Office 1: 1950:584–97.

1229. Rumian AP, Draper ER, Wallace AL, et al. The influence of the mechanical environment on remodelling of the patellar tendon. J Bone Joint Surg Br 2009;91:557–64.

1230. Russo CR, Lauretani F, Seeman E, et al. Structural adaptations to bone loss in aging men and women. Bone 2006; 38:112–8.

1231. Saal JA, Saal JS. Intradiscal electrothermal treatment for chronic discogenic low-back pain: a prospective outcome study with minimum 1-year follow-up. Spine 2000;25:2622–7.

1232. Saal JA, Saal JS. Intradiscal electrothermal treatment for chronic discogenic low-back pain: prospective outcome study with a minimum 2-year follow-up. Spine 2002;27:966–73; discussion 73–4.

1233. Saarakkala S, Julkunen P, Kiviranta P, et al. Depth-wise progression of osteoarthritis in human articular cartilage: investigation of composition, structure and biomechanics. Osteoarthritis Cartilage 2010;18:73–81.

1234. Sackett DL, Strauss SE, Richardson WS, et al. Evidence-based medicine. How to practise and teach EBM. Edinburgh: Churchill Livingstone; 2000.

1235. Sahar T, Cohen MJ, Uval-Ne'eman V, et al. Insoles for prevention and treatment of back pain: a systematic review within the framework of the Cochrane Collaboration Back Review Group. Spine 2009;34:924–33.

1236. Saifuddin A, Braithwaite I, White J, et al. The value of lumbar spine magnetic resonance imaging in the demonstration of annular tears. Spine (Phila Pa) 1998;23:453–7.

1237. Sales de Gauzy J, Vadier F, Cahuzac JP. Repair of lumbar spondylolysis using Morscher material: 14 children followed for 1–5 years. Acta Orthop Scand 2000;71:292–6.

1238. Salminen JJ, Erkintalo-Tertti MO, Paajanen HE. Magnetic resonance imaging findings of lumbar spine in the young: correlation with leisure time physical activity, spinal mobility, and trunk muscle strength in 15-year-old pupils with or without low-back pain. J Spinal Disord 1993;6: 386–91.

1239. Salminen JJ, Erkintalo MO, Pentti J, et al. Recurrent low-back pain and early disc degeneration in the young. Spine 1999;24: 1316–21.

1240. Sambrook PN, MacGregor AJ, Spector TD. Genetic influences on cervical and lumbar disc degeneration: a magnetic resonance imaging study in twins. Arthritis Rheum 1999; 42:366–72.

1241. Sanchez-Zuriaga D, Adams MA, Dolan P. Is activation of the back muscles impaired by creep or muscle fatigue? Spine (Phila Pa) 2010;35:517–25.

1242. Sanchez D, Adams MA, Dolan P. Spinal proprioception and back muscle activation are impaired by spinal 'creep' but not by fatigue. J Biomechanics 2006; 39:S33.

1243. Sandhu HS, Sanchez-Caso LP, Parvataneni HK, et al. Association between findings of provocative discography and vertebral endplate signal changes as seen on MRI. J Spinal Disord 2000;13: 438–43.

1244. Sandstrom J, Esbjornsson E. Return to work after rehabilitation. The significance of the patient's own prediction. Scand J Rehabil Med 1986;18: 29–33.

1245. Sargeant AJ, Dolan P. Human muscle function following prolonged eccentric exercise. Eur J Appl Physiol 1987;56:704–11.

1246. Sarzi-Puttini P, Atzeni F. New developments in our understanding of DISH (diffuse idiopathic skeletal hyperostosis). Curr Opin Rheumatol 2004;16: 287–92.

1247. Sasaki N, Odajima S. Elongation mechanism of collagen fibrils and force-strain relations of tendon at each level of structural hierarchy. J Biomech 1996;29:1131–6.

1248. Sasso RC, Foulk DM, Hahn M. Prospective, randomized trial of metal-on-metal artificial lumbar disc replacement: initial results for treatment of discogenic pain. Spine (Phila Pa) 2008;33:123–31.

1249. Sato H, Kikuchi S. The natural history of radiographic instability of the lumbar spine. Spine 1993;18:2075–9.

1250. Sato K, Kikuchi S, Yonezawa T. In vivo intradiscal pressure measurement in healthy individuals and in patients with ongoing back problems. Spine 1999;24:2468–74.

1251. Saur PM, Ensink FB, Frese K, et al. Lumbar range of motion: reliability and validity of the inclinometer technique in the clinical measurement of trunk flexibility. Spine 1996;21: 1332–8.

1252. Savage RA, Whitehouse GH, Roberts N. The relationship between the magnetic resonance imaging appearance of the lumbar spine and low-back pain, age and occupation in males. Eur Spine J 1997;6:106–14.

1253. Savigny P, Kuntze S, Watson P, et al. Low-back pain: early management of persistent non-specific low-back pain, NICE clinical guideline 88. London: National Collaborating Centre for Primary Care and Royal College of General Practitioners; 2009.

1254. Sawa AG, Crawford NR. The use of surface strain data and a neural networks solution method to determine lumbar facet joint loads during in vitro spine testing. J Biomech 2008;41:2647–53.

1255. Sawney P. Current issues in fitness for work certification. Br J Gen Pract 2002;52:217–22.

1256. Sawney P, Challenor J. Poor communication between health professionals is a barrier to rehabilitation. Occup Med (Lond) 2003;53:246–8.

1257. Schechtman H, Bader DL. In vitro fatigue of human tendons. J Biomech 1997;30:829–35.

1258. Schechtman H, Bader DL. Fatigue damage of human tendons. J Biomech 2002;35:347–53.

1259. Scheel IB, Hagen KB, Herrin J, et al. Blind faith? The effects of promoting active sick leave for back pain patients: a cluster-randomized controlled trial. Spine 2002;27:2734–40.

1260. Scheel IB, Hagen KB, Oxman AD. Active sick leave for patients with back pain: all the players onside, but still no action. Spine 2002;27:654–9.

1261. Schellhas KP, Pollei SR, Gundry CR, et al. Lumbar disc high-intensity zone. Correlation of magnetic resonance imaging and discography. Spine 1996;21:79–86.

1262. Schendel MJ, Wood KB, Buttermann GR, et al. Experimental measurement of ligament force, facet force, and segment motion in the human lumbar spine. J Biomech 1993;26:427–38.

1263. Schmid G, Witteler A, Willburger R, et al. Lumbar disk herniation: correlation of histologic findings with marrow signal intensity changes in vertebral endplates at MR imaging. Radiology 2004;231:352–8.

1264. Schmidt H, Heuer F, Claes L, et al. The relation between the instantaneous center of rotation and facet joint forces – A finite element analysis. Clin Biomech 2008;23:270–8.

1265. Schmidt H, Kettler A, Heuer F, et al. Intradiscal pressure, shear strain, and fiber strain in the intervertebral disc under combined loading. Spine 2007;32:748–55.

1266. Schmidt H, Kettler A, Rohlmann A, et al. The risk of disc prolapses with complex loading in different degrees of disc degeneration – a finite element analysis. Clin Biomech 2007;22:988–98.

1267. Schmidt H, Shirazi-Adl A, Galbusera F, et al. Response analysis of the lumbar spine during regular daily activities – a finite element analysis. J Biomech 2010;43:1849–56.

1268. Schmidt MB, Mow VC, Chun LE, et al. Effects of proteoglycan extraction on the tensile behavior of articular cartilage. J Orthop Res 1990;8:353–63.

1269. Schmidt TA, An HS, Lim TH, et al. The stiffness of lumbar spinal motion segments with a high-intensity zone in the annulus fibrosus. Spine 1998;23:2167–73.

1270. Schmoelz W, Huber JF, Nydegger T, et al. Dynamic stabilization of the lumbar spine and its effects on adjacent segments: an in vitro experiment. J Spinal Disord Tech 2003;16:418–23.

1271. Schollmeier G, Lahr-Eigen R, Lewandrowski KU. Observations on fiber-forming collagens in the annulus fibrosus. Spine 2000;25: 2736–41.

1272. Schollum ML, Robertson PA, Broom ND. ISSLS prize winner: Microstructure and mechanical disruption of the lumbar disc annulus: part I: a microscopic investigation of the translamellar bridging network. Spine 2008;33: 2702–10.

1273. Schonstein E, Kenny DT, Keating J, et al. Work conditioning, work hardening and functional restoration for workers with back and neck pain. Cochrane Database Syst Rev 2003: CD001822.

1274. Schonstrom N, Lindahl S, Willen J, et al. Dynamic changes in the dimensions of the lumbar spinal canal: an experimental study in vitro. J Orthop Res 1989;7: 115–21.

1275. Schrader PK, Grob D, Rahn BA, et al. Histology of the ligamentum flavum in patients with degenerative lumbar spinal stenosis. Eur Spine J 1999;8: 323–8.

1276. Schultz AB, Haderspeck-Grib K, Sinkora G, et al. Quantitative studies of the flexion-relaxation phenomenon in the back muscles. J Orthop Res 1985;3: 189–97.

1277. Schultz AB, Warwick DN, Berkson MH, et al. Mechanical properties of human lumbar spine segments. Part 1. Response in flexion, extension, lateral bending and torsion. J Biomech Eng 1979;101:46–52.

1278. Schwab F, Lafage V, Boyce R, et al. Gravity line analysis in adult volunteers: age-related correlation with spinal parameters, pelvic parameters, and foot position. Spine 2006;31:E959–67.

1279. Schwarzer AC, Aprill CN, Bogduk N. The sacroiliac joint in chronic low-back pain. Spine 1995;20: 31–7.

1280. Schwarzer AC, Aprill CN, Derby R, et al. Clinical features of patients with pain stemming from the lumbar zygapophyseal joints. Is the lumbar facet syndrome a clinical entity? Spine 1994;19:1132–7.

1281. Schwarzer AC, Aprill CN, Derby R, et al. The prevalence and clinical features of internal disc disruption in patients with chronic low-back pain [see comments]. Spine 1995; 20:1878–83.

1282. Schwarzer AC, Derby R, Aprill CN, et al. Pain from the lumbar zygapophyseal joints: a test of two models. J Spinal Disord 1994;7:331–6.

1283. Schwarzer AC, Wang SC, Bogduk N, et al. Prevalence and clinical features of lumbar zygapophyseal joint pain: a study in an Australian population with chronic low-back pain. Ann Rheum Dis 1995;54:100–6.

1284. Schwarzer AC, Wang SC, O'Driscoll D, et al. The ability of computed tomography to identify a painful zygapophyseal joint in patients with chronic low-back pain. Spine 1995;20:907–12.

1285. Screen HR, Lee DA, Bader DL, et al. An investigation into the effects of the hierarchical structure of tendon fascicles on micromechanical properties. Proc Inst Mech Eng [H] 2004;218: 109–19.

1286. Sedlin ED, Hirsch C. Factors affecting the determination of the physical properties of femoral cortical bone. Acta Orthop Scand 1966;37:29–48.

1287. Seidler A, Bolm-Audorff U, Siol T, et al. Occupational risk factors for symptomatic lumbar disc herniation; a case-control study. Occup Environ Med 2003;60: 821–30.

1288. Seki S, Kawaguchi Y, Chiba K, et al. A functional SNP in CILP, encoding cartilage intermediate layer protein, is associated with susceptibility to lumbar disc disease. Nat Genet 2005;37: 607–12.

1289. Selim AJ, Fincke G, Berlowitz DR, et al. Comprehensive health status assessment of centenarians: results from the 1999 large health survey of veteran enrollees. J Geron tol A Biol Sci Med Sci 2005;60:515–9.

1290. Seroussi RE, Krag MH, Muller DL, et al. Internal deformations of intact and denucleated human lumbar discs subjected to compression, flexion, and extension loads. J Orthop Res 1989;7:122–31.

1291. Seroussi RE, Pope MH. The relationship between trunk muscle electromyography and lifting moments in the sagittal and frontal planes. J Biomech 1987;20:135–46.

1292. Seroussi RE, Wilder DG, Pope MH. Trunk muscle electromyography and whole body vibration. J Biomech 1989;22:219–29.

1293. Setton LA, Chen J. Cell mechanics and mechanobiology in the intervertebral disc. Spine 2004;29:2710–23.

1294. Setton LA, Zhu W, Weidenbaum M, et al. Compressive properties of the cartilaginous end-plate of the baboon lumbar spine. J Orthop Res 1993;11:228–39.

1295. Sevastik J, Burwell RG, Dangerfield PH. A new concept for the etiopathogenesis of the thoracospinal deformity of idiopathic scoliosis: summary of an electronic focus group debate of the IBSE. Eur Spine J 2003;12:440–50.

1296. Shamji MF, Setton LA, Jarvis W, et al. Proinflammatory cytokine expression profile in degenerated and herniated human intervertebral disc tissues. Arthritis Rheum 2010;62: 1974–82.

1297. Shapiro F, Koide S, Glimcher MJ. Cell origin and differentiation in the repair of full-thickness defects of articular cartilage. J Bone Joint Surg Am 1993;75:532–53.

1298. Shaw WS, van der Windt DA, Main CJ, et al. Early patient screening and intervention to address individual-level occupational factors ('Blue Flags') in back disability. J Occup Rehabil 2009;19:64–80.

1299. Shea KG, Ford T, Bloebaum RD, et al. A comparison of the microarchitectural bone adaptations of the concave and convex thoracic spinal facets in idiopathic scoliosis. J Bone Joint Surg Am 2004; 86-A:1000–6.

1300. Shea M, Takeuchi TY, Wittenberg RH, et al. A comparison of the effects of automated percutaneous diskectomy and conventional diskectomy on intradiscal pressure, disk geometry, and stiffness. J Spinal Disord 1994;7:317–25.

1301. Shine KM, Simson JA, Spector M. Lubricin distribution in the human intervertebral disc. J Bone Joint Surg Am 2009;91:2205–12.

1302. Shirado O, Kaneda K, Tadano S, et al. Influence of disc degeneration on mechanism of thoracolumbar burst fractures. Spine 1992;17:286–92.

1303. Shirazi-Adl A. Strain in fibers of a lumbar disc. Analysis of the role of lifting in producing disc prolapse. Spine 1989;14:96–103.

1304. Shirazi-Adl A. Finite-element evaluation of contact loads on facets of an L2-L3 lumbar segment in complex loads. Spine 1991;16:533–41.

1305. Shirazi-Adl A. Finite-element simulation of changes in the fluid content of human lumbar discs. Mechanical and clinical implications. Spine 1992;17:206–12.

1306. Shirazi-Adl A. Biomechanics of the lumbar spine in sagittal/ lateral moments. Spine 1994;19:2407–14.

1307. Shirazi-Adl A. Nonlinear stress analysis of the whole lumbar spine in torsion – mechanics of facet articulation. J Biomech 1994;27:289–99.

1308. Siegmund GP, Davis MB, Quinn KP, et al. Head-turned postures increase the risk of cervical facet capsule injury during whiplash. Spine (Phila Pa) 2008;33:1643–9.

1309. Sigurdsson G, Halldorsson BV, Styrkarsdottir U, et al. Impact of genetics on low bone mass in adults. J Bone Miner Res 2008;23:1584–90.

1310. Simpson AK, Biswas D, Emerson JW, et al. Quantifying the effects of age, gender, degeneration, and adjacent level degeneration on cervical spine range of motion using multivariate analyses. Spine 2008;33:183–6.

1311. Simpson EK, Parkinson IH, Manthey B, et al. Intervertebral disc disorganization is related to trabecular bone architecture in the lumbar spine. J Bone Miner Res 2001;16:681–7.

1312. Simunic DI, Robertson PA, Broom ND. Mechanically induced disruption of the healthy bovine intervertebral disc. Spine 2004;29:972–8.

1313. Sinaki M, Mikkelsen BA. Postmenopausal spinal osteoporosis: flexion versus extension exercises. Arch Phys Med Rehabil 1984;65:593–6.

1314. Sinaki M, Nwaogwugwu NC, Phillips BE, et al. Effect of gender, age, and anthropometry on axial and appendicular muscle strength. Am J Phys Med Rehabil 2001;80:330–8.

1315. Sinclair SM, Shamji MF, Chen J, et al. Attenuation of Inflammatory Events in Human Intervertebral Disc Cells with a Tumor Necrosis Factor Antagonist. Spine (Phila Pa) 2011.

1316. Singh K, Masuda K, Thonar EJ, et al. Age-related changes in the extracellular matrix of nucleus pulposus and annulus fibrosus of human intervertebral disc. Spine 2009;34:10–6.

1317. Sinkjaer T, Andersen JB, Nielsen JF, et al. Soleus long-latency stretch reflexes during walking in healthy and spastic humans. Clin Neurophysiol 1999;110:951–9.

1318. Sipila S, Taaffe DR, Cheng S, et al. Effects of hormone replacement therapy and high-impact physical exercise on skeletal muscle in post-menopausal women: a randomized placebo-controlled study. Clin Sci (Lond) 2001;101:147–57.

1319. Sitte I, Kathrein A, Pfaller K, et al. Intervertebral disc cell death in the porcine and human injured cervical spine after trauma: a histological and ultrastructural study. Spine 2009;34:131–40.

1320. Sivan SS, Tsitron E, Wachtel E, et al. Age-related accumulation of pentosidine in aggrecan and collagen from normal and degenerate human intervertebral discs. Biochem J 2006;399:29–35.

1321. Sivan SS, Tsitron E, Wachtel E, et al. Aggrecan turnover in human intervertebral disc as determined by the racemization of aspartic acid. J Biol Chem 2006;281:13009–14.

1322. Sivan SS, Wachtel E, Tsitron E, et al. Collagen turnover in normal and degenerate human intervertebral discs as determined by the racemization of aspartic acid. J Biol Chem 2008;283:8796–801.

1323. Skaggs DL, Weidenbaum M, Iatridis JC, et al. Regional variation in tensile properties and biochemical composition of the human lumbar annulus fibrosus [see comments]. Spine 1994;19:1310–9.

1324. Skinner HB, Barrack RL, Cook SD. Age-related decline in proprioception. Clin Orthop Relat Res 1984:208–11.

1325. Skinner HB, Wyatt MP, Hodgdon JA, et al. Effect of fatigue on joint position sense of the knee. J Orthop Res 1986;4:112–8.

1326. Skrzypiec D, Tarala M, Pollintine P, et al. When are intervertebral discs stronger than their adjacent vertebrae? Spine 2007;32:2455–61.

1327. Skrzypiec DM, Pollintine P, Przybyla A, et al. The internal mechanical properties of cervical intervertebral discs as revealed by stress profilometry. Eur Spine J 2007;16:1701–9.

1328. Smeathers JE. Some time dependent properties of the intervertebral joint when under compression. Eng Med 1984;13:83–7.

1329. Smeathers JE, Joanes DN. Dynamic compressive properties of human lumbar intervertebral joints: a comparison between fresh and thawed specimens. J Biomech 1988;21:425–33.

1330. Smedley J, Inskip H, Buckle P, et al. Epidemiological differences between back pain of sudden and gradual onset. J Rheumatol 2005;32:528–32.

1331. Smedley J, Trevelyan F, Inskip H, et al. Impact of ergonomic intervention on back pain among nurses. Scand J Work Environ Health 2003;29:117–23.

1332. Smidt GL, McQuade K, Wei SH, et al. Sacroiliac kinematics for reciprocal straddle positions. Spine 1995;20:1047–54.

1333. Smidt GL, Wei SH, McQuade K, et al. Sacroiliac motion for extreme hip positions. A fresh cadaver study. Spine 1997;22:2073–82.

1334. Smith BM, Hurwitz EL, Solsberg D, et al. Interobserver reliability of detecting lumbar intervertebral disc high-intensity zone on magnetic resonance imaging and association of high-intensity zone with pain and annular disruption. Spine (Phila Pa) 1998;23:2074–80.

1335. Smith Jr GN, Brandt KD. Hypothesis: can type IX collagen 'glue' together intersecting type II fibers in articular cartilage matrix? A proposed mechanism. J Rheumatol 1992;19:14–7.

1336. Smith JW, Walmsley R. Factors affecting the elasticity of bone. J Anat 1959;93:503–23.

1337. Smith L, Garvin PJ, Gesler RM, et al. Enzyme dissolution of the nucleus pulposus. Nature 1963;198:1311–2.

1338. Smyth MJ, Wright,V. Sciatica and the intervertebral disc. An experimental study. J Bone Joint Surg 1959;40 A:1401–18.

1339. Snook SH, Webster BS, McGorry RW. The reduction of chronic, nonspecific low-back pain through the control of early morning lumbar flexion: 3-year follow-up. J Occup Rehabil 2002;12:13–9.

1340. Snook SH, Webster BS, McGorry RW, et al. The reduction of chronic nonspecific low-back pain through the control of early morning lumbar flexion. A randomized controlled trial. Spine 1998;23:2601–7.

1341. Soler T, Calderon C. The prevalence of spondylolysis in the Spanish elite athlete. Am J Sports Med 2000;28:57–62.

1342. Solomonow M, He Zhou B, Baratta RV, et al. Biexponential recovery model of lumbar viscoelastic laxity and reflexive muscular activity after prolonged cyclic loading. Clin Biomech 2000;15:167–75.

1343. Solomonow M, Zhou B, Baratta RV, et al. Neuromuscular disorders associated with static lumbar flexion: a feline model. J Electromyogr Kinesiol 2002;12:81–90.

1344. Solomonow M, Zhou BH, Baratta RV, et al. Biomechanics of increased exposure to lumbar injury caused by cyclic loading: Part 1. Loss of reflexive muscular stabilization. Spine 1999;24:2426–34.

1345. Solomonow M, Zhou BH, Harris M, et al. The ligamento-muscular stabilizing system of the spine. Spine 1998;23:2552–62.

1346. Solovieva S, Lohiniva J, Leino-Arjas P, et al. COL9A3 gene polymorphism and obesity in intervertebral disc degeneration of the lumbar spine: evidence of gene-environment interaction. Spine 2002;27:2691–6.

1347. Sornay-Rendu E, Allard C, Munoz F, et al. Disc space narrowing as a new risk factor for vertebral fracture: the OFELY study. Arthritis Rheum 2006;54:1262–9.

1348. Spangfort EV. The lumbar disc herniation. Acta Orthop Scand 1973;(Suppl. 142).

1349. Speciale AC, Pietrobon R, Urban CW, et al. Observer variability in assessing lumbar spinal stenosis severity on magnetic resonance imaging and its relation to cross-sectional spinal canal area. Spine 2002;27:1082–6.

1350. Spitzer WO. Scientific approach to the assessment and management of activity-related spinal disorders. A monograph for clinicians. Report of the Quebec Task Force on Spinal Disorders. Spine 1987; 12(Suppl):1–59.

1351. Spivak JM. Degenerative lumbar spinal stenosis. J Bone Joint Surg Am 1998;80:1053–66.

1352. Staal JB, Hlobil H, van Tulder MW, et al. Return-to-work interventions for low-back pain: a descriptive review of contents and concepts of working mechanisms. Sports Med 2002; 32:251–67.

1353. Staal JB, Hlobil H, van Tulder MW, et al. Occupational health guidelines for the management of low-back pain: an international comparison. Occup Environ Med 2003; 60:618–26.

1354. Stairmand JW, Holm S, Urban JP. Factors influencing oxygen concentration gradients in the intervertebral disc. A theoretical analysis. Spine 1991;16:444–9.

1355. Stanton TR, Henschke N, Maher CG, et al. After an episode of acute low-back pain, recurrence is unpredictable and not as common as previously thought. Spine (Phila Pa) 2008;33:2923–8.

1356. Stanton TR, Latimer J, Maher CG, et al. How do we define the condition 'recurrent low-back pain'? A systematic review. Eur Spine J 2010;19:533–9.

1357. Steffen T, Baramki HG, Rubin R, et al. Lumbar intradiscal pressure measured in the anterior and posterolateral annular regions during asymmetrical loading. Clin Biomech 1998;13:495–505.

1358. Steffen T, Rubin RK, Baramki HG, et al. A new technique for measuring lumbar segmental motion in vivo. Method, accuracy, and preliminary results. Spine 1997;22:156–66.

1359. Steindler A, Luck JV. Differential diagnosis of pain low in the back: allocation of the souce of pain by procain hydrochloride method. Jama 1938;110:106–12.

1360. Steinmann J, Tingey CT, Cruz G, et al. Biomechanical comparison of unipedicular versus bipedicular kyphoplasty. Spine 2005;30:201–5.

1361. Stewart TD. The age incidence of neural arch defects in Alaskan natives – considered from the standpoint of aetiology. J Bone Joint Surg [Am] 1953;35:937–50.

1362. Stokes IA. Surface strain on human intervertebral discs. J Orthop Res 1987;5:348–55.

1363. Stokes IA. Bulging of lumbar intervertebral discs: non-contacting measurements of anatomical specimens. J Spinal Disord 1988;1:189–93.

1364. Stokes IA, Aronsson DD. Disc and vertebral wedging in patients with progressive scoliosis. J Spinal Disord 2001;14:317–22.

1365. Stokes IA, Bevins TM, Lunn RA. Back surface curvature and measurement of lumbar spinal motion. Spine 1987;12:355–61.

1366. Stokes IA, Counts DF, Frymoyer JW. Experimental instability in the rabbit lumbar spine. Spine 1989;14:68–72.

1367. Stokes IA, Gardner-Morse M. Muscle activation strategies and symmetry of spinal loading in the lumbar spine with scoliosis. Spine 2004;29:2103–7.

1368. Stokes IA, Gardner-Morse M, Henry SM, et al. Decrease in trunk muscular response to perturbation with preactivation of lumbar spinal musculature. Spine 2000;25:1957–64.

1369. Stokes IA, Wilder DG, Frymoyer JW, et al. 1980 Volvo award in clinical sciences. Assessment of patients with low- back pain by biplanar radiographic measurement of intervertebral motion. Spine 1981;6: 233–40.

1370. Stokes IA, Windisch L. Vertebral height growth predominates over intervertebral disc height growth in adolescents with scoliosis. Spine 2006;31:1600–4.

1371. Stokes M, Young A. The contribution of reflex inhibition to arthrogenous muscle weakness. Clin Sci 1984;67:7–14.

1372. Stokes MJ, Cooper RG, Morris G, et al. Selective changes in multifidus dimensions in patients with chronic low-back pain. Eur Spine J 1992;1:38–42.

1373. Stoll TM, Dubois G, Schwarzenbach O. The dynamic neutralization system for the spine: a multi-center study of a novel non-fusion system. Eur Spine J 2002;11(Suppl 2):S170–8.

1374. Storr-Paulsen A. ['The body-consciousness in school' – a back pain-school.] Ugeskr Laeger 2002;165:37–41.

1375. Stuart M, Butler JE, Collins DF, et al. The history of contraction of the wrist flexors can change cortical excitability. J Physiol 2002;545:731–7.

1376. Stubbs M, Harris M, Solomonow M, et al. Ligamento-muscular protective reflex in the lumbar spine of the feline. J Electromyogr Kinesiol 1998;8:197–204.

1377. Sturesson B. Movement of the sacro-iliac joints: a fresh look. In: Vleeming A, Mooney V, Snijders CJ, et al, editors. Movement, Stability and Low-back Pain. Edinburgh: Churchill Livingston; 1997.

1378. Sturesson B, Selvik G, Uden A. Movements of the sacroiliac joints. A roentgen stereophotogrammetric analysis. Spine 1989;14:162–5.

1379. Sullivan A, McGill SM. Changes in spine length during and after seated whole-body vibration. Spine 1990;15:1257–60.

1380. Sullivan JD, Farfan HF. The crumpled neural arch. Orthop Clin North Am 1975;6:199–214.

1381. Sullivan MS, Dickinson CE, Troup JD. The influence of age and gender on lumbar spine sagittal plane range of motion. A study of 1126 healthy subjects. Spine 1994;19:682–6.

1382. Sumida K, Sato K, Aoki M, et al. Serial changes in the rate of proteoglycan synthesis after chemonucleolysis of rabbit intervertebral discs. Spine 1999;24:1066–70.

1383. Summers GC, Merrill A, Sharif M, et al. Swelling of articular cartilage depends on the integrity of adjacent cartilage and bone. Biorheology 2008; 45:365–74.

1384. Suwito W, Keller TS, Basu PK, et al. Geometric and material property study of the human lumbar spine using the finite element method. J Spinal Disord 1992;5:50–9.

1385. Svensson MY. Injury biomechanics. In: Gunzburg R, Szpalski M, editors. Whiplash Injuries. Philadelphia, U.S.A.: Lippincott-Raven; 1998.

1386. Swanepoel MW, Adams LM, Smeathers JE. Human lumbar apophyseal joint damage and intervertebral disc degeneration. Ann Rheum Dis 1995;54:182–8.

1387. Swanepoel MW, Adams LM, Smeathers JE. Morphometry of human lumbar apophyseal joints. A novel technique. Spine 1997;22:2473–83.

1388. Swanepoel MW, Smeathers JE, Adams LM. The stiffness of human apophyseal articular cartilage as an indicator of joint loading. Proc Inst Mech Eng 1994;208:33–43.

1389. Sward L, Hellstrom M, Jacobsson B, et al. Disc degeneration and associated abnormalities of the spine in elite gymnasts. A magnetic resonance imaging study. Spine 1991;16:437–43.

1390. Sward L, Hellstrom M, Jacobsson B, et al. Back pain and radiologic changes in the thoraco-lumbar spine of athletes. Spine 1990;15:124–9.

1391. Swinkels A, Dolan P. Spinal position sense is independent of the magnitude of movement. Spine 2000;25:98–104; discussion 5.

1392. Syczewska M, Oberg T, Karlsson D. Segmental movements of the spine during treadmill walking with normal speed. Clin Biomech 1999;14:384–8.

1393. Symmons DP, van Hemert AM, Vandenbroucke JP, et al. A longitudinal study of back pain and radiological changes in the lumbar spines of middle aged women. II. Radiographic findings. Ann Rheum Dis 1991;50:162–6.

1394. Symonds TL, Burton AK, Tillotson KM, et al. Absence resulting from low-back trouble can be reduced by psychosocial intervention at the work place. Spine 1995;20:2738–45.

1395. Symonds TL, Burton AK, Tillotson KM, et al. Do attitudes and beliefs influence work loss due to low-back trouble? Occup Med (Lond) 1996;46:25–32.

1396. Szebenyi B, Hollander AP, Dieppe P, et al. Associations between pain, function, and radiographic features in osteoarthritis of the knee. Arthritis Rheum 2006;54:230–5.

1397. Szpalski M, Michel F, Hayez JP. Determination of trunk motion patterns associated with permanent or transient stenosis of the lumbar spine. Eur Spine J 1996;5:332–7.

1398. Taimela S, Kankaanpaa M, Luoto S. The effect of lumbar fatigue on the ability to sense a change in lumbar position. A controlled study. Spine 1999;24: 1322–7.

1399. Takahashi I, Kikuchi S, Sato K, et al. Mechanical load of the lumbar spine during forward bending motion of the trunk-a biomechanical study. Spine 2006;31:18–23.

1400. Takahashi N, Yabuki S, Aoki Y, et al. Pathomechanisms of nerve root injury caused by disc herniation: an experimental study of mechanical compression and chemical irritation. Spine 2003;28: 435–41.

1401. Tamcan O, Mannion AF, Eisenring C, et al. The course of chronic and recurrent low-back pain in the general population. Pain 2010;150:451–7.

1402. Tampier C, Drake JD, Callaghan JP, et al. Progressive disc herniation: an investigation of the mechanism using radiologic, histochemical, and microscopic dissection techniques on a porcine model. Spine 2007;32:2869–74.

1403. Tanaka M, Nakahara S, Inoue H. A pathologic study of discs in the elderly. Separation between the cartilaginous endplate and the vertebral body. Spine 1993;18:1456–62.

1404. Tanaka Y. A radiographic analysis on human lumbar vertebrae in the aged. Virchows Arch A Pathol Anat Histol 1975;366:187–201.

1405. Taylor JR. Growth of human intervertebral discs and vertebral bodies. J Anat 1975;120:49–68.

1406. Taylor JR, Twomey LT. Age changes in lumbar zygapophyseal joints. Observations on structure and function. Spine 1986;11:739–45.

1407. Taylor JR, Twomey LT, Corker M. Bone and soft tissue injuries in postmortem lumbar spines. Paraplegia 1990;28:119–29.

1408. Teichtahl AJ, Wluka AE, Forbes A, et al. Longitudinal effect of vigorous physical activity on patella cartilage morphology in people without clinical knee disease. Arthritis Rheum 2009;61:1095–102.

1409. Teitz CC, Garrett WE, Miniachi A, et al. Tendon problems in athletic individuals. J Bone Joint Surg [Am] 1997;79:138–52.

1410. Tesch PA, Komi PV, Hakkinen K. Enzymatic adaptations consequent to long-term strength training. Int J Sports Med 1987; 8(Suppl. 1):66–9.

1411. Tesh KM, Dunn JS, Evans JH. The abdominal muscles and vertebral stability. Spine 1987;12:501–8.

1412. Tew SR, Kwan AP, Hann A, et al. The reactions of articular cartilage to experimental wounding: role of apoptosis. Arthritis Rheum 2000;43:215–25.

1413. Thambyah A, Broom N. On how degeneration influences load-bearing in the cartilage-bone system: a microstructural and micromechanical study. Osteoarthritis Cartilage 2007;15:1410–23.

1414. Thambyah A, Broom N. How subtle structural changes associated with maturity and mild degeneration influence the impact-induced failure modes of cartilage-on-bone. Clin Biomech 2010;25:737–44.

1415. Thayer R, Collins J, Noble EG, et al. A decade of aerobic endurance training: histological evidence for fibre type transformation. J Sports Med Phys Fitness 2000;40:284–9.

1416. Thompson JP, Pearce RH, Schechter MT, et al. Preliminary evaluation of a scheme for grading the gross morphology of the human intervertebral disc. Spine 1990;15:411–5.

1417. Thompson KJ, Dagher AP, Eckel TS, et al. Modic changes on MR images as studied with provocative diskography: clinical relevance – a retrospective study of 2457 disks. Radiology 2009;250:849–55.

1418. Thomsen K, Christensen FB, Eiskjaer SP, et al. 1997 Volvo Award winner in clinical studies. The effect of pedicle screw instrumentation on functional outcome and fusion rates in posterolateral lumbar spinal fusion: a prospective, randomized clinical study. Spine 1997;22: 2813–22.

1419. Thorstensson A, Hulten B, von Dobeln W, et al. Effect of strength training on enzyme activities and fibre characteristics in human skeletal muscle. Acta Physiol Scand 1976;96:392–8.

1420. Tischer T, Aktas T, Milz S, et al. Detailed pathological changes of human lumbar facet joints L1-L5 in elderly individuals. Eur Spine J 2006;15:308–15.

1421. Tkaczuk H. Tensile properties of human lumbar longitudinal ligaments. Acta Orthop Scand 1968;(Suppl):115.

1422. Tobias D, Ziv I, Maroudas A. Human facet cartilage: swelling and some physico-chemical characteristics as a function of age. Part 1: Swelling of human facet joint cartilage. Spine 1992; 17:694–700.

1423. Tokuhashi Y, Matsuzaki H. Repair of defects in spondylolysis by segmental pedicular screw hook fixation. A preliminary report. Spine 1996;21:2041–5.

1424. Tooms RE, Griffin JW, Green S, et al. Effect of viscoelastic insoles on pain. Orthopedics 1987;10:1143–7.

1425. Torzilli PA, Bhargava M, Park S, et al. Mechanical load inhibits IL-1 induced matrix degradation in articular cartilage. Osteoarthritis Cartilage 2010;18:97–105.

1426. Torzilli PA, Grigiene R, Borrelli Jr J, et al. Effect of impact load on articular cartilage: cell metabolism and viability, and matrix water content. J Biomech Eng 1999;121:433–41.

1427. Toursel T, Stevens L, Granzier H, et al. Passive tension of rat skeletal soleus muscle fibers: effects of unloading conditions. J Appl Physiol 2002;92:1465–72.

1428. Trafimow JH, Schipplein OD, Novak GJ, et al. The effects of quadriceps fatigue on the technique of lifting. Spine 1993;18:364–7.

1429. Tran-Khanh N, Hoemann CD, McKee MD, et al. Aged bovine chondrocytes display a diminished capacity to produce a collagen-rich, mechanically functional cartilage extracellular matrix. J Orthop Res 2005;23: 1354–62.

1430. Tranquille CA, Blunden AS, Dyson SJ, et al. Effect of exercise on thicknesses of mature hyaline cartilage, calcified cartilage, and subchondral bone of equine tarsi. Am J Vet Res 2009;70: 1477–83.

1431. Trotter JA. Functional morphology of force transmission in skeletal muscle. A brief review. Acta Anat 1993;146:205–22.

1432. Trotter JA, Purslow PP. Functional morphology of the endomysium in series fibered muscles. J Morphol 1992;212:109–22.

1433. Trout JJ, Buckwalter JA, Moore KC, et al. Ultrastructure of the human intervertebral disc. I. Changes in notochordal cells with age. Tissue Cell 1982;14: 359–69.

1434. Truchon M, Fillion, L. Biopsychosocial determinants of chronoc disability and low-back pain: a review. J Occup Rehabil 2000;10:117–42.

1435. Trudelle-Jackson E, Fleisher LA, Borman N, et al. Lumbar spine flexion and extension extremes of motion in women of different age and racial groups: the WIN Study. Spine (Phila Pa) 2010;35: 1539–44.

1436. Tschoeke SK, Hellmuth M, Hostmann A, et al. Apoptosis of human intervertebral discs after trauma compares to degenerated discs involving both receptor-mediated and mitochondrial-dependent pathways. J Orthop Res 2008;26:999–1006.

1437. Tse KY, Macias BR, Meyer RS, et al. Heritability of bone density: regional and gender differences in monozygotic twins. J Orthop Res 2009;27:150–4.

1438. Tsuji H, Hirano N, Ohshima H, et al. Structural variation of the anterior and posterior annulus fibrosus in the development of human lumbar intervertebral disc. A risk factor for intervertebral disc rupture. Spine 1993;18:204–10.

1439. Tulder van MW, Assendelft WJ, Koes BW, et al. Spinal radiographic findings and nonspecific low-back pain. A systematic review of observational studies. Spine 1997;22:427–34.

1440. Tullberg T, Blomberg S, Branth B, et al. Manipulation does not alter the position of the sacroiliac joint. A roentgen stereophotogrammetric analysis. Spine 1998;23:1124–8; discussion 9.

1441. Turner CH, Takano Y, Owan I. Aging changes mechanical loading thresholds for bone formation in rats. J Bone Miner Res 1995;10:1544–9.

1442. Tveit P, Daggfeldt K, Hetland S, et al. Erector spinae lever arm length variations with changes in spinal curvature. Spine 1994;19:199–204.

1443. Tveito TH, Hysing M, Eriksen HR. Low-back pain interventions at the workplace: a systematic literature review. Occup Med (Lond) 2004;54:3–13.

1444. Twomey L, Taylor J. Flexion creep deformation and hysteresis in the lumbar vertebral column. Spine 1982;7:116–22.

1445. Twomey L, Taylor J. Age changes in lumbar intervertebral discs. Acta Orthop Scand 1985;56:496–9.

1446. Twomey LT, Taylor JR. Sagittal movements of the human lumbar vertebral column: a quantitative study of the role of the posterior vertebral elements. Arch Phys Med Rehabil 1983;64:322–5.

1447. Twomey LT, Taylor JR. Age changes in lumbar vertebrae and intervertebral discs. Clin Orthop 1987:97–104.

1448. Twomey LT, Taylor JR, Taylor MM. Unsuspected damage to lumbar zygapophyseal (facet) joints after motor- vehicle accidents. Med J Aust 1989;151:210–2, 5–7.

1449. Tyrrell AR, Reilly T, Troup JD. Circadian variation in stature and the effects of spinal loading. Spine 1985;10:161–4.

1450. UKBEAM Trial Team. U.K. back pain exercise and manipulation (UK BEAM) randomised trial: cost-effectiveness of physical treatments for back pain in primary care. BMJ 2004;329:1381–5.

1451. UKBEAM Trial Team. U.K. back pain exercise and manipulation (UK BEAM) randomised trial: effectiveness of physical treatments for back pain in primary care. BMJ 2004;329:1377–80.

1452. Ulrich JA, Liebenberg EC, Thuillier DU, et al. ISSLS prize winner: repeated disc injury causes persistent inflammation. Spine 2007;32:2812–9.

1453. Umehara S, Tadano S, Abumi K, et al. Effects of degeneration on the elastic modulus distribution in the lumbar intervertebral disc. Spine 1996;21:811–9; discussion 20.

1454. Urban JP. The chondrocyte: a cell under pressure. Br J Rheumatol 1994;33:901–8.

1455. Urban JP, Holm S, Maroudas A, et al. Nutrition of the intervertebral disk. An in vivo study of solute transport. Clin Orthop 1977:101–14.

1456. Urban JP, McMullin JF. Swelling pressure of the lumbar intervertebral discs: influence of age, spinal level, composition, and degeneration. Spine 1988;13:179–87.

1457. Urban JP, Roberts S. Degeneration of the intervertebral disc. Arthritis Res Ther 2003;5:120–30.

1458. Urban JP, Smith S, Fairbank JC. Nutrition of the intervertebral disc. Spine 2004;29:2700–9.

1459. Urban RJ, Bodenburg YH, Gilkison C, et al. Testosterone administration to elderly men increases skeletal muscle strength and protein synthesis. Am J Physiol 1995;269:E820–6.

1460. Ursin H. Sensitization, somatization, and subjective health complaints. Int J Behav Med 1997;4:105–16.

1461. US Preventive Services Task Force. Primary care interventions to prevent low-back pain in adults: recommendation statement. Rockville, MD: Agency for Healthcare Research and Quality; 2004.

1462. Vaccaro AR, Hulbert RJ, Patel AA, et al. The subaxial cervical spine injury classification system: a novel approach to recognize the importance of morphology, neurology, and integrity of the disco-ligamentous complex. Spine 2007;32:2365–74.

1463. Valli M, Leonardi L, Strocchi R, et al. 'In vitro' fibril formation of type I collagen from different sources: biochemical and morphological aspects. Connect Tissue Res 1986;15:235–44.

1464. van den Eerenbeemt KD, Ostelo RW, van Royen BJ, et al. Total disc replacement surgery for symptomatic degenerative lumbar disc disease: a systematic review of the literature. Eur Spine J 2010;19:1262–80.

1465. van der Roer N, Ostelo RW, Bekkering GE, et al. Minimal clinically important change for pain intensity, functional status, and general health status in patients with nonspecific low-back pain. Spine 2006;31:578–82.

1466. van der Veen AJ, van Dieen JH, Nadort A, et al. Intervertebral disc recovery after dynamic or static loading in vitro: Is there a role for the endplate? J Biomech 2007;40:2230–5.

1467. van Kleef M, Barendse GA, Kessels A, et al. Randomized trial of radiofrequency lumbar facet denervation for chronic low-back pain. Spine 1999;24:1937–42.

1468. van Poppel MN, Koes BW, Smid T, et al. A systematic review of controlled clinical trials on the prevention of back pain in industry. Occup Environ Med 1997;54:841–7.

1469. van Tulder M. The project of European guidelines on LBP. Acta Orthop Scand 2002;73:20–5.

1470. van Tulder M, Becker A, Bekkering Tea et al. European guidelines for the management of acute nonspecific low-back pain in primary care. EC Cost Action B13. Available online at: www.backpaineurope.org. 2004.

1471. van Tulder MW, Assendelft WJ, Koes BW, et al. Spinal radiographic findings and nonspecific low-back pain. A systematic review of observational studies. Spine 1997;22:427–34.

1472. Vandervoort AA. Aging of the human neuromuscular system. Muscle Nerve 2002;25:17–25.

1473. Vanharanta H, Floyd T, Ohnmeiss DD, et al. The relationship of facet tropism to degenerative disc disease. Spine 1993;18:1000–5.

1474. Vanharanta H, Sachs BL, Spivey MA, et al. The relationship of pain provocation to lumbar disc deterioration as seen by CT/discography. Spine 1987;12:295–8.

1475. Vascancelos D. Compression fractures of the vertebra during major epileptic seizures. Epilepsia 1973;14:323–8.

1476. Veldhuizen AG, Wever DJ, Webb PJ. The aetiology of idiopathic scoliosis: biomechanical and neuromuscular factors. Eur Spine J 2000;9:178–84.

1477. Venner RM, Crock HV. Clinical studies of isolated disc resorption in the lumbar spine. J Bone Joint Surg [Br] 1981;4:491–4.

1478. Verbeek JH, van der Weide WE, van Dijk FJ. Early occupational health management of patients with back pain: a randomized controlled trial. Spine 2002;27:1844–51; discussion 51.

1479. Veres SP, Robertson PA, Broom ND. ISSLS prize winner: Microstructure and mechanical disruption of the lumbar disc annulus: part II: how the annulus fails under hydrostatic pressure. Spine 2008;33:2711–20.

1480. Veres SP, Robertson PA, Broom ND. The morphology of acute disc herniation: a clinically relevant model defining the role of flexion. Spine (Phila Pa) 2009;34:2288–96.

1481. Verhoof OJ, Bron JL, Wapstra FH, et al. High failure rate of the interspinous distraction device (X-Stop) for the treatment of lumbar spinal stenosis caused by degenerative spondylolisthesis. Eur Spine J 2008;17:188–92.

1482. Vernon-Roberts B. Disc pathology and disease states. In: Ghosh P, editor. The Biology of the Intervertebral Disc. Boca Raton, Florida: CRC Press; 1988. p. 73–119.

1483. Vernon-Roberts B, Fazzalari NL, Manthey BA. Pathogenesis of tears of the annulus investigated by multiple-level transaxial analysis of the T12–L1 disc. Spine 1997;22:2641–6.

1484. Vernon-Roberts B, Moore RJ, Fraser RD. The natural history of age-related disc degeneration: the influence of age and pathology on cell populations in the L4–L5 disc. Spine 2008;33:2767–73.

1485. Vernon-Roberts B, Pirie CJ. Healing trabecular microfractures in the bodies of lumbar vertebrae. Ann Rheum Dis 1973;32:406–12.

1486. Verzijl N, DeGroot J, Thorpe SR, et al. Effect of collagen turnover on the accumulation of advanced glycation end products. J Biol Chem 2000;275:39027–31.

1487. Videman T, Battie MC. The influence of occupation on lumbar degeneration. Spine 1999;24:1164–8.

1488. Videman T, Battie MC, Gibbons LE, et al. Associations between back pain history and lumbar MRI findings. Spine 2003;28:582–8.

1489. Videman T, Battie MC, Gill K, et al. Magnetic resonance imaging findings and their relationships in the thoracic and lumbar spine. Insights into the etiopathogenesis of spinal degeneration. Spine 1995;20:928–35.

1490. Videman T, Battie MC, Parent E, et al. Progression and determinants of quantitative magnetic resonance imaging measures of lumbar disc degeneration: a five-year follow-up of adult male monozygotic twins. Spine 2008;33:1484–90.

1491. Videman T, Leppavuori J, Kaprio J, et al. Intragenic polymorphisms of the vitamin D receptor gene associated with intervertebral disc degeneration. Spine 1998;23:2477–85.

1492. Videman T, Levalahti E, Battie MC. The effects of anthropometrics, lifting strength, and physical activities in disc degeneration. Spine 2007;32:1406–13.

1493. Videman T, Levalahti E, Battie MC, et al. Heritability of BMD of femoral neck and lumbar spine: a multivariate twin study of Finnish men. J Bone Miner Res 2007;22:1455–62.

1494. Videman T, Nurminen M. The occurrence of annular tears and their relation to lifetime back pain history: a cadaveric study using barium sulfate discography. Spine 2004;29:2668–76.

1495. Videman T, Sarna S, Battie MC, et al. The long-term effects of physical loading and exercise lifestyles on back-related symptoms, disability, and spinal pathology among men. Spine 1995;20:699–709.

1496. Vingard E, Mortimer M, Wiktorin C, et al. Seeking care for low-back pain in the general population: a two-year follow-up study: results from the MUSIC-Norrtalje Study. Spine 2002;27:2159–65.

1497. Viola S, Andrassy I. Spinal mobility and posture: changes during growth with postural defects, structural scoliosis and spinal osteochondrosis. Eur Spine J 1995;4:29–33.

1498. Virgin WJ. Experimental investigations into the physical properties of the intervertebral disc. J Bone Joint Surg [Br] 1951;33:607–11.

1499. Vleeming A, Albert HB, Ostgaard HC, et al. European guidelines for the diagnosis and treatment of pelvic girdle pain. Eur Spine J 2008;17:794–819.

1500. Vleeming A, Pool-Goudzwaard AL, Stoeckart R, et al. The posterior layer of the thoracolumbar fascia. Its function in load transfer from spine to legs. Spine 1995;20:753–8.

1501. Vleeming A, Snijders CJ, Stoeckart R, et al. The role of the sacroiliac joints in coupling between spine, pelvis, legs and arms. In: Vleeming A, Mooney V, Snijders CJ, et al, editors.

Movement, Stability and Low-back Pain. Edinburgh: Churchill Livingstone; 1997.

1502. Vleeming A, Stoeckart R, Volkers AC, et al. Relation between form and function in the sacroiliac joint. Part I: Clinical anatomical aspects. Spine 1990; 15:130–2.

1503. Vleeming A, Volkers AC, Snijders CJ, et al. Relation between form and function in the sacroiliac joint. Part II: Biomechanical aspects. Spine 1990;15:133–6.

1504. Von Korff M, Moore JC. Stepped care for back pain: activating approaches for primary care. Ann Intern Med 2001;134:911–7.

1505. Vuillerme N, Anziani B, Rougier P. Trunk extensor muscles fatigue affects undisturbed postural control in young healthy adults. Clin Biomech 2007;22:489–94.

1506. Waddell G. 1987 Volvo award in clinical sciences. A new clinical model for the treatment of low-back pain. Spine 1987; 12:632–44.

1507. Waddell G. The back pain revolution. 2nd ed. Edinburgh: Churchill Livingstone; 2002.

1508. Waddell G, Aylward M, Sawney P. Back pain, incapacity for work and social security benefits: an international literature review and analysis. London: Royal Society of Medicine Press; 2002.

1509. Waddell G, Burton AK. Occupational health guidelines for the management of low-back pain at work – evidence review. London: Faculty of Occupational Medicine; 2000.

1510. Waddell G, Burton AK. Occupational health guidelines for the management of low-back pain at work: evidence review. Occup Med (Lond) 2001;51: 124–35.

1511. Waddell G, Burton AK. Concepts of rehabilitation for the management of common health problems. Norwich: The Stationery Office; 2004.

1512. Waddell G, Burton AK. Concepts of rehabilitation for the management of low-back pain. Best Pract Res Clin Rheumatol 2005;19:655–70.

1513. Waddell G, Burton AK. Is work good for your health and well-being? London: TSO; 2006.

1514. Waddell G, Burton AK, Kendall NAS. Vocational rehabilitation: what works, for whom, and when? London: TSO; 2008.

1515. Waddell G, Burton AK, Main CJ. Screening to identify people at risk of long term incapacity for work. London: Royal Society of Medicine Press; 2003.

1516. Waddell G, Main CJ, Morris EW, et al. Normality and reliability in the clinical assessment of backache. Br Med J (Clin Res Ed) 1982;284:1519–23.

1517. Waddell G, O'Connor M, Boorman S, et al. Working Backs Scotland. A public and professional health education campaign for back pain. Spine 2007;32:2139–43.

1518. Waddell G, Sell P, McGregor AH, et al. Your back operation. London: The Stationery Office; 2005.

1519. Wagner DR, Reiser KM, Lotz JC. Glycation increases human annulus fibrosus stiffness in both experimental measurements and theoretical predictions. J Biomech 2006;39:1021–9.

1520. Wai EK, Roffey DM, Bishop P, et al. Causal assessment of occupational bending or twisting and low-back pain: results of a systematic review. Spine J 2010; 10:76–88.

1521. Wai EK, Roffey DM, Bishop P, et al. Causal assessment of occupational carrying and low-back pain: results of a systematic review. Spine J 2010; 10:628–38.

1522. Wai EK, Roffey DM, Bishop P, et al. Causal assessment of occupational lifting and low-back pain: results of a systematic review. Spine J 2010; 10:554–66.

1523. Walker BF. The prevalence of low-back pain: a systematic review of the literature from 1966 to 1998. J Spinal Disord 2000;13:205–17.

1524. Walsh AJ, Lotz JC. Biological response of the intervertebral disc to dynamic loading. J Biomech 2004;37:329–37.

1525. Walsh K, Cruddas M, Coggon D. Low-back pain in eight areas of Britain. J Epidemiol Community Health 1992;46:227–30.

1526. Walsh TR, Weinstein JN, Spratt KF, et al. Lumbar discography in normal subjects. A controlled, prospective study. J Bone Joint Surg Am 1990;72:1081–8.

1527. Walter BA, Korecki CL, Purmessur D, et al. Complex loading affects intervertebral disc mechanics and biology. Osteoarthritis Cartilage 2011;19:1011–8.

1528. Wang DL, Jiang SD, Dai LY. Biologic response of the intervertebral disc to static and dynamic compression in vitro. Spine 2007;32:2521–8.

1529. Wang M, Dumas GA. Mechanical behavior of the female sacroiliac joint and influence of the anterior and posterior sacroiliac ligaments under sagittal loads. Clin Biomech 1998;13:293–9.

1530. Wang N, Hikida RS, Staron RS, et al. Muscle fiber types of women after resistance training – quantitative ultrastructure and enzyme activity. Pflugers Arch 1993;424:494–502.

1531. Wang Y, Battie MC, Boyd SK, et al. The osseous endplates in lumbar vertebrae: thickness, bone mineral density and their associations with age and disk degeneration. Bone 2011;48: 804–9.

1532. Wasiak R, Pransky G, Verma S, et al. Recurrence of low-back pain: definition-sensitivity analysis using administrative data. Spine 2003;28:2283–91.

1533. Wassen MH, Lammens J, Tekoppele JM, et al. Collagen structure regulates fibril mineralization in osteogenesis as revealed by cross-link patterns in calcifying callus. J Bone Miner Res 2000;15:1776–85.

1534. Waters TR, Putz-Anderson V, Garg A, et al. Revised NIOSH equation for the design and evaluation of manual lifting tasks. Ergonomics 1993;36:749–76.

1535. Watson PJ, Booker CK, Main CJ, et al. Surface electromyography in the identification of chronic low-back pain patients: the development of the flexion relaxation ratio. Clin Biomech 1997;12:165–71.

1536. Watters 3rd WC, Baisden J, Gilbert TJ, et al. Degenerative lumbar spinal stenosis: an evidence-based clinical guideline for the diagnosis and treatment of degenerative lumbar spinal stenosis. Spine J 2008;8:305–10.

1537. Waxman R, Tennant A, Helliwell P. Community survey of factors associated with consultation for low-back pain. BMJ 1998; 317:1564–7.

1538. Weaver JK, Chalmers J. Cancellous bone: its strength and changes with aging and an evaluation of some methods for measuring its mineral content. J Bone Joint Surg Am 1966;48:289–98.

1539. Webb R, Brammah T, Lunt M, et al. Prevalence and predictors of intense, chronic, and disabling neck and back pain in the UK general population. Spine 2003; 28:1195–202.

1540. Weber H. The natural history of disc herniation and the influence of intervention. Spine 1994;19:2234–8; discussion 3.

1541. Weber H, Burton AK. Rational treatment of low-back trouble? Clin Biomech 1986;1:160–7.

1542. Wedderkopp N, Kjaer P, Hestbaek L, et al. High-level physical activity in childhood seems to protect against low-back pain in ealry adolescence. Spine J 2009;9:134–41.

1543. Weightman B. Tensile fatigue of human articular cartilage. J Biomech 1976;9:193–200.

1544. Weiler C, Nerlich AG, Zipperer J, et al. 2002 SSE Award Competition in Basic Science: expression of major matrix metalloproteinases is associated with intervertebral disc degradation and resorption. Eur Spine J 2002;11:308–20.

1545. Weiner BK, Fraser RD. Spine update lumbar interbody cages [published erratum appears in Spine 1998 Jun 15;23(12):1428]. Spine 1998;23:634–40.

1546. Weiner BK, Fraser RD, Peterson M. Spinous process osteotomies to facilitate lumbar

decompressive surgery. Spine (Phila Pa) 1999;24:62–6.

1547. Weinfeld RM, Olson PN, Maki DD, et al. The prevalence of diffuse idiopathic skeletal hyperostosis (DISH) in two large American Midwest metropolitan hospital populations. Skeletal Radiol 1997;26:222–5.

1548. Weinstein JN, Lurie JD, Tosteson TD, et al. Surgical versus nonoperative treatment for lumbar disc herniation: four-year results for the Spine Patient Outcomes Research Trial (SPORT). Spine 2008;33:2789–800.

1549. Weishaupt D, Zanetti M, Hodler J, et al. Painful Lumbar Disk Derangement: Relevance of Endplate Abnormalities at MR Imaging. Radiology 2001;218: 420–7.

1550. Welle S, Thornton C, Jozefowicz R, et al. Myofibrillar protein synthesis in young and old men. Am J Physiol 1993;264: E693–8.

1551. Wenger KH, Schlegel JD. Annular bulge contours from an axial photogammetric method. Clin Biomech 1997;12:438–44.

1552. Wergeland EL, Veiersted B, Ingre M, et al. A shorter workday as a means of reducing the occurrence of musculoskeletal disorders. Scand J Work Environ Health 2003;29:27–34.

1553. Westgaard RH, Winkel, J. Ergonomic intervention research for improved musculoskeletal health: A critical review. Industrial Ergonomics 1997;20:463–500.

1554. Wetzel FT, LaRocca SH, Lowery GL, et al. The treatment of lumbar spinal pain syndromes diagnosed by discography. Lumbar arthrodesis. Spine 1994;19:792–800.

1555. Wheeldon JA, Pintar FA, Knowles S, et al. Experimental flexion/extension data corridors for validation of finite element models of the young, normal cervical spine. J Biomech 2006;39:375–80.

1556. White III AA, Bernhardt M, Panjabi MM. Clinical biomechanics and lumbar spinal

instability. In: Szpalski M, Gunzburg R, Pope MH, editors. Lumbar segmental instability. Philadelphia, U.S.A.: Lippincott Williams & Wilkins; 1999.

1556a. WHO. International classification of functioning, disability and health. Geneva: World Health Organisation; 2001. www.who.int/icf/icftemplate/cfm.

1557. Wiberg G. Back pain in relation to the nerve supply of the intervertebral disc. Acta Orthop Scand 1947;19:211–21.

1558. Wiersema BM, Wall EJ, Foad SL. Acute backpack injuries in children. Pediatrics 2003;111:163–6.

1559. Wild A, Jager M, Webb JK. Staged reposition and fusion with external fixator in spondyloptosis. Z Irthop Ihre Grengeb 2001;139:152–6.

1560. Wilder DG, Aleksiev AR, Magnusson ML, et al. Muscular response to sudden load. A tool to evaluate fatigue and rehabilitation. Spine 1996;21:2628–39.

1561. Wilder DG, Pope MH. Epidemiological and aetiological aspects of low-back pain in vibration environments – an update. Clin Biomech 1996;11:61–73.

1562. Wilk V. Pain arising from the interspinous and supraspinous ligaments. Australas Muscuskel Med 1995;1:21–31.

1563. Wilke DR. Institute of Biology, Studies in Biology No 11: Muscle. 2nd ed. London: Edward Arnold; 1979.

1564. Wilke HJ, Claes L, Schmitt H, et al. A universal spine tester for in vitro experiments with muscle force simulation. Eur Spine J 1994;3:91–7.

1565. Wilke HJ, Neef P, Caimi M, et al. New in vivo measurements of pressures in the intervertebral disc in daily life. Spine 1999;24:755–62.

1566. Wilke HJ, Wolf S, Claes LE, et al. Stability increase of the lumbar spine with different muscle groups. A biomechanical in vitro study [see comments]. Spine 1995;20:192–8.

1567. Will RE, Stokes IA, Qiu X, et al. Cobb angle progression in adolescent scoliosis begins at the intervertebral disc. Spine (Phila Pa) 2009;34:2782–6.

1568. Willett TL, Labow RS, Lee JM. Mechanical overload decreases the thermal stability of collagen in an in vitro tensile overload tendon model. J Orthop Res 2008;26:1605–10.

1569. Williams FM, Manek NJ, Sambrook PN, et al. Schmorl's nodes: common, highly heritable, and related to lumbar disc disease. Arthritis Rheum 2007;57:855–60.

1570. Williams IF, Craig AS, Parry DAD, et al. Development of collagen fibril organization and collagen crimp patterns during tendon healing. Int J Biol Macromol 1985;7:275–82.

1571. Williams K, Abildso C, Steinberg L, et al. Evaluation of the effectiveness and efficacy of Iyengar yoga therapy on chronic low-back pain. Spine (Phila Pa) 2009;34:2066–76.

1572. Williams M, Solomonow M, Zhou BH, et al. Multifidus spasms elicited by prolonged lumbar flexion. Spine 2000;25:2916–24.

1573. Williams MM, Hawley JA, McKenzie RA, et al. A comparison of the effects of two sitting postures on back and referred pain. Spine 1991;16:1185–91.

1574. Williams P, Simpson H, Kyberd P, et al. Effect of rate of distraction on loss of range of joint movement, muscle stiffness, and intramuscular connective tissue content during surgical limb-lengthening: a study in the rabbit. Anat Rec 1999;255:78–83.

1575. Williams P, Watt P, Bicik V, et al. Effect of stretch combined with electrical stimulation on the type of sarcomeres produced at the ends of muscle fibers. Exp Neurol 1986;93:500–9.

1576. Williams PE, Goldspink G. Longitudinal growth of striated muscle fibres. J Cell Sci 1971;9:751–67.

1577. Williams PE, Goldspink G. Connective tissue changes in immobilised muscle. J Anat 1984;138:343–50.

1578. Wilmink J, Wilson AM, Goodship AE. Functional significance of the morphology and micromechanics of collagen fibres in relation to partial rupture of the superficial digital flexor tendon in racehorses. Res Vet Sci 1992;53:354–9.

1579. Wilson AM, Goodship AE. Exercise-induced hyperthermia as a possible mechanism for tendon degeneration. J Biomech 1994;27:899–905.

1580. Wiltse LL. The etiology of spondylolithesis. J Bone Joint Surg [Am] 1962;44:539–60.

1581. Wiltse LL, Bateman JG, Hutchinson RH, et al. The paraspinal sacrospinalis-splitting approach to the lumbar spine. J Bone Joint Surg Am 1968;50:919–26.

1582. Wiltse LL, Newman PH, Macnab I. Classification of spondylolisis and spondylolisthesis. Clin Orthop Relat Res 1976:23–9.

1583. Wiltse LL, Rothman LG. Spondylolisthesis: classification, diagnosis and natural history. Semin Spinal Surg 1993;5:264–80.

1584. Winkelstein BA, Weinstein JN, DeLeo JA. The role of mechanical deformation in lumbar radiculopathy: an in vivo model. Spine 2002;27:27–33.

1585. Wognum S, Huyghe JM, Baaijens FP. Influence of osmotic pressure changes on the opening of existing cracks in 2 intervertebral disc models. Spine 2006;31:1783–8.

1586. Wong BL, Kim SH, Antonacci JM, et al. Cartilage shear dynamics during tibio-femoral articulation: effect of acute joint injury and tribosupplementation on synovial fluid lubrication. Osteoarthritis Cartilage 2010;18:464–71.

1587. Wood DJ. Design and evaluation of a back injury prevention program within a geriatric hospital. Spine 1987;12:77–82.

1588. Wood KA, Standell CJ, Adams MA, et al. Exercise training to improve spinal mobility and back muscle fatigability: a possible prophylaxis for low-back pain? In: Physical Medicine Research Foundation symposium; 1997; Prague; 1997.

1589. Wood PHN, Badley EM. Epidemiology of back pain. In: Jayson MIV, editor. The lumbar spine and back pain. 2nd ed. Tunbridge Wells: Pitman Medical; 1980. p. 29–55.

1590. Wu HC, Yao RF. Mechanical behavior of the human annulus fibrosus. J Biomech 1976;9:1–7.

1591. Wu J, Qiu Y, Zhang L, et al. Association of estrogen receptor gene polymorphisms with susceptibility to adolescent idiopathic scoliosis. Spine 2006;31:1131–6.

1592. Wuertz K, Godburn K, MacLean JJ, et al. In vivo remodeling of intervertebral discs in response to short- and long-term dynamic compression. J Orthop Res 2009;27:1235–42.

1593. Wynne-Jones G, Dunn KM, Main CJ. The impact of low-back pain on work: a study in primary care consulters. Eur J Pain 2008;12:180–8.

1594. Yahia L, Rhalmi S, Newman N, et al. Sensory innervation of human thoracolumbar fascia. An immunohistochemical study. Acta Orthop Scand 1992;63:195–7.

1595. Yahia LH, Audet J, Drouin G. Rheological properties of the human lumbar spine ligaments. J Biomed Eng 1991;13:399–406.

1596. Yamamoto E, Paul Crawford R, Chan DD, et al. Development of residual strains in human vertebral trabecular bone after prolonged static and cyclic loading at low load levels. J Biomech 2005.

1597. Yamamoto E, Paul Crawford R, Chan DD, et al. Development of residual strains in human vertebral trabecular bone after prolonged static and cyclic loading at low load levels. J Biomech 2006;39:1812–8.

1598. Yamamoto I, Panjabi MM, Oxland TR, et al. The role of the iliolumbar ligament in the lumbosacral junction. Spine 1990;15:1138–41.

1599. Yamashita M, Ohtori S, Koshi T, et al. Tumor necrosis factor-alpha in the nucleus pulposus mediates radicular pain, but not increase of inflammatory peptide, associated with nerve damage in mice. Spine 2008;33:1836–42.

1600. Yamashita T, Cavanaugh JM, Ozaktay AC, et al. Effect of substance P on mechanosensitive units of tissues around and in the lumbar facet joint. J Orthop Res 1993;11:205–14.

1601. Yamashita T, Minaki Y, Oota I, et al. Mechanosensitive afferent units in the lumbar intervertebral disc and adjacent muscle. Spine 1993;18:2252–6.

1602. Yamashita T, Minaki Y, Ozaktay AC, et al. A morphological study of the fibrous capsule of the human lumbar facet joint. Spine 1996;21:538–43.

1603. Yamauchi K, Inoue G, Koshi T, et al. Nerve growth factor of cultured medium extracted from human degenerative nucleus pulposus promotes sensory nerve growth and induces substance p in vitro. Spine (Phila Pa) 2009;34:2263–9.

1604. Yang G, Marras WS, Best TM. The biochemical response to biomechanical tissue loading on the low-back during physical work exposure. Clin Biomech 2011;26:431–7.

1605. Yang KH, King AI. Mechanism of facet load transmission as a hypothesis for low-back pain. Spine 1984;9:557–65.

1606. Yao JQ, Seedhom BB. Mechanical conditioning of articular cartilage to prevalent stresses. Br J Rheumatol 1993;32:956–65.

1607. Yarasheski KE, Zachwieja JJ, Bier DM. Acute effects of resistance exercise on muscle protein synthesis rate in young and elderly men and women. Am J Physiol 1993;265:E210–4.

1608. Yassi A, Cooper JE, Tate RB, et al. A randomized controlled trial to prevent patient lift and transfer injuries of healthcare workers. Spine 2001;26:1739–46.

1609. Yasuma T, Arai K, Yamauchi Y. The histology of lumbar intervertebral disc herniation. The significance of small blood

vessels in the extruded tissue. Spine 1993;18:1761–5.

1610. Yasuma T, Koh S, Okamura T, et al. Histological changes in aging lumbar intervertebral discs. Their role in protrusions and prolapses. J Bone Joint Surg Am 1990;72:220–9.

1611. Yates JP, Giangregorio L, McGill SM. The influence of intervertebral disc shape on the pathway of posterior/posterolateral partial herniation. Spine (Phila Pa) 2010;35:734–9.

1612. Yates JP, McGill SM. The effect of vibration and posture on the progression of intervertebral disc herniation. Spine (Phila Pa) 2011;36:386–92.

1613. Yingling VR, Callaghan JP, McGill SM. Dynamic loading affects the mechanical properties and failure site of porcine spines. Clin Biomech 1997;12:301–5.

1614. Yoganandan N, Larson SJ, Gallagher M, et al. Correlation of microtrauma in the lumbar spine with intraosseous pressures. Spine 1994;19:435–40.

1615. Yoganandan N, Myklebust JB, Wilson CR, et al. Functional biomechanics of the thoracolumbar vertebral cortex. Clin Biomech 1988;3:11–8.

1616. Yoganandan N, Pintar FA, Stemper BD, et al. Level-dependent coronal and axial moment-rotation corridors of degeneration-free cervical spines in lateral flexion. J Bone Joint Surg Am 2007;89:1066–74.

1617. Yoganandan N, Ray G, Pintar FA, et al. Stiffness and strain energy criteria to evaluate the threshold of injury to an intervertebral joint [see comments]. J Biomech 1989;22:135–42.

1618. Yoshizawa H, O'Brien JP, Smith WT, et al. The neuropathology of intervertebral discs removed for low-back pain. J Pathol 1980;132:95–104.

1619. Young AE, Wasiak R, Phillips L, et al. Workers' perspectives on low-back pain recurrence: 'It comes and goes and comes and goes, but it's always there'. Pain 2011;152:204–11.

1620. Yu J, Fairbank JC, Roberts S, et al. The elastic fiber network of the annulus fibrosus of the normal and scoliotic human intervertebral disc. Spine 2005;30:1815–20.

1621. Yu J, Tirlapur U, Fairbank J, et al. Microfibrils, elastin fibres and collagen fibres in the human intervertebral disc and bovine tail disc. J Anat 2007;210:460–71.

1622. Yu SW, Haughton VM, Sether LA, et al. Annulus fibrosus in bulging intervertebral disks. Radiology 1988;169:761–3.

1623. Yu W, Gluer CC, Grampp S, et al. Spinal bone mineral assessment in postmenopausal women: a comparison between dual X-ray absorptiometry and quantitative computed tomography. Osteoporos Int 1995;5:433–9.

1624. Zhai G, Hart DJ, Kato BS, et al. Genetic influence on the progression of radiographic knee osteoarthritis: a longitudinal twin study. Osteoarthritis Cartilage 2007;15:222–5.

1625. Zhang J, Wang JH. Mechanobiological response of tendon stem cells: implications of tendon homeostasis and pathogenesis of tendinopathy. J Orthop Res 2010;28:639–43.

1626. Zhang Y, Hunter DJ, Nevitt MC, et al. Association of squatting with increased prevalence of radiographic tibiofemoral knee osteoarthritis: the Beijing Osteoarthritis Study. Arthritis Rheum 2004;50:1187–92.

1627. Zhao F, Pollintine P, Hole BD, et al. Discogenic origins of spinal instability. Spine 2005;30:2621–30.

1628. Zhao FD, Pollintine P, Hole BD, et al. Vertebral fractures usually affect the cranial endplate because it is thinner and supported by less-dense trabecular bone. Bone 2009;44:372–9.

1629. Zheng S, Xia Y, Bidthanapally A, et al. Damages to the extracellular matrix in articular cartilage due to cryopreservation by microscopic magnetic resonance imaging and biochemistry. Magn Reson Imaging 2009;27:648–55.

1630. Zhou H, Hou S, Shang W, et al. A new in vivo animal model to create intervertebral disc degeneration characterized by MRI, radiography, CT/discogram, biochemistry, and histology. Spine 2007;32:864–72.

1631. Zigler J, Delamarter R, Spivak JM, et al. Results of the prospective, randomized, multicenter Food and Drug Administration investigational device exemption study of the ProDisc-L total disc replacement versus circumferential fusion for the treatment of 1-level degenerative disc disease. Spine (Phila Pa) 2007;32:1155–62; discussion 63.

1632. Zioupos P. Accumulation of in vivo fatigue microdamage and its relation to biomechanical properties in ageing human cortical bone. J Microsc 2001; 201:270–8.

1633. Zioupos P, Hansen U, Currey JD. Microcracking damage and the fracture process in relation to strain rate in human cortical bone tensile failure. J Biomech 2008;41:2932–9.

1634. Ziv I, Maroudas C, Robin G, et al. Human facet cartilage: swelling and some physicochemical characteristics as a function of age. Part 2: Age changes in some biophysical parameters of human facet joint cartilage. Spine 1993;18: 136–46.

1635. Zmuda JM, Cauley JA, Glynn NW, et al. Posterior–anterior and lateral dual-energy x-ray absorptiometry for the assessment of vertebral osteoporosis and bone loss among older men. J Bone Miner Res 2000;15: 1417–24.

1636. Zou J, Yang H, Miyazaki M, et al. Dynamic bulging of intervertebral discs in the degenerative lumbar spine. Spine (Phila Pa) 2009;34: 2545–50.

1637. Zucherman JF, Hsu KY, Hartjen CA, et al. A multicenter, prospective, randomized trial evaluating the X STOP interspinous process decompression system for the treatment of neurogenic intermittent claudication: two-year follow-up results. Spine 2005;30:1351–8.

1638. Balague F, Mannion AF, Pellise F, et al. Non-specific low back pain. Lancet 2012;379(9814): 482–91.

1639. Wang Y, Videman T, Battie MC. Lumbar vertebral endplate lesions: associations with disc degeneration and back pain history. Spine 2012 (in press).

Index

Page numbers followed by "f" indicate figures, "t" indicate tables, and "b" indicate boxes.

Index